Case Management

A Practical Guide for Education and Practice

FOURTH EDITION

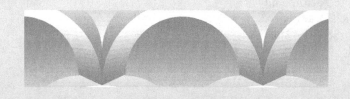

Case Management

A Practical Guide for Education and Practice

FOURTH EDITION

Suzanne K. Powell, RN, MBA, CCM, CPHQ

Editor-in-Chief
Professional Case Management: Leading Evidence-Based
Practice Across Transitions of Care
Lippincott Williams & Wilkins
Philadelphia, Pennsylvania

Hussein M. Tahan, PhD, RN, FAAN

System Vice President of Nursing Professional Development
and Workforce Planning
MedStar Health
Columbia, Maryland

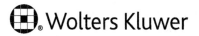

Philadelphia • Baltimore • New York • London
Buenos Aires • Hong Kong • Sydney • Tokyo

Acquisitions Editor: Nicole Dernoski
Editorial Coordinator: Lauren Pecarich
Marketing Manager: Linda Wetmore
Production Project Manager: Barton Dudlick
Design Coordinator: Stephen Druding
Manufacturing Coordinator: Stacie Gantz
Prepress Vendor: S4Carlisle Publishing Services

Fourth Edition

9 8 7 6 5 4 3

Printed in the United States of America

Library of Congress Cataloging-in-Publication Data

Names: Powell, Suzanne K., author. | Tahan, Hussein M., author.
Title: Case management: a practical guide for education and practice /
   Suzanne K. Powell, Hussein M. Tahan.
Description: Fourth edition. | Philadelphia: Wolters Kluwer Health, [2019] |
   Includes bibliographical references and index.
Identifiers: LCCN 2017059967 | ISBN 9781496384256
Subjects: | MESH: Case Management
Classification: LCC RT90.7 | NLM W 84.7 | DDC 362.17/3068—dc23 LC record available
   at https://lccn.loc.gov/2017059967

LWW.com

DRC0722

This textbook is dedicated to my husband, James,
and
to the memory of my father, Harry, my mother, Leah,
and
my brother, David

—Suzanne

This book is dedicated to my parents, family, and friends,
and
to those who make a difference in people's lives every day

—Hussein

We also dedicate this textbook to the patients and families we serve—may your
quality of life be optimized because of case management services;
to our wonderful friends and colleagues who always encourage us to achieve our
dreams and remind us to have fun along the way; and
to the current and future case managers who give their lives every day to
those in need—may God bless you!

FOREWORD

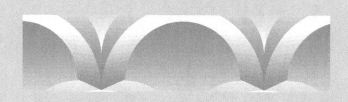

The foundational wisdom of case management is fluid and mirrors an equally fluid health and behavioral health industry. This wisdom is vibrant, with a unique synergy that encompasses both basic and advanced varieties of shifting perspectives across ever-expanding practice settings, health disciplines, roles, and around the globe. Although the learning curve for all health care professionals is particularly steep, case managers are challenged daily with the need to possess and demonstrate proficiency. It is common to feel that the best strategy for successful knowledge acquisition involves placing the key resources under your pillow each night hoping to absorb the content via osmosis.

Case managers must be well versed in the latest generation of knowledge. The scope is vast, including a wide range of topic areas. There are reimbursement models that speak to value-based fiscal imperatives. Innovative treatment and modes of care delivery are only surpassed in complexity by the technology that supports them. A steady stream of legislative mandates guides the actions of all involved professionals, with heightened legal and ethical accountability at every turn. In addition, professional regulations, standards of practice, and ethical codes speak to the vast parameters and scope of case management practice. Lifelong learning is the norm, with performance metrics to delineate professional responsibility for distinct goals and objectives on an individual, departmental, and organizational basis. White papers and journal articles are published on specialized topics and trends (e.g., health literacy, behavioral health integration, electronic communication, workplace violence, legal issues), each informing stakeholders of key points for consideration. New interventions are being implemented to promote patient engagement, treatment adherence, as well as improved outcomes (e.g., motivational interviewing, SBIRT [screening, brief intervention, and referral to treatment]).

The role of the case manager is intricate in design. The role itself reflects a workforce that is transdisciplinary in scope and interprofessional in its practice. The diverse expertise of each discipline merges to accurately address the complexities of distinct populations. Mutual collaboration and respect guide the efforts of care coordination teams,

each unified toward achieving patient-centered goals. Basic and advanced tools are warranted to guide each element of the case management process. Exquisitely woven together is an indispensable core of knowledge, theories, and competencies endemic to all case managers: timeless, yet open to expansion and evolution. Going forward, through technology and industry influences, case management will grow and change as it has before. Education and the inspiration that comes from academia will complement our core curriculum, standards of practice, and whatever the future holds.

We, case managers, are fortunate to have two visionaries who represent decades of experience and practical application, Dr. Hussein Tahan and Suzanne Powell. The first edition of *Case Management: A Practical Guide for Education and Practice (then titled Case Management: A Practical Guide to Success in Managed Care,* by Suzanne K. Powell) appeared in 1996. In this updated 4th edition, the dynamic duo of Tahan and Powell have incorporated advancements, improvements, and, along with other subject matter experts, provided content to reflect our ever-changing world and workforce: one that speaks to students plus seasoned case managers. The central tenets of this book have stood the test of time.

We are two professionals who come from the most diverse of backgrounds: one a registered nurse, attorney, and professional case manager and the other a social worker and professional case manager; both authors are educators and leaders in their respective professions. We are honored and privileged to call the authors of this book our respected colleagues, mentors, and friends. Together, we have seen case management grow and with the benefit of this revised book, the upcoming generation of case managers will have a reliable resource to begin and refresh their case management knowledge.

Lynn S. Muller, JD, BA-HCM, RN, CCM
Partner, Muller and Muller

Ellen Fink-Samnick, MSW, ACSW, LCSW, CCM, CRP
Principal, EFS Supervision Strategies, LLC

PREFACE

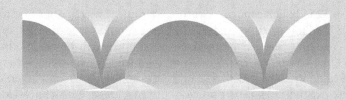

The late Dr. John Miller was an old-fashioned physician in the truest sense. With a medical practice typical of those of the 1960s and 1970s, he was devoted to his patients and always looked out for their best interests. He was accustomed to making patient decisions and dispensing curatives in a single-handed fashion. Conversely, he was not used to being second-guessed or "policed" by insurance companies. When the face of healthcare began to change in the early 1980s, it was difficult for Dr. Miller to come aboard. When "managed care"—with its ominous implied restrictions—no longer loomed as a threat, but became reality, he fought back. In classic Gandhi-like tradition, Dr. Miller carried out his own brand of "civil disobedience," leaving his patients in the hospital longer than what was becoming acceptable by utilization management standards. He also penned his disapproval of the "new ways" to several large newspapers and got himself bounced out of favor with a few managed care insurance plans. As a self-professed "medical dinosaur," he did a lot of charity work, made frequent house calls, and exemplified patient advocacy.

The older physicians, who remembered "how it used to be," felt frustrated because of a severing of the patient–physician relationship; many of those physicians have since retired. It seemed that case managers were evolving as the link between the beleaguered healthcare system and the crucial need for patient advocacy. There is a "Dr. Miller" in virtually every healthcare organization and/or professional discipline across the continuum of care. The constantly changing dynamics of care delivery warrant careful attention to the impact these changes have on the individual health professional, the interdisciplinary care team, the healthcare leader, and the people we care for. Case management practice and case managers have been traditionally, and continue to be today, applied as proactive strategies to undergo effective change, enhance the patient care experience, and engage the various members of healthcare teams. The value of case management today, more than ever, has been demonstrated in financial terms, in quality and safety outcomes (inclusive of patient's experience of care), in health professional role satisfaction and engagement, and in many other ways. These prompt the need to maintain and enhance our knowledge for case management practice and, therefore, the continued publication of the *Case Management: A Practical Guide for Education and Practice* textbook.

The first edition of this textbook was initiated in the early 1990s. At that time, case management was poorly defined; in fact, many health professionals could not yet distinguish between the concepts of "case management" and "managed care." It was becoming crystal clear that case managers were a critical asset to what was termed the *healthcare crisis*, but their impact was diluted by poor training, unavailable scientific evidence demonstrative of their value, quick burnout (and subsequent turnover of case managers), and lack of a standardized definition and nationally recognized practice guidelines.

By the late 1990s, case management had grown at an astounding rate. Not only were there peer-reviewed journals, textbooks, seminars, and college courses about case management, but there were now professional associations, nationally recognized standards of practice, care guidelines, accreditation opportunities, specialty board certifications, and credentials with increasing credibility. Clearly, the earlier editions of this book no longer needed some of the "baby steps," but it did require a tremendous amount of new information to guide case management practice into the adolescent and adult evolutionary stages. In fact, the case management knowledge became so profuse that textbooks on advanced case management practice published by various agencies are a testament to the enormous development that case management had gone through in a few short years.

In addition to the core elements of the first edition, the second edition included information on evaluation and steps to create or change your current case management model; trends in international case management and case management academia; the *Case Management Code of Ethics and Professional Conduct*; and an entire chapter on credentials, organizations, and standards. The second edition also included information necessary for the case manager to function with all the new managed care, legal, and insurance changes, including the Balanced Budget Act of 1996; updated versions of utilization management modalities that incorporated "through the continuum" concepts; case management approaches to expedited and standard appeals, reconsiderations, and grievances; and critical ethical issues that have surfaced since the early 1990s. The intent was that the second edition would function as a teaching tool and useful reference on pertinent issues for case managers from all health professions.

Many of healthcare's problems have shifted, but they still represent an inequitable and raging economic tidal wave. The price tag for US healthcare has been rising for the past several decades; in 1980, it was $255 billion compared with $721.4 billion in 1990, $1.37 trillion in 2000, and $2.6 trillion in 2010. During the same time periods, the annual per-capita healthcare expenditure has arisen from $1,108 in 1980 to $2,843 in 1990, $4,855 in 2000, and $8,412 in 2010. The attribution of these expenditures as percentage of the nation's gross domestic product (GDP) were 8.9% in 1980, 12.1% in 1990, 13.3% in 2000, and 17.4% in 2010.* The US healthcare spending has continued to grow; in fact, it has experienced a 4.3% increase in 2016 as compared with the 2015 expenditure, reaching a staggering $3.34 trillion or $10,348 per person annually and 17.9% of the nation's GDP. Spending is projected to continue to grow at an average of 5.6% per year between 2016 and 2025 and at 4.7% per year on a per-person basis, while the healthcare percent GDP is expected to reach 19.9% by 2025.† The need is still great, and case management remains an exciting challenge, because case managers are in a unique position to continue to be recognized for their contributions to healthcare quality, safety, and economic stewardship.

We had decided to publish the third edition of this textbook for several reasons, among which were, at the time, the increasing popularity of case management as a strategy for ensuring that individuals receive quality, safe, and cost-effective healthcare services; the continued confusion about case management models and roles; and a limited number of available training and education programs for case managers. We also, however, had education and practice in mind and a special return to the basics of case management practice. We felt such focus was lacking in the industry then and would enhance the practice of case management.

We had noticed that most of the available case management literature fell in the "advanced" knowledge category; the number of academic and training programs in case management had been declining; and more health professionals were expressing interest in becoming case managers but uncomfortable with their knowledge of case management practice. Therefore, we decided to contribute a case management textbook that addressed those concerns—one that would be an invaluable resource for those who desired to become case managers as well as those who were interested in enhancing their case management knowledge, skills, and competencies. In addition,

our intent was to offer case management experts involved in training, educating, or mentoring others a textbook equipped with up-to-date information about case management. A major characteristic of the third edition was the approach we had taken to enhance the development of case management knowledge and advance the field. The list of objectives at the beginning of each chapter framed the learning opportunities. The list of key terms assisted case managers to become familiar with the case management language spoken in the various practice settings and highlighted the essential aspects of learning the chapter addressed. The study questions at the end of each chapter were thought to enhance learning through reflection and practical application. Those study questions were meant to encourage readers to reflect on the content they reviewed in the chapter and ask them to apply the gained knowledge into practice. Finally, the posttests for each chapter that were available at the end of the textbook also were meant to further the learning opportunity and at the same time to reward the reader with continuing education credits. One was expected to complete the posttest and submit the answers to Wolters Kluwer/Lippincott Williams & Wilkins to receive education credits that could, for example, be used toward recertification.

The last chapter in the third edition focused on *problem-based learning* (PBL) to allow health professionals to practice case management by proxy. Different from the traditional approach to learning, this chapter was designed for teamwork: a group of individuals could gather in a formal or informal setting and work through a PBL case. Through interaction, discussion, questioning, curiosity, and sharing of knowledge and past experiences, group members could begin to mentor each other, or a case management expert can facilitate group learning with an ultimate goal of spreading the knowledge through active exchange of experiences, information, skills, and competencies.

Because the healthcare environment is constantly transforming, it was a natural expectation that we update the textbook to reflect the current dynamics and case management practices. Therefore, we embarked on the fourth edition. By now our names as authors and case management experts are well recognized in the industry, and with that we owe it to you, the case management community and professional case managers, that we maintain our legacy of service, contribution, and dissemination of knowledge: to keep the *Case Management: A Practical Guide for Education and Practice* alive and of great utility. With the enactment of the Patient Protection and Affordable Care Act of 2010; increased focus on value-based care; expected transparency with the public regarding quality, safety, and financial outcomes of care; and the patient's experience of care being at the center of healthcare delivery, it was necessary that we update this textbook.

In this edition, we have enhanced the knowledge, innovations, and practical tools we had shared in the past and added new topics to reflect current practice and anticipated

*Centers for Medicare & Medicaid Services. (2016). *National healthcare expenditure summary including share of gross domestic product, calendar year 1960–2016* [Online]. Retrieved January 2, 2018, from https://www.cms.gov/Research-Statistics-Data-and-Systems/Statistics-Trends-and-Reports/NationalHealthExpendData/NationalHealthAccountsHistorical.html
†Centers for Medicare & Medicaid Services. (2016). *National healthcare expenditure data, NHE fact sheet: Historical NHE, 2016* [Online]. Retrieved December 10, 2017, from https://www.cms.gov/research-statistics-data-and-systems/statistics-trends-and-reports/nationalhealthexpenddata/nhe-fact-sheet.html

near-future changes. For example, in this edition we discuss, among many other topics, the impact of the Patient Protection and Affordable Care Act and value-based purchasing/value-based care in the field of case management. We also discuss the roles of the case management leader and the case management support associates, interprofessional practice and provision of team-based care, interdisciplinary patient care rounding and its invaluable contribution to care coordination, and safe transitions of care across the continuum of health and human services. In addition, we review clinical documentation improvement (CDI) and the CDI specialist role, use of case management information systems and health information technology including digital communication tools and tele-case management, and meaningful use for their role in quality, cost-conscious, and safe care. Moreover and as the title of the textbook implies, we have updated the chapter on PBL and expanded this full chapter to include learning practices, training programs, and professional development of the case management team. This chapter now features topics such as competency management, preparation of case managers for their roles, training curricula and orientation programs, and experiential learning inclusive of simulation. Finally, we provide essential information about case management accreditation agencies and standards and specialty board certifications,

and we have continued to emphasize important legal and ethical considerations for case management practice and summarize use of evidence-based guidelines and standards practice. Lastly, we would like to acknowledge Lynn S. Muller for her contribution of Chapter 8: Legal Considerations in Case Management Practice to this edition.

Similar to the past editions, it is our hope that the fourth edition of this textbook, coupled with a solid training program, will help develop professional case managers both who are new to the practice and who have demonstrated peak job performance. Another benefit that can be realized by healthcare institutions and providers is developing a new case management model (or improving the conditions of an existing one) that can ensure quality and safe patient care practices and improve the satisfaction of those who receive health services—the patients and their families/caregivers. It will also ensure the satisfaction of those who provide these services—the professional case managers and their colleagues who will be recognized as shining lights, pulling the fragmented pieces of healthcare together, for the utmost benefit of the patient and family.

Suzanne K. Powell
Hussein M. Tahan

CONTENTS

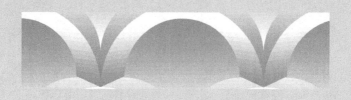

PART 1

Introduction to Case Management Practice

"Foolish is the doctor who despises the
knowledge acquired by the Ancient."

HIPPOCRATES, C. 460-C. 377 B.C.

CHAPTER 1

Overview of Case Management

"The names of the patients whose lives we save can never be known. Our contribution will be what did not happen to them. And, though they are unknown, we will know that mothers and fathers are at graduations and weddings they would have missed, and that grandchildren will know grandparents they might never have known, and holidays will be taken, and work completed, and books read, and symphonies heard, and gardens tended that, without our work, would never have been."

DONALD M. BERWICK, MD

LEARNING OBJECTIVES

Upon completion of this chapter, the reader will be able to:

1. Define case management.
2. List four milestones in the history and evolution of case management systems.
3. Describe the difference between the dyad and triad models of case management.
4. Describe the role of the nurse versus the social worker in case management.
5. Recognize five strategies in ensuring the effectiveness of case management models.
6. Determine the value of telehealth and information systems in the practice of case management.

ESSENTIAL TERMS

Acute Care Case Management • Admission Case Management • Beyond-the-Walls Case Management • Care Management • Case Management • Case Management Code of Professional Conduct • Case Management Model • Case Manager • Community-Based Case Management • Complex Case Management • Disease Management • Dyad/Triad Models of Case Management • Emergency Department (ED) Case Management • Entrepreneurial Case Management • Home Health Case Management • Homebound Criteria • Hospice Case Management • Hospitalist • Improvement Standard • Insurance Case Management • Integrated Case Management • Intermittent Care • International Case Management • Managed Care • Medical Necessity • Nurse Case Manager • On-site Case Management • Palliative Care Case Management • Patient-Centered Medical Home • Perioperative Case Management • Population Health Management • Reasonable and Necessary • Rehabilitation Specialist • Skilled Nursing Facility Case Manager • Social Worker Case Manager • Telehealth • Telephonic Case Management • Third-Party Payor • Vocational Case Management • Within-the-Walls Case Management • Workers' Compensation Case Management

▶ THE REALITY OF THE HEALTHCARE ENVIRONMENT

When the first edition of this book was written over 25 years ago, the reality of healthcare looked very different than it does today. And at the end of 2017, history will show that healthcare is in the midst of tremendous turmoil again. However, there are some tenets that remain clear and eternal, and these are standards that all case managers practice;

1. The patient and family are the center of the healthcare universe, where advocacy and patient choice is key;
2. With the above in mind, stewardship, the fiscally thoughtful management of resources, is necessary; and

3. Quality and safety of the provisions of health-care and the case management plan of care are foundational.

Balancing the choices of the patient/family, with stewardship, and making sure the quality of care is optimum, is not an easy task. But it is, and will be, the prime directive of case management. This will not change.

This chapter will answer some of the basic questions that new case managers will ask, and seasoned case managers may bypass. "What is case management?" "What is a case manager?" "What is managed care?" We are asked these questions weekly by staff nurses, attending physicians, residents, interns, patients, families, other healthcare professionals, and nursing students, who are especially eager to learn about their future career options. Often, what is being asked is "What does a case manager do?"

This question is not easily answered, given the plethora of job descriptions, licensures, certifications, and models of case management available. Lack of standardization and the void of widely agreed-on definitions have made answering such a question more complex and challenging. However, this book attempts to describe what a case manager does, keeping in perspective the diversity of case management practice and the roles assumed by case managers. For over three decades, we sometimes see the terms *case management*, *nursing case management*, and *managed care* still being used interchangeably, even though case management experts agree that they are not synonymous. Add to these terms all the other expressions for this endeavor (such as care management, care coordination, case coordination, service coordination, transitional planning, and continuity coordination), and much confusion results.

In the more recent past, the titles of a case manager and the licensure have been challenged. Whenever these other terms are used, always ask what the job roles and responsibilities are; what is the required licensure; and what practice settings are included. With more case managers working across healthcare settings, clarification of these questions may be critical to one's license. There are some good journal articles on licensure protection, and the reader is encouraged to study them.

To answer the basic question in the novice, the difference between managed care and case management is simple and complex at the same time:

▶ *Managed care* is *systems* oriented and focuses on health insurance plans and the management of member benefits.
▶ *Case management* is *people* oriented and negotiates the managed care systems in a way that, ideally, benefits everyone, particularly the patient.

Managed care was a natural response to a healthcare system of waste and expanding, expensive technology. In the 1950s and 1960s, healthcare was paid for on a fee-for-service basis; essentially, this meant that a bill was rendered and paid without limitation of any kind. In the 1970s and 1980s, Medicare reimbursement changed to the Diagnosis-Related Groups (DRGs)/Inpatient Prospective Payment System, which set the following standard: each diagnosis carried with it a set prearranged reimbursement, whether a patient stayed in the hospital 2 days and cost the hospital $1,000 or stayed 2 weeks and cost the hospital $15,000. This system changed the face of healthcare forever. With new limitations being placed on reimbursement for care, everyone started scrambling to improve the management of that care. Even now—three decades later—the ripple effects are still being felt by everyone: the payor, the provider, and the recipient of care.

Managed care systems sprang up in insurance companies and hospitals and in virtually all agencies affected by healthcare dollars. Health maintenance organizations (HMOs), preferred provider organizations (PPOs), and traditional healthcare plans began to manage the care through various forms of restrictions such as prior authorization for services, use of networks or panels of providers, preadmission authorization, utilization management and review, capitation, DRG reimbursement, per diem payments, and gatekeeping.

Managed care is a mutating and dynamic force—economically driven—that is constantly trying out new delivery systems. The goal of managed care is to encourage consumers, providers, and payors to all become accountable for the wise use of limited and ever-expensive healthcare resources. The definitions of managed care—perhaps because they are changing at such a velocity—often focus on strategies used in managed care and the restrictions placed on healthcare dollars. This is exemplified in the following three definitions:

1. Managed care is the provision of services or strategies designed to improve access to care, quality of care, and the cost-effective use of health resources. Managed care services include, but are not limited to, case management, utilization management, peer review, disease management, and population health (Case Management Society of America [CMSA], 2016).
2. Managed healthcare, according to Kongstvedt (2003), is a regrettably nebulous term. At the very least, it is a system of healthcare delivery that attempts to manage the cost of healthcare, the quantity and quality of that healthcare, and access to that care. Common denominators include a panel of contracted providers (network of participating providers) that is less than the entire universe of available providers; some type of limitations on benefits to subscribers (enrollees or consumers of care) who use noncontracted providers (unless authorized to do so); and some type of authorization system (certification for

services prior to their provision). Managed healthcare is actually a spectrum of systems, ranging from so-called managed indemnity to PPOs, point of service (POS), open-panel HMOs, and closed-panel HMOs.

3. "Managed care is defined as a set of techniques used by or on behalf of purchasers of healthcare benefits to manage healthcare costs by influencing patient care decision making through case-by-case assessments of the appropriateness of care prior to its provision. The implementation of managed care strategies follows a series of other cost control measures including insurance benefit limitations and exclusions, prepaid health plans, prospective payment systems, and fee schedules" (Williams & Torrens, 1993, p. 226).

Managed care conjures up different images to different people: some see it as an over-bureaucratization, which will lead to rationing of services, limitations on access to care, poor quality of care, and loss of choice and autonomy. Others see managed care as a necessary evil that will provide healthcare coverage to a larger segment of the U.S. population. The simple days when the physician decided on patient care, ordered it, billed for it, and was paid are over. The new reality of requirements, restraints, restrictions, authorizations, gatekeeping, and rationales has catapulted the healthcare environment into ever-increasing complexity. Issues never before thought of must now be addressed. Such issues include the following:

▶ What services will Patient A's health insurance company allow? When and by whom?
▶ What will Patient B's pharmacy benefit cover, and which pharmacy must he or she use?
▶ What patient is reimbursed under a DRG versus a risk contract or a per diem rate?
▶ What extended care facility or home health agency can be used?
▶ What physician is contracted with the health insurance plan?
▶ Is the Medicare coverage of the traditional type or a risk contract type?
▶ How can the case manager provide a safe discharge plan if the insurance company wants the patient discharged quickly and while the patient is supposedly still ill?
▶ How can the case manager secure necessary durable medical equipment if it is not covered in the health plan?

And safe answers to those issues are what case management is all about.

▶ CASE MANAGEMENT

Nursing was quick to recognize the constraints healthcare was under, and nurses viewed the dilemma as an opportunity to expand their practice and patient advocacy roles.

They became the response to managed care. The nature of managed care dictates that healthcare services are limited; it is economics driven. Case management balances this concept by ensuring caring, access, and quality. For this reason, case managers are proving themselves to be the most effective equalizers to managed care.

Historically, the definitions of case management found in the literature often confused, rather than clarified, the issue for several reasons. Some of these reasons still exist today and contribute to case management role confusion and in some instances role overload.

▶ There are numerous models of case management; in fact, there are as many models and definitions as there are healthcare organizations in the United States. Each model looks at case management from the organization's own perspective and therefore defines its own goals, processes, and type/context of case management rather than supplying a definition that applies universally. Often, this definition describes what works for that particular facility or setting.
▶ The definition often merely restates the case management process—what a case manager does—rather than contributing a definition.
▶ Many still simply confuse case management with a discharge planner or utilization reviewer.
▶ Some definitions make it difficult to differentiate between individual case management functions. As with managed care, the case management role is evolving and dynamic. Once a purer role, the case manager is now often a hybrid of the clinical care provider, utilization reviewer, and quality improvement specialist-case manager.
▶ Some definitions are influenced by the specialty or profession of the person who assumes the role of case manager. For example, nursing primarily reflects management of clinical care in its case management practice; social work focuses on psychosocial counseling and brokerage of community resources; utilization management emphasizes resource consumption and allocation; and vocational rehabilitation stresses return to work.
▶ Many terms that are supposed to be interchangeable with "case management" have surfaced in the past decade:
  ▶ Client (or Patient) Navigator
  ▶ Patient Advocate
  ▶ Healthcare Coach
  ▶ Care Coordinator
  ▶ Guided Health Nurse
  ▶ Medical Home Coordinator
  ▶ Clinical Resource Coordinator
  ▶ Resource Coordinator
  ▶ Transition Coach
  ▶ Utilization Manager
  ▶ Discharge Planner

To prevent confusion, some professional case management organizations continue to advocate for national and standardized definitions of case management. The CMSA, the Commission for Case Management Certification (CCMC), the American Case Management Association (ACMA), and the National Association of Social Workers (NASW) are four organizations that have done much work over the years to bring clarity to case management.

The CMSA, a multidisciplinary organization, defines case management as:

> a collaborative process of assessment, planning, facilitation, care coordination, evaluation and advocacy for options and services to meet an individual's and family's comprehensive health needs through communication and available resources to promote patient safety, quality of care, and cost-effective outcomes (CMSA, 2016).

The CCMC, established in 1992 to administer the first certification exam in case management, the Certified Case Manager (CCM) credential, defines case management as:

> a collaborative process that assesses, plans, implements, coordinates, monitors, and evaluates the options and services required to meet the client's health and human service needs. It is characterized by advocacy, communication, and resource management and promotes quality and cost-effective interventions and outcomes (CCMC, 2017).

The NASW defines case management as:

> a process to plan, seek, advocate for, and monitor services from different social services or health care organizations and staff on behalf of a client. The process enables social workers in an organization, or in different organizations, to coordinate their efforts to serve a given client through professional teamwork, thus expanding the range of needed services offered. Case management limits problems arising from fragmentation of services, staff turnover, and inadequate coordination among providers. Case management can occur within a single, large organization or within a community program that coordinates services among settings (NASW, 2013).

The ACMA defines case management as:

> a collaborative process that facilitates recommended treatment plans to ensure the appropriate medical care is provided to disabled, ill or injured individuals. It refers to the planning and coordination of health care services appropriate to achieve the goal of medical rehabilitation. Case management may include, but is not limited to, care assessment, evaluation of a medical condition, development and implementation of a plan of care, coordination of medical resources, communication of health care needs to the patient and/or family members, monitoring of an individual's progress, and promotion of cost-effective care (ACMA, 2016).

By combining aspects of these definitions, the reader can focus on a bigger picture of what case management is all about. Case managers are the pivotal, prime movers of the managed and healthcare environment. Their presence adds humanity to an otherwise overwhelming system. More important than the definition of case management or what case managers accomplish is the heart of their role: the holistic, advocacy, and humane care of both patients and their families.

Case management and *care management* are two terms that tend to be used interchangeably; however, they are not exactly the same. Case management is a way of managing unique and high-risk health conditions, often associated with costly acute care and hospital stay. Patients who require case management services are of diminished/compromised self-capacity and have complex medical conditions. Care management, on the other hand, is a system of care for patients with particular conditions where services are delivered across the continuum of care; it ensures seamless transition to the right provider at the right time. In case management, healthcare services are delivered primarily applying the medical model; in care management, services are delivered applying the psychosocial model. In either model, care is facilitated by a case manager (Bodie-Gross & Tahan, 2008).

▶ CONSUMER DEFINITION OF CASE MANAGEMENT

Case managers continually come across patients/clients (and practitioners) who are unclear about the case management role. We need a good "elevator speech," simple definition. Several years ago, the Case Management Leadership Coalition (CMLC) developed a consumer-friendly definition of case management. This emerged after comprehensive research of the varied definitions published in the case management literature as well as the views of experts in case management, including a few public advocates. The main purpose of this research effort was to develop a definition the consumer of healthcare services (including case management services) would understand. This development was an important milestone in the evolution of case management. Case managers are encouraged to share this definition with their patients and their families when attempting to explain what case management is and what case managers do. The CMSA (2007) definition is as follows:

> Case management assists people to navigate through the healthcare and community systems to find solutions that work.

▶ HISTORICAL PERSPECTIVE

Case management concepts and approaches to healthcare delivery and resources are not new. However, as a healthcare delivery system, case management is a fairly recent phenomenon. It has been in use for almost a century (Display 1-1). In the early 1900s, case management was applied by public health nurses and social workers in the form of

display 1-1

▼▼ SELECT MILESTONES IN THE EVOLUTION OF CASE MANAGEMENT

Early 1900s (turn of the 20th century)—Coordination of healthcare services in the public health sector by public health nurses and community social workers.

1920s—Coordination of services for chronically ill behavioral health patients by psychiatric specialists and social workers in the outpatient care setting.

1930s—Community-based case management approaches applied by public health visiting nurses in the community care setting.

Early 1940s—Case management approaches used as cost-saving measures in workers' compensation.

Post-World War II—Coordination of services by insurance companies for soldiers with complex injuries or health conditions and requiring multispecialty services.

1970s—Workers' compensation insurers develop and implement case management programs focusing on "return-to-work."

1970s—Coordination of services (health and human/medical and social services) by social workers and human service specialists in the community care setting funded through Medicare and Medicaid demonstration projects.

1978—Older Americans Act authorizes the use of case management services for elder patients through Area Agencies on Aging.

1980s—Case management of the catastrophically ill or injured with the main focus on cost containment.

Mid-1980s—Case management programs in acute care settings mainly as a nursing initiative.

1990s—Hospital-based case management programs became multidisciplinary in nature and similar programs proliferated into other care settings.

Late 1990s to Early 2000s—Case management is practiced in every setting across the healthcare continuum and in almost every healthcare organization. Role of the case manager is performed by various healthcare professionals, including nurses, social workers, physical therapists, vocational rehabilitation counselors, pharmacists, and physicians.

2009—Number of case managers exceeds 100,000, at least one-third of whom hold a certification in case management.

coordination of healthcare services and resources for patients and families while in the community-based setting. In the 1920s, professionals in the fields of psychiatry and social work applied case management concepts in the management of the care of the behavioral health patients, especially in the ambulatory/clinic and community-based settings.

Case management practice and models as we know them today proliferated in the mid-1980s after the implementation of the prospective payment system (i.e., the DRG system) in the acute care setting. They witnessed increased popularity in the 1990s as a result of the rise in managed care organizations and the use of capitation as the desired reimbursement method for healthcare services. Today, case management models are applied in almost every healthcare organization or setting regardless of type (acute, subacute, rehabilitation, ambulatory, community-based, long-term care, home health, palliative and hospice care, etc.). Case management practices flourished as a result of the implementation of prospective payment systems beyond the acute care setting (e.g., acute and subacute rehabilitation facilities, long-term care, and nursing homes) as well as because of their proven value in healthcare quality and safety.

▶ WHO SHOULD BE CASE MANAGERS?

It is 2017, and case management pioneers are still astounded by the frequency with which this question continues to be asked. The answer is still the same as it has been in previous editions of this textbook.

Every discipline today seems to have case managers. Depending on the agency, the educational preparation varies from a high school diploma (General Education Development [GED] acceptable) to master's level and beyond. The level of academic completion continues to be a hotly debated topic in some circles. The professional license is the other issue defining who should be a case manager. In today's healthcare market, the main and most common contenders for the role of case manager are nurses and social workers; however, that is broadening to include many other professional disciplines. Traditionally, social workers held the position of discharge planners in most hospitals until the mid- to late 1980s. With the advent of the prospective payment system and managed care (i.e., with the goal of getting the patient through the cost-intensive acute care setting as efficiently as possible), the trend in that level of care is the use of nurses as case managers. Nevertheless, the "nurse versus social worker as case manager" debate still remains a touchy subject. Turf wars have broken out over it, articles have been written about it, and jobs have been lost over it.

▶ Who is More Appropriate for the Role of Case Manager?

Critical to answering this question is assessing the type of population needing case management. This will help to determine the professional background that will most suitably meet the patients' needs. For example, foster children as the target population reflect a predominantly social model, thus needing the expertise of a social worker case manager. Respiratory therapists have been hired as case managers for patients with chronic pulmonary diseases such as cystic fibrosis, chronic obstructive lung disease, or asthma. The cognitively fragile population may also benefit from the use of social workers or from psychiatrically experienced registered nurses (RNs). Rehabilitation facilities may use RNs, social workers, or physical/occupational therapists individually or as teams. Gerontology practitioners may be best suited for the fragile elderly. In the workers' compensation arena, where the main focus is return to work of the injured employee, vocational rehabilitation or disability managers are best fitted for the case manager role.

Getting more specific, in a disease management program for diabetes, dietitians have been effectively utilized. Certified Diabetes Educators (CDE) have successfully managed that population for years. In an asthma program, respiratory training is invaluable; in behavioral health programs, social worker case managers have been successful.

Acute hospital care, at first glance, appears to be a purely medical model; thus, at that level of care, the obvious choice would appear to be professional registered nurses. Consider some of the responsibilities of a hospital-based case manager:

- Astute assessment skills are necessary to aid in recognizing ominous changes in medical status, whereby timely interventions can forestall an impending medical crisis; often, these changes in patient status may also necessitate a change in the service plan.
- Thorough systems assessment, documentation, and placement into utilization management language are needed for insurance authorization and reimbursement purposes.
- Descriptions of wounds and surgical interventions often must be reported to the insurance company for negotiating hospital stay authorization.
- Coordination of durable medical equipment and other resources for home use will often necessitate a medical perspective. For example, tracheostomies may require a range of supportive equipment from suction catheters and suction machines to home oxygen or aerosol masks. Colostomies require colostomy bags and skin care products. Diabetes monitoring needs blood glucose monitoring devices and related supplies.
- Knowledge of medications and of the safe and appropriate time to change from an intravenous route to an oral route is important.
- The meaning of various laboratory and test results must be understood when looking at the total medical picture.
- Teaching may include any aspect of medical care, from teaching the patient (and or family/caregiver) the side effects and correct administration of specific medications to suctioning a tracheostomy or packing and redressing a wound in a sterile manner.
- Understanding of patient flow and throughput is a necessary skill for today's case managers. Flow and throughput focus on assessment and evaluation of patients' conditions and treatment plans in an effort to ensure that care is received in the most appropriate setting, that is, the patient is provided care at the necessary level. For example, patients may transition from the emergency department to

the intensive care unit (ICU) or from the telemetry unit to a regular floor as their conditions warrant.
- Knowledge of insurance plans and health benefits is essential and allows case managers to be effective at utilization management, assuring that acute care is the most appropriate level of care for the patient based on his or her health condition and required care.
- Identification of actual or potential delays in care or treatment allows them to be addressed with the goal of resolving the issues and preventing deterioration in the patient's condition, thereby improving outcomes of care and enhancing the patient's satisfaction.
- Command of outcomes measurement and evaluation of the provision of care and services, including core measures, quality and safety indicators, regulatory requirements, and accreditation standards.

Although nursing may be the first thought when reading the foregoing, in reality, the acute care setting is not a purely medical model. Trauma units routinely overflow with various patients, from those who have been in motor vehicle accidents to those who have sustained gunshot wounds, to those who have been victims of gang violence. ICUs house patients who have attempted suicide or drug overdoses. Personnel on medical floors treat cellulitis and abscesses from intravenous drug abuse; those on obstetric floors routinely witness "babies having babies"—14-year-olds who are already multigravida moms. Staff on all units treat catastrophic conditions and diseases that can bring the strongest families to their knees. All inpatient care units need the assistance of social workers as well—for social assessments, psychosocial counseling, and social discharge planning. However, the intensity of involvement of the social worker in care is dependent on the individual patient/family need. Often, the social worker case manager tends to focus on the patient's social, financial, and complex discharge planning needs.

A person's professional training elicits its own unique perspective; a nurse case manager and a social worker each have a different point of view about what a patient's needs might be on discharge. Both contribute important data for a patient's successful rehabilitation, illustrating that perhaps the best solution is a nurse case manager–social worker team approach. This is ideal in many settings, not only in acute care but also at subacute levels such as hospice or spinal cord rehabilitation centers.

▶ WHAT MAKES THE NURSE CASE MANAGER–SOCIAL WORKER TEAM WORK?

Superimposing nurse case managers on already existing social worker-discharge planners has created turf wars in the past; such is overcome only after until both professionals realize their importance and necessity. The nurse case manager–social worker team members may initially appear to have some overlapping roles as well as their more obvious, distinctly separate responsibilities. However, these overlapping gray areas do not necessarily mean duplication. Good communication within the team and mutual trust regarding follow-through can eliminate the risk of wasted effort from repetition. Some nurse case manager–social worker teams have had difficult times because of attitudes about roles "carved in stone" or an individual need to "do it all." These attitudes make one of the basic tenets of teamwork—pitching in for one another—very difficult. Ensuring that the most qualified professional gets involved in the care of a patient is important. One way of achieving this objective is by having the nurse case manager provide case management services if the patient's prevailing needs are clinical or educational in nature and a social worker case manager do so if the prevailing needs are financial or social.

The case management–social worker team has now had several years to test its efficacy. It has proven to be essential in many settings. Important suggestions given by facilities with five or more years of this team (dyad) model are as follows:

1. Strategically place case managers and social workers under one department; this will minimize territorial issues.
2. Teach and facilitate the team concept. Success is reflective of the team effectiveness rather than the individual contribution alone.
3. Stress the three "Cs"—communicate, communicate, communicate. Communication is the key to success.
4. Document, in writing, the basic components of each job description. However, there are many gray areas that overlap because of covering for one another or because of the sequence of events in an individual's case. "How to" and resource manuals specific to the local cultures, community resources, and facilities should be kept updated. This includes updating addresses, telephone numbers, contacts, and any new resources. This also will allow for more independence of the team members.
5. Outline the selection criteria for nurse versus social worker case manager. For example, a nurse case manager may be needed for teaching the patient and family about complex wound care, whereas a social worker case manager gets involved in counseling a family regarding their coping pattern in response to their premature newborn. Even when such criteria are spelled out, there will always be situations where both the nurse and the social worker case managers are involved, as when a patient and family conference is conducted or during interdisciplinary patient care management rounds.
6. Implement in-service programs. This is a good strategy to keep the team current. For example, social workers require training in the basics of utilization review; case managers require more in-depth practice in grief counseling; both case managers and social workers need to know the latest changes in regulatory and legal issues.

Perhaps the element most responsible for making nurse case manager–social worker teams work best is the elusive factor known as chemistry. When all the components of a good nurse case manager–social worker team are in place, the patient wins, the family wins, the facility wins, the healthcare team is pleased, job satisfaction peaks, and managed care becomes quality, cost-efficient care.

In the adage that "everything old is new again," a "triad model" has resurfaced. It is not a secret that the utilization management burden is growing, with health insurance companies carving out both level of care denials and specific day denials. In several facilities, the aforementioned nurse case manager and social worker dyad model remain; they are the care coordination arm of the triad model. The third arm of the triad model is where the utilization management role becomes a separate role. This has worked in many facilities because it allows the care coordination portion of the model to focus more fully on the patient/family needs.

The utilization management arm has a major role to play. Whereas the team in front of the patient and family pulls the patient through the system and works toward efficient, quality transitions, the utilization management portion focuses on the following responsibilities:

▶ The patient must meet evidence-based criteria to be in the right status and the correct level of care. This also can identify risk or quality issues before they become problematic.
▶ Compliance with Centers for Medicare & Medicaid Services (CMS) regulations (including all the changes in those regulations) and payor protocols are actively adhered to.
▶ Communication with the payors, so that procedures, hospitalizations, and transitions to other care are authorized. This must be done when (or before) the payors request clinical reviews.
▶ Communication with the rest of the team to help manage the patient in an efficient manner.
▶ Communication with the physician practices to find out plans of care and match them with the correct status or payor authorizations.

By the astute practice of the tasks and good communication with the team members, the utilization managers make sure the insurance coverage is maximized and the rate of denials of care is minimized. Further, quality of care is enhanced and avoidable hospital days and avoidable readmissions are reduced.

▶ CASE MANAGEMENT CODE OF PROFESSIONAL CONDUCT

Case managers are expected to act on the basis of case management-related ethical principles and standards as well as those of their original profession or specialty. For example, in addition to the case management code of ethics, nurse case managers would also adhere to the nursing code of ethics, and social work case managers would comply with the social work code of ethics. Those who abide by the professional code of ethics are able to protect the best interest of their patients, are accountable and responsible, are effective advocates, and recognize ethical dilemmas and address them.

In 1996, the Commission for Case Manager Certification (CCMC, 2015) adopted a Code of Professional Conduct for Case Managers. Compliance with this code is mandatory for all applicants of the CCM certification examination and those already holding the CCM credential. The code can be obtained from CCMC's website (www.cmcertification.org). This code was written to protect the public and represents another step needed for credibility and accountability of case management. The Code of Professional Conduct for Case Managers has been revised multiple times since 1996, most recently in 2015.

The code consists of these sections:

1. Preamble.
2. Scope of Practice for Case Managers.
3. Principles (fundamental assumptions to guide professional conduct).
4. Rules of Conduct (prescribe the level of conduct required of every CCM).
5. Guidelines for Professional Conduct (offer information with regard to various aspects of an individual's professional conduct).
6. Guidelines and Procedures for Processing Complaints.

The objective of the code is to protect the public interest, is ethically oriented, and, according to CCMC enforcement, offers the following advantages:

▶ It constitutes a response to the professional obligation to provide only quality services to clients.
▶ It safeguards clients by identifying unethical practitioners and disciplining them through censure or, when warranted, the revocation of their professional credential.
▶ It serves as a form of self-regulation that helps protect practitioners from ill-considered or overly restrictive regulations that might be imposed by other entities.
▶ It protects the public interest by providing guidance to both the public at large and case managers as to what constitutes ethical conduct, how to adhere to ethical practice, and what to do in case ethical standards and principles were overlooked.

With all the complexities of case management, including ethical and legal dilemmas, Codes of Conduct in whatever licensure you have serve as another reminder of staying focused on the patient or family while maintaining professional responsibilities. There is another necessity for understanding specific codes of conduct. As lawsuits increase, there is always a chance that a case manager may end up in court; in such situations, standards, codes, and protocols can always be held up as a "sword or a shield." Whether a code of conduct, or *Standards of Practice for Case Management*, are protective may depend on a case manager's knowledge of these texts and adherence to them.

▶ OPPORTUNITIES IN CASE MANAGEMENT

As the managed care environment tightens, more positions for case managers are becoming available in both the public and the private domains. The massive changes in reimbursement strategies in the late 1990s by the Health Care Financing Administration (HCFA, known today as the CMS) served to increase the opportunities for case managers not only in the acute care settings, but at the postacute level as well. Because managed care strategies are constantly changing, it is reasonable to speculate that some of the current case management job responsibilities may become more diverse, some may no longer be considered necessary, and new ones may be emphasized. At any rate, the basic functions of case management—ensuring quality of and access to care in a cost-efficient manner—will not become less relevant.

Case management began as either a community-based model with a focus on the community or a hospital-based model with a focus on one acute episode of care. Now the trend is managing the patient through the continuum of care, which includes acute and postacute levels of care, including the patient's home. In this integrated system, there is more continuity for the patient when a single case manager oversees all levels of care. Disease management, or managing a patient population that is defined by a specific medical condition, is a good example of case management that follows a patient throughout the continuum of care and services. The multidisciplinary team for a single patient includes all the key players in the patient's individual case, although some of the players may change depending on the patient's needs. The team may also include case managers from various portions of the care plan such as insurance companies, third-party payors, skilled nursing facilities (SNFs), hospices, physician groups, hospitals, home healthcare agencies, the patient's employer (if the case has to do with workers' compensation), and the family or caregiver.

Some medical soothsayers predict that in the near future, hospital care will consist mainly of ICU treatments, and the trend does appear to be going in that direction. Recently, it was joked that craniotomies will soon be 'drive-by'—witness the many craniotomy patients who are now discharged on postoperative day one and the mastectomy patients who are outpatient and discharged within 23 hours. The trend is pervasive.

The largest portion of every healthcare dollar is spent in acute hospitals, which provides the financial incentive to move care out of the costly hospital setting and into the community. Therefore, new models of case management continue to be generated. The vision of keeping patients out of the hospital may become a reality through still unexplored case management strategies.

Case management across all levels of care has several advantages:

▶ Its primary focus is on wellness and optimization of a person's quality of life, autonomy, independence, and patient or family functioning.
▶ Potential problems can be avoided through preventive practices.
▶ There may be foreseeably fewer readmissions to the acute level of care (inpatient or emergency department episodes of care).
▶ There may be less acuity when a patient is readmitted through early identification of medical changes, thus resulting in less costly hospitalizations and reduced lengths of stay.
▶ Unnecessary admissions may be prevented. These may include low-acuity admissions or those known as "social admissions," primarily for disposition problems.
▶ A contact person is provided for patients to help them access and navigate the complex healthcare system.
▶ Careful medical monitoring may decrease complications.
▶ There may be fewer visits to emergency departments and fewer 911 calls.

When a case manager (in any setting) follows patients in this way, many emergency department visits are appropriately avoided. A study performed in 1992 by the U.S. Department of Health and Human Services revealed that of the 90 million emergency department visits that year, only 45% were deemed urgent or emergent (Anonymous, 1994). Almost as many people went to emergency departments for coughs and sore throats as for chest pain and level I traumas. These trends continue to be evident today. Rather than sending a patient to an emergency department, a case manager—on assessment—may send the patient to his or her primary care provider (PCP) or an ambulatory care site, or may call in an extra home health nurse visit, a respiratory professional, a social worker, or a psychiatric nurse to visit the patient. Perhaps the far-sighted payor source is contracted with one of the new, futuristic, entrepreneurial physician groups who specialize in the age-old activity of house calls. Surely, even a physician-assisted house call is less expensive than a 911 ambulance charge plus the emergency department treatment charges.

▶ MATCHING PERSONAL GOALS AND BELIEFS WITH THE APPROPRIATE CASE MANAGEMENT MODEL

There are many types of case management models in the contemporary healthcare environment. Those interested in case management as an employment opportunity are advised to evaluate the job description and responsibilities carefully to see whether the model of case management offered is compatible with personal beliefs and professional goals. Some might prefer the episodic version of case management, whereas others would find long-term relationships with patients very satisfying. If home-based case management services are included in your job description, would you be at ease going into others' homes and assessing their medical and psychosocial needs? Are you comfortable and effective with issues such as self-neglect, noncompliance, or abuse (child or elder)? Are you clinically astute enough to safely triage a patient at home and make appropriate care decisions? If you have a nursing specialty that you find gratifying, perhaps a disease management or population health position in that area would be a perfect fit, especially if you also like to follow "your" patients throughout the continuum of care.

Another issue for your discernment is whether you feel that direct care is part of the nursing case management role. In varying degrees, some nursing case management delivery systems, although rare today, combine the nursing case management role with bedside nursing care. In this combined role, the case management–bedside nurse may assess acute care and discharge planning needs for the patient. A plan of care would be developed by the nurse; included in it would be the required clinical interventions that are based on the patient's condition as well as the postacute care or services required on the patient's discharge back to the home setting or transfer to a less-acute-care facility. The plan of care would then be sent to the multidisciplinary team for additional recommendations and then sent back to the nurse for evaluation. The team assists the nurse in the implementation and evaluation of the plan.

Variations on this type of case management–staff nurse model exist, but universal acceptance of this style of case management is lacking. Case management experts tend to feel strongly that case managers should not perform direct bedside nursing care. Combining these roles may present a main cause of frustration, burnout, and the eventual demise of the case management model; however, with limited resources, especially in small, rural hospitals, this may occur. A combined role may risk having the bedside nurse busy with direct care provision while important aspects of case management such as discharge planning activities for a patient with a complex health condition and needs are delayed until the bedside nurse is free enough to tackle such activities. An example is following up on the need to discharge a patient to an SNF setting and the patient or family needs to review available options and decide on a choice of facility.

When assessing job openings in case management, note that many employment opportunities are available for various aspects of the total case management role; these are not the whole picture but can provide valuable experience in the management aspects of healthcare. Some of these areas are preadmission case management, utilization management, quality improvement, risk management, telephone triage, and transitional planning. When interviewing or during a preinterview telephone call, it is wise to ask about the expected job responsibilities because some job advertisements may be misleading. For example, an advertisement for utilization reviewers may actually be more akin to a case management position or vice versa.

Experience in the above roles is important, because considerable skills and an extensive knowledge base are useful to perform case management functions well. In the evolving role of what a case manager *is* and *does,* more of these functions are being included in the hybrid interpretation of a case manager. Many case managers who come into the profession with utilization management or quality improvement backgrounds have made the transition with more ease than even the most clinically competent staff nurses. All experiences are valuable and will add to your knowledge, skills, and competencies. They are also essential for career advancement and professional development.

▶ MODELS OF CASE MANAGEMENT

It is not the intent of this section to describe various case management models in detail or to present a comprehensive list of all the models that exist today. Current models are well detailed in some of the invaluable case management journals that are available. Innovative case management models are being attempted in every phase and setting of healthcare delivery, and current publications describe them and articulate their successes and barriers to success.

Case management models have been broadly described in either of two approaches: within-the-walls and beyond-the-walls case management. Within-the-walls case management models are those that are implemented in the acute care/hospital setting and focus primarily on managing the care of patients during an acute episode of illness. Beyond-the-walls case management models are those that are implemented in settings other than acute care such as outpatient, community, payor-based, and long-term care. The role of the case manager in these models varies depending on the settings in which it is implemented. For example, the case manager in within-the-walls models plays

an active role in transitional or discharge planning; in the outpatient and community settings, he or she may focus more on management of chronic illness and prevention of disease progression; in the long-term settings, the focus may be more on supportive or rehabilitative care; while in the payor-based setting, case management may emphasize management of member benefits and triaging patients to the appropriate level of care when needed.

It is recommended that those who develop a new case management department review the current literature for ideas and lessons learned to avoid committing similar mistakes or wasting their efforts. More importantly, it is essential that each organization evaluate its individual needs and the population it serves before instituting a specific case management model. This is key to case management success. The right case management model will maximize reimbursement, lower the total costs of providing care, and satisfy an organization's internal and external customers (i.e., patients, patients' families, and payors). A case management model that does not complement the internal structure and satisfy identified critical needs is likely to fail.

The proliferation of case management models is not without problems. The integration of case managers continues to be an emerging challenge. Historically, acute care case managers performed their responsibilities in an episodic manner, focusing on the safe discharge of a patient to the natural next level of care. Case managers external to the acute care setting performed their job responsibilities according to their job descriptions. There was essentially no communication between the two except for, perhaps, a brief time during the actual "handing over" of the patient. Like managed care, case management became very fragmented.

Problems with this fragmented case management model ensued, and "through the continuum" case management models developed, especially when an organization had integrated systems. There are still multiple coordination challenges about who does what, where, and when. When all case managers are under one organizational umbrella, however, it makes it easier to coordinate the communication; in such a setting, the patient benefits with more continuity of case management coverage. In those organizations without the integrated systems of acute care, home healthcare, SNF care, ambulatory and rehabilitation care, and so on, case management still remains fragmented. Now that there are so many external and internal case managers, an emerging challenge is to find an efficient method of everyone working together.

One suggestion for complex and integrated systems is that one case manager must assume accountability and responsibility for being the central point of contact. If an integrated system includes HMO case managers, acute care case managers, home health case managers, rehabilitation case managers, and SNF case managers, the model still remains fragmented, unless, for example, the HMO case manager is accountable for the coordination of the big picture of care; the other case managers (or "attending case manager") will manage the crises and details while that patient resides in their respective levels of care.

In this instance, the HMO case manager is chosen as the primary case manager. Other case managers can also take on the role of the coordinating case manager; a payor-based case manager or a case manager for a group of several self-funded health plans may be the primary case manager. This case manager is responsible for ensuring that the care meets acceptable standards, that the care is within the benefits guidelines of the health plan, and that the care is provided through a PPO when possible. This case manager essentially becomes the consultant for the case, coordinating all levels of care and overseeing the resource utilization. Nevertheless, this case manager cannot provide all the aspects of care needed at all levels of care; the time-intensive responsibility of coordinating the day-to-day care, education, and social services will go to the case manager of whatever setting the patient resides in.

It is imperative that at the beginning of a patient's case, all case managers agree on the coordination efforts. Whether the pivotal case manager will be called the primary case manager, the case management consultant, or the case management coordinator, is something that will work itself out in case management history. The important thing is that the assignment is made. If this case management challenge is not attended to, case management will eventually get a reputation as being a cause, rather than the cure, of healthcare fragmentation, poor quality, and unsafe experiences or medical errors. In general, the consultant case manager will assist the other case managers with important issues with which only one who has followed the patient through the chronic illness may be familiar. In addition to issues such as allowable benefits and PPO providers, this case manager will supply others with patient-specific information on important psychosocial and financial aspects of the case or areas in which the patient needs more education and instruction about the illness, injury, or disability.

The assignment is a bit more complex than just choosing the "least busy" case manager. The choice has legal and regulatory ramifications. For example, CMS regulations state that a hospital's personnel are responsible for the safe discharge of its patients; therefore, it is the responsibility of the hospital social work–case management team to provide this service. *The Conditions of Participation for Medicare Hospitals—CMS Discharge Planning Regulations* (CMS, 2011, No. 482.43) state that the hospital must arrange for the initial implementation of the patient's discharge plan. In this instance, the HMO or payor-based case manager will communicate with other case managers by providing the names of PPO facilities or speaking with the patient or family. However, this may be further complicated if there is an HMO-risk Medicare plan (as an example); the hospital–HMO contract may require the HMO case manager to perform the discharge planning duties. Does the regulatory or contractual agreement take precedence? This is a decision for the hospital administration to make. In general:

1. First, assess contractual and regulatory agreements. If administration or legal counsel needs to be involved, get their expertise and advice.
2. Second, if there are no legal restrictions, then communication is the key. Always keep focused on the bottom line: the patient.

The following reflect some of the general classifications of case management models that are available in our contemporary healthcare environment. Broadly stated, case management models can be differentiated by setting, disease type, and domain (the provider domain and the payor domain). Providers include hospitals, nursing homes, subacute and rehabilitation facilities, physician offices, home health agencies, hospices, or mental health settings. Payors include any insurance setting (workers' compensation, HMOs, PPOs, Medicare, Medicaid, employer groups, etc.). Regardless of where case management is practiced along the healthcare continuum, the complexity, intensity, and major characteristics of the model depend on the following factors: the care setting or level of care, patient population, reimbursement methods, and the care provider (Display 1-2).

In addition to being common case management models, the following also represent potential areas of case management employment.

---

display 1-2

FACTORS THAT IMPACT MODELS OF CASE MANAGEMENT

1. The CONTEXT of the care setting where case management is practiced; for example, ambulatory, community-based, acute care, subacute/rehabilitation, long-term care, telephonic, and nursing homes.
2. The PATIENT POPULATION served and its needs; for example, critical/acute episode of illness, specific disease such as asthma or heart failure, long-term supportive care, or chronic illness.
3. The REIMBURSEMENT METHOD applied; for example, managed care, capitation, discounted rate, prospective payment system, accountable care.
4. The CARE PROVIDER needed for care provision; for example, generalist, specialist, individual, multidisciplinary team, internal or external to the healthcare agency.

Adapted from Tahan, H. (2008). Case management practice settings and throughput. In S. Powel & Tahan (Eds.), *CMSA core curriculum for case management* (2nd ed., pp. 39–73). Philadelphia, PA: Wolters Kluwer/ Lippincott Williams & Wilkins.

▶ Acute Care Case Management

Acute care case management is usually time limited, episodic nursing case management at the hospital level. This model integrates clinical care management, utilization management, and transitional planning functions. Acute care case management may be managed in at least five different ways. First, it may be unit based, in which case managers manage patients while on a particular unit such as ICU, orthopedic, medicine, or telemetry. In a second scenario, acute care case management may mean that case managers follow patients from admission to discharge regardless of the levels of care the patient transitions through (for example, admitted to intensive care, transitions to telemetry and then a regular inpatient unit, and ultimately discharged to the home setting). These case managers often do prehospital teaching if the admission is nonemergent and planned. The same case manager will follow up with a patient in whatever level of care or unit is required, thus ensuring continuity of care. Third, acute care case management may be disease based, following up with patients according to their primary illness. Each setting requires unique components, skills, and knowledge for effective care. Fourth, case management may be practiced on the basis of an individual physician or group of physicians within a specialty. In this case, the case manager follows patients who are cared for by such physician(s) regardless of diagnosis or unit with the hospital where care is provided. Finally, acute care case management may be represented through primary nursing case management.

Case managers may also practice hands-on care of the patient. They identify acute care needs and discharge needs as well as help develop the treatment plan with the multidisciplinary team. This is not an either/or phenomenon; successful hospitals have found that a combination of case manager roles best meets the needs of the organization and patients.

Case managers in acute care settings are frequently registered professional nurses. Most often and at a minimum, they are prepared at the bachelor's degree level. In recent times, more and more graduate-level case managers have been produced. The combination of nurse and social worker case managers is another more recent occurrence in the acute care setting; in fact, such a combination is not popular in other healthcare settings.

Adjunctive to acute care, many facilities are recognizing the importance of providing throughput areas such as the emergency department, admitting office, and perioperative services, with designated case managers. This case manager can steer a patient into a more appropriate setting before admitting him or her into acute care; the process of case management should begin at the earliest possible time.

EMERGENCY DEPARTMENT CASE MANAGEMENT

Since the emergency department is, perhaps, the most common entry point to the hospital setting, it is important for case managers to provide gatekeeping oversight there. In the emergency department case management model, the case manager interfaces with physicians, nurses, social workers, admitting office staff, payor-based case managers, and others to ensure cost-effective and medically necessary care. Emergency Department case managers deal with various groups of patients, including those who are to be treated and released, admitted to the hospital, discharged but require services such as home care, and observed for a period of time before a final decision is made whether to admit or release. They are also involved in the care of patients who present mainly with social rather than medical problems, such as homelessness and domestic violence or abuse. Since the advent of the Medicare two-midnight rule, Emergency Department case managers are frequently tasked with ensuring the correct status of any admissions (observations, inpatient, etc.).

ADMISSION CASE MANAGEMENT

Today's mature case management models of the acute care settings recognize the importance of gatekeeping at the point of admission to the hospital. Case managers in the admitting office evaluate the patient's condition (primary and secondary reasons for admission to the hospital) and the preliminary expected plan of care (e.g., type of diagnostic and therapeutic procedures) and intended length of stay for appropriateness for care provision in the acute setting. These case managers may also be responsible for assessing out-of-state (or out of country) admissions to their facility.

The main focus of the case manager's assessment here is the patient's severity of illness and intensity of services requirement. If the patient's condition does not meet the standard or criteria for admission to the acute care setting, the patient is diverted to an alternate level of care that is more appropriate to the patient's condition and the needed services. The case manager in this case contacts the patient's physician, explains the situation, including the findings of the assessment, and negotiates agreement on the alternate care setting. The use of the admitting office case manager has proven effective in reducing reimbursement denials or the conversion of an acute hospital stay to an observation status instead.

PERIOPERATIVE SERVICES CASE MANAGEMENT

Another common entry point into the hospital are the surgical suites. With ever-changing regulatory issues, having a case manager in this department can avoid lack of payment and denials. This type of case manager is known as the PACU case manager (post anesthesia care unit [PACU]). The PACU case manager may or may not care for surgical patients during the preadmission testing phase, the day of surgery as the patient goes through the surgical phase, and/or in the recovery area postsurgery and during recovery from anesthesia. This PACU case manager ensures that the patient has been authorized for surgery by the health insurance plan, underwent appropriate preadmission testing and was deemed ready for surgery, received medical clearance for surgery, signed necessary consents, and had no questions that remained unanswered.

These case managers are imperative for positively impacting the revenue cycle of the hospital. Several examples of the work these case managers do are in Chapter 5. Medicare's regulatory issues define an 'inpatient only' surgery versus an outpatient surgery. If the PACU case manager assesses it wrong, the hospital will not get paid. Many acute care facilities have learned the hard way after not getting reimbursed for an 'inpatient only' surgery (think of very intense, expensive procedures).

▶ Complex Case Management

In another type of service-based case management, known as complex case management, the case selection includes patients who are at risk for extremely high healthcare costs (e.g., patients with AIDS; premature infants in neonatal ICUs; and patients with possible kidney/liver/heart/bone marrow transplant, high spinal cord injury, or end-stage renal disease receiving hemodialysis). Almost any setting can support a complex case management model: insurance companies, hospitals, disease management carve-outs, home health, rehabilitation facilities, and so on.

Complex case management focuses, not only on patients with chronic illness, but also on those with disabilities and catastrophic illnesses who require intensive short- or long-term management of services. The focus of the case manager in these populations is rehabilitation (physical and vocational), occupational therapy, return to work, prevention of deterioration in the patient's condition, and management of healthcare resources.

▶ Disease Management/Population Health Management

Disease management, more recently called population health management, and sometimes referred to as chronic care management, is an arrangement that gives the healthcare agency responsibility for ensuring that a given population receives a defined set of services in a coordinated and continuous fashion. Ultimately, the services should improve the health of the population by appropriately managing the existing disease entity (e.g., heart failure or diabetes), preventing or delaying the progression of disease and the need for acute care and, therefore, reducing the cost and improving the quality of care.

Unlike case management for a particular condition or disease in the acute care setting (and, therefore, for only one episode of illness), disease managers/population health managers follow their population through all levels of care. Some disease managers/population health managers are required to follow their patients for a limited time, as in high-risk pregnancy. Others may follow their patients, such as those with cancer or heart failure, for longer periods. Disease management/population management programs are often developed in sites such as physician practices or insurance companies.

In disease management/population management models, case managers apply evidence-based guidelines or protocols. These protocols are nationally recognized standards of care that describe the necessary care and treatments (diagnostic and therapeutic interventions) for patients with a specific chronic health condition such as heart failure or end-stage renal disease and that are based on the severity of illness. These protocols also include the expected outcomes of care that are easily measured and tracked over time. Case managers assess patients and classify them, according to specific criteria, into low-, moderate-, or high-risk groups. They then manage the care of the patients, applying treatments and interventions indicated by their risk group. Treatments include medications, lifestyle changes, and health education. Such models of care have proven effective in preventing the need for emergency department visits or acute care hospital stays.

▶ Insurance (Third-Party Payor) Case Management

Case managers must balance quality of care and patient advocacy with the responsibility for carefully shepherding that health plan's dollars. If there is a conflict between the expectations of the insurance company and the facility to which the member is currently admitted for care, the case manager must depend on communication and negotiation skills in resolving the conflict. The case manager is the company's liaison. Third-party payor case managers often have the power to authorize services and levels of care. Their main focus is managing members' benefits effectively and ensuring that members receive healthcare services in the most appropriate level of care or setting justified by the presenting health condition. Case managers may perform their job responsibilities in two ways: telephonically and on-site.

TELEPHONIC CASE MANAGEMENT

Some case managers for large insurance companies have patients all over the United States and must rely on telephone interviews. Because their assessment and planning are only as good as the information they can extract from the facility/member, they must be skilled in asking tough, pertinent questions. If they do not get the right answers, coverage for a hospital admission (or specified days) may be denied.

ON-SITE CASE MANAGEMENT

On-site case management is often preferable to telephonics. The member's medical record can be reviewed, members of the involved healthcare team can be interviewed, if necessary, and the patient (health plan member) can be seen and assessed. Proximity to the patient is an advantage. It allows the case manager to develop a therapeutic relationship, see a patient's condition firsthand, and make personal observations when assessing the patient's interactions with family members for discharge assessment purposes. Sometimes a picture is worth a thousand words.

Regardless of whether insurance-based case managers perform their job responsibilities telephonically or on-site, the focus of the role is the same. Case managers in this model assess the patient's condition, determine the type and level of setting in which the patient should receive care, and ensure that the discharge plan (postepisode care) matches the patient's and family's needs. In addition, they manage the patient's health benefits as stipulated in the health plan and promote compliance with the standards and procedures of the insurance company and as agreed on in the plan.

▶ Palliative Care, End-of-Life Care, and Hospice Case Management

Case managers in the palliative care, end-of-life care, and hospice case management model coordinate the care and comfort of the dying patients and their families. Often, the nurse becomes the primary manager of the case; the physician becomes a consultant. A special focus in this model is the care of patients who are suffering from a terminal illness and who have a limited life expectancy, that is, care at the end of life. Case managers here deal with the complex consequences of illness as the patient's death nears, as well as postdeath during the family's bereavement stage.

From a palliative care perspective, case managers care for patients who have chosen supportive rather than curative care and services. Such services are offered either in a hospitalized setting, in the patient's home, or on an ambulatory basis. Hospice care, on the other hand, takes place either in an institutional setting (e.g., hospital, SNF, or medical hospice facilities) or in the patient's home. In either setting, the focus of the case management model is the same: respectful, comfortable, and dignified death.

▶ Home Health Case Management

In home health case management, case managers serve the needs of the chronically ill in the home setting. Coordination of several therapeutic modalities may be necessary in an individual case. These may include wound care, infusion therapy services, physical therapy, speech therapy, occupational therapy, coordination of durable medical equipment, tube feeding, medication monitoring, assessments, tube/tracheostomy care—almost anything done in hospitals. If the patient is stable, home care can also include such intensive services as ventilator assistance. These case managers monitor for early warning signs, contact the patient's primary physician for treatment, and can thereby prevent or lessen the severity of exacerbation of the illness and reduce the frequency of readmissions to

the hospital. The therapeutic home health case manager's relationship usually begins and ends with insurance authorization. However, acting as a patient advocate, the case manager can help to extend authorization from the insurance company if tangible reasons can be cited and the case manager is adept at negotiation.

▶ Physician Groups/Patient-Centered Medical Homes

As large physician practice groups become more common, case management positions in this area are being seen more frequently. Clinical nurse specialists or highly experienced nurses are often placed in a case management role in physician specialist offices (e.g., cardiology, pulmonary, neurology, gastroenterology, oncology, or orthopedics).

Patient-centered medical homes (PCMH) are the evolution of case managers in a physician practice. These may be referred to as a primary care medical home or a patient-centered health home. This model may be found within a community clinic, physician group, or ambulatory facility. A medical home model provides accessible, continuous, coordinated, and comprehensive patient-centered care. It is managed centrally by a PCP with the active involvement of a nonphysician case manager. Providers that have been deemed a medical home may receive supplemental payments to support operations expected in a medical home, such as case managers. To be deemed a medical home, physician practices are often required to improve practice infrastructure and meet certain eligibility conditions (CMSA, 2016; Tahan & Treiger, 2017).

▶ Skilled Nursing Facility Case Management

When patients' self-care needs exceed their self-care capabilities after an episode of acute illness, SNF placement may be necessary. Some SNF case managers act as liaisons between the acute care and subacute care levels, assisting during the convalescent period by determining appropriate needs and services and obtaining required payor funds for the SNF care. Many other responsibilities that resemble those of an acute care case manager may be required during the patient's SNF admission. This level of care has opened up case management opportunities in large numbers because of the federal reimbursement changes that have taken place (e.g., implementation of the prospective payment systems) and that continue to occur. Gerontologists, nurses, physical or occupational therapists, and social workers are good choices for this case management position.

▶ Integrated Case Management

Traditionally, case management has been separated by medical conditions versus mental or behavioral health. Integrated case management is designed to collapse the silos between these two important aspects of humanity. This type of case management requires special training and skills, and some consider it to be advanced practice (Tahan & Treiger, 2017). However, given the sociopolitical trends today, the fortunate patient has no behavioral components. Conversely, case managers are having to attend to growing numbers of patients with horrendous trauma, both physically and mentally.

▶ Public Health/Community-Based Case Management

This model helps families and patients access appropriate services needed for independent functioning. A wide range of target populations may receive services, depending on the focus of the agency. Community health nursing, such as that on Indian reservations or with high-risk/low-income maternal or child health, has long been taking care of families' health on a case-by-case basis. Other areas or populations needing case managers include mental health, geriatrics, catastrophic diseases such as AIDS, homeless families, or substance abuse patients. Some populations can be well served with a social service professional; others require medical knowledge, especially in the HIV and geriatric populations. As is the case with home health nursing, community-based case management also works to prevent exacerbations of illnesses by early assessment of changes in patients' conditions and early interventions.

▶ Rehabilitation Specialists

Many rehabilitation units (both freestanding and those in acute or subacute care facilities) have discovered the efficacy of the case manager–social worker team concept. Patients enter rehabilitation units for many reasons, such as cerebral vascular accidents, motor vehicle accidents, traumas, gunshot wounds, head injuries, and spinal cord injuries. Most patients are not even allowed on rehabilitation units unless they are functioning at a low enough level to require intensive rehabilitation services. Inherent in the criteria for acceptance onto this unit is a precipitating illness or event that requires a full-scale biopsychosocial assessment, planning, and intervention. The goal is to bring that person back to a functional level that matches his or her baseline level as much as possible. Depending on the precipitating event, this type of case management may require the utmost in creativity, pulling in both private and community resources.

▶ Vocational Case Management

Vocational case management may be a component of rehabilitation case management, a part of workers' compensation case management, or a separate form of employment. Vocational case managers assist patients (usually injured workers or those who have acquired a work-related illness) in returning to meaningful employment, given their new limitations as a result of injury or disease in the work setting. A thorough knowledge of disability and workers' compensation laws and excellent assessment skills (both of functional and cognitive ability and employability) are necessary. A special focus on vocational case management is rehabilitation of the patient, which addresses job retraining, modification, adjustment, and reentry to the work setting.

▶ Workers' Compensation

Case management is the key strategy in management of workers' compensation cases. The goals are to proactively prevent injuries, when possible, and to manage injuries when they occur. Workers' compensation case management stresses early recognition and referral of the injured patient and provides a comprehensive evaluation, assessment, and care plan. The primary focus of workers' compensation case management is return-to-work. Another aspect of case management is prevention of work-related injuries or illnesses. As in all types of case management, workers' compensation lends itself to abuses; therefore, the case manager must be aware of the red flags of malingering while maintaining a strong patient advocate role.

▶ Case Management Firms

Case managers working in private case management agencies need a national network of resources. Patients are often willing to travel to receive the best care for their particular illness. Case managers may need to identify the most up-to-date treatment for a specific disease and locate the facility that offers that treatment. Patients may be admitted to hospitals anywhere in the United States or even worldwide. This type of case management holds the same limitations as telephonic reviews (i.e., reliance on asking the right questions and receiving accurate information from a nurse on the other end of the line, who may have little time to spare for telephone consultation).

Private case management focuses on managing the care and resources of patients with chronic illnesses, disabilities, or injuries that have resulted in long-term and complex physical, cognitive, or psychosocial problems. Patients with such conditions tend to consume expensive healthcare resources and require care that is intensive and time consuming. Their conditions are long-term; most often, they are not resolved and sometimes last until the patient's death.

▶ Entrepreneurial Case Management

Several brave nurses have been willing to risk starting their own case manager businesses. Also known as case management consultants, these independent case managers may be contracted by patients, family members, physicians, or insurance companies. Entrepreneurial case managers need good business skills and the ability to work autonomously. There are some perils involved in this type of case management; if a patient sustains a poor outcome from a referred physician or treatment, the company may be sued for liability. On the positive side, independent case managers often have increased freedom to fulfill the patient's desires and needs, especially if the patient has funds to supplement private insurance. Without financial constraints and insurance policy restrictions, patient choices can be implemented to the benefit and satisfaction of the patient, family, and physician.

As in other forms of case management, independent case managers coordinate all aspects of care, in the home and in any level of care needed. Specialties such as geriatrics or rehabilitation may dominate a professional group practice, depending on the skill and experience of the case managers. Patients may reside in various parts of the country, and travel may be part of the job description.

Before considering entrepreneurial case management, assess whether you have both the background skills required for the job and the personality makeup. Successful case managers benefit from some of the entrepreneurial characteristics listed in Display 1-3 (Tassel, 1994, pg. 143).

In 1990, some entrepreneurial nurses employed by St. Mary's Hospital in Tucson, Arizona, seized an opportunity to contract case managers and community nursing services to a medical HMO, forming a nursing HMO group. Their vision included a better way to manage patients, enter the managed care arena, strengthen business opportunities for case managers, and advance the nursing profession (Michaels, 1992). With the fast-changing healthcare climate, opportunities for entrepreneurship abound. An unselfish vision in the proper hands can benefit the patient, the nursing profession, and all those touched by the dilemmas inherent in the managed care arena.

---

display 1-3

ENTREPRENEURIAL CHARACTERISTICS

▶ *Opportunist*—Sees opportunities but also the risk involved in pursuing them.
▶ *Risk taker*—Accepts risk and attempts to manage it effectively and proactively.
▶ *Visionary*—Sees a better way of doing things and takes advantage of the situation.
▶ *Actor*—Is action oriented with little patience for frequent committee meetings.
▶ *Strategist*—Focuses on the best solutions, especially those that ensure meeting the goals.
▶ *Innovator*—Is unafraid to try a new way of doing something.
▶ *Learner*—Is open-minded and asks questions to develop new strategies and advance own knowledge.
▶ *Confident*—Assesses opportunities comfortably, confidently, and produces favorable changes and results.
▶ *Flexibility*—Adapts to fast-paced changes and is able to rearrange priorities.

Tassel, M. V. (1994, August). Case managers use entrepreneurial skills. *Hospital Case Management*, 143.

▶ Hospitalists

Although not a case management model per se, this current hospital structure has shown success in many locations and is another type of case management model. Most often, there is at least one case manager on each hospitalist team; a social worker is included in the more evolved models and where the patient population managed by hospitalists is of increased acuity and complexity. Hospitalists are physicians who take over care for the primary care provider (PCP) when the PCP's patients are admitted to the hospital. Many physicians like this arrangement because they can then focus on their office patients without running from their office to a hospital on the west side of town, then to another on the east side of town. It also allows physicians to get some rest, because there are physicians in-house at the hospital during the day and night to handle medication changes or emergencies. However, there are some problems, as with all new innovations. Not all patients feel secure without their "own" physician, and not all physicians are willing to "give up" their patients during hospitalizations. Much variation exists among those trying out this model. Case managers act in a capacity similar to that of any hospital-based case manager.

▶ EVALUATION OF A CASE MANAGEMENT MODEL

Evaluation of the case management needs of your organization and the patient population is germane to both the development of new case management departments and to situations where the current case management department is not meeting its goals. This strategic planning activity will direct the organization toward the target and possibly save time, money, resources, and staff burnout from unnecessary failure.

One large inner-city hospital identified case management services as a means of responding to changes in reimbursement strategies. They appeared to do all the right things; they reviewed the literature, visited other hospitals and studied what worked for those sites, and appointed a multidisciplinary team to implement the chosen model. What they did not do was evaluate their needs and match a model that worked with a similar population of patients. They were in a big city, and most of their patients had a low income with little family or financial support. The model hospital that they chose to emulate was a small community hospital with affluent patients and sufficient family and financial support. When choosing a case management model or evaluating one that is less than satisfactory, consider the following areas in your organization:

▶ The geographic location. An organization/facility in a large city with adequate acute, postacute, and community services support has very different needs than does a rural organization/facility with limited or distant resources.

▶ The demographics of the patient population served. In the preceding example, one hospital had very different patient needs than the other it attempted to emulate. The inner-city hospital likely had more Medicaid and Medicare patients; the community hospital likely had more private insurance patients. Transitional and discharge planning also might have posed different challenges. The inner-city hospital had a greater number of emergency department visits because a lower percentage of its admissions were managed care patients who had PCPs. Denied reimbursement levels were crippling, high-risk patients were not being expediently identified, and disease management programs were not available.

This scenario will change with the growing numbers of managed care Medicare and Medicaid plans, but it clearly illustrates the importance of evaluating your patients' demographics.

▶ Collect and analyze data.
  1. Discern the patient mix.
  2. Assess the payor mix commonly seen in your organization or facility and the percentage each type accounts for: Medicare, Medicaid, private pay, workers' compensation, private insurance.
  3. Evaluate the major types of reimbursement: Managed Medicare versus fee-for-service, DRG reimbursement, capitation, per diem, and so on.
  4. Discern which diseases or medical conditions (e.g., traumas, organ transplantation) compose a large proportion of the patient population. List the high-volume, high-cost, high-risk diagnoses encountered.
  5. Assess recidivism. Which patients with which diseases frequently get readmitted to the hospital, go to the emergency department, call or visit the physician? What is the acuity and chronicity of the population?

▶ Assess gaps in staff education and training. A well-trained case management staff will contain all the ingredients for success. To case manage in an environment that yields quality care, the case manager must be clinically astute. To affect patient, provider, and payor satisfaction, the case manager must be adept in communication and negotiation skills and be knowledgeable in all areas covered in this text. To develop the best strategies for maximum reimbursement with minimal denials, case managers must clearly understand the ramifications of insurance benefit designs and reimbursement systems.

▶ Set organizational goals. It is important that the organization is clear about what it wants to achieve with case management services. Set short-term, intermediate, and long-range goals as part of a strategic planning activity.

▶ Consider the standards of regulatory agencies. Regulatory and accreditation agencies play a major role in the decisions a healthcare provider or administrator makes. Case management can fulfill many requirements for several of these agencies, while also improving quality and satisfaction as well as balancing costs and revenue.

▶ Operationalize case management at the patient level; that is, ensure that the model is patient- and family centered and would apply to the care of every patient regardless of location in the organization: Clinic, ICU, regular floor, observation in the emergency department, home setting, and so on. To achieve this, all staff must be familiar with the model and trained in its implementation while they are involved in care delivery to their patients. One important aspect of the model is that it must be relevant to all patient populations served to facilitate consistency and conformity in care provision.

▶ Redesign implementation processes. Because the implementation of the case management model impacts the way care is delivered and its related context and processes, redesigning these processes is essential. Otherwise, it may appear that the model is implemented in a vacuum, presenting the staff with great challenges in implementation. For example, staff, including physicians, must be aware of the role of the case manager and its contribution to patient care management. Examples of the processes that would require redesign are care provision or management such as transitional or discharge planning, financial processes such as resource allocation and utilization review and management, and quality or outcomes measurement such as compliance with core measures and reporting of significant events to the risk management department.

▶ Determine the system of measurement of the effectiveness of the case management model. It is important to identify the metrics to be used for evaluation of the model prior to implementation. It is also advisable to determine the process of data collection, analysis, and reporting. The metrics should be determined on the basis of the goals and expectations of the model; translate each goal into a measurable objective. This avoids unnecessary and costly efforts, especially if the metrics identified can serve multiple purposes. For example, core measures, if chosen, are also required by CMS.

▶ SUGGESTED STEPS FOR CHOOSING OR CHANGING YOUR CASE MANAGEMENT MODEL

1. Develop your organizational compass by listing important goals. Perhaps your organization decided on the following goals:
   ▶ To balance the cost of care with the reimbursement.

▶ To be a world-class hospital or managed care organization or home health agency (other) by achieving clinical and administrative benchmarks in selected areas.

▶ To develop an integrated system for a seamless flow of patients across the continuum of care.

▶ To ensure superior quality and safety outcomes as well as patient experience of care.

2. Prioritize the goals that are most important to the organization. Balancing the cost of care with available reimbursement is essential for survival, so your organization may choose this as its first goal. Clinical excellence is also important, so the organization may choose this goal as its second goal. A seamless, integrated system may be on the "wish list" for the future. When prioritizing goals, consider regulatory and accreditation requirements.

3. Evaluate your present strengths and weaknesses because they affect your ability to accomplish those goals. There are many avenues to increase cost-efficiency, decrease waste, and continuously improve quality of services and care. What are your current systems that are good or salvageable? Use the evaluation data you gathered earlier to address this step. For your first goal, you may determine that you already have a preadmissions nurse or a solid utilization management department. However, your length of stay is long because of weakness on the transitional or discharge planning end. Unreimbursed care and denials are a serious problem. Do you have readmissions in a few targeted conditions? Will you benefit from a disease management structure in these specialties? Do you have staff expertise that can fill needed roles? Do you have the technology to support the changes planned, or will this be a major expense that must be budgeted?

Decide which goals can be accomplished with minimal changes versus those that may be in your future. Do not try to do everything at once; for example, before community integration is attempted, hospital-based or internal case management should be well defined and operational. The internal case management system should be developed with a vision of ultimately extending its scope into the community and caring for the patient throughout the continuum of care.

Consider the example of the large inner-city hospital that tried to use a small community hospital model; it did not fail in its case management attempt but rather learned some very important lessons. It continued with a new, customized case management pilot program that included training case managers in transitional or discharge planning; educating physicians, nurses, and other staff members in the case management process; and implementing aspects of disease management for targeted patient populations such as individuals with asthma.

4. Evaluate future trends that will affect patient care and reimbursement. Are you expecting more Medicare and Medicaid managed care patients? Are the demographics of your community changing? Are you well positioned to get enough business in the healthcare future?

5. Plan how you will monitor for success. In the large inner-city hospital, monitoring was done in several ways:

   ▶ Lag days were identified and monitored.

   ▶ Areas tracked to ascertain if there was improvement included denied payments, recidivism rate for identified patient populations, and length of stay for targeted DRGs.

   ▶ Satisfaction with the case management process was measured for physicians, nurses, and other care providers.

6. Adapt aspects of current case management models to your needs and requirements. Customize what you see and read to best meet the needs of your organization and patients. Apply various designs of case management and disease management if that will move you toward your goals of quality and cost-efficiency. When possible, improve the model. Anything that is done can be done better. If your organization has requirements that have not been addressed by others, be creative! Go where no healthcare organization has gone before, and your facility may write the next "best practice" article on case management models.

▶ INFORMATION TECHNOLOGY AND CASE MANAGEMENT

Historically, case managers kept track of their daily activities using a "paper and pencil" approach, which was a manual and laborious process. Their work was viewed as "top secret"; they documented their involvement in patient care in a file that was kept out of the patient's medical record; no one had access to the file except for the case management program administrators. The primary focus then was utilization review and reimbursement for care rendered. Now, contributions of case managers in patient care are no longer secret; in fact, they are transparent to all who are directly or indirectly involved in patient care, and the role has expanded beyond utilization management. In addition, the documentation of case managers' activities is kept permanently in the patient's medical record and accessed daily by other members of the healthcare team.

With "meaningful use" mandates, the use of the "paper and pencil" approach to case management documentation is a thing of the past. Accreditation and regulatory agencies require a seamless multidisciplinary approach to patient care planning and management, with evidence of compliance present in the patient's medical record. Health information technology companies began to address this issue over a decade ago; however, the software applications developed only recently are becoming useful to case managers, with an accurate depiction of what case management practice is about.

Recently, the use of information technology in case management practice has been on the rise and is integrated into major medical record documentation software applications. Initially, case management information technology development focused on the utilization review and management aspect of transitional the role of the case manager; today, however, applications have grown to allow effective approaches to clinical care management; discharge planning; quality and patient safety; variance management; patient flow management; cost analyses; and data collection, aggregation, and reporting. Such improvement in case management information technology is evidence of the maturation of case management programs and their value in healthcare delivery and management.

In the absence of case management information technology, case managers engaged in numerous manual and labor-intensive activities that were considered "busy work" or "clerical work" and resulted in increased job-related stress and dissatisfaction. Examples of these activities are duplicate documentation; photocopying parts of the medical record to keep in own files or share with others; using a "to do list" or placing stickers (Post-It notes) everywhere as reminders to complete certain activities, or for others, asking them to follow up on things or answer certain questions; filing of forms; and using a list/tool for tracking delays in care (i.e., variances).

McGonigle and Mastrian (2008) claim that case management information technology presents case managers with solutions to these problems. It allows them to be more efficient and efficacious in their role. For example, information technology facilitates data collection (e.g., variances, outcomes measures), report generation, and dissemination. It also functions as an effective tool for bringing people, data, and procedures together for the betterment of patient care, especially in the area of managing information to support case management functions and decision making at the individual, team, and organization levels.

The benefits of case management information technology are numerous, as the following examples illustrate (McGonigle & Mastrian, 2008):

1. *Work flow*: Support of case management process; reduction of duplicate documentation; elimination of double data entry; improvement of data entry, retrieval, access, storage, and dissemination; generation of reminders of due tasks; and generation of alerts, especially those that are patient-safety oriented.
2. *Patient care*: Keeping patients safe, monitoring progress, use of best practices and evidence-based care, use of nationally recognized standards and guidelines, standardization of care patterns, reduction or elimination of medical errors, and compliance with core measures.
3. *Organizational*: Improving the efficiency of care activities, better job satisfaction, increased accountability, improved relationships among care providers, and return on investment measures for case management.

▶ TELEHEALTH AND CASE MANAGEMENT

The use of telehealth is not new; however, its application in case management is fairly recent. When telehealth approaches are used in case management practice, it is referred to as *tele-case management*. Tele-case management is simply the provision and management of healthcare services from a distance. It has become more common because of disease management or population management programs that require the use of telecommunication technologies for improving patients' adherence to medical regimens, health education, and psychosocial or emotional support (e.g., congestive heart failure patients). The evolution of telehealth to provide direct patient care is rapidly becoming the norm (did the patient have a stroke? Does the patient need to come to a stroke center from the rural facility he or she is currently in?).

The use of tele-case management also means the sharing of information with others for the better management of patient care and employing telecommunication technologies such as the telephone, fax machines, and electronic communication via the Internet. Sharing of information in this fashion was the first aspect of tele-case management used by case managers, especially after an increase in the use of managed care health insurance plans. Examples of tele-case management activities include authorizations of services, telephone triage, concurrent reviews of patient care and progress, and handling of reimbursement of denials and appeals.

Care must be taken when using telehealth, because there still remain licensure limitations across state lines; there is still a lack of national policy for interstate practice. This can be different for various licensures and from one state to the next. Further, security and privacy risks cannot be understated (Tahan & Treiger, 2017).

▶ A DAY IN THE LIFE OF A CASE MANAGER

This section, beginning with the next paragraph, narrates the experiences of a hospital case manager in the early 1990s. We tell the story of this case manager using the first person pronoun just to keep it real and personal. This case manager describes her story as follows:

For several years, I have case managed clients (patients) belonging to self-insured plans in a five-state area. Although sometimes this is on-site, it is mostly telephonic—and very different from case management within facilities. The pace is not as intensive; however, the knowledge base of each client's benefit package must be exact. Each model of case management has its challenges and its joys.

Several years ago, I attended a case management seminar given by one of the pioneer case management teams in the southwestern United States. When the speakers asked for audience questions, I asked each speaker to describe a typical workday. Their stories were interesting and educational, but what surprised me was how varied their individual experiences were. Only one case manager's day resembled my own! After some reflection, I realized that even my own tasks differ dramatically from day to day. As I listened, I realized that there are many forms of case management, with different managers laying emphasis on different facets of the case management system. To some, discharge planning is a priority. Others act as utilization review nurses. One nurse case manager appeared to be involved with basic staff nursing (direct patient care) but had strong ties to the multidisciplinary team. No singular set of role definitions could describe this group. Soon I discovered the reason: case management was in its adolescence, complete with identity crisis and a growing, awkward form. Case managers attempt to do everything for everyone—an impossible task—while insurance regulations, state laws, and professional standards are ever changing.

I believe our identity as case managers will arise out of our own field. Certification examinations are already a reality, and standards on case management practice as well as legal and ethical guidelines will be written to guide us through life as case managers.

I am a hospital case manager. My patient population is a medical mix, with some surgical patients. My patients are all ages and may have multisystem failure, pulmonary disease, HIV, suicide gestures, gastrointestinal bleeding, cancer, pancreatitis—in other words, almost any medical problem. When other units are full, orthopedic, neurologic, obstetric, cardiac, surgical, or even older pediatric patients may appear in my ward and need case managing.

▶ An Ideal Day in the Life of a Case Manager

An ideal day in my life would be to use the morning to review patient charts, especially new admissions, input utilization management data, check on any quality of care issues, set up transfers and equipment needs, and elicit plans from physicians during their morning rounds and then pass these on to insurance company liaisons (perhaps third-party payor case managers) and others who are part of the plans.

After these preliminaries are handled and as needs arise, I would visit patient rooms, talk to patients, and catch family members for brief consultations. Then I would, if I was lucky, enjoy an ideal 30-minute lunch without shop talk.

The afternoon would be the time to tie up loose ends, finish utilization review from the morning, complete transfers to other facilities, and do patient rounds. Patient rounds are room-to-room visits designed for introduction, initial assessment of possible discharge needs or further plans for discharge, patient education on various topics, emotional support for impending invasive procedures or surgeries, assessment of patient satisfaction, and handling the many different issues that pop up unexpectedly.

This is my ideal day, not my typical day.

▶ An Actual Day in the Life of a Case Manager

I have picked a day to share that is without long meetings, because such a day would not provide the educational intent of this section, which is to draw a clear picture of the case manager serving on the front lines. However, long meetings are often a vexing reality; therefore, setting daily priorities is essential.

6:30 AM—I log on to the computer and peruse my assigned patient census. I quickly look at new admissions for ages and admitting diagnoses and log in obvious and necessary social service referrals. Then, I attend to the notes taped to my door!

7:00 AM—Shift report/Huddle. I set my first priority list for the day, which frequently changes. Today's list looks like this:

- ▶ Speak to physicians about a do-not-resuscitate (DNR) order for Mrs. Adams—impending code.
- ▶ Visit Mr. Innes—multicomplaints to staff.
- ▶ Transfer Mr. Block to SNF. Dr. T to follow.
- ▶ Transfer Mrs. Cohn to SNF. Find a physician to follow.
- ▶ Call mental health agency—is it possible to do an involuntary transfer of Ms. Diamond today? Make sure psychiatric sitters are available.
- ▶ Possibly transfer Mrs. Elliot to SNF tomorrow. Finish plans.
- ▶ Review arterial blood gas values for Mr. Frank. Does he need home oxygen?
- ▶ Put in for social work referrals for Mrs. Garrett and Mr. Harris.
- ▶ Talk with physical therapist about Mr. Harris—is it safe for him to go home?
- ▶ Probably discharge Mr. Johns today or tomorrow. Arrange for home intravenous antibiotics; get authorization from insurance company.

7:45 AM—I leave hurriedly to attend a short daily case manager meeting. I ask the charge nurse to please make a notation to ask Mrs. Adams' physicians (if they come by) about the DNR order. (If they do not show up by the time I get back, I will call them.)

8:10 AM—Back on the unit. The physicians called Mrs. Adams' daughter. She wants "everything done." I expect the worst in this case (i.e., that she will code shortly) but hope that my gut feelings are wrong.

I am moving along on my priority list:

▶ I look at Mr. Block's chart. His temperature spiked last night. Physicians wish to hold patient transfer and culture blood and urine. This may take 24 to 48 hours. The following calls need to be made about change of plans:
1. Patient/family.
2. Social worker.
3. SNF—will they hold the bed? (yes, thanks! Or maybe . . .).
4. Transportation—cancel stretcher van.
5. Insurance company—need hospitalization coverage for additional hospital days.
▶ I document all of the above in the medical record.

The psychiatric nurse phones me. The mental health agency has completed the paperwork for an involuntary admission to a mental health facility for Ms. Diamond. The sheriff should be arriving to pick her up around 9:30 AM (not much time!). Ms. Diamond is unaware of the plan. Her physicians feel it is not in her best interest to tell her beforehand because she has a history of suicide attempts and adamantly refuses help. The psychiatric nurse will be there but recommends a call to security, because this procedure sometimes gets "ugly." I alert security and the attending and resident physicians of the plans. All are relieved that after 4 days in this hospital Ms. Diamond will finally be in a proper setting for her issues.

The unit secretary gives me Mr. Frank's arterial blood gas results, which show a PO_2 of 49. I call the physician for a verbal order for home oxygen, then the durable medical equipment company for delivery of two portable oxygen tanks to the hospital for Mr. Frank's ride home (he lives 50 miles away). I coordinate the home oxygen setup with the company and the patient's family.

Better check to see whether Mrs. Cohn is stable for transfer. Yes. I have not yet found a physician to follow her up at the nursing home. Priority: find one!

Now facing me are four large men in civilian clothes. They are here to "escort" Ms. Diamond to the mental health facility. They have come early. Why four? They explain that two are in training. Ms. Diamond is a fragile, petite woman; I do not want her to be frightened. I ask "the boys" to be patient, then call the psychiatric nurse, who arrives to speak with Ms. Diamond about the plan. I call security. Ms. Diamond is visibly upset, crying. She is making loud accusations, heard throughout the unit, toward the staff and her significant other. I comfort the significant other, realizing that he has tried to do what is

best. Meanwhile, the psychiatric nurse works magic in calming the patient. Finally, Ms. Diamond, escorted by the four deputies, leaves peacefully, quietly crying. We are all left with a little sadness. Ms. Diamond is a pretty, intelligent, young woman in a lot of emotional pain. I document each detail into the computer.

Back to Mrs. Cohn. Which physician goes to the SNF? I look in my files and pick one with whom I often have success.

Emergency! Before I have a chance to make the call, I hear a Code Blue. It is for Mrs. Adams! I run to her room. Compressions have already started. I cut open the code cart while the code team rushes in. I begin recording. We get a fleeting heartbeat 5 and 8 minutes, then lose it. Every advanced cardiac life support medication is used. The chaplain, already alerted, has called Mrs. Adams' daughter, who is on her way to the hospital. I ask the chaplain to try to stop the daughter before she arrives at the room. At 20 minutes, the heartbeat is erratic, but Mrs. Adams is intubated. A bed in the ICU is available. (Thank goodness the daughter did not walk in on this.) Mrs. Adams is transferred to ICU. I look up to see the physician speaking to Mrs. Adams' daughter. In tears, she accompanies him to the ICU. I document the transfer into the computer.

Back to the nurses' station. I hear someone say, "Is this a full moon?"

Another answers, "It looked full last night."

A resident physician turns his head skyward and howls like a wolf. Laughter breaks some of the tension.

10:30 AM—Back to finding a physician for Mrs. Cohn. I page the physician I have chosen. He calls back and agrees to follow up Mrs. Cohn at the nursing home. Relief! (Sometimes finding a physician to follow up at an SNF is an all-day task.) I call the resident to write transfer orders and dictate the discharge summary. I call the family; they are pleased with the transfer news. The SNF is close to home, making visiting easy. Mrs. Cohn also is happy to be "graduating" from the hospital. The social worker sets up transportation; I inform the SNF of the physician's name and phone number, Mrs. Cohn's health status today, and her time of departure. The charge nurse and staff nurses are told of the transfer and time. I document.

I am starting to feel pressured because I have not yet done any utilization review or looked at my new patient charts.

Mr. Johns' physician tells me that he can leave the hospital today if I can set up twice-daily intravenous ceftriaxone at home. The physician has already spoken with his patient about leaving today, and Mr. Johns will not take "tomorrow" for an answer! Okay. I can do that! I check the facesheet for the name of the insurance company and call them. The insurance representative likes the idea of sending him home; it saves 5 hospital days. I am also given the okay to use our hospital's home health agency. I call the home health agency, and the agency's coordinator does the rest. I enter Mr. Johns' room and tell him to be patient and that we will get him out as soon as possible. Does he have transportation home? No problem. I document.

I look at my list again—social service referrals. These will take only a few minutes, so I get them done.

Finally, I have time to do some "admission" reviews on my new patients. I add a few thoughts to my priority list: one patient may not be able to return to independent living; another is being worked up for probable new diagnosis of cancer, with possible referrals to chaplain services and oncology life enrichment; another patient is a 19-year-old new admission, entering for diabetic ketoacidosis (new diabetic diagnosis). I make a note to call the diabetic nurse educator to start teaching. I document everything.

The charge nurse lets me know Mr. Frank's oxygen has not arrived. I make another call; it is in the truck, on its way.

From overhead, I hear: "Any trauma surgeon to medical ICU." I call to see whether this is about Mrs. Adams. Yes. She coded again in the ICU. She has one chest tube inserted and needs another. The daughter still wants every effort made. It looks grim.

12:00 PM—Telephone call for me. Lunch, already! Ready in 15 minutes. I want to squeeze in some admission reviews, then a quick lunch. The luncheon rule is no shop talk allowed. It seeps through at times, anyway. I sit down and take a deep breath. At what time this morning did I stop breathing?

12:30 PM—Back to the front lines. I had better see to Mr. Innes' multicomplaints while I am refreshed. Mr. Innes has chronic obstructive pulmonary disease, and the staff knows him from previous, recent hospital admissions. Usually a pleasant patient, this time he is different. He also has a new diagnosis—severe anemia. I review Mr. Innes' chart for updates: at admission, his hemoglobin and hematocrit levels were very low. He received 3 units of blood, and his condition is fairly stable now. After several procedures and tests, no source of bleeding can be identified. Mr. Innes recognizes me when I enter. I tell him that I hear that he is unhappy with some aspects of his care and suggest that perhaps I can help. Mr. Innes has many concerns, ranging from the wrong diet on his meal trays to too much noise from the nearby nurses' station. Other, more important, clues to his discontent emerge subtly as we continue our talk. He is concerned about how his debilitated wife is getting along, with his being so often in the hospital. Finally, after so many tests, "Why won't they tell me what's wrong?"

We take each issue one at a time. A call to the dietary department (actually, three calls) fixes the dietary problem. I suggest a room change (if available) to a quieter part of the unit. He is pleased with this idea. Together, we call his wife, and they agree to have home nurse and social worker visits. With the approval of their family physician, I set this in motion. The next major hurdle is Mr. Innes' health concerns. I ask him if he feels that no one is telling him the truth. He answers, "Yes," and expresses fear that bad news is on the way. I know that his tests are negative. I explain that it may feel like he is not being told the truth, but the tests truly do not show a bleeding source anywhere. I also explain that his laboratory test values are stable; he is doing well. He agrees to allow me to discuss his concern with his physician, which I do. The physician then spends time with him, showing him the written test results and making plans for further workups if his hematocrit and hemoglobin levels drop again. The complaints stop; Mr. Innes seems more relaxed and remains that way for the remainder of his stay.

1:00 to 2:00 PM—Weekly multidisciplinary patient rounds. Each patient on the unit is discussed. The focus is on the entire range of needs for each patient and how well we (as a team) are meeting these needs.

I call back down to the ICU. Mrs. Adams has a grim prognosis, with three chest tubes now in place. There are no family members present at this time.

I recheck Mr. Frank's oxygen. It has arrived, and he has departed.

I recheck Mrs. Cohn's transfer. The transport team is in the room now.

I recheck Mr. Johns. Home health intravenous antibiotics are set up, and he is a happy guy.

I review Mrs. Elliot's chart; she is scheduled for possible transfer to SNF tomorrow. Her chart looks good. I call the SNF; her bed is available. Social services can call for transportation tomorrow. A taxi is appropriate, relevant to discussions with the physician, patient, and family. I document and proceed to the next priority.

I check Mr. Harris' chart; is it safe for him to go home? I look at the physical therapist's notes—excellent progress today. Perhaps one more day of physical therapy. I did not think Mr. Harris would do this well. He is spunky, though!

A family member finds me and needs to talk. We go into the family room. Dad is deteriorating more each month. He has Parkinson's disease, and the family is feeling overwhelmed with the care. This family feels guilty about putting Dad in a nursing home. What other options do they have? We explore insurance benefits, financial ability to get home health aide care, increase in respite care time, and family/neighbor/church support. I ask the social worker to speak to this family about possible community resources. We plan to have a family meeting the next day with the social worker to explore options further. This gives me time to find out more about insurance benefit possibilities. I add this patient to my priority list.

I review more charts until it is time for my 3:00 PM monthly case managers' meeting.

▶ Discussion

The nature of the written word necessitates telling a story in a linear fashion. However, I can attest to the fact that many of these events actually occur simultaneously during a busy day. What this account does not depict are the many other interactions and interruptions: support for staff members; answering telephone calls and pages; discussing patient plans with dozens of physicians, nurses, social service personnel, physical therapists, home health professionals, and more. Each day, there are reports to and negotiations with insurance companies regarding length of stay and patient needs. Education of patients in areas pertaining to their own individual needs is a key component. Also, many individual problems and concerns arise that are unique to an individual patient's diagnosis and life support.

The pace is often breakneck. Boredom is not in a case manager's dictionary. I frequently look at the clock and wonder what happened to the day. This type of case management is not for everyone and could leave some on the ragged edge. I once overheard a job description in which the employee appeared to be able to do one activity at a time. Discussing it with the charge nurse on the unit, I said that it was a unique concept, doing one thing at a time. She smiled at me and said, "Don't get any ideas. You love this pace." She was right.

Although this account was written back in the 1990s, it continues to be relevant and depict a day in the life. With shortening length of stay in hospitals, pressure to comply with the utilization management practices of insurance companies (especially managed care), and increasing demands from accreditation and regulatory agencies, the pace of case management has turned from fast to faster and now fastest. Multidisciplinary patient care rounds have become a daily rather than weekly occurrence; complex discharge planning is evident in every patient currently seen in the hospital setting; and the need to carefully review and manage compliance with publicly reported quality data such as acute myocardial infarction, heart failure, and pneumonia core measures has only increased the complexity of the role of the case manager and filled the day in the life with competing priorities and activities that cannot be managed in a linear fashion, but require resolution in the most efficient and effective manner despite the time and resource constraints case managers may face while caring for their patients.

▶ CONFUSING TERMS AND DEFINITIONS

In 1996, a class action lawsuit was filed in a district court, claiming that the HCFA (now known as CMS), arbitrarily and capriciously interpreted Medicare's "confined to home" requirement to deny severely disabled Medicare beneficiaries needing home health services (Bureau of National Affairs, 1998). This is not surprising, given the ambiguous definitions that abound in many areas of healthcare. This is certainly one trend that will change; healthcare terminology must become more distinct and accurate to avoid lawsuits. In many ways, insurance-related definitions that are still open to interpretation drive the authorization of healthcare services. Nebulous terminology can no longer be acceptable when more adverse outcomes are entering the courtrooms. The case manager, as a patient advocate, must be alert to vague interpretations of benefits. Recent attempts at improving this situation have been made, and specific criteria are now being attached to some of the more vague definitions. Time, and possibly litigation, will define this trend.

▶ Improvement Standard

Here is one recent change in definition that did require litigation to clarify. Not long ago, Medicare beneficiaries could receive extended home health or SNF services only if they could prove these services made an improvement in their condition. Unfortunately, many people with chronic diseases such as Lou Gehrig disease or multiple sclerosis could not get the help they required to maintain improvement made and subsequently deteriorated further. This injustice was first voiced in the early 2000s by the Centers for Medicare Advocacy.

On February 16, 2017, the *Jimmo v. Sebelius* court approved a corrective statement to be used by the CMS to affirmatively disavow the use of an "Improvement Standard" for Medicare coverage. The standard now explains that skilled nursing services would be covered when they are necessary to maintain the patient's current condition or prevent or slow further deterioration (Centers for Medicare Advocacy, 2017a). However, it is imperative that case managers know about this, because some home health agencies and SNFs are not aware of this nuance of an old Medicare benefit.

▶ Medical Necessity

Sometimes, care is denied on the grounds that it is "not medically necessary." This is a time bomb that case managers have dealt with since the birth of managed care. Often the basis for medical necessity is political or economic rather than clinical reasons. Because the definition of medical necessity has caused more than a few problems, it has evolved a bit further than some other managed care definitions. Over the years, evidence-based criteria have surfaced and are now used in place of this vague wording. However, despite these criteria, insurance companies still use this, because not every case can fit into the criteria but still requires a specified level of care.

This trend will thus continue with other vague wording. The detail to which it will evolve is a matter of practicality; in this example, it would not be practical to specify the following criteria for every service or equipment that is covered in the benefit design. That would truly be "cookbook medicine" and would not allow for new developments in disease treatment without a major overhaul in the benefit design.

Several definitions of medical necessity can be found in the literature and benefit books. The most comprehensive of them, and considered a classic, included the following criteria (Anonymous, 1998):

▶ The services or equipment were consistent with the individual's diagnosis or medical condition.
▶ The services or equipment were prescribed or rendered by a physician or other qualified healthcare professional.
▶ The services or equipment were generally accepted as effective (that is, consistent with nationally accepted and recognized standards of practice).
▶ The services or equipment were not primarily based on the recipient's convenience.
▶ The more economical choice (rent vs. buy) is chosen when there is more than one alternative available.

From a case management standpoint, it must be realized that there is an economic benefit to the insurance company if the claim for medical necessity is *not* appealed. If a patient or family strongly feels that a service or piece of equipment should be covered, explain the appeals process according to the state laws and insurance policy and procedures. This frees the case manager from a potential legal mess; it shows good faith. It also frees the case manager from an ethical tangle; if the case manager is also an employee of the insurance company making the rules, at least there is another step that can be provided while acting on behalf of the patient.

Reasonable and Necessary

This one piggybacks on the medical necessity concept. The intention may have been to supplement somewhat the definition of the term *medical necessity* (and it did), but very little useful information was actually added. According to one expert, if a treatment meets the following conditions, it will rarely provoke an argument about being reasonable and necessary, except in cases in which it returns the patient to a lesser quality of life (Banja, 1997).

▶ A general agreement exists on the meaning of the treatment's or service's success.
▶ The treatment or service in question not only results in an outcome meeting that definition, but does so most or all of the time.
▶ The treatment or service is affordable or inexpensive.

The efficacy of treatments and services is being scientifically determined and defined through the many disease management and outcomes management projects occurring throughout the United States and the rest of the world. As empirical results are agreed on, vague definitions will be replaced by best practice criteria.

This concept opens up an ethical Pandora's box. According to John Banja, PhD, "no treatment is reasonable if delivering it imposes intolerable burdens on others. Thus it

would not be reasonable for a hospital to routinely deliver treatments whose costs could not be recovered because doing so would propel the hospital to bankruptcy" (Banja, 1997, p. 35). At what point is the cost or the burden unreasonable? I had one patient who needed a heart transplant. No one could refute the necessity or the reasonableness; she did not have enough left ventricular ejection fraction to sustain life. She also had a stipulation in her insurance policy that excluded heart transplants.

Reasonable and necessary treatment has changed numerous times throughout the centuries. What were considered best practices in the 1800s would be considered "witchcraft" today or malpractice; what is considered unscientific and unconventional today may be the key to true health in a few short decades. Reasonable care today means that healthcare services are provided on the basis of the patient's medical condition, acuity, and severity of the illness and that the course of treatment conforms to what is nationally recognized and agreed on as the standard of care.

Intermittent Services

Intermittent services is another term that gets confused. It is used mainly in the home health setting and means that care is provided on a part-time basis, for portions of the time such as a few hours in a day and for a few days of the week.

Skilled versus Nonskilled Care

There continues to be confusion among healthcare professionals as to what constitutes skilled or nonskilled care and services. Some agencies commit the mistake of confusing aspects of care that require the involvement of a licensed professional or care provider and those that do not. Skilled healthcare services are those that require delivery by a licensed professional such as a registered nurse; a social worker; or a physical, occupational, or speech therapist (e.g., wound care, vital signs assessment and monitoring, physical rehabilitation). Nonskilled healthcare services are those that can be provided by an unlicensed healthcare paraprofessional such as a home health aide or a homemaker (e.g., bathing, feeding, preparing meals).

Activities of Daily Living

Traditionally, activities of daily living (ADLs) have focused on the basics of functional life: eating, dressing, bathing, toileting, and other life essentials of self-care. ADLs are often defined according to range of motion, muscle strength, or mental clarity. Case managers have broadened this definition to include other important aspects of a patient's life. Is the ability to participate in chosen spiritual activities less important than the ability to bathe oneself? However, few benefit designs allow support for this one critical example, and there are many more like it.

▶ Homebound

Under Medicare guidelines and for purposes of the statute, an individual shall be considered "confined to the home" (homebound) *if the following two criteria are met*:

1. *Criteria-One*: The patient must, because of illness or injury, need the aid of supportive devices such as crutches, canes, wheelchairs, and walkers; the use of special transportation; or the assistance of another person in order to leave their place of residence, OR the patient must have a condition such that leaving his or her home is medically contraindicated.

If the patient meets one of the criteria in Criteria-One, then the patient must ALSO meet two additional requirements defined in Criteria-Two.

2. *Criteria-Two*: There *must* exist a normal inability to leave home, AND leaving home *must* require a considerable and taxing effort.

In 2011, CMS published this new proposed policy as "Clarification to Benefit Policy Manual Language on 'Confined to the Home' Definition." Unfortunately, the proposed policy change was included with unrelated materials and went unnoticed by beneficiary and consumer advocates until November 1, 2013. The 2011 explanation for the policy change was stated as:

Medicare considers beneficiaries homebound, if, because of illness or injury, they have conditions that restrict their ability to leave their places of residence. Homebound beneficiaries do not have to be bedridden, but should be able to leave their residences only infrequently with "considerable and taxing effort" for short durations or for healthcare treatment (Centers for Medicare Advocacy, 2017b).

This criterion still leaves a wide area for interpretation. Essentially, the spirit of the guidelines states that it would be a hardship for the homebound person to leave the home to get medical care.

One patient had multiple sclerosis. At the time she was admitted to case management, she was essentially bedbound; with much difficulty, she could transfer to the wheelchair. The primary insurance company repeatedly stated that she was not homebound because she was able to get to her physician appointments every other month. However, this was done only at great hardship and some risk. The definition of homebound as interpreted by this company was that it was "impossible to leave the home; as long as there was a way to transport the patient, the patient was not homebound." This company's definition of homebound would not hold up and with the aid of some education and negotiation, the patient was authorized to receive home care.

▶ Adequate Patient Education

Adequate patient education is defined as the provision of appropriate teaching or transmission of pertinent information to meet the patient's needs, including any necessary postoperative instructions, lifestyle changes (healthy behaviors), and activity or nutritional counseling. These activities must always be reflected in the patient's medical record. This is a key role in case management. It is critical for good and desirable outcomes in disease management or chronic care programs. Many accreditation agencies require case management programs to provide adequate patient education. Criteria that are specific to the education desired must be added to make accreditation more meaningful and compliance with the standards more manageable.

▶ Care or Lack of Care

This is defined as inappropriate or untimely assessment, intervention, or management of care. Again, this is too vague to hold up. "Inappropriate" and "untimely" may mean different things to different people.

▶ In a Timely Manner

The ability to receive care or appeal decisions in a timely manner is a basic patient right. Specific, set time frames for obtaining services are the ideal, but not always the reality. In the absence of predetermined intervals, the case manager should look for unreasonable delays in obtaining care or precertification for care. This problem is becoming more common, and even the best case managers have probably been personally frustrated at some point while caring for patients. However, when the situation is endangering a patient's health, action must be taken. More providers are receiving accreditations from such organizations as The Joint Commission (TJC), the American Accreditation Healthcare Commission/Utilization Review Accreditation Commission (URAC), and the National Committee for Quality Assurance (NCQA). Within the standards of many accreditations are strict time frames that must be adhered to; accreditation status depends on it.

Access to care is also a standard that is scrutinized during some accreditations and directly related to providing care in a timely manner; providers are accountable for reasonableness in providing access to care in a timely manner. All this also directly relates to customer satisfaction. There are customer satisfaction reports published for all to see; the media can be a powerful tool to ensure that patients receive attention in a timely manner, or consumers will merely pick another provider.

▶ INTERNATIONAL PERSPECTIVE ON CASE MANAGEMENT

There was a time in the mid-1990s when some experts thought that case management had a life span of about 5 more years; they were more than a little bit wrong. In the United States, case management has become the link between managed care, other type payors, and patient care. It is not only here to stay, but is expanding internationally, as evidenced by numerous publications in case management that are of an international nature.

We believe that the United States has some of the best—and the most complicated—care in the world. Many countries have more socialized medical healthcare structured systems than the United States. Three important characteristics of the socialized medicine approach are that the systems (1) usually provide universal coverage for basic healthcare needs, (2) are relatively simple to administer, and (3) are, therefore, inexpensive. Great Britain has a national health service; France has a national insurance system; The Netherlands has a system based on private practice physicians, community- and church-affiliated hospitals, and nonprofit and for-profit insurers; and Australia has publicly funded universal coverage for basic medical services with approximately 30% of the population also carrying private insurance for access to private hospital services and other services not covered by public funding. However, as the private, for-profit insurers penetrate the healthcare industries of the various countries, more complex healthcare rules can be expected. In Australia, an increasing percentage of public services are being provided by for-profit healthcare corporations. In almost every country, all services (both public and private) are coming under increasing pressure to provide high-quality and cost-effective care, leading to increasing complexity and cost-consciousness; therefore, case management systems and models are needed. In fact, most of these countries either have already implemented case management demonstration projects or are in the process of examining the value of such programs.

Healthcare complexity was the major catalyst for case management's growth in the United States; the complex insurance benefit packages and reimbursement rules that overtook our healthcare industry led to the use of nurses and other licensed professionals as case managers. Unlike the "good old days," physicians do not have the time to juggle all the necessary aspects of a patient's case; they sincerely appreciate the efforts of case managers sorting out the benefit designs and discharge planning possibilities.

Many countries are looking to the United States for lessons (both positive and negative) that are applicable in their own rapidly changing environments. Universal coverage is common in other countries, which often do not actively promote health or disease prevention but rather specifically exclude services unless they are "curative." However, significant health promotion programs were provided, yet were not always tied to health insurance. Although the rank order may be slightly different, most countries have the same major disease epidemiology, including cardiovascular disease, cerebrovascular disease, cancer, depression/mental health, and infectious diseases. This has led to a growing interest internationally in evidence-based disease management programs that integrate all aspects of health. As a consequence of the economic imperatives in

the United States, considerable work has been done here in research and evaluation. Consequently, as interest in this area grows and as successes in disease and chronic care management programs become more public, the international exchange of evidence-based information has become an ongoing occurrence.

The Dutch healthcare system has been chosen as one example demonstrating similarities and differences among other countries' healthcare systems and is discussed in detail below. The Dutch started with a social structure like many other countries, attempted many models, learned some of the same lessons, and responded to some of the same challenges as did the United States, England, Australia, and others. Australia, New Zealand and Canada are also highlighted.

The Dutch are a healthy population, as a whole, and are capable of delivering the most modern forms of healthcare. Historically, the issue of "rights" was rarely discussed; rather, The Netherlands had a system of "obligations." Essentially, there is an obligation that physicians, hospitals, and other providers care for all patients; there is also an obligation that all patients pay for the care rendered (through various public and private systems). Persons with high incomes are obligated to purchase health insurance, with some employer contributions; persons with low incomes are also obligated to purchase insurance, and their employers contribute to the fund. The bottom line in The Netherlands is that all members of society receive care, all providers receive compensation for their efforts, and all people with limited means can afford insurance.

In The Netherlands, general practitioners fulfill a gatekeeper role like the PCP in managed care. Patients are free to choose their general practitioner but must have a referral before seeing any specialist. The patient can then choose any physician within the licensure of the referral specialty; hospitals are another free choice in this model.

Healthcare has been facing changes and challenges in The Netherlands. There are essentially three systems of insurance in The Netherlands: sickness funds, private insurance, and the Exceptional Medical Expenses Act. This has created administrative complexities when coordinating services for the elderly, the chronically ill, and other groups such as the mentally ill. Upper-income elderly persons are subject to very high insurance premiums. Some programs are funded by the local government out of direct tax revenue and are not part of any of the three insurance systems, causing the fragmentation we know so well in America. On the other hand, "mergers" among sickness funds and private insurance systems are occurring. These alliances are resulting in selective contracts with specialists and hospitals. The capitated agreements with the health insurers are being shared with the specialists and hospitals (risk sharing), and specialists and hospitals have formed umbrella organizations not unlike America's physician hospital organizations (PHOs). Patients pay higher out-of-pocket expenses if generic medications are not used.

At this time and in the traditional healthcare system, formal referrals to home care services are not needed; the patients initiate contact themselves. An initial visit for assessment purposes commences. Then a care plan is developed that includes care or treatment goals and a listing of services and frequency of the visits planned. The assessment visits are often done by a team composed primarily of nursing and social work professionals. Even this does not go on without resistance and turf battles.

Demographically, Dutch healthcare and home care face challenges similar to those in other countries: the population is aging, the number of single family households is rising, and more women are working outside the home, leading to less available family support. The challenges cross all country boundaries: structural and financial changes, risks of potentially misaligned incentives, increasing costs of healthcare, and fragmentation. As a result of the changes, many countries are more focused on patient rights.

In 1994, a concept called *transmural care* was introduced in The Netherlands. This is similar to the *shared care* of England and the *integrated care delivery* of the United States. The concept of an integrated delivery system was especially challenging to The Netherlands, a country that has traditional divisions between hospital and primary and specialist care delivery systems. In addition, the population, as in the United States, was becoming increasingly demanding about what they expected from a healthcare system. Technology was allowing minimally invasive surgeries and safer equipment in the home setting, and the resulting trend toward shorter lengths of stay in the hospital was another inevitable change. The Dutch leaders recognized that something had to be done, and transmural care was chosen as a means to realize more efficient, higher-quality healthcare.

In 1995, the National Advisory Council on Health-Care defined transmural care as care geared to the needs of the patient, provided on the basis of cooperation and coordination between general and specialized caregivers, with shared responsibility and specifications for delegated responsibilities (Van der Linden & Rosendal, 2002). Transmural care can range from merely improving patient transfers from hospital to home, to a complete redesign of a specific patient group. There are essentially seven categories of transmural projects; each project is reminiscent of case management, either through coordination of care efforts or by working toward an efficient length of stay in hospitals. Most probably, the lessons learned from these projects would be something all countries can relate to as well as benefit from.

1. *Home health*: The evolution of home care technology has advanced the use of home healthcare in lieu of hospital stays. This is similar to home health models everywhere, with the exception that in The Netherlands (and possibly in other countries),

general practitioners also receive special training to handle the bedside technology for patients. Specially trained nurses provide the around-the-clock care, with these physicians on call as backup.

2. *Before-and-after care in the primary care setting*: These transmural projects focused on performing prehospital diagnostic workups to shorten lengths of stay and increasing the use of home care postoperatively. It was found that this approach increased patient privacy and often led to a more rapid recovery.

3. *Consultation of medical specialists in the primary care setting*: These projects moved specialists outside the walls of hospitals and into diagnostic centers. These centers demonstrated a 35% reduction in laboratory tests.

4. *Specialized transmural nurses*: These projects developed specialized training programs for nursing that are very similar to case management/disease management as it is evolving everywhere. These nurses are responsible for care that had traditionally been in the general practitioner's domain. For example, in diabetic outpatient clinics, the transmural nurses would provide diabetic education to patients. Other types of clinics may see cancer or asthma patients. Cancer patients would receive various intravenous therapies from nurses, and asthma patients would receive respiratory treatments by specialty nurses.

5. *Rehabilitation units/wards*: In many countries, posthospital care requires lengthy waiting lists or complex admission procedures. In an attempt to streamline transfers for patients requiring posthospital care, a growing number of hospitals have either opened their own rehabilitation wards or facilitated special contracts with nursing homes.

6. *Discharge planning*: Specialized "liaison" or "transfer" nurses were promoted to facilitate expedited discharges. These nurses are actively involved in identifying high-risk or potentially difficult discharges.

7. *Pharmacologic transmural care*: Pharmacy boundaries widened in these transmural projects, ranging from provision of medications posthospitalization to a model similar to specialty pharmacy companies that provide mail-in medications for either patient or home nurse administration.

The transmural care projects opened up a Pandora's box that is probably familiar to most people working in the healthcare sector of any country. Some of the challenges include:

▶ *Cooperation issues*: Transmural care involved a new way of healthcare professionals working together. Traditionally, general practitioners and specialists have operated independently of each other, without much direct communication. New skills were required to work effectively in multi-disciplinary teams.

▶ *Training programs*: As with case management, transmural care has been added to and currently is being offered in training programs.

▶ *Development of transmural care protocols*: As is the case with clinical pathways in specific settings and through-the-continuum, The Netherlands realized that transmural care requires new protocols and practice standards.

▶ *Length of stay challenges*: When utilization review became a constant companion of the managed care industry in the United States, the lengths of stays shortened; the patients in acute care came in sicker and were discharged sicker; families were burdened with these responsibilities; and the sicker patients led to increased workload for hospital staff, often leading to higher employee turnover. The story and the lessons are the same all over. Some Dutch experts looked on transmural care as a self-defeating system. How many case managers have not felt that way about managed care, from time to time?

▶ *Financial incentives*: The staff is working harder, discharging patients quicker. The families are more burdened. The general practitioners are losing autonomy. The challenges and after-effects of transmural care continued on an ever-increasing scale. Nevertheless, the reimbursement system did not support any incentives for all this trouble. Empty beds and/or increased production did not produce revenues. Until 1995, medical specialists were paid on a fee-for-service basis; therefore, they were inclined to see patients longer rather than sending them back to the general practitioner.

Initially, healthcare experts in The Netherlands seemed skeptical that anyone other than physicians needed to be case managers. There has been some conflict between the general practitioners and specialists about patient control and case management. The general practitioners are paid a capitated wage. They feel it is their role to be the managers of their patients and are supporting the idea of treating fewer patients and getting reimbursed at a higher capitated rate. This would give them the time to do case management or disease management, without a lower overall salary. Some Dutch experts were skeptical of the experience with trained transmural nurses. Nevertheless, the interest in disease management, case management, occupation and workplace wellness, quality improvement, and quality assurance in the health system is growing. On an optimistic note, the Dutch—as a society—value collaboration; this is an excellent foundation for their goals.

The Dutch experience is similar to the evolving healthcare industry globally. However, attitudes about case management differ. The welcome that case management receives varies widely within any healthcare system, usually depending on the observer's role within the system and what people think case management is. For example, in Australia there is a reasonable degree of interest and acceptance of case management, but there is a great deal of resistance to managed care. The interest in and acceptance and recognition of case management's potential value have been positive in Australia, and one consequence of this has been the development of a postgraduate course in case management at the University of Melbourne (one of Australia's most prestigious universities). The course is taught over the Internet and has attracted students from as far away as New Zealand, Australia, Japan, and South Korea. New Zealand, Israel, Spain, Canada, Puerto Rico, South Africa, Argentina, and the Pacific Rim send representatives to U.S. case management annual conferences, both as speakers and attendees.

The primary focus of case management may be different in various countries. The catalyst for case management as a strategy occurred in the United States because of managed care challenges, but the initial bottom line was cost containment, with quality and safety being a close second. Perhaps this rank order has changed, at least in some organizations, but the reality is that healthcare is expensive and must be contained within a budget. Because of differing reimbursement structures in other countries, cost-containment strategies were not always the primary reason for case management. In Australia, which spends approximately half as much on healthcare per capita compared with the United States, the emphasis has been more on quality. This is not to say that cost issues are being ignored, but as a result of a different financial structure and overall lower expenditure, the incentives are quite different from those in the United States. Some private hospitals are looking to case management not so much to save money as to increase the satisfaction of patients, which will in turn help attract people to the private system. Public hospitals in Australia have been looking to case management as a way of performing better in an environment that has (in most areas) shifted to a case-mix funding base. In Australia the largest area for growth in case management is in the community-based aged care sector, where for at least the past 20 years, significant efforts and public resources have been invested into helping people stay at home longer. This has included a significant commitment to case management as the way of coordinating and organizing these services.

In England, New Zealand, and Australia, community case management occurred first, followed by hospital case management; they are distinctly different case management roles. Perhaps community case management evolved first because these countries have had community nursing for decades. For example, in New Zealand, community case management merely added service accessing and coordination functions to the job descriptions of the nurse specialists already practicing in the community setting (Litchfield, 1998).

Even with different reimbursement structures, varying perspectives of nursing, and diverse demographic and geographic needs, case management definitions evolving in other countries do not fall far from those currently promulgated in the United States, such as the CMSA's official case management definition. In New Zealand, case management as practiced by the Professional Nurse Case Manager (PNCM) is described as "a scheme for professional nursing practice in which the client is pivotal, a caring partnership between the client and the case manager is essential, and where attending to client's health as expression of the whole life process is the norm. The organization and management of case management provide for continuity and integration of healthcare services crossing primary, secondary, and tertiary settings, attending to the diversity of people's need where it arises or is anticipated" (Litchfield, 1998, p. 31). Although this is a more nursing-based definition, it emphasizes the patient as being of pivotal importance and management of the needs of the patient throughout the continuum of care as essential.

▶ CASE MANAGEMENT IN CANADA

The following was written by Genelle Leifso, RN, BSN, CPN(C), Senior Nurse Advisor for the Workers' Compensation Board (WCB) of British Columbia (BC). Both similar and different perspectives on case management are provided here as with the Dutch healthcare experience. It is exciting to see case management evolving globally in such a caring and balanced way.

The Canadian healthcare system operates under a federally enacted law referred to as the Canada Health Act of 1984. This legislation enshrined the principles of a universal, accessible, portable, comprehensive, and nonprofit/publicly funded healthcare system that is now as synonymous with Canada as apple pie is with America. Universal means that all Canadians are covered, and accessible means that no particular area or region will be deprived of routine service. Canadians moving from one province to another are provided for because their coverage is portable, and the care is comprehensive because everything except that which is deemed cosmetic is covered. The entire system is publicly funded, and any province instituting user fees is penalized.

Taxes are collected federally, and proportional transfer payments are made to the provinces that are charged with disbursements and implementation of healthcare services. This level of healthcare has required increasing amounts of the Canadian gross domestic product (GDP). In 1975 it required 7.1%; in 1980 it went to 9.1%; in 2006 it was 10.4%; in 2008, it was 10.8%, in 2016 it was 11.1%, and it is expected to continue to rise. Provincial governments currently spend one-third of their budgets supporting healthcare. In Canada, each province has a

Workers' Compensation Act; the provincial WCB develops its own policy and guidelines that interpret the Act. Thus, coverage can differ from province to province. Each Board is fully funded by that province's employers.

Increasing interest in efficient, cost-effective healthcare delivery has led to the development of centers of excellence. The intent is to avoid expensive service duplication when possible. In BC, the government has focused on "closer to home" service delivery in the past several years. This has resulted in the increased need for community-based services and home care—services that the United States is still struggling to provide adequately.

Resource allocation at the WCB of BC is determined by the nature or seriousness of the injury and the preinjury salary of the injured worker. The case manager at the WCB of BC operates within established guidelines that determine how many treatments will be covered (e.g., chiropractic, physiotherapy). Likewise, vocational rehabilitation consultants provide input geared to reestablishing preinjury salaries. Case managers do not prescribe treatment; therefore, the worker's attending physician (who is considered to be the PCP) is consulted, and approval is sought for proposed treatment plans. At the WCB of BC, the development of a case management model has been driven by the need to improve the quality of service to injured workers in the province in a more cost-effective fashion.

Case managers deal with several cultural issues that affect their ability to provide service. BC has a large immigrant population, with many of the new arrivals coming from the Far East. For many, fluency in English takes some time to develop. If a member of this population is injured, ongoing interpretation needs to be provided to ensure service delivery and to aid in identifying all the barriers to successful problem resolution. We must also be sensitive to those cultural perspectives related to injury and rehabilitation. Certain cultures have particular ways of viewing disfigurement or disability. For example, a South Asian man with a partially amputated hand has immense culturally driven body image problems, which often separate him from the social supports (i.e., temple activities) that contribute to ongoing stability in the life of a newer immigrant. In addition, different cultural groups have preferred treatment modalities. At the WCB of BC, injured workers from an Asian background often have requests for acupuncture approved as a culturally sensitive therapy even if, in those circumstances, current medical literature would not support its use.

Case management is practiced under many other monikers in Canada. In hospital settings, nurse clinicians, clinical nurse specialists, or clinical resource nurses are involved in ongoing case management of their specific patient or client groups. In some facilities, utilization review is being done in collaboration with physicians. Currently, it is a politically sensitive area with nurses involved in the day-to-day work, and physicians doing the "enforcing" with their peers. Nurses and, in some settings, social workers are also involved in discharge planning—another form of case management. Similarly, in a community health environment, nurses may share the case management role with social workers.

In the WCB of BC setting, there is multidisciplinary provision of case management services. Although the medical advisors, nurse advisors, and psychologists may develop the actual clinical care plan that will be the "critical pathway" for the worker's return-to-work plan, the adjudicator (at the WCB this person is called the case manager), vocational rehabilitation consultant, and therapists (e.g., occupational, physiotherapy) who are part of the treatment or rehabilitation network, and the individual's PCP are all considered members of the case management team.

Recruitment of new case managers entails targeting professionals with bachelor's degrees in health or social science fields. There was no such requirement for adjudicators who have been grandfathered into this new and demanding role. It is difficult to say how many case managers are in Canada. Titling of practitioners as case managers differs from that in the United States. Therefore, some hospital staff members who would be called clinical nurse specialists in Canada would be called case managers in the United States. Within the WCB of BC, the claims adjudicators all became case managers in 1997. Current recruitment is trying to attract individuals with a health science background (e.g., nursing, occupational therapy, kinesiology). In Ontario, the WCB has recruited and hired a large number of nurses who are trained as case managers.

Canadians are afraid of the managed care concept. Managed care is equated with cookie-cutter medicine, which is quite different from the evidence-based, clinical guideline–driven care that case management advocates. There is resistance among current medical and claim staff members who lack understanding of these different concepts and fail to see the need for, or benefit from, the change into case management models. Further, case management outcomes measurement is not being done; however, nurse advisors are continuing to explore ways to track the success of their interventions.

Case management is a solution to the Canadian healthcare system and its challenges when it can:

- Offer earlier intervention;
- Avoid service duplication;
- Provide a primary point of contact for injured workers and their healthcare providers; and
- Offer efficiencies to the employer community and an earlier return-to-work for their injured workers.

A case management association was present in Canada for several years: the National Case Management Network (NCMN) published several articles in case management journals. Although this nonprofit organization could not sustain the membership and ceased business operations in 2014, the documents they produced, *Canadian Standards of Practice for Case Management* and the *Canadian Core Competency Profile for Case Management Providers*, continue to influence excellence and professionalism for the process of case management and the role of case management providers in Canada. Academic institutions, employers, and government agencies are using both these documents to optimize Canada's health workforce under the increasingly demanding and complex healthcare needs of Canadians. They can be retrieved at http://www.ncmn.ca (National Case Management Network, 2015).

▶ TRENDS IN CASE MANAGEMENT

There are exciting trends in case management. First, it has become a healthcare strategy in its own right and is an integral aspect of any healthcare delivery environment today. Professional credentials have added credibility; the work of the CMSA, CCMC, NASW, and ACMA has moved case management into international waters; accreditation of case management programs or models has also added consistency and accountability; and the outcomes movement will sustain case management through the consumer and employer demands for documented "results."

Educational opportunities in case management are more specified and appropriate than they were any time in our history. A case manager no longer needs to learn "by the seat of their pants," as the pioneers did. In many healthcare environments, the orientation process for case managers has now become a thorough education, often complete with simulation (SIM) training and useful tools by the aforementioned organizations.

The healthcare environment in which case management is practiced, and thus case management itself, is in major transition. Although no one can say what healthcare will look like in the coming years, case managers can count on change in the way case management is viewed and practiced.

Case management opportunities are expanding. The case management trend is from individual case management to managing a population-specific practice. An advanced-level nursing degree may fill this need in the future. Major changes in both human demographics and healthcare funding and reimbursement will open up opportunities inclusive of all areas of healthcare. The coordination skill of case management is needed everywhere: hospitals, SNFs, insurance companies, physician hospital organizations (PHOs), HMOs, home health agencies, rehabilitation hospitals, and so on. The older segment of the population is expected to increase sevenfold from 1980 to 2050. The pattern of illness and disease has undergone a dramatic change from predominately infectious disease in the early 1900s to diseases that require case/disease management (chronic diseases). These chronic conditions, coupled with managed Medicare and Medicaid, make a perfect marriage for the skills of a trained case manager. The future looks very rewarding for case management.

Regardless of the healthcare changes that occur, certain tenets of patient care will not change and will remain important: the patient/family is the center of our concern. The patient will and must become more engaged in his or her healthcare. Patient advocacy will be foundational. The evolved question healthcare professionals will ask is no longer "what is the matter with the patient?" but rather "what matters to the patient?" (Bowen, 2015).

▶ REFERENCES

American Case Management Association. (2016). *Compass: Directional training for case managers. Version 3.0*. Little Rock, AR: Author.

Anonymous. (1998, Spring). Not medically necessary. *Rehabilitation Review, 37*, 4

Banja, J. (1997). Reasonable and necessary care. *The Case Manager, 8*(6), 34–36.

Bodie-Gross, E., & Tahan, H. (2008). Roles and functions of case managers. In S. Powell & H. Tahan (Eds.), *CMSA Core curriculum for case management* (2nd ed., pp. 159–176). Philadelphia, PA: Wolters Kluwer/Lippincott Williams & Wilkins.

Bowen, D. J. (2015). FUTURESCAN™ 2015 healthcare trends and implications 2015–2020. Retrieved February 22, 2017, from http://www.americangovernance.com/education/symposia/2015/winter/files/feb15bowen.pdf

Bureau of National Affairs. (1998). Homebound Medicare beneficiaries file lawsuit against HCFA for denial of benefits. *BNA's Medicare Report, 9*(20), 513.

The Canada Health Act, CIR 94-4E. (2005, May 16 revised). The Canada Health Act: Overview and options. Retrieved from https://lop.parl.ca/content/lop/researchpublications/944-e.htm

Case Management Society of America. (2007). Case management leadership coalition adopts consumer definition of case management. Retrieved November 12, 2017, from http://dev.cmsa.org/Employer/NewsEvents/PressReleases/tabid/271/ctl/ViewPressRelease/mid/1004/PressReleaseID/19/Default.aspx

Case Management Society of America. (2016). *Standards of practice for case management*. Little Rock, AR: Author.

Centers for Medicare Advocacy (2017a). *Federal court approves CMS corrective statement to enforce Jimmo settlement*. Retrieved June 11, 2017, from http://www.medicareadvocacy.org/medicare-info/improvement-standard/

Centers for Medicare Advocacy (2017b). *New CMS proposed homebound policy would leave medicare beneficiaries without coverage*. Retrieved June 11, 2017, from http://www.medicareadvocacy.org/new-cms-proposed-homebound-policy-will-leave-medicare-beneficiaries-without-coverage/

Centers for Medicare & Medicaid Services. (2011). Condition of participation: Hospital discharge planning. Federal register 42 CFR §482.43. Retrieved November 12, 2017, from https://www.gpo.gov/fdsys/pkg/CFR-2011-title42-vol5/pdf/CFR-2011-title42-vol5-sec482-43.pdf

Commission for Case Manager Certification. (2015). *Code of professional conduct for case managers, with standards, rules, procedures, and penalties*. Rolling Meadows, IL: Author. Retrieved June 10, 2017, from https://ccmcertification.org/sites/default/files/downloads/2015/0000.%20Code%20of%20Professional%20Conduct_FINAL%20%26%20APPROVED_January%202015.pdf

Commission for Case Management Certification. (2017). *Definition and philosophy of case management*. Retrieved June 10, 2017, from https://ccmcertification.org/about-us/about-case-management/definition-and-philosophy-case-management

Kongstvedt, P. R. (2003). *Essentials of managed health care* (4th ed.). Gaithersburg, MD: Aspen Publishers.

Litchfield, M. (1998). Case management and nurses. *Nursing Praxis in New Zealand, 13*(2), 26–35.

McGonigle, D., & Mastrian, K. (2008). Information systems and case management. In S. Powell & H. Tahan (eds.), *CMSA core curriculum for case management* (2nd ed., pp. 292–323). Philadelphia, PA: Wolters Kluwer/Lippincott Williams & Wilkins.

Michaels, C. (1992). Carondelet St. Mary's nursing enterprise. *Nursing Clinics of North America, 27*(1), 77–85.

National Association of Social Workers. (2013). *NASW standards for social work case management*. Retrieved June 10, 2017, from https://www.socialworkers.org/practice/naswstandards/casemanagementstandards2013.pdf

National Case Management Network. (2015). *Canadian standards of practice for case management* and *Canadian core competency profile for case management providers*. Retrieved June 11, 2017, from http://www.ncmn.ca

Tassel, M. V. (1994, August). Case managers use entrepreneurial skills. *Hospital Case Management*, 143.

Tahan, H. M., & Treiger, T. M. (Eds.). (2017). *CMSA core curriculum for case management* (3rd ed.). Philadelphia, PA: Wolter Kluwer.

Van der Linden, B. A., & Rosendal, H. (2002). The birth of transmural care in the 1990s. In E. van Rooij, L. Droyan Kodner, T. Rijsemus, & G. Schrijvers (Eds.), *Health and health care in the Netherlands. A critical self-assessment of Dutch experts in medical and health sciences* (pp. 191–197). Maarssen, The Netherlands: Elsevier Gezondheidszorg.

Williams, S. J., & Torrens, P. R. (1993). *Introduction to health services*. New York: Delmar.

Roles, Functions, and Preparation of Case Management Team Members

"Imagine a proactive process that begins with how a case management job description is crafted and the case managers for that position are recruited. Consider including competencies endemic to professional case management practice that flow across each element of a case manager's role and functions that appear on the job description. In addition, the competencies are woven into the outcomes done for the department, which are consistent with overall department plus organizational goals. Now envision a career ladder to guide a case manager's career trajectory within the organization, which is actively discussed as a fluid dialogue with the department manager during quarterly meetings. Ultimately, the performance metrics by which the case managers are measured align with the case management specific competencies. The process described is not illusion or fantasy; it is the reality of the new age of proactive performance management for professional case management."

TREIGER AND FINK-SAMNICK (2017)

LEARNING OBJECTIVES

Upon completion of this chapter, the reader will be able to:

1. Explain five optimal and five undesired outcomes of case management.
2. Describe the roles and responsibilities of case managers.
3. Differentiate between a case manager's leadership roles and personality traits.
4. Describe the difference between hard and soft savings.
5. List three ways to prepare for a case conference.
6. List two reasons patient advocacy is important to case management.

ESSENTIAL TERMS

Accountability • Advocacy • Advocate • Assertiveness • Clinical Documentation Specialist • Collaboration • Complementary and Alternative Medicine (CAM) • Confidentiality • Conflict Resolution • Coordinator of Care • Cost-Benefit Analyst • Crisis Intervention • Critical ThiWnking • Educator • Hard Savings • Insurance Benefit Analyst • Leadership • Levels of Care • Multidisciplinary Patient Care Rounds • Negotiator • Optimal Outcomes • Performance Management • Privacy • Role and Function Study • Soft Savings • Transition Plan • Utilization Manager • Value-Based Purchasing

▶ CASE MANAGEMENT: ROLES, FUNCTIONS, AND GETTING OPTIMAL OUTCOMES

"Care management" is an umbrella term used to include care coordination, case management, and transitional care. These are not new concepts to healthcare or nursing, but now they often correspond to new roles in new settings. Case management evolved from legislative and payment reform as early as the 1980s and focused attention on utilization

review (UR) and the appropriate use of resources in the acute care setting (Powell & Tahan, 2010).

Research on case management roles, responsibilities, and functions has evolved over the past 25 years. Much of that research has been done using scientific research methods by the Commission for Case Managers Certification (CCMC). Case management roles and functions have changed, and these survey results have become more crucial to training and education. The CCMC conducts a national practice analysis study every 5 years to assure the most updated information (Bankston-White & Birmingham, 2015a). The results have been further confirmed by smaller studies such as the one in Utah (Luther, Marc-Aurel, & Barra, 2017).

Roles differ in various settings. But, make no mistake, in all settings case managers are essential to patients/clients. Whether the latter are receiving initial information about their medical conditions or are in hospital undergoing surgery or treatment, they are often afraid. It is here that you, as a case manager, play a large role in their lives, and your ability to execute your skills thoroughly and meaningfully is critical.

This chapter will highlight the latest informational overview about the roles and functions of case managers. Updates will occur in peer-reviewed journals as new data are gathered. This chapter will also detail specific roles for new (or seasoned) case managers to understand; it will detail a section on the roles of directors/managers of case management departments.

Please note, however, that even "new" case managers are likely not new to their healthcare profession. In the 2014 survey for the Role and Function study from the CCMC, nearly half of the respondents (46.91%) were between the ages of 51 and 60 years, the largest age group being 56 to 60 years (24.69%). Another 14.3% were aged 61 to 65 years, and 4.7% were over 65 years. These statistics reveal an important insight: case management is not an entry-level role; rather, it is a specialty or advanced practice. Those who become case managers have had a number of years in prior roles, such as nursing, social work, or vocational rehabilitation (Tahan, Watson, & Sminkey, 2015).

Being a competent case management professional translates into doing things well and taking responsibility for the outcomes. Patricia Benner's book *From Novice to Expert* discusses competence and expertise using the Dreyfus Model of Skill Acquisition (Benner, 1984). This model theorizes that a health professional such as a registered nurse must pass through five levels of proficiency when acquiring and developing a skill. Stage I describes those just beginning to learn the role and gain theoretical knowledge but having no experience yet. They are referred to as Novices. Stage II, the Advanced Beginners, describes those who have little or limited experiences from which to draw when performing their new responsibilities. For example, this stage may describe a staff nurse who enters the role of case management with little understanding of insurance principles, utilization modalities, quality issues, or transitional planning.

The other three stages—Competent, Proficient, and Expert—describe a progression of advanced skills and perceptions. This holistic understanding goes beyond a merely analytical response to a situation to an intuitive grasp of the events taking place. According to Benner, an intuitive grasp is not wild guessing; it is a direct comprehension of a situation that is available only when a broad base of knowledge, experience, and a deep understanding has been encountered. Therefore, advanced competency is often more visible in its absence and thus may go unnoticed and unrewarded. Experienced case managers learn to organize, plan, and coordinate multiple patient needs and requests and to reshuffle their priorities in the midst of constant patient changes (Benner, 1984, p. 149).

▶ CCMC Role and Function Study 2014

In 2015, the CCMC released its latest survey results from its 2014 practice analysis research study. Practicing case managers are surveyed every 5 years; the 5-year research cycle is purposeful and necessary to allow changes in the field to evolve and become routine practice expectations. This survey identifies common activities and knowledge areas necessary for competent and effective performance of case managers; from this, the certified case manager (CCM) certification examination is born. Of special note is the emergence of specific activity and knowledge domains in the area of case management ethical, legal, and practice standards during this latest survey (Tahan et al., 2015).

The essential activity domains cited in the CCMC Role and Function Study (Tahan, Watson, & Sminkey, 2016) include the following:

- *Delivering case management services*: This activity domain includes vast subsets of over fifty-five functions. It includes the basic activities of the case management process and delivery or healthcare services to patients and their families.
- *Accessing financial and community resources*: This domain includes the identification of specific patient cases that would benefit from case management and some additional types of services as well as the facilitation of patients' access to those programs, services, and funding resources.
- *Delivering rehabilitation services*: This domain highlights the facilitation of optimal wellness, functioning, or productivity and all the detailed activities required to be done, especially after a serious acute illness or injury.
- *Managing utilization of healthcare services*: The details of this domain include over/underutilization of services and resources, education of providers about the appropriate use of resources and health insurance concepts, and advocating what is in the best interest of the patient and family.
- *Evaluating and measuring quality and outcomes*: This activity domain includes the assessment, monitoring, collection of outcomes data, and evaluation of patient-related outcomes. It also emphasizes the use of evidence-based practice guidelines in the development of the case management plans.
- *Adhering to ethical, legal, and practice standards*: This domain includes adherence to legal, regulatory,

ethical, professional conduct, and accreditation requirements that are pertinent to case management practice and a patient's case (e.g., informed consent, Health Insurance Portability and Accountability Act, and Americans with Disabilities Act) and to the health education of the client on appeal rights. Additionally, this domain addresses the need for case managers to apply and adhere to the standards of case management practice such as those advocated for by the Case Management Society of America.

To ensure effective execution of case management activities, case managers apply specific knowledge and skills in their practice. Therefore, the CCMC's practice analysis study also identifies the core knowledge areas case managers apply for effective, safe, optimal, and competent performance. These knowledge domains as gleaned from the CCMC survey include (Tahan et al., 2016):

▶ *Care delivery and reimbursement methods*: Some of the knowledge topics in this domain include adherence to care regimen; case management process and tools; cost-containment principles; factors used to identify client's acuity or severity of illness and levels of care; goals and objectives of case management practice; management of patients with multiple chronic illnesses; negotiation techniques; and transitions of care.

This domain also addresses the *continuum of care/continuum of health and human service*: A few of the topics in this area are healthcare delivery systems; hospice, palliative, and end-of-life care; interdisciplinary care team; levels of care and care settings; management of acute and chronic illness and disability; medication therapy management and reconciliation; managed care concepts; reimbursement and payment methodologies (e.g., bundled, case rate, prospective payment systems, and value-based purchasing); and utilization management principles and guidelines.

▶ *Psychosocial concepts and support systems*: This knowledge domain includes topics such as behavioral change theories and stages; client activation, engagement and empowerment; conflict resolution strategies; health coaching and counseling; interview techniques such as motivational interviewing; support systems, including family and community-based services; resources for the uninsured or underinsured; abuse and neglect (e.g., emotional, psychological, physical, and financial); crisis intervention strategies; end-of-life issues (e.g., hospice, palliative care, withdrawal of care, and do not resuscitate); multicultural, spiritual, and religious factors that may affect the patient's health status; and spirituality as it relates to health behavior.

▶ *Rehabilitation concepts and strategies*: Topics in this domain include vocational and rehabilitation service delivery systems; assistive devices; functional capacity evaluation; job modification and adjustment; postinjury rehabilitation, including disability management and life care planning; and return to work.

▶ *Quality and outcomes evaluation and measurement*: Some of the topics in this knowledge domain include accreditation standards and requirements; cost-benefit analysis; data interpretation and reporting; program evaluation and research methods; and quality and performance improvement concepts. Additionally, this domain includes knowledge related to types of outcome indicators and their relationship to regulatory reporting and pay for performance.

▶ *Ethical, legal, and practice standards*: This evolving (and relatively new) knowledge domain includes topics such as case recording and documentation; ethics related to care delivery (e.g., advocacy, experimental treatments and protocols, end-of-life care, and refusal of treatment/services); ethics related to professional practice (e.g., professional behavior, code of conduct, veracity, patient autonomy, and patient's right to self-determination); healthcare and disability-related legislation (e.g., Americans With Disabilities Act, Occupational Safety and Health Administration regulations, and Health Insurance Portability and Accountability Act [HIPAA]); legal and regulatory requirements; privacy and confidentiality; risk management; and critical pathways, standards of care, practice guidelines, and treatment guidelines.

How much time is spent on various roles and responsibilities was cited in Luther et al. (2017). In their survey, which included case management respondents from various settings, they found that the most common roles were:

▶ Direct patient interaction (DPI), including assessment and patient care plan development, determining a patient's level of self-management, medication management, health coaching strategies, and end-of-life care planning;

▶ Utilization management;

▶ Transitional care processes, including participation in and coordination of transitional care issues;

▶ Population health management, including steps of patient risk stratification and accordingly providing important case management services and resources;

▶ Interprofessional communication and collaborative relationships within and between healthcare systems and providers.

Data from Luther et al.'s (2017) study revealed that, on average, respondents spent most of their time (35%) on DPI. When analyzing the data by patient setting, outpatient respondents reported that, on average, they spent 40% of their time on DPI. In contrast, inpatient respondents reported an average of 24%.

The study by Luther et al. (2017) also revealed that the second highest category comprised time spent on utilization management (UM) activities. On average, the respondents reported spending 28% of their time on UM, with outpatient respondents spending an average of 25% and inpatient respondents spending an average of 36% performing UM activities. Interestingly, the last major category measured was transitional care, on which all respondents spent an average of 11% of their time.

Luther et al. (2017) also saw a relatively new trend—a good deal of "discharge planning" was performed in inpatient *and* outpatient settings. Both inpatient and outpatient care managers were preparing patients and their families for admissions and following up on patient needs after discharge. In the recent past, the care management activity of preparing patients for admissions was conducted in silos, with neither of the care management teams of the two care setting was aware of the planning and preparation of the other. Transitions are often episodes of uncoordinated and fragmented care known to place patients at a much higher risk for medical errors and suboptimal care if not managed effectively and carefully. The findings of the study by Luther et al. (2017) suggest that care managers are working in concert across care settings to identify discharge needs and prepare patients during admissions and transition episodes; with the extension of more bundled care processes and payment structures, this is an important trend.

Examination of the survey by Luther et al., the CCMC Role and Function studies, and future practice analyses are vital to developing the future case management workforce. The job of developing this workforce involves a concerted effort between educational and professional organizations, moving forward to discover new pathways of education for new care managers, as well as promoting the skills of leadership for experienced case managers (Luther et al., 2017).

▶ Optimal versus Inadequate Case Management Outcomes

It is necessary to be clear about the purpose of case management and its related outcomes to understand the context of the case manager's roles, responsibilities, and required skills and knowledge. Three main target goals (or tenets) of case management are quality care, access to healthcare services, and cost efficiency. Many smaller goals contribute to these ultimate aims and, when achieved, culminate in "good case management." When these goals are not met, the consequences are suboptimal quality of care or poor and costly utilization of healthcare resources. The CCMC 2014 Role and Function Study supports the need for excellent case management and good outcomes.

Unmet case management goals may occur for many reasons. The following are some examples:

- No formal case management program in the healthcare facility or agency;
- Unclear roles and responsibilities of case managers and other professionals impacted by the introduction of case management;
- Case manager's role conflict, confusion and/or overload;
- Poorly trained case managers;
- Inadequate case management staffing;
- Inadequate social service staffing to support the psychosocial aspect of the care needed and the patient with complex social determinants of health issues;
- Case loads that are too heavy to permit case managers to adequately attend to the patients with diverse and complex health needs;
- Patient/family resistance;
- Staff resistance;
- Patients who are incorrigibly noncompliant (versus nonadherent) with care regimen and medications;
- Unrelenting patient/family dissatisfaction;
- Lack of cooperation from the payor source;
- Lack of, or inadequate, payor resource;
- Lack of understanding among members of the healthcare team regarding case management principles.

Tables 2-1 through 2-6 included in this chapter display outcomes of case management. On the left of each table are optimal outcomes—characteristics resulting from competent case management practice. The right side of each table lists consequences that could occur when those objectives are lacking or inadequately met. As the issues and game rules of the healthcare environment change, the goals must also transform to match new priorities. It is certain, however, that quality, effectiveness, and efficiency must never be compromised in any situation.

▶ TABLE 2-1   Quality of Care Issues

OUTCOMES FROM OPTIMAL CASE MANAGEMENT	OUTCOMES FROM INADEQUATE CASE MANAGEMENT
▶ Increased patient/family satisfaction and rewarding care experience	▶ Patient/family dissatisfied with care; possible increase in lawsuits
▶ Optimal clinical outcomes through monitoring of and adherence to quality standards of care	▶ Increased quality of care issues; medical errors and unsafe experiences of care; possible risk management scenarios, complaints, and grievances
▶ Comprehensive and accurate assessment of clients' deficits, needs, health status, resources, formal and informal support systems, and outcomes	▶ Care plans lacking focus on the specific and desired needs of the patient/family; unresolved or unimproved health conditions; increased complications/ineffective care, medical errors, and unsafe situations
▶ Matching assessed needs to valuable services/resources	▶ Duplication, fragmentation or gaps in services, and unmet client's needs
▶ Continuity of care emphasized, thus reducing or eliminating fragmentation, duplication, or gaps in treatment plan and/or services	▶ Fragmented, inefficient, duplicative, and costly care; wasted services and resources
▶ Careful monitoring of safety issues and prevention of complications, suboptimal care, or medical errors	▶ Missed risk factors that lead to risk management issues (e.g., falls, avoidable deterioration in health condition); avoidable complications requiring return to acute care
▶ Reduced adverse patient outcomes	▶ Increased adverse outcomes and errors
▶ Proactive: prevention of adverse occurrences when possible or initiation of interventions quickly if prevention is not possible, thereby minimizing poor outcomes	▶ Adverse occurrences maximized before anyone recognizes them
▶ Maximum recovery; minimum complications	▶ Minimal recovery; maximum complications

▶ TABLE 2-2   Collaboration among Healthcare Team Members/Professionals

OUTCOMES FROM OPTIMAL CASE MANAGEMENT	OUTCOMES FROM INADEQUATE CASE MANAGEMENT
▶ Physician satisfaction with the case management process and the quality of patient care	▶ Alienation and frustration of physicians; undesired outcomes
▶ Healthcare team member satisfaction with the case management process and the quality of care	▶ Lack of teamwork; uncooperative clinicians; undesired outcomes
▶ Roles are clearly defined	▶ Role conflict or confusion; frustrated professionals
▶ Effective collaboration and coordination strengthened among all members of the healthcare team	▶ Treatment delays; fragmented care; frustrated and obstructed efforts to improve health status of the patient
▶ Communication enhanced among the multidisciplinary team	▶ Each discipline singing in a different key, resulting in discordant care for the patient; miscommunications and misunderstandings among the team alienate team members
▶ Case manager's engaged and satisfied with their roles; role recognition and interest	▶ Case manager's are discouraged and dissatisfied with their roles; role burden and stress

▶ TABLE 2-3   Fiscal Responsibilities

OUTCOMES FROM OPTIMAL CASE MANAGEMENT	OUTCOMES FROM INADEQUATE CASE MANAGEMENT
▶ Provider-payor satisfaction	▶ Uncooperative providers
▶ Balancing fiscal responsibility for the client, the healthcare facility/agency, and the reimbursement source	▶ Conflicts of interest; mixed or inequitable loyalties; poor or unethical allocation of resources; ineffective reimbursement
▶ Appropriate and efficient use of benefits and resources; health services provided at the appropriate level and care setting	▶ Suboptimal use of healthcare resources; unnecessary waste; over- or underutilization of resources
▶ Cost-efficient care through timely use of appropriate level of care for the client's needs	▶ Expensive and inappropriate level of care; may not be reimbursed by payor source; may leave facility or patient fiscally responsible for excess payment
▶ Appropriately reduced length of hospital stays; services provided at the correct level of care and in the correct status	▶ Increased length of hospital stays; denials for services rendered; wrong status and overutilization of levels of care
▶ Reduced visits to emergency department and planned visits to clinic/primary care providers	▶ Increased number of emergency department or unscheduled clinic visits
▶ Unnecessary readmissions prevented; acuity on admission reduced; number of admissions reduced	▶ Preventable readmissions; higher acuity upon admission; frequent and unnecessary readmissions
▶ Careful identification and matching of clients' needs with resources available (both public and private resources, especially those available in the community)	▶ Suboptimal use of healthcare system and public or private resources; patients remain unconnected to key community-based resources
▶ Maximizing reimbursed services at all levels of care by meeting established criteria, performing precise utilization reviews, accurate and thorough documentation, and timely patient discharges or transitions to other levels of care	▶ Healthcare agencies/facilities at increased financial risk because of lost revenue for the facility from uncompensated patient care; unnecessary or unjustified delays in discharge from acute care or transitions to another level of care; increased charges to patients; patients unable to pay or left financially destitute
▶ Successful negotiation of cases with the payor source for appropriate continuation of lengths of stays or extension of services	▶ Healthcare agencies/facilities at increased financial risk because of lost revenue for the facility from uncompensated patient care; increased denials for services rendered; increased charges to patients; patients unable to pay or left financially destitute
▶ Accurate interpretation of benefits for the patient and the healthcare facility	▶ Healthcare agencies/facilities at increased financial risk because of lost revenue for the facility from uncompensated patient care; increased charges to patients; patients unable to pay or left financially destitute; increased bad debts

▶ TABLE 2-4   Patient and Family Advocacy

OUTCOMES FROM OPTIMAL CASE MANAGEMENT	OUTCOMES FROM INADEQUATE CASE MANAGEMENT
▶ Personal attention in a large, complex, and perhaps impersonal healthcare system	▶ The patient and family feel left alone, frustrated, and afraid; lack of sensitivity and compassion in care provision
▶ Case manager as advocate for patient/family	▶ No one to advocate for patient/family; what is in the best interest of the patient/family is inconsistently upheld
▶ Patient's quality of life and well-being, autonomy, and, if possible, independence optimized through thoughtful, appropriate placement at discharge from an episode of care	▶ Patients warehoused in inappropriate environments; poor quality of life and well-being; unsafe discharges or transitions from an episode of care
▶ Fostering educated, independent choices in all aspects of care and services	▶ Uninformed decisions; lack of knowledge of health condition, plan of care, and care regimen
▶ Education on disease processes, allotted services, rehabilitation techniques, self-care management; education matched to individual needs	▶ Poor health education resulting in noncompliance with treatment plan, "out-of-control" feelings, decreased self-care capabilities, and inability to avoid or allay the disease process; disengaged from own healthcare
▶ Patient and family empowerment through participation in informed decision making	▶ Paternalism; decreased freedom of choice; decreased autonomy of patient

▶ TABLE 2-4 Patient and Family Advocacy (*continued*)

OUTCOMES FROM OPTIMAL CASE MANAGEMENT	OUTCOMES FROM INADEQUATE CASE MANAGEMENT
▶ Optimal function of patient-family unit	▶ Frightened, exhausted, stressed-out patient and family
▶ Optimizing self-care capabilities by assisting patient to become fully functional as quickly as possible; if return to independence is not possible, assisting family unit and client in obtaining supportive care	▶ Minimal time for patient to become independent and optimally healthy; family may become exhausted or dysfunctional and utilize excessive healthcare services
▶ Ensuring patient/family understand the direction of the plan of care and knowledge of the disease process and red flags through education, clinical pathways, and so on	▶ Confusion, anxiety, and out-of-control feelings of patient and family; lack of knowledge contributing to a lack of adherence to care regimen
▶ Careful monitoring of and advocating for a clinically appropriate treatment plan	▶ Duplication of services; gaps in treatment plan; wasteful services; inappropriate levels of care; excess costs being billed to patient
▶ Activated patient/family and engagement in self-care and oversight of own health	▶ Ineffective healthy lifestyle; limited self-care management resulting in lack of adherence to care regimen
▶ Assisting patient/family in accessing the complex healthcare system, thus utilizing available and necessary resources	▶ Underutilization of resources, leaving some patient needs unmet; services ordered not covered by the health insurance plan, creating wasted effort and possibly extensions of hospital stays because of delays in accessing needed services for a safe discharge or transition
▶ Finding solutions to noncovered services; accessing charitable agencies and services	▶ Families' funds exhausted through noncoverage of services, necessitating private payment; ineffective use of community-based resources

▶ TABLE 2-5 Outpatient/Community-based Care Management

OUTCOMES FROM OPTIMAL CASE MANAGEMENT	OUTCOMES FROM INADEQUATE CASE MANAGEMENT
▶ Thorough identification of discharge needs, including medical, educational, durable medical equipment, and social support	▶ Frustrated patient and exhausted family that is suboptimally caring for the patient
▶ Facilitation of timely, coordinated, safe, and appropriate discharges or transitions to another level of care or provider	▶ Unsafe, incomplete disposition; lack of postdischarge resources/services and improper level of care or provider
▶ Linking the patient with appropriate level of care and services: acute, subacute, supervisory, homebound, or community-based services	▶ Service gaps; higher readmission rates and emergency department visits
▶ Linking the patient with appropriate healthcare provider and services: primary care, specialty care, community-based resources	▶ Service gaps; delay in care and avoidable readmission to acute care or access to emergency services
▶ Comprehensive and consistent posthospital or post–extended-care facility follow-up	▶ Complications during convalescent phase of care with setbacks and possibly avoidable readmissions for acute hospital care
▶ Optimal outpatient management that reduces or avoids acute hospital readmissions through early identification of health status changes or changes in self-care capabilities	▶ Poor outpatient management leading to increased complications and unexpected deterioration of condition, premature progression of health condition, and increased utilization of acute facilities
▶ Chosen level of care for patient matches the patient's needs and financial capability	▶ Patient's/family's financial resources are prematurely exhausted through nonreimbursed placement of patient in an expensive care facility

▶ TABLE 2-6   Professional Case Management Practice

OUTCOMES FROM OPTIMAL CASE MANAGEMENT	OUTCOMES FROM INADEQUATE CASE MANAGEMENT
▶ Promotion of professionalism by creatively and proactively finding solutions to the problems facing the healthcare system	▶ Case management in a subordinate and supportive role, rather than in a collaborative partnership with other healthcare professionals
▶ Enhanced research opportunities about efficient, effective care for the chronically and acutely ill	▶ Diminished credibility because of lack of serious research
▶ Increased job satisfaction and engagement	▶ Job stress and burnout
▶ Established scientific base for case management practice; evidence-based practice	▶ Unclear science behind effective case management practice; outdated practice
▶ Innovation in case management practice	▶ Practice that is not cutting edge and that lacks innovation or relevance
▶ Dissemination of best practices; case managers feel the need to disseminate knowledge and share their experiences with others	▶ Best practices kept within individual organizations; lack of desire to share knowledge with others
▶ Increased membership in case management–related professional organizations; strong and well-respected professional societies	▶ Weak case management professional organizations

▶ ESSENTIAL ROLES AND FUNCTIONS OF CASE MANAGERS

A generation ago, the task of case management belonged to the family physician. Choices were simple; insurance companies usually paid for the services that the physicians deemed necessary. Enter the age of convoluted health insurance plans, multiple specialists for a single patient, absent primary owner of care (or lack of a case manager), multidisciplinary teams that include dozens of members of varied backgrounds, the rush to get patients through the system and into less cost-intensive settings, increasing chronicity and acuity of health problems, ethical dilemmas, increased patient and family expectations, and the list goes on.

As Figure 2-1 shows, the case management role is a pivotal one. This chapter discusses essential roles and responsibilities that affect how well the case manager performs the role. Although the list is extensive, it should be noted that the role of the case manager continues to evolve and, therefore, the list may still be incomplete or may vary from one organization to another. Because case management responsibilities are extensive, on some days, case managers may feel that they are "dancing as fast as they can!"

The roles and responsibilities of case managers continue to change and evolve similar to the way our healthcare system is constantly changing. Case management roles also vary according to the patient population being served, the setting in which the case manager is employed, and the case management perspective (i.e., program structure, vision, goals, objectives, and processes). The job priorities of each case management position must also be weighed.

A hospital case manager may have a perspective (e.g., clinical care management) that is different from the one who is employed by an insurance company (e.g., member benefits management); a case manager for a private insurance company may encounter different issues than another who works for Medicaid or long-term care. An entrepreneurial case manager may have a different point of view and priority set compared with another who works for a privately owned or state-run company; a case manager who is responsible for patients across a continuum of healthcare settings may have a different perspective from the one who is responsible for episodic (i.e., one episode of illness and one care setting) case management.

Roles and responsibilities also differ because of the case mix of patients for whom the case manager is responsible. For example, geriatric patients have needs that are different from those of high-risk obstetric, AIDS, cancer, or cystic fibrosis patients; virtually each clinical category has its own needs. At times, the case manager may find the various roles complementary and necessary; at other times, conflicting. As a patient advocate, the case manager wants the best of everything for the patient and family; as the procurer of healthcare resources, the case manager may not be able to obtain all that the patient wants or needs. Perhaps a service is not covered or the patient has already used up that particular benefit; perhaps the insurance company does not feel the patient is entirely homebound and denies home nursing services, claiming the services are unnecessary and unjustified. Fortunately, however, other resources can come to the rescue. Knowledge of alternative and community resources—and the case manager's own creativity—can often ease such situations or ethical dilemmas and offer some options.

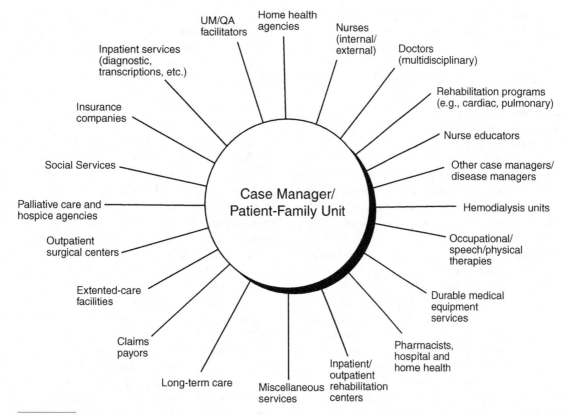

Figure 2-1 Case manager/patient-family unit.

After considering all the diverse roles, responsibilities, and challenges listed in the first two chapters of this book, it is no wonder that student or novice case managers have difficulty seeing "the big picture" of what case management is all about. As sometimes happens, within the question lies the answer. The question is "What is the big picture of case management?" The answer is "Case management is the big picture of the patient's entire universe!" Often, some professionals have traditionally been task oriented; the physician writes the orders, and the nurses have to finish all the tasks on all their patients within the allotted time. If the tasks are accomplished within the time specified, using the correct method and applying the correct amount, to the correct patient, the nurse can then go home and sleep peacefully. Case management is not task oriented in the same way. The case manager must look at the big picture—an expanded version of the whole universe of the patient. This includes the patient's past capabilities (physical, cognitive, emotional, financial, and psychosocial), the patient's current condition, and an anticipation of the patient's future needs and abilities. It includes not only the patient, but all those closely affected by the patient's current and future world—the family, caregiver, friends, care aides, or significant other. Lastly, a case manager must also take into consideration everything that could affect the patient: the strength or lack of psychosocial support, financial support, insurance benefits, cognitive abilities,

physical condition, and all other important aspects of the patient's universe.

The following case management skills are important strengths to develop and will greatly aid all case management daily activities, no matter what the setting. Not everyone is organized or is a "detail person" or a "top-notch" negotiator, and not every case manager needs all these characteristics. Many excellent case managers are weak in some areas and compensate adequately with other talents. Nevertheless, if any shortcoming is causing problems, the case manager should look for ways to grow; all of the roles can be enhanced or developed if desired. Not all the roles and responsibilities that follow may apply to one's clinical area of expertise, practice, or type of case management; yet, many are essential in every form of case management. Some of these roles are so complex that one or more chapters would be required to describe them, for example, UM, insurance issues, risk management, legal and ethical practice, and transitional and discharge planning. Critical elements of some of the roles are discussed in this chapter, for example, cost-benefit analysis, negotiation skills, and assertiveness. Discussions of many of these roles will overlap throughout the textbook, as case management is not a set of distinct job actions but rather a tapestry of many aspects of life woven together.

It should be noted that the roles, functions, and responsibilities of case managers are also defined by professional organizations such as the Case Management Society of America (CMSA), the American Case Management Association (ACMA), the American Nurses' Association (ANA), and the National Association of Social Workers (NASW); they are validated by research, including the current and past CCMC Role and Function studies and the ANA's practice analyses, which give direction to potential case management competencies and required knowledge for practice. All are defined on the basis of scientific evidence, experiences and opinions of case management experts, and the lessons learned from organizations that have implemented case management programs for quite some time. Roles and responsibilities of case managers are also found in the designed job descriptions of the employing agency or the healthcare facility.

A note about job descriptions: there is no standard or nationally recognized case management job description at this time. The literature published on this topic, similar to this textbook, tends to list all possible roles and responsibilities; however, an organization's specific job description lists those responsibilities it finds relevant to its program of case management and priorities. That said, a job description is a vital part of a well-run case management department and should connect with any performance management metrics of the staff. A well-written job description should have the basics, such as salary grade, reporting structure, educational degrees/certification required, and key functions. In fact, it should also contain many of the skills, roles, and functions/responsibilities listed in this chapter; this will set case managers up for success, as they would know the desired outcomes and expectations of the employer.

The Activity and Knowledge Domains articulated earlier, and those roles described in the remainder of this chapter, should be used as a guide for understanding or designing the role of a case manager. They should be studied carefully and considered on the basis of what is required or essential for a specific care setting or case management practice.

▶ The Patient Advocate

Think for a moment about a time when you felt especially vulnerable, when few elements of your life were within your control. Perhaps you were told you had an inoperable tumor, or the dreaded test came back positive, or a loved one was seriously ill. Times such as these leave people feeling overwhelmed, uncertain, emotionally drained, and afraid. Those who can ask pertinent questions are already on their way to healing, but many are too overcome with the enormity of their situations to even articulate their needs; they become paralyzed.

The role of a patient advocate is one of the most important of the case manager's charges; it is also one of the greatest challenges. Advocacy is integral to every action case managers take and every decision they make, regardless of the care settings or the patients in their care.

It is most necessary when dealing with patients and families who are unable to speak for or represent themselves. Historically, nurses and social workers have always acted as patient advocates to some extent. Today's healthcare climate presents some challenges to that role. "Advocacy for the patient was given highest priority unless it conflicted with advocacy for the physician or advocacy for the employing institution" (Leddy & Pepper, 1989, p. 378). Today, advocacy for the payor source (which may also be the employer) often muddies the issue. It is the case manager's primary responsibility—an obligation, if you will—to remember that the patient is the most relevant unit, not the payor, not the utilization modality, not the service offered or not offered, not the other providers of care, and not the healthcare institution. Advocacy is being patient/family-centered and focused in one's approach to care where the patient/family is the top priority, if not the only priority.

How does a case manager act as a patient advocate? In a sense, this entire textbook readies the case manager for that role. By understanding the principles and functions of case management, the case manager can best position the patient to maximize his or her chances for optimal services, outcomes, quality of life, and well-being.

One tenet of advocacy is to assist patients to achieve autonomy and self-determination, to help them become empowered and independent. This is done by supporting patients or families in caring for an incapacitated family member, for example, to articulate their views and choices, and to make informed decisions. The case manager is obligated to act in the patient's best interest, but the patient will determine what the definition of "best interest" will be, according to personal wishes, beliefs, needs, and values. There are times when patients and families do not know what they need, what is available to them, or even what they want, because their situation is simply too overwhelming. Eliciting preferences and priorities from patients or their families is a great relief to them; it also steers the case manager in the right direction. In turn, the case manager keeps the family/patient unit updated and informed on how plans are progressing. Changes and detours can be discussed when the need arises.

Autonomy in decision making, informed consent, and self-determination also require informational support. The quality and relevance of the information are important, and the quantity of data must be delicately balanced. Giving information that the patient did not seek and is not ready to hear and that is too detailed—causing information overload—violates the basic principles of patient advocacy. Giving too little information may be considered paternalistic and prevents self-determination and informed consent.

One of the biggest challenges the case manager often has to face is the ethical dilemma of the conflicting roles of patient advocate versus gatekeeper. It is difficult to balance the demands of these two strict taskmasters—one necessitates optimal patient care and services, and the other demands cost containment and stringent allocation of resources. Wise allocation of resources fulfills the requirement for the role of the gatekeeper, but may violate the concepts of advocacy. On the other hand, if case managers can successfully perform the role of patient advocate, they can often become the balancing force for inequities in the system. The best way to deal with such dilemmas is by asking yourself, "What is in the best interest of the patient and family?" Answer such questions by always ensuring that the patient's and family's autonomy and freedom of decision making are maintained, their needs/wishes/interests are met, and their rights are protected. This confirms your role as an effective patient advocate.

The essence of advocacy is caring for another human being. Caring involves being concerned about another's welfare; it is the root of the role of patient advocacy and the heart of nursing, social work, and other helping professions. Caring between the case manager and the patient requires reciprocal communication, trust, respect, understanding, and commitment. Almost every task a case manager performs is done out of involvement with, and caring for, the quality of care and patient safety. Negotiations to achieve the optimal resources for a patient and the scrutiny of the case for quality of care and safety issues are expressions of caring.

Establishing a caring connection may be the first line of case management business, because "people don't care how much you know until they know how much you care." One basic tenet of case management, and a very caring part of the job description, is facilitating patient autonomy, empowerment, and involvement in own care. To assist others in building self-reliance in their own lives is one of the greatest gifts a case manager can give.

If we lived in a perfect healthcare world where everyone had equal access to healthcare resources and patients were knowledgeable and engaged players in their own care, advocacy may not be necessary. The reality is that inequities exist in our healthcare environment, and a majority of the population do not have the knowledge or the savvy to access this convoluted system. Case management is not a job for the meek. In fact, it involves quite a bit of risk-taking. At times, being a patient advocate requires going toe to toe with everyone from physicians to insurance companies. Through the case manager's caring, attention, and support, perhaps one more patient will be prevented from "slipping through the cracks," will receive the help needed for one more try at independent living, or will have a last wish acknowledged and granted. Supporting a patient's own choices with available means and services is the gift of advocacy. Examples of how a case manager engages in patient advocacy activities are presented in Display 2-1.

▶ Protector of Privacy and Confidentiality

In today's age of technology, including telephonics, electronic communications, telehealth, and social media, maintaining

---

display 2-1

EXAMPLES OF CASE MANAGER'S ADVOCACY ACTIVITIES

1. Doing the right thing, at the right time, by the right health professional, and in the right amount
2. Maintaining the patient's and family's privacy and confidentiality, and protecting their rights, especially to choice and informed consent
3. Educating the patient and family about healthcare services, benefits, medical condition, and medical regimen
4. Seeking the patient's and family's informed consent to treatment
5. Seeking the patient's and family's involvement in care planning and selection of treatment options
6. Making referrals to necessary services on behalf of the patient
7. Informing members of the healthcare team of the patient's and family's wishes, interests, and needs.
8. Assuring authorizations by the patient's health insurance company (payor) for services to be rendered to avoid denials and appeals
9. Ensuring provision of evidence-based care
10. Coordinating a case conference to resolve conflict between a patient and family members and to solve problems
11. Facilitating the patient's access to needed services and resources
12. Identifying variances (delays) of care and addressing them as indicated; preventing the occurrence of variances
13. Ensuring that care provision is fair, just, timely, and equitable
14. Coordinating services across the continuum of care, health and human services, and settings
15. Providing the patient and family with emotional support and psychosocial counseling, especially during situations of anxiety, apprehension, uncertainty, and confusion
16. Answering the patient's and family's questions and guiding them through the healthcare maze

---

privacy and confidentiality is no easy task. It seems as if everyone has access to the patient's medical record, including many types of medical caregivers, quality improvement specialists, health insurance companies, auditors, billers, case managers, governmental representatives, and others.

The reader is referred to Chapter 8 for recommendations on the preservation of privacy and confidentiality. New problems are arising because of electronic documentation, and fail-safe ways must be provided to keep patients' medical records from computer hackers, employers, and others without a right or a need to know. Hackers seem to break the best firewalls and security infringement barriers, and virus or ransomware is always a threat.

The case manager has an obligation—as a patient advocate—to protect the patient's privacy as much as possible. By doing so, the case manager is protecting that person's dignity, is practicing within the ethical standards and scope of care, and adhering to the case management professional code of conduct. Case managers in their daily practice ensure that the involved in the patient's care and access the medical record are appropriate involved healthcare professionals based on the patient's health condition and treatment plan, and that the patient has agreed to their involvement. These case manager's also adhere to the HIPAA regulation when engaged in a release of information activity.

▶ The Coordinator of Care

Coordination of care is the umbrella role under which all other roles fall; it is the foundation of case management. If done well, case management provides a seamless and smooth-running system in which everyone benefits: patient, family, provider, and payor. If done poorly, case management is a rough ride, with team members colliding into one another and desired outcomes remaining unmet. Coordinating with many care providers (with their different perspectives, orders, suggestions, and roles), facilitating collaboration among these professionals, and then matching it all to the patient's agreement and payor's authorization for care are no small tasks. The "what," "when," "how," and "why" of the coordination of services make up an individual sequence that depends on the nature of each patient's illness and health condition, psychosocial support network, health insurance coverage, and many other factors.

Procuring resources and services is sometimes called "brokering of services;" it is part of the overall coordination of care role. The first place to look for resources that will meet the patient's needs is the patient's own support system. If skilled services are required, most health insurance companies cover them. However, there are limits either in the number of home care visits allowed or in a dollar cap. Community resources may be needed to fill in gaps that the family and insurance company cannot cover. However, many people lack the support of family, friends, or church; some do not have health insurance. Sometimes the only option is charity care or privately paid support. Persistence and creativity eventually yield enough services for a safe patient discharge or transition. Here, the case manager acts as a general problem solver. To have an experienced, knowledgeable social worker on board is probably the closest thing to case management heaven. The social, emotional, or socioeconomic problems of many patients are overwhelming, and many would benefit from a good social worker's expertise. However, if social service support is unavailable, the case manager's knowledge of community resources, including ways to access them, is a necessity.

▶ The Utilization Manager

Historically, utilization review has been referred to as the process of monitoring intensity of service and severity of illness (see "InterQual" in Chapter 5: Utilization Management), medical necessity, and appropriateness of the level of care the patient has been receiving. However, case managers do not simply monitor or review the utilization of services; they manage them. Thus, the more appropriate terminology to be used is *utilization management*. The use of utilization tools, such as Milliman Care Guidelines (MCG), clinical pathways, or InterQual, reveals the patient's changing condition and the necessary level of care and setting. For acute care case management, this changing condition provides a cue for the case manager to speed up a discharge plan if the patient is doing exceptionally well or change a discharge plan if the patient is deteriorating or remains debilitated. Tools correspond to different healthcare environments. Many organizations are experimenting with tools that follow a patient through a continuum of care; these tools have shown some success, although they present several challenges, as seen in the case management literature.

UM is the term that an insurance company can understand; authorization for extensions of hospital days is often based on utilization modalities (see Chapter 5). UM functions in another capacity, too: reviewing for appropriate utilization of services and resources can reveal overutilization of tests, procedures, and services. Overutilization may arise from many causes, including the following:

- ▶ The facility is a teaching hospital or an academic medical center in which medical students, interns, and residents are trying to find the balance between good and complete care.
- ▶ Patients insist on expensive, high-tech procedures.
- ▶ Physicians are cautious if a litigious event arises (e.g., a patient falls).
- ▶ Physicians practicing defensive medicine overcautiously order multiple tests to prevent lawsuits.
- ▶ A test has a duplicate order and no one noticed it.
- ▶ The monitoring frequency (e.g., of hemoglobin/hematocrit or prothrombin/partial thromboplastin time) can be changed because of the patient's stability, but no one has done so.
- ▶ A medication given intravenously can be changed safely to an oral route.
- ▶ Routine tests ordered and completed without supportive evidence for their indication of benefit, just because they have always been done that way.

There are also situations where resources are underutilized, and they include the following:

- ▶ Delays in performing a necessary test or procedure.
- ▶ Denial of certain services by health insurance companies even when clinicians feel those services are warranted.
- ▶ Lack of monitoring of a patient's response to treatment resulting in lack of performing indicated tests (e.g., assessing hemoglobin/hematocrit levels after administering blood and blood product transfusions, assessing prothrombin/partial thromboplastin time when patients are on anticoagulation therapy).
- ▶ Not placing a patient on skin care precaution although he or she is at risk for skin breakdown.

▶ Transferring a patient to subacute rehabilitation when he or she could benefit from acute rehabilitation services.

The UM role can be touchy. Conflicts may arise if the physician feels the case manager is telling him or her what to do or is "policing" the patient and patient care. Utilization tools such as clinical pathways and evidence-based practice guidelines are sometimes helpful in that regard. When a care plan goes off the path, that clinical pathway—and the patient—can become the focus of discussion, which directs the conversation away from any personal physician practice and maintains the focus on the patient.

▶ Facilitator for Changes in Level of Care

Many case managers have entered the world of case management through the role of either discharge planner or utilization reviewer. Regardless, these tasks require an assessment of the total medical, psychosocial, and financial needs of each patient. Although some cases may be similar, no two are exactly alike. Discharge and transitional planning should be started at the time of admission or, if possible, during preadmission screening.

Examples of discharge planning that involve transitional changes in levels of care are discharges from a hospital to a skilled nursing facility or to home, or from a subacute facility to home. Other examples include the transfer of a patient from an intensive care unit to a regular unit in a hospital or from a primary to a specialty care provider such as general medicine to cardiology. Sometimes, the level of care may move to a more acute phase. If a home care patient is found to be quickly deteriorating, will a skilled nursing facility prevent further decline and avoid an acute hospitalization? Or does the patient require acute rehabilitation?

Case managers must also be alert to a patient's medical readiness to change the levels of care, such as transfers from the intensive care unit to a step-down unit or a standard patient floor. In today's hospital care environment, the case manager must alert and prompt the physicians that the patient may be ready for this change; more health insurance companies today are issuing specific denials, even as explicit as a level of care denial for X number of days, because medically, the patient could have been cared for at a lesser level sooner. As case managers coordinate the transition of patients from one level of care to another, they rely on their knowledge and skills in utilization management to appropriately manage these transitions.

Changes in the level of care can go in either direction. If a home health case manager finds the patient's condition deteriorating and the home situation is no longer safe, a call to the physician may elicit some home modalities to be attempted, an order for a move to a skilled nursing facility, or a hospital admission, or a visit to the emergency department. Home care case managers often facilitate the change from home healthcare to hospice care when appropriate and when the patient and family are ready.

▶ The Health Insurance Benefit Analyst

Many types of case management require an intensive analysis of benefit allowances. This is especially true for entrepreneurial case managers and for those working with union groups, self-funded plans, or payor-based organizations. This skill is least important for acute care case management; essentially, as long as a patient requires acute care, most plans cover the expense. However, other case managers, and certainly those who follow a patient through all levels of care and home, must be aware of benefit limitations.

Case managers often describe this role as that of a *gatekeeper or game keeper*. Each insurance company has its own rules, covered services, interpretation of UM modalities, and types of reimbursement. To obtain the full hospital stay authorization, to maximize the chance of a successful discharge plan, to minimize last-minute surprises, and to be legally correct in any type of case management, *know the game rules for your patient's insurance plan*.

Consider home health benefits. Some plans allow sixty visits per year; others allow $10,000 per year; still others may allow a set dollar amount per visit or any combination of these. For this case management responsibility, a call to the claims payor or a careful study of the most recent benefit book is the safest route. Each health insurance plan design is unique, and patient care must be customized to adhere to the set of rules and regulations of the plan to which the patient belongs. Case managers must know every detail of the benefit book. It is essential that case managers understand the strategies behind health insurance structures.

Another important consideration for case management is that in the realm of insurance benefits, case managers are often looked to for new trends in reimbursement. Sometimes, case managers are not aware of why they are asked for their "opinions." Early in the 1990s, one payor requested that the case manager research preventive screening for high-risk colon cancer patients. During the conversation, it became clear that this company's benefit design allowed for preventive screening for high-risk beneficiaries for prostate cancer and breast cancer; it disallowed the same consideration for beneficiaries with a high risk for colon cancer. This situation was remedied after detailed information on this topic was provided and the necessary organizational protocol initiated. Over the years, we know of case managers who fought for a particular service to save a patient's life. Although that life was not always spared, benefits changed and future patients were offered the benefits. Did these pleas, telephone calls, and meetings really help future patients? Something changed the minds of those who make the rules—perhaps credible case managers and court judgments were the right combination.

▶ The Cost–Benefit Analyst

Beyond analyzing insurance benefits, many case managers are asked to do a cost analysis of a case. Occasionally, family members need comparative financial information, or insurance companies (inclined to refuse payment for a requested plan if they feel that a less cost-intensive solution is available) may request prices. Many case managers are required to make a formal documentation of savings per case for accounting purposes. Disease or chronic care management case managers may be required to contribute to the savings information for an entire population of disease-specific patients such as a population of patients with heart failure.

Many case managers shun this responsibility. There may be several reasons for doing so:

▶ They do not go into a "warm and fuzzy" helping profession to do accounting work. Case managers improve the quality and safety of a patient's life.
▶ Case managers already know that they improve care quality and safety, and reduce costs per case; justifying their existence is someone else's responsibility or considered unnecessary.
▶ It is difficult to understand accounting and budgeting concepts.
▶ It is often tedious and time-consuming to address and report financial details.

Apart from these "reasons", case managers are as real an expense to the payors and healthcare facilities that hire them as are physician services, hospital costs, and medications. Everything has its price and must prove its worth in the business world; "warm and fuzzy" case managers are no exception. In fact, this skill is so important that basic accounting, or a course in analyzing costs in healthcare, should be a case management curriculum item. It is understandable that case managers are not always comfortable doing this task; the main licenses that comprise case managers certainly do not stress accounting principles. It is also very time-consuming to justify how dollars were saved in a case for reporting purposes, and time is a commodity that few case managers have in excess.

Case managers must periodically write reports on each case they manage. At times, when costs were clearly saved (often in huge amounts), this budgetary portion of the report is felt to be fun, almost exhilarating; at other times, when payors want dollars saved more than they want improvement in the quality of life, this part of the report usually is a challenge and felt to be stressful. To understand cost-benefit analysis, it is necessary to distinguish between the nuances of "hard" versus "soft" savings on a case.

HARD SAVINGS

Costs that are clearly saved or avoided in a case are the *hard savings* or *avoided costs*. A new patient once asked the case manager to attempt negotiation on a large hospital bill that was several months old and in another state. The patient and case manager agreed that it was a long shot. Knowing that some companies extend contracted rates to specific facilities in other states, they did some homework. As luck would have it, this was a match! The new patient

saved more than $78,000 on the hospital bill, and case management time was less than 2 hours. This is hard savings—the result of strong case management.

Some examples of hard savings are the following. Please note that insurance companies are also looking at these, and will deny reimbursement for the "wrong" level of care, length of stay, unauthorized benefits, and so on. And also see the section on "Avoidable Days/Delays" in Chapter 5.

▶ Change in level of care facilitated by the case manager to one that is most appropriate based on the patient's condition and treatment plan;
▶ Change in length of stay facilitated by the case manager;
▶ Change to a contracted preferred provider organization healthcare professional facilitated by the case manager;
▶ Negotiation of price of services, supplies, equipment, or per diem rates facilitated by the case manager;
▶ Negotiation of frequency of services facilitated by the case manager;
▶ Negotiation of duration of services facilitated by the case manager;
▶ Prevention of unnecessary bed days, supplies, equipment, services, or charges facilitated by the case manager;
▶ Discovery of unauthorized charges that are unwarranted.

SOFT SAVINGS

Soft savings are also called *potential savings* or *potential costs/charges*. If a case manager is *not* assigned to a patient, the potential costs incurred might be much higher than with case management. Soft savings are not as concrete as hard savings. They are, however, very real savings; they represent costs that are avoided, most likely because of case management intervention and follow-up by the case manager. The reason they are not considered hard savings is that no one can be absolutely certain what the outcome of the case would have been if a case manager had not been on board. These are the savings that take time and patience to document. High-risk pregnancy case management is a good example. If a 16-year-old pregnant teenager who is a known substance user and a diabetic is not case managed, the baby could end up in the neonatal intensive care unit (NICU) upon birth for 2 months at a minimum cost of $1,000,000 or more. However, with support and intervention, there is also a chance that the baby could be fairly healthy and may require only a short period of hospitalization.

Case managers are not always comfortable playing the "what if" scenario. It is more challenging and time-consuming to document these types of cases. With hard savings, it is a simple equation: *the total hospital bill minus the contracted rate that should have been billed equals the hard savings*. With soft savings, each case manager must research potential charges to document potential avoided costs. The potential charges are often specific to a location, type of facility, and contracted rates the payor would have allowed had the services been provided. Then the case manager must guesstimate factors such as the length of time in the NICU (how premature was this baby?). Each case is unique, and so are the potential savings. Therefore, each cost-benefit report for soft savings will require a customized set of numbers. It helps to keep a file of these numbers and use them for reference in future cases. As more outcomes data on case/disease management become available, case managers will be clearer about what is actually a case management impact.

Some examples of soft savings are the following:

- ▶ Avoidance of potential hospital readmissions (Note that, depending on the case review, this could also be either a hard savings or a potential missed opportunity.)
- ▶ Avoidance of potential emergency department visits
- ▶ Avoidance of potential medical complications
- ▶ Avoidance of potential legal exposure
- ▶ Avoidance of potential costs (equipment, supplies, etc.)
- ▶ Avoidance of potential acute care days
- ▶ Avoidance of potential home health visits
- ▶ Avoidance of unscheduled clinic visits
- ▶ Prevention of medical errors.

Other soft savings relate to quality and satisfaction. It is difficult to put a dollar amount on these, and they are sometimes priceless to the patient and family. Examples may include the following:

- ▶ Improved quality of care and outcomes
- ▶ Improved patient/family satisfaction with case management services and care experience
- ▶ Improved patient adherence to the care regimen
- ▶ Patient's improved quality of life and well-being
- ▶ Patient's improved social support network.

The detailed research is the tough part; the math is quite simple.

1. How much did the care cost? $20,000.
2. How much would the care have cost without case management services? $30,000.
3. Subtract number two from number one. The difference is the costs saved. $30,000 − $20,000 = $10,000 saved.
4. Lastly, consider all miscellaneous costs and subtract them from the costs saved. What other costs did the payor incur for the case management fee, physician fees, and other expenses? $1,500.

Total costs saved: $10,000 − $1,500 = $8,500 savings *because case management was involved*.

There is a small, but growing, amount of research about cost efficiencies and savings resulting from case management services. When the published literature is reviewed, one may observe that such research is not generalizable and that it is limited to the setting where it has been conducted. Additionally, such research lacks standardized approaches, which prevents its replicability in other settings. Despite these concerns, case management experts have been able to document the value of the programs to their organizations and have been able to sustain these services. Healthcare organizations that employ case managers save money and improve their bottom line as a result of the unnecessary hospital days, ambulatory visits, or healthcare resources case managers prevent every day. This translates into millions of dollars annually for each organization. These numbers are important for case management survival. Case managers work hard for cost savings; documentation of the results of these efforts will continue to ensure the future of case management by speaking in terms that business people can understand. For those who resist this accounting skill, remember that sometimes case managers have saved much more than a 30:1 ratio, and the savings were in terms dearer than dollars.

▶ The Case Management Negotiator

In the current healthcare environment of scarce resource availability and declining benefits, the art of negotiation is extremely important. Negotiation is essentially a communication exchange for the purpose of reaching an agreement. It is a daily activity of case managers and used with all parties: patients/families, payors, care providers (internal or external to a healthcare organization), vendors of durable medical equipment, transportation agents, community service providers, and so on. Cost containment, often through negotiation skills, was one of case management's well-known attributes. However, with the proliferation of contracted rates, negotiation opportunities are diminishing and are shifting from a primary focus on cost to a focus on value, quality, and safety. It is important to continue to look for these opportunities and have the skills to make each negotiation opportunity count. Some people are natural-born negotiators, and to become an expert and effective negotiator requires practice. The effort is well worth it, because advocating for a patient's needs frequently requires this skill. Things will rarely happen for a patient unless the case manager makes them happen, and that usually takes negotiation.

Negotiation serves the following important purposes:

- ▶ It facilitates reaching an agreement. Case managers use negotiation to solve problems and conflicts as they arise in the course of caring for a patient and family.
- ▶ It has the capacity to control costs—one of the primary reasons case managers negotiate.

▶ It has the capacity to gain medically necessary benefits for the patient that the patient would otherwise not receive. This is the other primary reason case managers negotiate: access to services.

▶ It can avoid chaos. Many case managers attempt to obtain services or equipment for a patient, knowing full well that the patient needed what was being requested to maintain stability. Many case managers live through frustration and chaos when the patient's condition deteriorates, at least partly because the negotiation for the requested service or equipment is denied or treatment is delayed.

▶ It can be a learning experience. Case managers may learn why the request is denied (sometimes there *is* a valid reason). They may also reveal weaknesses in the "No" argument, which could further strengthen the case manager's negotiation stance.

▶ It can improve the quality of care. Case managers frequently assess a patient's needs and monitor care and services. When a potential delay in treatment, test, or procedure is identified, such as a delay in completing an MRI, the case manager negotiates expedition of such a test. This ultimately provides clinicians with the ability to better diagnose a health problem and to institute appropriate action.

▶ It can improve the patient's or family's experience of care. Case managers are caring and compassionate care providers. They are sensitive to the patient/family needs, desires, and cultural values and belief system. They spend a considerable amount of time getting to know the patient and family; understanding their needs; and developing a respectful, trusting, and therapeutic relationship. Ultimately, such a relationship allows for improved patient and family care experience where the patient feels comfortable speaking up and sharing sensitive yet important information that when withheld, may result in suboptimal care outcomes or delay the progress toward meeting care goals.

▶ It can improve communication. As case managers negotiate, they interact with members of the healthcare team (formally or informally). During such interactions, case managers keep the team well informed of the status of the patient's plan of care, decisions of insurance companies (payors) about authorizations for care to be provided, and changes in the patient's condition (progress or deterioration). Additionally, the interactions ensure that all team members are on the same page with the plan of care, the goals of treatment, and outcomes to be achieved.

Some case managers are hesitant to take on the "big guys." There are five stages of negotiation that will take some of the fear out of this task.

1. Do your homework. Be optimally prepared to present the facts clearly. Before negotiation begins, it is wise to do some research and understand the other side. For example, know what services are covered, know the approximate readmit rates if a patient does not receive a particular service, and be prepared to ask for a supervisor—by name, if possible—if you feel strongly about a particular service need. Establish standards of care and practice, written protocols, written criteria, and community care guidelines before the first telephone call or contact. Also, assess yourself for any hidden agendas that may push the negotiation into conflict.

2. Start your engines. Negotiation starts by stating the problem(s) and the goal and stating what is needed to solve the problem. For example, explain the reasons why the services are imperative and the benefits of the services to all concerned (i.e., less costly readmissions to the acute care setting). State the request in a positive and thorough way. Be courteous to the other party; negotiation is a two-way street and facts need to be shared. Areas in which there is agreement can be put aside temporarily; then, begin to search for mutual compromise.

3. Use the three "Cs"—communicate, communicate, and communicate. Always have clear, factual, and pertinent data to share and avoid losing sight of the goal of negotiation while communicating. Cultivate an interactive, collaborative relationship rather than an antagonistic one. Wait for the right moment to make your pitch and avoid talking too much. Use active listening and acknowledge the other side's concerns; ask how some of the problems may be overcome. Unless there is some indication that a message has been received, true communication has not taken place. Common mistakes can create a defensive environment not conducive to negotiation. Some behaviors that may be problematic include poor listening skills, poor use of questions, improper disclosure of ideas, mismanagement of issues, becoming emotional, inappropriate stress reactions, too-quick rejection of alternatives, misuse of a negotiating team member, failure to disclose true feelings, improper timing, and being aggressive rather than assertive. Sometimes, if the flames are getting too hot, it is time to take a break and resume at a later date.

4. Be realistic. Attempting to negotiate for a service, medical equipment, or a price that absolutely will not be covered wastes everyone's time and energy. Approach negotiation as a process, not as an event or one-time task. Focus on interests rather than positions. Appreciate small wins; they are as important as the large ones. Always have alternate solutions or options for use when necessary.

5. Put it in writing. Once an agreement has been reached, write it down and have all parties sign

it. This can avoid future problems when, months down the road, the claims payor calls you with a question about this situation or the other party "forgot" what was agreed.

Another reason that case managers are sometimes reluctant to start negotiations is that they have run up against some rather unreasonable characters. There are two types of negotiators: the aggressives and the cooperatives. Aggressive negotiators use psychological maneuvers such as intimidation and threats to make their "opponent" feel disparaged. Cooperative negotiators try to establish trust. Knowledge of the differences can arm a case manager in powerful ways. If, to your dismay, your negotiation tactics resemble the more aggressive or manipulative model, study the weaknesses and evaluate yourself.

THE AGGRESSIVE NEGOTIATOR

▶ The aggressive negotiator moves psychologically against his or her "opponent." Note the key word *psychologically*. If the case manager feels that something is amiss, that he or she is being toyed with, the case should be brought back to facts.
▶ Common tactics include intimidation, accusation, threats, sarcasm, playing games, and ridicule.
▶ There is an overt or covert claim that the aggressive negotiator is superior and never loses a negotiation.
▶ The aggressive negotiator makes extreme demands and few concessions.
▶ There are frequent threats to terminate negotiations.
▶ False issues are brought up time and again. Once more, the case manager needs to bring the case back to the facts.

STRENGTHS OF THE AGGRESSIVE MODEL Any
perceived strengths are diminished by a lack of trust in future negotiations. Often, aggression is perceived as coercive; however, perseverance allows for achieving desired goals.

WEAKNESSES OF THE AGGRESSIVE MODEL Some
weaknesses include:

▶ It is more difficult to be a successful aggressive negotiator.
▶ Tension and mistrust that develop may increase the likelihood of misunderstandings.
▶ Deadlock over one trivial issue may escalate other issues.
▶ The "opponent" may develop "righteous indignation" and pursue the case with more vengeance.
▶ One's reputation as an aggressive negotiator will hurt future negotiations.
▶ Aggressive tactics increase the number of failed negotiations.
▶ The trial rate for aggressive negotiators is more than double.

THE COOPERATIVE NEGOTIATOR

▶ The cooperative negotiator moves psychologically toward his or her "opponent."
▶ The cooperative negotiator establishes a common ground. For case managers, the common ground is the patient.
▶ This negotiator is trustworthy, fair, objective, open-minded, and reasonable. This is very important. Respect and trustworthiness are critical for negotiations.
▶ This negotiator works to establish credibility and unilateral concessions. The attitude is one of win-win.
▶ This negotiator seeks to obtain the best joint outcome for everyone. This requires respect, empathy, and active listening as described in other sections of this text.
▶ Future negotiations are made easier.

STRENGTHS OF THE COOPERATIVE METHOD Some
strengths include:

▶ The cooperative method promotes mutual understanding.
▶ Agreement is generally produced in less time than with the aggressive approach.
▶ There is a larger percentage of agreement in cases than with aggressive approaches.
▶ The cooperative method often produces a better outcome than do aggressive strategies.
▶ The percentage of "successful" negotiations is much higher.

WEAKNESSES OF THE COOPERATIVE METHOD
Some weaknesses are:

▶ Aggressives view cooperatives as weak, so they push harder.
▶ Cooperative negotiators risk being manipulated or exploited because of the assumption that "If I am fair and trustworthy and make decisions with all parties in mind, then the other side will feel an irresistible moral obligation to reciprocate."

If negotiations start sounding like something from a professional wrestling match, use the following techniques to overcome the deadlock. Try resummarizing ideas, discussing the remaining alternatives, asking hypothetical questions, evaluating the differing points of view, and analyzing past and future needs of all concerned. When some people feel angry and have their backs against the wall, they say nothing; unexpressed emotions can result in misunderstandings and detours. Always remember that *the most important focus is the patient and family and what they require for safety and health purposes.* When negotiating, case managers can increase the likelihood of achieving desired outcomes by avoiding the behaviors listed in Display 2-2.

BEHAVIORS TO AVOID DURING A NEGOTIATION

1. Making the other side feel guilty, distrusted, or disrespected
2. Using sarcasm, cynicism, or put-down statements
3. Becoming emotional or losing one's temper
4. Threatening the other side
5. Rushing the process or becoming impatient with progress or the lack thereof
6. Playing games or tricks
7. Distorting the facts
8. Jumping at the first offer
9. Refraining from asking questions for fear of appearing stupid
10. Losing sight of the bottom line, the long-term goal
11. Cultivating an aggressive, antagonistic relationship
12. Talking too much
13. Giving up prematurely
14. Appearing unprepared

▶ Facilitate a Reputation of Follow-Up and Follow-Through

Although case managers who work in silos still exist, fewer case managers perform strictly episodic case management every year because the trend is toward case management through a continuum of care. Episodic case management involves following the patient through a single episode of acute illness. An increasing number of case managers follow up their patients wherever they reside, whether acutely ill in a hospital or chronically stable at home. Others perform intermittent postdischarge hospital follow-up on a need-to basis. How often a case manager needs to follow up after discharge depends on the agency's case management model and workflow, and the acuteness or chronicity of the patient's condition. Some questions to ask that may also facilitate how and when to follow up include:

▶ Is the care optimal? Is the patient receiving quality care? Is the patient receiving the services that were brokered prior to discharge?
▶ Does the patient's condition still match the level of care he or she is receiving?
▶ Is the patient/family still satisfied with the arrangement and care, or is modification needed?
▶ Are the treatment goals being met, or are new goals needed? Are the desired outcomes achieved?
▶ Are the appropriate care providers involved in the delivery of care and services?

Following patients through the continuum of care is becoming common practice. However, there will always be acute care case managers or case managers whose jobs are to follow the patient wherever he or she may be. The type and extent of follow-up will depend on the job description of the case manager, the practice setting, and the organization's case management program design.

A related skill for a case manager is good follow-through. Gaining either patient or physician trust is not always easy, but perhaps the most important activity as an inroad to trust is follow-through once a plan has been finalized. If something impedes the plan, a telephone call to the patient or physician to discuss the problem and to offer a potential solution or new course of action keeps the trust level high.

▶ The Clinical Edge

Keeping yourself up-to-date on new treatments and technologies in your area of case management is a necessary edge, and it is important to update clinical knowledge regularly through seminars and texts. It is impossible to completely case manage in a medical environment without clinical expertise. Many extra days have been authorized by health insurance companies because important clinical data have been provided by the case manager. Accurate assessment of discharge needs depends on knowledge of the disease process and treatment regimens. Practice standards also change as safer and improved methods are discovered. A clinically sharp case manager has an important advantage over others, and it is necessary to apply up-to-date knowledge, evidence, and standards to the care of your patients.

Clinical expertise and critical thinking are expected of case managers. The disease-specific case manager must have an intimate knowledge of the population he or she is serving. In essence, a disease management case manager is a case management specialist in a particular clinical area or disease entity. The case manager is familiar with the pathophysiology of the disease, its progression, diagnostic and therapeutic tests and procedures, treatment options, and desired outcomes. All of this knowledge benefits the patient and family.

▶ Knowledge of Complementary and Alternative Medicine

What started out as a grassroots movement in the early 1970s is now big business, and case managers must be aware of the ramifications of their patients' use of complementary and alternative medicine (CAM). Some modalities such as acupuncture have been used for thousands of years in other cultures. Herbal medicine has been proven to assist in many chronic conditions. Magnetic therapy is being studied by credible organizations. As with Western medicine, CAM is powerful and must be respected. Many of the complementary modalities are an excellent adjunct to Western medicine. Sometimes, the two traditions do not coexist harmoniously. This is such a complex situation that the famous *Physician's Desk Reference* has come out with a herbal version. It is well documented that many patients use complementary medicine without informing their healthcare provider. The reason is often fear of ridicule; physicians have traditionally balked at non-Western approaches to healthcare. This has dramatically changed in the past decade; however, some patients are still not comfortable telling their physicians about their own "trial and error" methods of CAM.

The use and acceptance of CAM is one of the most far-reaching changes in healthcare. Insurance plans are already covering certain modalities, and the changes have just started taking place. The National Institutes of Health (NIH) has allocated millions of dollars for the Office of Alternative Medicine's budget. The White House Commission on Complementary and Alternative Medicine Policy has also done the same. Well-respected healthcare systems, including the Cleveland Clinic and Mayo Clinic, use alternative modalities. These credible forums promote scientifically rigorous research into various modalities. The results may change the face of healthcare.

Case managers, as patient advocates, promote what is in the best interest of their patients. Doing so means that the case manager respects the patient's wishes, values, and beliefs, including his or her attitudes about CAM. If a patient is using any CAM modality, it must be communicated to the healthcare team (with permission), incorporated in the plan of care, and considered for its impact on care progression and options.

▶ Critical Thinker and Problem Solver

In nursing, this skill is often referred to as critical thinking; in business, the same type of skill is referred to as problem-solving. In both, it is being a creative thinker, having the ability for clinical reasoning, or "thinking outside the box." Critical thinking is the ability to:

▶ Put together the known components of the problem,
▶ Anticipate the potential issues and concerns,
▶ Research possible solutions,
▶ Find a way to improve the condition, and
▶ Be mindful of the impact of your actions on achieving desired outcomes.

Critically thinking case managers have the capacity to examine the patient's clinical record, walk into a patient's room, look at the patient, perhaps ask a question or two, and then make an emergency move that could save a patient's life. This relates to clinical expertise and effective reasoning; it is also problem-solving. Such case managers are able to put together all the known components, add medical knowledge and intuition, identify a problem, and initiate a solution.

This skill of critical thinking may be an intrinsic part of a case manager's performance metrics, as case managers are assigned to patients/clients with complex

medical, cognitive and behavioral, functional, and social needs. Critical thinking serves as a trigger to the mental calisthenics required to engage the case management process; it starts with assessment and problem identification and goes through to the case management stages of termination, if not postdischarge transition and/or follow-up (Treiger & Fink-Samnick, 2017).

Critical thinking is a methodical and analytical process, fostering a case manager's ability to work through complex situations and provide a strategic means to advance professional case management interventions across the practice setting. Critical thinking must incorporate the following (Treiger & Fink-Samnick, 2017):

▶ Suspend judgment,
▶ Deconstruct the situation,
▶ Reflect on individual actions, and
▶ Synthesize thoughts.

Thinking on one's feet may be needed in many situations case managers face. Components of a case management problem may be complex, and the sheer number of considerations that must be taken into account may be dizzying. Case managers must have this ability to function in the complex world of healthcare.

▶ Knowledge of Legal and Quality Issues, and Standards of Practice

Quality outcomes are a main goal of case management. Astute case managers routinely avert potential disasters by recognizing potential problems and resolving them before they get too far out of line. Related to this is the responsibility to monitor quality of care or risk management issues. Monitoring for quality of care issues is required in all aspects of patient care. Some of the main tenets of case management are provision of quality and safe care and identifying deviations from standards of care or practice, which is an important obligation. Case managers, being on the front lines, often pick up potential or actual variances (e.g., delays, errors, or omissions) from standards of care; this is another potential way in which case managers can avert a full-blown crisis (see Chapters 7 and 8).

▶ We Are All Accountable

Competency and accountability go hand in hand. The simplest definition of accountability is "being responsible." Case managers are responsible for a myriad of outcomes (results) from the case management interventions they perform daily.

Dennis O'Leary, former president of The Joint Commission, discusses the "cascade of accountability." This cascade can begin with an individual who, through a union contract or some other leverage, holds his or her employer accountable for offering a range of high-quality healthcare coverage options. The employer, in turn, holds the health plan accountable; the health plan holds the provider organization accountable for delivering services that result in good outcomes. The provider organization will hold physicians, case managers, and other clinicians accountable to the individual patient . . . and make no mistake, the latter healthcare group will be held accountable in a court of law (see Chapter 8).

▶ Preparation of Case Management Team Members

Chapter 5 discusses the various members of the case management team; however, this entire textbook prepares you for the case manager's role. In general, the key players in the case management team include:

- ▶ Nurse Case Manager
- ▶ Social Worker
- ▶ Physician Advisor
- ▶ Clinical Documentation Specialist
- ▶ Denials and Appeals Manager
- ▶ Care (or Case) Management Assistant
- ▶ Physician Practices/Attending Physicians

However, other critical ad hoc professionals may have pertinent information and are responsible for certain care activities, without which the team cannot make a thorough and informed decision. These may include family members/ significant others, physical/occupational/speech therapists, rehabilitation staff/physicians, pharmacists, health insurance or payor case managers, representatives from home health or skilled nursing facility, agents of community-based resources, even the primary care physician . . . the list is unique to every situation and individual patient/family.

Before your conversation begins, each member must have an accurate and thorough clinical assessment of the situation. When the stress level gets high (as it sometimes does), emotional IQ cannot be overstated. Be colloquial and not adversarial in your approach; gain a reputation for solving problems. Personal or organizational agendas may be lurking, and it is imperative to be aware of any of these possibilities prior to the case meeting. This has been said many times, but focusing on the patient is always the best approach. It moves the emotions away from any hidden foci and allows everyone to focus on the same goal.

Often, these case conferences are called for because of transitional planning barriers or conflicting thoughts about the plan of care among patients and their family members. The goal is to synthesize the current situation and discuss potential "next steps" to move the patient forward. When discussing discharge or transfer plans, make sure you have the patient's/family's cooperation in a plan; this can save time and potentially wasted attempts at transition plans.

A word about the actual discussion. Many of us have been involved in meetings that are hijacked by an individual who may take more than his or her fair share of "dialogue space." Be succinct and to the point about your needs and concerns. Everyone is busy and often may have a low tolerance for rambling conversations. And, finally, keep lines of communication open, and follow through on what is discussed. More trust will be gained because of good follow-through than from any other approach you may use.

▶ The Facilitator of Multidisciplinary Patient Care Rounds

Various types of multidisciplinary rounds may take place; these include daily rounds with physician groups and other healthcare professionals, PRN (pro re nata, a Latin phrase which means "as needed") huddles as new changes or knowledge becomes known, weekly rounds discussing all cases on the case manager's caseload, and patient care conferences that focus on one particular patient with extensive needs or special problems. The case manager is often responsible for facilitation and coordination of these rounds. A few tips for well-coordinated rounds/huddles are included in Display 2-3.

---

display 2-3

TIPS FOR PATIENT CARE ROUNDS

1. Know the case/medical histories of the patients being discussed in as much detail as possible. You must be able to give a good overview of the patients' present status and state the priority problems that need discussion clearly and completely.

2. Focus on the plan of care, including the transitional and discharge plans. Communicate outcomes of interactions with payor-based case managers.

3. Involve everyone on the patient's healthcare team. Each member knows the patient from a different perspective, and the sum total of all the perspectives allows a more complete picture of care. As the patient advocate, do not forget the patient's and family's perspective, and communicate what is in their best interest.

4. Try not to allow interruptions during conferences with the healthcare team. If possible, hold calls and pagers until the completion of rounds.

5. Anticipate problems that might arise with all the solutions discussed, and have a second possible course ready in case the first one falls through.

6. Bring each case to closure with a plan with which everyone can work, if possible. Be in the habit of making rounds an effective use of time.

7. Set time limits to help make rounds an efficient use of time.

8. Conclude the rounds after making sure that items that require follow-up have been delegated among the team members and that each item had a designated responsible party. Ensure that expectations are made clear.

▶ It Is a Multidisciplinary (Interdisciplinary) World

This is a multidisciplinary world; all players are important. Currently, in the healthcare environment, several types of teams are required for the practice of case management, accreditation, and quality initiatives. A team is a group of people who have come together for a specific purpose such as provision of safe and quality care to patients and their families. Ideally, teams are empowered to assess problems, institute actions, initiate changes, and evaluate the impact of those actions and changes. Case managers are well acquainted with multidisciplinary (interdisciplinary) teams. Quality improvement teams and cross-functional teams have a different focus and are often run quite differently than patient care teams. For example, patient care teams may be planned for daily, weekly, or biweekly meetings depending on the patient population and care setting. The agenda and purpose is focused around patient care. Sometimes, patient care conferences are impromptu, almost emergent, in their timing. Often, the team members depend on which patients need attention and what the underlying problems may be; this necessitates a constant changing of important team players.

A quality team, on the other hand, most often has a set schedule, a specific goal or goals (i.e., to reduce readmissions in patients with congestive heart failure), an assigned group of team members (with occasional experts called in on an ad hoc basis) that will change only infrequently, and the initial luxury of a meeting or two to get to know the team members and establish meeting guidelines. The cross-functional team members can include almost anyone (physicians, case managers, biostatisticians, computer programmers, data analysts, administrators, financial personnel, etc.), depending on the reason for the initiation of the team. The team members are chosen for their ability to contribute to solving problems.

▶ Stellar Case Managers have Strong Interpersonal Communication Skills

The case manager, as the hub of the wheel (Fig. 2-1), must channel information to and from all other parties. Almost every case management task requires some form of communication. This is a mandatory, not to be compromised, case management skill. The ability to communicate and work well with people is a characteristic that many employers place among their top three priorities when hiring case managers; therefore, many case management firms assess applicants for these skills. Each patient may have several agencies on board and many individuals involved in the care plan. The case manager must not only work with all of these agency members, but also coordinate with them and the services they represent. This is not always easy when there are conflicting ideas and priorities about what is right and best for the patient.

Communication can be verbal, nonverbal, or written. There are four primary purposes of communication: (1) to inquire, (2) to inform, (3) to persuade, and (4) to entertain. Communicating to entertain is uncommon in case management practice. The other three purposes are essential in the case management process. Inquiring, informing, or persuading can be done through written communication or verbally, either in person or by telephone. Written communication must be succinct and unambiguous; verbal communication (which also should be succinct and unambiguous) often involves tact and diplomacy.

Informational communication forms a large part of case management transactions. Insurance companies must be informed and updated about their members' health conditions, treatment plans, and progress; thoroughness and creative persuasion are often important here. Patients need information about their disease process and treatments. An important case management communication skill is the ability not only to understand complex and technical information, but to be able to translate this information into layman's terms so that it is understandable to a patient or family. This is not always easy, because other factors may block the exchange of information. The patient may have suboptimal receptive and retention abilities because of shock, illness, high anxiety level, fear, depression, developmental age, language, or cultural barriers, already experiencing "information overload" or harboring an "I don't care" attitude.

Murphy's Law of medicine says that the more medical specialists on a case, the less they speak to one another. The case manager is often the integrator and collaborator of the fragmentation of care caused by this situation. The complexity and increased acuity and need for intense resources of patients who are selected by the case manager for case management services make it necessary that multiple healthcare professionals (sometimes including several physicians) be involved in the care. Add to this scenario the payor-based professionals (e.g., case manager) and other external agents such as those from medical transportation companies, skilled nursing facilities, home care agencies, and so on, with whom case managers interact daily regarding coordinating care for these patients. Keeping the lines of communication open across these professionals and agencies is a monumental task that, if not coordinated properly, may result in poor patient outcomes and unsafe experiences. The role of the case manager as integrator is a necessary responsibility in these situations. Not having a designated person to assume this role is a "recipe for failure," with its poor results experienced primarily by the patient and family.

According to some experts, nonverbal communication sometimes relays more of the message than the verbal component does. Posture, tone of voice, facial expressions, and nervous mannerisms provide clues that enhance or confuse the message. This information may assist the case manager in "reading" the real message. Nonverbal gestures may also help or hinder the case manager in his or her role. Ask coworkers to critique your style and record yourself to assess this powerful element of communication.

Perhaps the most important act of communication is that of listening. A wise person once directed, "listen twice as much as you speak. That is why you have two ears and one mouth." The ability to listen sends a message that the case manager places the needs of the patient before his or her own needs or those of the organization.

▶ Assertiveness Skills

Assertiveness skills are an important part of the case manager's communication repertoire. Not infrequently, case managers are placed in tense situations; any case manager who has *never* been told off by a physician is either an expert at assertiveness or is topping the scale of wishy-washy passivity. Historically, those in the helping professions have always tried to please everyone. "We hate to offend anyone. We pride ourselves on being fair, flexible and open-minded. Someone quipped that we try to be so open-minded our brains fall out" (Chenevert, 1988, p. 69). Flexibility is necessary in some situations; backbone is necessary in others. Passive behavior (e.g., giving up your seat when a doctor enters the room) is no longer applauded or condoned.

Substituting self-doubt with self-assurance is the first step in assertiveness and takes patience and practice; after changing your attitude, you can change your behavior. First, an understanding of the differences among passive behavior, aggressive behavior, and assertive behavior is helpful.

- ▶ In passive behavior, you may violate your own rights by ignoring them (i.e., self-denying) and allowing others to infringe on you; doing as you are told can lead to feelings of anxiety, helplessness, and depression.
- ▶ In aggressive behavior, others may be violated, dominated, humiliated, intimidated, or put down; one usually is taking advantage of another or enhancing oneself at the expense of the other (i.e., self-enhancing). Aggressive behavior may lead to feelings of guilt, bitterness, and loneliness.
- ▶ In assertive behavior, one is direct, honest, and lacking in excuses. One usually pushes hard without attacking and is expressive and able to influence the results and effect desirable outcomes. To be assertive, you must trust your feelings, like yourself, respect your own hunches and feelings, and be willing to accept the consequences of your assertive behavior.

Assertiveness is a tool, not a weapon (Chenevert, 1988). It is a desired communication style for the case manager. Fundamental to assertiveness practice is the substitution of "I" messages for "you" messages. "You"

messages often put the recipients on the defensive. Simple questions such as "Why did you. . .," "When do you plan to. . .," "What did you intend by. . ." immediately cause people to put on their armor.

"I" messages such as "I feel. . .," "I understand that. . .," "I want. . .," "I expect. . .," "I choose. . .," "I plan. . .," or "I am. . ." provide a clear, honest, and direct expression of one's feelings, thoughts, opinions, and beliefs. Other verbal techniques include choosing words carefully, speaking clearly, using a full, well-modulated voice, and projecting the message boldly, confidently, positively, frankly, and concisely. Nonverbal techniques include good posture, head held up, good eye contact, and hands quiet and relaxed (Chenevert, 1988).

Assertiveness allows you to act instead of react in a given situation. It is the perfect tool to get not only your own needs met, but also those of your patients; it is the perfect tool for the patient advocate to use. A rule of thumb is "focus on the patient and you will be amazed at how the petty, peripheral things will float away, and your work will seem less complicated and cluttered" (Chenevert, 1988, p. 156).

▶ Conflict Resolution Expert and Referee

Fear and anger are emotions commonly expressed by patients and families. Attentive listening is often all that is needed to defuse the anger. Some simply need validation or a bit of control over their seemingly uncontrollable situation. Honest and thorough answers are often what are required. The skills used for crisis intervention and conflict resolution may be similar. However, crisis intervention often revolves around pure grief, whereas conflict resolution requires detective work to get to the core problem, which is often hidden behind various acting-out behaviors. Also, the case manager should be prepared to play referee when conflict enters the multidisciplinary team; patients and families are not the only dispensers of acting-out behaviors. The case manager needs to stay objective and bring the focus back to the patient.

Use of diplomacy is both a skill and an art. When several of the team players are singing in different keys, the case manager must possess the tact and finesse to bring the group through negotiation and help them to decide which key is best for the patient.

▶ Hey Coach!

Lest this list starts to sound like an athletic arena, case managers coach, counsel, and support their patients on a daily basis. Consider complex and chronic conditions such as diabetes. Several times a day, small invasive procedures (e.g., finger sticks for monitoring blood glucose level) must be performed. Aspects of life such as diet and exercise that many people take for granted must be scientifically balanced against insulin and other factors that impact diabetes. Nonadherence to medical regimens is often the result of this daily battle. The case manager realizes that approximately 95% of a diabetic's care is self-care; for true empowerment, the patient is the center of the universe, with the case manager as a supportive coach and a catalyst for change in the individual's lifestyle.

Case managers also coach members of the healthcare team. They share with them the latest information about a patient's condition and plan of care. They teach them about the procedures and reimbursement methods of insurance companies, transitional and discharge planning rules and regulations, hospital-related administrative procedures and standards, and so on. In some situations, they also mentor newly employed or novice case managers.

Seasoned case managers, or managers of case managers, may coach staff in ways that improve their chances of success. This may be as free-form as when a case manager "phones a friend" with a question, or one with more structure, as a written opportunity for improvement.

◗ You Will Need Organizational Skills and the Ability to Prioritize

With all the details that must be attended to, organizational skills are a must. Also, time is prime; time constraints are frequent, and often everything must be accomplished precisely and quickly. Since the evolution of the quality movement, seminars on organizational and leadership growth abound. Many case managers are already organized people; if you are not, or if your organizational skills need improvement, seek out these seminars. This may make or break your acceptance to a care management department during an interview.

The ability to prioritize is simply doing the most important task first. In general, successful and effective case managers excel at prioritizing. Each hour and each day has its own priorities. Meetings have been missed because of a change in a patient's medical condition requiring immediate attention, and interfacility transfers have been delayed to meet the safety needs of a suicidal patient. The ability to shift gears instantaneously is as important—knowing that case management priorities are moving targets. Priorities shift with changing conditions, needs, and interests of patients. Distinguishing between urgency and importance is vital. Urgent tasks must be attended to immediately, no matter what. Important tasks come next. The ability to decide what is important and what is more or less routine is often a matter of common sense. Staying close to the patient/family priorities and agreed-upon care goals allows you to provide care that is important to the patient/family and not just to the healthcare team. Having a "feel" for the pacing and sequencing of a case is important; sometimes intuition plays a role and pushes a case farther "up the list," which averts an urgent scenario later. For example, getting a code status or calling a family meeting may ward off a crisis

situation. Delegation of tasks often helps to get several tough jobs done.

Attention to detail belongs to this category of skills. If you are not a detail person, bone up. Each case has so many variables, multiplied by the number of patients you have, that your total amounts to perhaps thousands of details. Again, missed details can destabilize the whole case, compromise the outcome, and leave patients, families, and other healthcare professionals dissatisfied.

◗ Resourcefulness and Creativity Can Save the Day

Case managers must adapt to different units, facilities, doctors, patients' cultures, other case managers, changing medical conditions, and changing transitional plans. Sometimes a care plan must turn on a dime; this requires flexibility and creativity so that no hospital day or resource is wasted. Rigidity can lead to poor case management, bad outcomes, and stress or burnout.

When the case manager may be called on to provide everything from a translator for an obscure European dialect to a macrobiotic diet, flexibility may turn into creativity. Creativity is often the first key in solving unusual problems. Tenacity and persistence are the other keys. Creativity is the ability to think "outside the box." Case managers are challenged with unique situations every day, and their previous experiences may not be directly applicable to resolving these situations. Therefore, to think and act creatively is a necessary skill all case managers must possess.

Creativity is so important in case management that administrators who do the hiring may want to use a case management version of the Edison test of creativity. Before hiring engineers, Thomas Edison would hand the applicant a light bulb and ask how much water it held. Edison had at least two methods to obtain the answer. An engineer could use gauges, measure all the angles, and calculate the surface area; this took an average of 20 minutes. Or an engineer could fill the light bulb with water, pour the contents in a measuring cup, and get the answer in less than a minute. Edison politely thanked the first group for their time but hired the second group.

◗ Crisis Intervention/Grief Counselor

Most end-of-life and/or hospice case managers and social workers are well trained and prepared for playing the role of grief counselor, but some others may need to seek training. Not everyone is comfortable with this assignment; yet in the healthcare field, it is inevitable that case managers will be involved when the condition of a loved one deteriorates or when death occurs. Some situations may be more challenging for a particular case manager to feel comfortable with than others. We personally find it easier to comfort children of an aged parent than parents who have lost their child—no matter what the age of the child is. On some level, parents feel that for a child to die first is not the natural order of things. Yet pediatric patients, young trauma victims, and young AIDS patients are "disrespectful" of that order. Inherent in the populations that require case management are those who are dying. Case managers should attend seminars or peruse the literature on grief counseling to become more proficient in this area.

▶ Health Educator

The opportunities for case managers to teach are unlimited. Most often done in conjunction with the agency/hospital education staff, the topics for education of patients, families, or significant others are wide-ranging and varied. Some topics include medication administration and side effects, disease processes and treatment, insurance coverage and noncoverage, tube/catheter care, lifestyle changes/behavior modification, red flags to watch out for, and any other needs that have been individually assessed. Staff nurses often help with medical topics, but patients also ask questions related to insurance, such as what pharmacies they are allowed to use, how much is their deductible and copay, how can they change Medicaid plans, or whether they can change doctors. The case manager is looked to as the expert in these areas.

A careful assessment of teaching needs and the bridging of knowledge deficit leads to cost-effectiveness and greater patient satisfaction and adherence to medical regimen. Readmissions because of a lack of adherence are reduced when the patient understands the disease process and the importance of the treatment needed. If a patient suffers from a newly diagnosed health condition, it is critical to thoroughly educate the patient and family; insufficient understanding can lead to a deteriorated medical condition, more avoidable emergency department visits, complications, and hospital readmission.

Case managers often see patients who, after a long discussion with their physicians, are more confused than ever. The ability to clearly explain difficult concepts in simple, easy-to-understand, lay terminology is an asset to the case manager–patient relationship. It helps build trust, and the patient does not feel embarrassed or condescended to. A ready-made file of handouts and information is a time-saver; bilingual handouts are also needed while dealing with diverse populations.

The health teaching process may require repetition. However, other factors can hinder learning: too much information in too short a time, fear, anger, shock, depression, medications, or any number of painful experiences patients in hospitals routinely go through. When preadmission or preoperative teaching can be carried out, it turns out to be an excellent choice—and is now the norm rather than the exception. Some insurers attempt to deny readmission payments if they feel the hospitalization was caused by poor discharge preparation (i.e., education).

Education about what case managers do and what case management is can sometimes be the most challenging of topics. Patients are not the only ones who require education about case management; even payors who retain case management firms are at a loss to articulate what they want from case management in specific cases. Just as it is up to case managers to explain about their capabilities and limitations to patients, it is also up to them to do the same for companies that hire them.

▶ BASIC VERSUS ADVANCED CASE MANAGEMENT SKILLS

The skills discussed earlier cannot easily be separated into basic and advanced case management. Certainly, many of the aspects of case management discussed in this chapter are mandatory, even for a beginner. So what constitutes advanced case management skills? Does the individual with an advanced degree overshadow those with lesser degrees? The core licensure is determined by the best match to the patient population; it is not something to be placed in a hierarchy. It is true that some case managers attempt to define the difference between advanced and basic skills by level of academic degree rather than by experience and skill. However, those with doctorate degrees who have never practiced more than cursory case management (although well presented at case management seminars) may have difficulty handling an actual patient caseload. Certifications such as the CCM credential or the Accredited Care Manager (ACM) from the ACMA can be held by various levels of education degrees and by almost every healthcare licensee. (For more on certification, please see Chapter 10.)

Although it may be difficult to articulate what constitutes an advanced case management practice, advanced case managers have certain attributes and skills in common. Advanced case managers:

▶ Have published their works in magazines, peer-reviewed and non–peer-reviewed journals, trade publications, or textbooks. They are committed to advancing the case management industry with valid, pertinent, and useful information and evidence-based knowledge.

▶ Have a creative sense that allows thinking outside the box. This talent is a combination of experience, knowledge of outcomes, competence, expertise, and intuition.

▶ Typically have had case management experience in several healthcare settings (perhaps with health maintenance organizations (HMOs), hospitals, workers' compensation, and self-funded plans); they have case managed patients through a continuum of care, not just through an episode of illness.

▶ Understand the basic principles of management, leadership, outcomes (including how to put together a simple case management outcomes management project), and continuous quality improvement (CQI).

▶ Keep up with the upcoming trends in healthcare and plan strategies for future needs; this may range from the whirlwind increase in the use of CAM to regulatory and fiscal changes happening at the regional or national level.

▶ Possess a good working knowledge of technical support systems and use of digital care tools.

▶ Are the ones peers typically call on when assistance with difficult cases is needed.

▶ Often hold leadership positions in their organizations.

▶ Have thorough autonomy, as well as a thorough understanding and use of the core case management components (assessment, problem identification, planning, implementation, coordination, monitoring, evaluation, follow-up, and advocacy).

▶ Possess a core national specialty certification.

▶ Hold a bachelor's or master's degree in a healthcare field that is related to case management.

▶ Engage in the conduct of case management-related research and innovative practices, dissemination of findings or innovations, and the utilization of research outcomes in their own practices and for the benefit of patient care.

▶ Mentor novice case managers or those interested in becoming case managers. They also act as consultants to others interested in improving their case management programs.

After completing this list, it occurred to us why case management has grown so fast that many are uncomfortable with its vast expansion. It had to—for survival. No one else had taken up the flag and run with it, and the patients needed help. Just when people are most vulnerable, they are thrown into a complex and convoluted system with a reputation for rationing care that requires a tremendous amount of information to blaze through. We heard a joke at a case management conference that brings this point home: there was a group of NASA scientists trying desperately to work out a problematic area in the space program. After weeks of struggling, one of the rocket scientists threw up her hands and said, "Come on. It's not like this in *case management*!"

▶ Case Management and Leadership Skills

Case management requires a wide array of leadership and management skills: delegation, conflict resolution, crisis intervention, collaboration, consultation, coordination, identification, and documentation. However, case managers are no longer just managers of care; they are leaders—and there is a difference. *Managers manage systems; leaders lead people.* Case managers do both; they manage cases (patients'

care) and lead or guide people (the healthcare team). Leadership is one step up on the ladder of professional growth. As case management continues to grow in responsibility, leadership qualities will necessarily be presumed.

The jury is still out about whether leaders are born or made. However, experts have noticed specific attributes that successful leaders share, regardless of the type of organization they lead. Effective leaders exhibit the following characteristics:

▶ Promote a vision. People need a vision of where they are going. Leaders provide that vision.

▶ Inspire others. Leaders are charismatic and able to inspire others to follow them for a certain cause, a purpose, an objective, or a goal. As such, others then feel satisfied and accomplished and that they have made a difference.

▶ Follow the golden rule. Anyone who has been demeaned or treated with disregard knows what effect that treatment has on the work.

▶ Make others feel important. They emphasize the strengths and utilize the talents of others in the organization. Then they share in the success and give credit where it is due.

▶ Admit mistakes. Everyone makes them. According to Will Rogers, "We're all ignorant. Only on different subjects."

▶ State to others that they do not know something and seek assistance as necessary. They look for their team members to complement each other where the "whole is more than the sum of its parts."

▶ Praise others in public. Criticize others only in private.

▶ Stay close to the action. In case management, it is the administrator who goes to the "front lines" occasionally to get back to "reality." This also means that the leader is visible and accessible.

▶ Say, "I don't know" when confronted with a case management problem; then assist with a solution.

▶ Get the whole story before making a decision.

▶ Focus on what is right, not on who is right.

▶ Develop a plan and execute effectively.

▶ Think and act in a goal-oriented manner.

▶ The Case Management Director

Case management directors are sometimes called administrators, executives, leaders, or even managers, depending on the size and scope of the position. In this section, we refer to such individuals as "directors." New regulations and evolving models of care bring increased emphasis and focus to transitions of care, given that the role of the case management director continues to evolve, growing in importance and complexity. To operate most effectively, case management directors must understand the full range of their responsibilities and their impact. They must find opportunities for themselves and their departments to stay current because the regulatory environment continues to change. The process of listing the functions and responsibilities of directors is, by its very nature, also evolving (Bankston-White & Birmingham, 2015a, b).

Bankston-White and Birmingham (2015a, b) discuss the seven tracks of case management directors' responsibility. The operational and budgetary issues are critical for a successful care management department.

TRACK 1: STAFFING/HUMAN RESOURCES

The first task for a successful case management department or program is to hire the best staff. This is not always easy or transparent; we have all seen people who have interviewed well but have not met the expectations of the organization.

Staffing ratios are critical: too many and the department will not meet budgetary initiatives; too lean, and the work may remain undone, resulting in poor outcomes. Staffing ratios are tougher to predict. There are many variables to be considered in your particular system, including the volume and complexity of the patients served.

The director should know the metrics behind the workload; he or she should not only look at the caseload ratio, but also consider the whole picture of work to be done (Bankston-White & Birmingham (2015a). Some organizations hire Case Management Assistants (CMAs) for duties that pertain to more clerical or transactional work, such as giving Medicare Important Messages or medicare outpatient observation notice (MOON) to patients; assisting with sending clinical information to alternate levels of care; or faxing/sending clinical documentation to insurance companies. CMAs have added efficiencies to case management departments and are considered an important part of a care management team.

TRACK 2: COMPLIANCE AND ACCREDITATION

One of the most critical elements of the directors' scope is attending to compliance and accreditation requirements. The Centers for Medicare & Medicaid Services (CMS) develops conditions of participation (CoPs) and conditions for coverage (CfCs) that hospitals and healthcare organizations must meet in order to participate in the Medicare and Medicaid programs. The CoPs apply to the entire hospital and are not broken down into departments, but rather listed by "basic functions" that indicate that if a hospital (or another type of organization) intends to provide services to federal beneficiaries (Medicare and Medicaid), the organization must follow the CoPs (Bankston-White & Birmingham, 2015a). The director must review, and keep updated, all of the basic functions for the organization so that there can be a strong collaboration and accountability for meeting these minimum standards. Strong policies and procedures help the department to meet these regulatory

issues and other regulations (HIPAA, patient rights, and patient choice).

TRACK 3: DISCHARGE PLANNING (TRANSITIONAL PLANNING)

Although the case manager at the front lines is usually responsible for carrying out work, the director is accountable for orchestrating the right care management model for an efficient, effective team. Case management models have changed over the years and the medical literature is now full of good methods to try out and implement. Ultimately, the responsibility for selecting the best model for your population lies with your director and team; deciding on your model will take data, communication, and collaboration with other departments/units and a strong care management team.

TRACK 4: UTILIZATION MANAGEMENT

UM is detailed in Chapter 5; however, the director is accountable for the success and outcomes of the staff who are entrusted with this task. UM is a key element of the fiscal health of the organization. When payors deny medical care in whole or in part, the organization must bear the cost of care if the UM tasks are not done using evidence-based criteria. Further, denials and appeals take on a larger scope with the CMS discharge appeal rights (See Chapter 5).

TRACK 5: INTERNAL DEPARTMENTS

Directors of case management departments interact with almost every other unit of the hospital or agency. They serve on committees such as Ethics, Compliance, or Quality Assurance; they inform and develop relationships with physicians and physician advisors; they are important the work of the Health Information Technology (HIT) Teams; and they are often in close proximity to the legal department, as patient issues arise. Another important role relates to the system's managed care contracts, which must be understood by the director and the staff so that correct information is provided to the patients physicians and other health professionals. These are just a few of the many internal interactions a director has, and they are necessary and ubiquitous to the entire system.

TRACK 6: EXTERNAL ORGANIZATIONS

External organizational connections are necessary for a well-run care management department. The external relationship and the necessary work to be done are determined by the scope of the director's role functions, director. Healthcare systems may have "internal" home health agencies, skilled nursing facilities, acute rehabilitation centers, etc., which would require a different approach than when these postacute facilities are truly external. There also will always be external home health agencies, skilled nursing facilities, acute rehabilitation centers, veteran hospitals, psychiatric systems, child/adult protective agencies, etc.

External organizational relationships are critical. There are numerous examples of why "it takes a village" for a smooth transition of care. One example of metrics may be the length of stay (LOS) for patients who are referred to an skilled nursing facility (SNF). It does not depend solely on the efficiency of the hospital case manager. It can also depend on the response times of multiple organizations, including the SNF, the payor (if preauthorization is needed), and the ambulance company (if transport is required)—to name a few of the players (Bankston-White & Birmingham, 2015b).

With so many providers to be related to, the director may, for the sake of expediency, delegate many of these relationships to staff. However, the director is often the "face" of the department and plays a critical role in the matter of transitions of care.

TRACK 7: QUALITY AND PROGRAM OUTCOMES

Directors who are accountable for performance measures must be involved with the hospital-wide Quality Assurance and Risk Management programs, because case management is one of the central departments that affect the outcome of other departments and the hospital as a whole. Often, the director is a member of several quality teams within the agency or hospital. One of the clearest measures of success for a director of case management is how he or she impacts the bottom line (Bankston-White & Birmingham, 2015b).

Metrics are essential for the director to demonstrate that the department is worthy of the cost involved in running a care management program or service. The impact that the case management department can have on the hospital's revenue cycle is enormous, in terms of patient safety and satisfaction, in the quality of care, and in the reduction of avoidable days and readmissions. The cost of case management and its impact on the revenue cycle must be a balanced equation.

Therefore, demonstrating program outcomes—outcomes management—is a complex and integrated role of the director. Outcomes are results. Case management outcomes are the results of case management interventions. Outcomes management is a scientific system of assessing, evaluating, and managing the results; the results demonstrate the effectiveness of the actions. Case managers are intimately involved in many of these mandated requirements and are increasingly requested to participate in these projects.

The director may also oversee the clinical documentation improvement specialists; these are staff who facilitate an accurate representation of healthcare services through complete and accurate reporting of diagnoses and procedures. All this is tied to value-based purchasing and, certainly, the revenue cycle. Value-based purchasing is a method of reimbursement that links financial incentives to providers' performance on a set of defined measures; how the medical records are thoroughly and accurately documented is vital.

The need to be a strong leader for staff, systems, and processes has never been more important. The work of the director and his or her staff will influence performance and outcomes for both internal and external partners by developing strong working relationships, allowing for an open exchange of ideas, and creating an opportunity for improvement on all sides.

❱ PERFORMANCE MANAGEMENT/ METRICS

Directors of care management departments may delegate the task of performance review or appraisals of the staff to others in the department (e.g., managers, team leads). It is an important yet time-consuming task that is usually completed on an annual basis. In a best-practice department, a broad overview of necessary competencies in the department should first be spelled out in the job description. Once hired, a detailed list of the competencies should be used for training/orientation purposes; a solid training/orientation should be given to all new employees, and this could take months. And lastly, these skills, roles, and functions will appear in the performance review. This comprehensive approach yields employees set up for success, and the dreaded "employee performance review" is a thing of the past.

The other common type of employee review is called a "360 degree assessment or appraisal." Challenges to this approach include the amount of training needed by reviewers to fully understand an employee's role, manipulation of ratings, and overall validity and reliability of the feedback. Employees often have a difficult time seeing this exercise as a partnership between the employee and the manager; they also cite the fact that the focus is more on the negatives and weakness than strengths (Treiger & Fink-Samnick, 2017).

Some strengths have, however, been noted in the 360 degree appraisals, and the following list should be considered by directors of case management departments (Treiger & Fink-Samnick, 2017):

❱ Improved feedback from additional sources,
❱ Team development,
❱ Personal and organizational performance development,
❱ Responsibility for career development,
❱ Reduced discrimination risk,
❱ Improved customer service, and
❱ Training needs assessment.

Workplace performance today is driven by skills, attitude, customer feedback, and team collaboration. High-quality performance management systems are driven by the development of strong skills as opposed to solely ranking an individual at a fixed moment in time (the old bell curve method of the twentieth century).

DISCUSSION QUESTIONS

1. Cite an example in which case management was done poorly. Explore reasons and illustrate ways in which improvements could be made in future.

2. Do the characteristics necessary for a case manager differ from those needed for a direct care nurse? If so, how?

3. How do the job responsibilities of case management differ from traditional direct care nursing?

4. Cite an example in which you demonstrated the role of patient advocate. What happened? Had you not advocated for the patient, what *could have* occurred?

5. Evaluate your own strengths and weaknesses in terms of essential characteristics of a case manager. How would you turn weaknesses into strengths?

6. What personality traits contribute to success as a case manager? Why? How does each trait add value to the case manager's role effectiveness?

7. What leadership skills are necessary for successful case management? How does each skill contribute to the case manager's role effectiveness?

8. List one activity that should *not be done* in a case conference.

▶ REFERENCES

Bankston-White, C., & Birmingham, J. (2015a). Case management directors how to manage in a transition-focused world: Part 1. *Professional Case Management Journal, 20*(2), 63–78.

Bankston-White, C., & Birmingham, J. (2015b). Case management directors how to manage in a transition-focused world: Part 2. *Professional Case Management Journal, 20*(3), 115–127.

Benner, P. (1984). *From novice to expert. Excellence and power in clinical nursing practice.* Menlo Park, CA: Addison-Wesley.

Chenevert, M. (1988). STAT—*Special techniques in assertiveness training for women in the health professions* (3rd ed.). St. Louis, MO: CV Mosby.

Leddy, S., & Pepper, M. (1989). Conceptual bases of professional nursing. Philadelphia, PA: Lippincott Williams & Wilkins.

Luther, B., Marc-Aurel, M., & Barra, J. (2017). A statewide survey report of roles and responsibilities in current Utah care management processes. *Professional Case Management Journal, 22*(3), 116–125.

Powell, S., & Tahan, H. (2010). *Case management: A practical guide for education and practice.* Philadelphia, PA: Wolters Kluwer Health.

Tahan, H., Watson, A., & Sminkey, P. (2015). What case managers should know about their roles and functions: A national study from the Commission for Case Managers Certification: Part 1. *Professional Case Management Journal, 20*(6), 271–296.

Tahan, H., Watson, A., & Sminkey, P. (2016). Informing the content and composition of the CCM Care Managers Certification Examination: A national study from the Commission for Case Managers Certification: Part 2. *Professional Case Management Journal, 21*(1), 3–21.

Treiger, T., & Fink-Samnick, E. (2017). Collaborate, Part IV. Ramping up competency-based performance management. *Professional Case Management, 22*(3), 101–115.

CHAPTER 3

Management of Resources and Reimbursement Systems

LEARNING OBJECTIVES

Upon completion of this chapter, the reader will be able to:

1. Describe the various methods of reimbursement for healthcare services.
2. Define prospective payment system.
3. Define managed care organizations.
4. Differentiate between governmental and private (commercial) health insurance plans.
5. Differentiate between Medicare and Medicaid benefit programs.
6. Determine the role of case managers in managed care contracting.
7. List five reimbursement-related responsibilities of case managers.

ESSENTIAL TERMS

Aid to Families with Dependent Children (AFDC) • CAP • Capitation • Carve-Out • Catastrophic Claims • Catastrophic Coverage • Catastrophic Reinsurance • Categorically Eligible • Centers for Medicare & Medicaid Services (CMS) • Coinsurance • Competitive Medical Plans • Consolidated Omnibus Reconciliation Act (COBRA) • Coordination of Benefits (COB) • Copayment • Coverage Gap • *Current Procedural Terminology,* 4th edition (CPT-4) • Days per Thousand • Deductible • Deferred Liability • Diagnosis-Related Groups (DRGs) • Direct Contract Model • Eligibility Worker • Employer Mandate • Fee-for-Service • Gatekeeper • Grievance • Group Model • Health Maintenance Organization (HMO) • Indemnity Plans • Independent Practice Association (IPA) • *International Classification of Diseases,* 10th revision—Clinical Modification (*ICD-10*-CM) • Lifetime Reserve Days • Long-Term Care (LTC) • Managed Care Contract (MCC) • Managed Care Organization (MCO) • Managed Indemnity Plans (MIP) • Management Information System • Medicaid • Medical Assistance Only (MAO) • Medically Needy/Medically Indigent (MN/MI) • Medicare • Medicare Benefits Periods • Medicare Advantage Plan (MAP or MA) • Medicare Part A—Hospital Insurance • Medicare Part B—Medical Insurance • Medicare Part C—Medicare Advantage Plans • Medicare Part D—Medicare Prescription Drug Coverage • Medicare Risk Contracts • Medicare SELECT • Medigap Plans • Network Model • Open Enrollment Period • Office of Prepaid Health Care Operations and Oversight • Other Weird Arrangement (OWA) • Outliers • Pay-for-Performance (P4P) • Physician Hospital Organization (PHO) • Point-of-Service (POS) • Preferred Provider Arrangements (PPA) • Preferred Provider Organization (PPO) • Premiums • Primary Care Physician (PCP) • Prospective Payment System (PPS) • Quality Improvement Organization (QIO) • Reinsurance • Sixth Omnibus Budget Reconciliation Act (SOBRA) • Specialist Care Provider (SCP) • Social Security Disability (SSD) • Social Security Income (SSI) • Spend Down • Staff Model • Stop Loss • Third Party • Third-Party Liability (TPL) • Tricare • Value-based Purchasing • Viatical Settlements • Workers' Compensation

Health insurance provides the financial motor that runs the medical/healthcare system. Although it may be the most confusing part of case management practice, it is perhaps one of the most important aspects of the role a case manager needs to understand. Each insurance company has its own rules, standards, procedures, and by-laws. Some companies carve these rules in stone, whereas others modify them slightly on a patient-by-patient basis, especially if they foresee a favorable chance of lessening the prospect of a future expensive acute or hospital admission. If at times the case manager feels like the master of ceremonies in the insurance game, he or she will be in good company. However, without a solid knowledge of health insurance benefits and covered services, the case manager's best intentions, plans, time, skills, and energy will be wasted if he or she hears the words "insurance refused to pay" for this plan (patient's plan of care), treatment, intervention, or service. It is better to know up front what is in and what the limitations are and to try to negotiate from there than to have to throw away a patient's entire plan of care.

Working closely with a knowledgeable social worker provides valuable information and may also prevent a true disaster for some patients. For example, consider the case of HIV-positive patients who enrolled in Medicare's Social Security Disability (SSD). More than one HIV-positive patient has been lured into accepting SSD category instead of the Social Security Income (SSI) category; the latter pays out less money. In these instances, when the financial statement was checked by Medicaid, it was found that those who were paid the SSD rate no longer qualified for medical insurance under Medicaid. Their monthly income was slightly higher than what qualifies a person for Medicaid coverage. Therefore, these ill members had no money to buy expensive medications, and if they needed hospitalization, it would have to be through hospital charity until they could spend down (see "Spend down" later in this chapter) into a Medicaid plan.

This type of scenario can be more than just confusing and financially troublesome. For some, it means life or death. Consider the case of a single mother in her late twenties from Arizona. The woman worked full-time as a clerk and went to school part-time to improve her future prospects for a better-paying job. When she was diagnosed with leukemia in 1992, she eventually qualified for the Arizona Health Care Cost Containment System (AHCCCS), Arizona's form of Medicaid. She was receiving Aid to Families with Dependent Children (AFDC), which allowed her the right to the state's Medicaid coverage and a chance at a bone marrow transplantation. However, when she became too ill to work and was persuaded to apply for SSD at $456.80 per month, the SSD payments put her and her son $86 over the limit for AFDC. She was taken off the AFDC rolls, and with it the AHCCCS rolls. Her chance for a bone marrow transplantation was gone, and she died of leukemia a short time later. Because of this type of outcome, there has been some reform in the rules; however, as a patient advocate the case manager must balance the requirements of the patient with the "rules of the game." Similar situations are still occurring today and the case manager must be astute about these issues to better counsel patients about what is best for them.

The information in this chapter does not cover all that a case manager must know about health insurance and reimbursement methods, because each health insurance plan has its own standards for coverage or interpretation of coverage and procedures. In addition, the rules change yearly or sometimes more frequently. When describing different types of plans such as a health maintenance organization (HMO) or a preferred provider organization (PPO), it must be understood that even their basic structures are constantly changing. As the health insurance company's vision of healthcare becomes clearer, the definitions of these plans become more blurred; this is in an effort to become more efficient.

From mathematics to physics, every classification of knowledge has its own terminology. Case managers learned to be fluent in "medical-ese" in nursing school. Now we must also be fluent in "insurance-ese"; therefore, some parts of this chapter are in glossary form. In their role as patient advocates, case managers must understand the convoluted system that insurance is. They also should be wary so that plans of care and services do not saddle patients and their families with unexpected bills or, worse, place them in Catch-22 scenarios like the bone marrow transplantation case and others mentioned earlier.

As seen in Chapter 1's section on "International Perspective on Case Management," each country has its own types of health laws and regulations, standards, insurance benefits, policies, and reimbursement methods. The United States has tried many reimbursement strategies, and each leads to a different incentive for plans of care. Other countries certainly have used strategies that the United States has borrowed and learned from; other countries have also learned from the United States (in terms both of what works and what may best be left alone).

▶ TYPES OF HEALTHCARE INSURANCE

The healthcare system in the United States includes two main broad types of insurance companies: commercial and governmental. Commercial insurance is also known as private insurance and includes programs such as the following:

1. *Liability insurance*: Benefits are paid for bodily injury, property damage, or both.
2. *No-fault auto insurance*: Benefits are paid for bodily injury, property damage, or both, incurred while driving a car. The policies and regulations of this type of insurance vary state by state.
3. *No-fault workers' compensation*: Benefits are paid for bodily injury or for a work environment–related illness. Benefits also include replacement of lost wages because of an injury or illness that occurred while in the workplace. This type of insurance is regulated by the state; in some states, it is regulated by the federal government.
4. *Accident and health insurance*: Benefits include payments for healthcare costs and may include short- or long-term disability. This type of insurance may have an annual or lifetime maximum benefit.
5. *Indemnity insurance*: Benefits are in the form of payments rather than healthcare services, provide security against possible loss or damages, and are paid on the basis of predetermined amounts in the event of covered loss.

6. *Stop-loss insurance*: Benefits are used to cover cases that are costly; that is, that may require a large dollar outlay (see "Protective Strategies for Insurance Companies" later in this chapter).

7. *Managed care insurance plans*: Provide a generalized structure for the management of use, access, cost, quality, and effectiveness of healthcare services, and link individual users of this benefit to providers of healthcare services. Reimbursement is based on the arrangement agreed upon between the insurance plan, the patient, and the provider of care, and is defined in the health insurance plan.

8. *Union health*: Offers coverage for healthcare services for the employee of one or a group of organizations where the employees belong to a collective bargaining unit.

9. *Consumer-driven insurance plans*: Offered primarily in an employer setting. These may include arrangements such as health savings accounts (HASs), health reimbursement accounts, high-deductible health plans (HDHPs), or similar medical payment options where members use these accounts to pay for routine healthcare expenses. The HDHP protects the consumer from catastrophic medical expenses. These plans are self-funded by the consumer and can be either pretax or tax benefit.

Government insurance plans are public programs and include Medicare, Medicaid, and Military.

1. *Medicare benefit program*: Financed by Social Security; benefits those age 65 or older, those under age 65 with certain disabilities, and those of any age with end-stage renal disease who are entitled to Social Security benefits. The Centers for Medicare & Medicaid Services (CMS) provides administrative oversight for this program and identifies mandated hospital services through its conditions of participation manual for hospitals.

   Medicare benefits consist of a number of options; Part A covers hospitalization, skilled nursing care, home care (other than custodial), and hospice care. Part B covers physician services, outpatient services, ambulance transport, clinical research, and mental health. Part D covers prescription drugs. Part C is the Medicare Advantage option, for example, Medicare Choice and Managed Medicare, which offers same services as those of Medicare at a minimum but in a context similar to that of managed care (commercial insurance).

2. *Medicaid benefit program*: Financed by state and federal governments through tax structures; benefits those who are considered indigent, with income at or below poverty levels, the uninsured, or those with inadequate medical insurance. Eligibility for Medicaid benefit depends on a person's income,

assets, and dependents. Some states may impose a copayment or a nominal deductible for certain services on the beneficiary.

Medicaid benefits are also available in the form of Managed Medicaid and are offered in a context similar to that of managed care health insurance plans (commercial insurance). The drivers for such offering are improved access to services by beneficiaries, quality and safe care, and cost containment. Services provided in such plans must include at a minimum those offered by traditional Medicare benefit plan. Some states require Medicare beneficiaries to enroll in a Managed Medicaid plan.

3. *Military benefits*: Benefits active duty and retired members of the military, their families, and survivors. It is in the form of either TRICARE, CHAMPVA, or Veterans Administration. TRICARE is offered in a managed care context to both active duty and retired military, and their families including survivors. CHAMPVA is available for eligible veterans and their families (dependents and survivors) and covers medical care.

4. *Federal employee*: Benefits current and retired federal employees and covered family members.

5. *Indian's health*: Benefits Indians; usually offered in the form of Indian Health Services, Tribal Health Program, or Urban Indian Health Program.

▶ REIMBURSEMENT AND PROTECTIVE STRATEGIES

▶ Cost-Sharing Strategies for Insurance Companies

The following four terms relate to cost-sharing strategies used by most health insurance companies. The beneficiary is usually responsible for copayments, coinsurance, and deductibles.

PREMIUMS

Premiums are the monthly fees that most health insurance companies charge the member (an enrollee) for insurance coverage. This fee is paid regardless of whether a beneficiary or plan member accesses healthcare services.

COPAYMENT

Copayment is a set amount of money specified by each health insurance plan that the member must pay at the time healthcare services are rendered (Kongstvedt, 2003). This out-of-pocket payment may range from $1 (for Medicaid recipients) to $25 or more. Pharmacy copayments also are common. They tend to be paid per prescription (e.g., $5 per prescription filled). Some patients are unable to pay even small copayments, so many physicians and emergency departments waive them.

COINSURANCE

Coinsurance is another type of out-of-pocket expense for the health insurance plan member. This type of cost-sharing limits the amount of coverage by a health plan to a certain percentage, commonly 80% (Kongstvedt, 2003). The member is responsible for the remaining 20%, but normally there is a ceiling dollar amount (usually $5,000). Private/indemnity plans often use coinsurance strategies.

DEDUCTIBLE

A third type of out-of-pocket expense for a health plan member is the medical deductible; typically, this must be paid every year before the health insurance becomes active for that year. In the 1990s, deductible amounts were frequently $100 to $300. With the rising cost of healthcare, high deductibles of $1,000 to $1,500 are now offered to keep monthly premiums lower. Deductibles are common in private health insurance plans (i.e., commercial) and PPOs; HMOs rarely use deductibles.

▶ Protective Strategies for Insurance Companies

CAP

Not to be confused with capitation, a CAP is the maximum dollar amount allowed in an insurance policy the health insurance plan assumes toward healthcare expenses incurred by the individual member. Some policies are capped at $25,000, whereas others are capped at $1 million or more for a lifetime. Yearly caps are occasionally (although rarely) specified. Some insurance sources have no maximum cap, such as most Medicaid plans.

REINSURANCE (AKA "STOP LOSS")

Reinsurance, or stop loss, is purchased by an insurance company to protect itself against extremely expensive cases. Just as an individual may purchase a health insurance plan with a $500 deductible for protection from high medical bills, health plans also purchase reinsurance with deductibles. A stop loss is a form of reinsurance that protects a health plan when a medical case exceeds (for example) $100,000 (Kongstvedt, 2003); any charges over $100,000 are paid at 80% from the reinsurance company. The remaining expenses (the 20%) are the responsibility of the health plan. Stop-loss amounts differ, just as an individual may purchase higher or lower deductibles on their insurance plan. These high-dollar claims are known as catastrophic claims. Because certain diagnoses or injuries carry proven statistics of being expensive cases, *catastrophe reinsurance* may be tied to diagnoses such as AIDS and human organ transplants.

DEFERRED LIABILITY

Deferred liability offers Medicaid plan protection in specific circumstances. Suppose a patient is admitted through the emergency department without medical insurance and spends down to a level at which he or she is eligible for membership in a Medicaid plan. Under deferred liability, a portion of the medical expenses is deferred by payments from federally funded offers. This helps the plan to maintain some financial control, especially if the new member is very ill. In many states, sick newborns (e.g., premature babies) are an automatic deferred liability category.

THIRD-PARTY LIABILITY

Third-party liability (TPL) can best be understood by an example. Suppose an automobile accident victim is admitted to the hospital. Mr Victim was sitting at a red light when Mr Careless hit him from behind while driving his car. Mr Victim had lacerations and facial swelling caused by his head hitting the steering wheel. He had to be monitored for a possible cardiac contusion. Mr Victim and Mr Careless both had medical and automobile insurance plans. Most likely, Mr Careless' auto insurance would be the liable third party for Mr Victim's hospital bill.

Insurance companies keep a close eye on certain red flags (warning signs or symptoms that warrant caution or careful attention) that may signal TPL. Some target diagnoses may include motor vehicle accidents, multiple trauma, near-drowning, and unnatural events such as explosions, burns, assaults, fractures, and lacerations. Insurance sources that may be liable include automobile, homeowners', workers' compensation, malpractice, and product liability insurance.

CARVE-OUT

A carve-out plan "carves out" or replaces a portion of the insurance coverage provided to beneficiaries (health insurance plan members). Carve-outs are usually explicitly excluded from a provider managed care contract (MCC) and tend to include expensive procedures or catastrophic conditions such as organ or bone marrow transplantation, or AIDS care coverage. Carve-out services are those covered through arrangements with other providers. Healthcare providers are not responsible for services carved out of their MCCs. The companies that provide the services usually have case managers managing expenses and members' benefits. However, it is wise to continue to oversee such cases. Many little rules for coverage in carve-out portions of a plan need attention. For example, in one plan autologous bone marrow transplants are covered. The policy starts 30 days before the actual transplant. This means that the bone marrow must be both harvested and transplanted within a 30-day time frame. On the other end, some policies will pay for all services, including medications for 12 months after the procedure. If an organ transplantation requires lifelong antirejection medications, the primary case manager must coordinate care after the carve-out policy expires.

LIMITS

Limits in a health insurance plan describe the types of services covered (including a list of providers an enrollee may use for healthcare services), delineate the enrollee choice for services (e.g., within or out-of-network), and explain the associated costs and premiums.

▶ Types of Reimbursement

PROSPECTIVE PAYMENT SYSTEM

In 1983, Social Security amendments initiated the Medicare Prospective Payment System. Under this system, hospitals are no longer reimbursed on a fee-for-services basis; that is, for inpatient services, on the basis of what services were performed, how long the patient stayed in the hospital, or the costs of care. Rather, hospitals are reimbursed for certain types of insurance, most notably Medicare, according to diagnosis-related groups (DRGs) (see discussion in the following section). DRGs set predetermined rates of reimbursement; the hospital is permitted to keep excess dollars if the patient does not incur the limit of cost. Conversely, the hospital is required to absorb losses for patients who are more resource intensive than given in the DRG allotment.

The DRG system also prospectively allocates the average number of days a patient will stay in the acute care setting; this allocation is stipulated by diagnosis or procedure. The predetermination of days also includes the minimum number of days of inpatient hospital stay to meet eligibility for reimbursement and an upper limit for the number of days a patient may stay in the acute care setting; again these are designated by diagnosis or procedure. Another aspect of the DRG system is a predetermined expected acuity (called relative weight) that is also by diagnosis or procedure, which together with the length of stay, impacts the amount of reimbursement a hospital receives for care and services rendered. It is important for the acute care/hospital case manager to manage a patient's length of hospital stay to ensure only those who meet acute care medical necessity criteria are hospitalized and their stay continues to meet such criteria, otherwise the hospital will face financial risk attributed to lack or reduced reimbursement.

The prospective payment system (PPS) has moved into almost all care settings, including the subacute care arena, long-term care (LTC), skilled care facilities, home care, rehabilitation, and others. This change has brought about the most far-reaching transformation in healthcare since the initiation of the PPS in 1983.

In the ambulatory care setting, the PPS is called "ambulatory payment classification (APC)." It originated in 2000 and includes a fee schedule for bundled outpatient services. It is encounter based and similar in philosophy to that of the hospital-based DRG system or inpatient PPS. However, unlike the DRG system, a single outpatient encounter may result in the payment of one or more APCs depending on the services provided. Each APC is composed of services that are similar in clinical intensity, resource utilization, and costs. When submitting claims for outpatient services rendered, the provider indicates the specific code(s) that correspond to the service(s). These codes are based on the Healthcare Common Procedure Coding System (HCPCS) derived from the American Medical Association's Current Procedural Terminology (CPT) coding system. An APC may consist of a number of HCPCS and has a designated relative weight or severity that informs the reimbursement amount. Because this payment is a prospective and "fixed" payment to the provider (e.g., hospital), the provider remains at risk for potential "profit or loss" with each APC payment it receives.

The APC system applies to outpatient surgery, outpatient clinics, emergency department services, observation services, and outpatient testing (e.g., radiology and nuclear medicine imaging) and therapies (e.g., intravenous infusion therapies and administration of blood and blood products). APCs for observation services cover extended assessments, procedures, and patient management activities.

In the rehabilitation care setting, the PPS is called "case mix groups (CMGs)." It requires a patient assessment instrument (PAI) that is completed for every rehabilitation patient. For rehabilitation patients in the inpatient setting (i.e., the inpatient rehabilitation facility [IRF] setting), the PAI is referred to as IRF-PAI. On the basis of that score, the patient is placed in a CMG. The CMG then establishes the reimbursement rate for care and services rendered. Like in the DRG system, CMG rates are predetermined and an organization is reimbursed that amount regardless of the cost incurred while caring for the patient. The CMG classification is determined on the basis of clinical and medical characteristics as well as expected resource consumption; those patients who have similar problems and require similar resources are grouped together into a CMG.

In the skilled nursing facility (SNF), the PPS is called "resource utilization groups (RUGs)." Minimum datasets for large numbers of SNF patients were reviewed to determine the RUG system. The final product was a system of 7 major categories and 44 RUG hierarchies. This system has been updated since; there are 5 major categories and 66 RUG hierarchies available today. Data reviewed to establish the RUG system included medical and clinical conditions, resources, and services required for care. The hierarchy and RUG are allocated a specific reimbursement rate that the SNF receives as reimbursement for the care rendered.

In the home care setting, the PPS is called "home health prospective payment system (HH PPS)" that is reimbursed on the basis of a classification referred to as home health resource groups (HHRGs). Currently there are 153 HHRGs available with varying acuity level or intensity of service and therefore different reimbursement rates. Reimbursement for home care services, unlike all other PPS systems, is determined on the basis of a nursing assessment that is completed at the time a patient is admitted (during first visit) into home care. Reimbursement is determined on the basis of a score the patient receives after the nurse completes the Outcomes and Assessment Information Set (OASIS). This instrument consists of clinical, financial, administrative, and service utilization data, as well as specific outcome indicators. The resulting score places a patient in one of the 80 HHRGs.

Each HHRG has a predetermined dollar amount associated with it and the home care agency is reimbursed that amount regardless of the actual number of visits rendered to a patient. Reimbursement occurs on the basis of a unit of payment that is defined by a 60-day episode of care. Usually upon a patient's admission into home care and completion of the OASIS assessment, the home care provider submits a Request for Anticipated Payment to the CMS. The provider also submits a claim to the CMS at the conclusion of the services. At this time the CMS reconciles these payments and finally reimburses the home care provider the permissible payments for the episode of care. For patients who require continued home care services beyond the initial 60-day episode, the home care provider submits a request for recertification as many times as the patient continues to require home health services and meet the eligibility criteria for such services.

DIAGNOSIS-RELATED GROUPS

A group of Yale researchers developed the DRG system in the 1970s on the basis of hospital-based historical data on thousands of patients. They were originally designed as a patient classification system and not as a reimbursement method (InterQual Inc., 1993). A total of 494 diagnoses are listed and divided into 25 major diagnostic categories. Several variables account for the choice of DRG for a patient, including the primary diagnosis, comorbidities (preexisting conditions), treatment procedures (including diagnostic or surgical), age, sex, complications, secondary diagnosis, secondary procedure, length of stay (LOS), and discharge status. Each DRG is scored according to its potential consumption and intensity of resources. Each DRG category has a specific expected acuity rating (or relative weight/rate) and an expected LOS that is presented as a range with a minimum LOS and an upper limit that is greater than 2 standard deviations from the mean.

A dollar amount is placed on each DRG, and hospitals are most often reimbursed a flat rate for all patients who fall within each DRG category. If a particular case has been extremely cost intensive or had a very long LOS (one that exceeds the upper range) when compared with other cases in the chosen DRG, extra reimbursement is possible for these outlier cases. Extra reimbursement is determined on the basis of the number of extra days a patient spends in the hospital, as long as these days are justified by the patient's health condition and the care/services required. For example, a simple appendectomy would not be considered an outlier case until the patient stayed for 15 days. Then the case may cost the hospital more than two times the DRG rate of payment, or $44,000, whichever is greater (Williams & Torrens, 1993). As a comparison, a case has a goal LOS for a simple appendectomy of 1 day; however, with abscess or peritonitis, the goal LOS is 4 days. The number of allocated days usually changes annually on the basis of historical data; sometimes it increases, other times it decreases.

Perhaps more than any other factor, DRGs provided the impetus for hospitals to utilize case managers. With the exception of the abovementioned outlier cases, the hospital will receive the same basic DRG reimbursement whether the case is managed well or poorly and regardless of the costs incurred.

Compare the two following cases:

1. Patient A with Medicare coverage came into the emergency department with abdominal pain. An ultrasound performed in the emergency department showed gallstones. An open cholecystectomy was performed on the evening of the patient's first hospital day. She was tolerating clear liquids on the evening of postoperative day 1 (POD 1). On POD 2, she tolerated full liquids and was ambulating short distances. Her diet was advanced as tolerated. On POD 3, she tolerated a soft diet, her bowels were functioning, and she was taking oral pain medications. She was discharged in the evening of POD 3, her fourth day in the hospital.
2. Patient B with Medicare coverage came into a different emergency department with abdominal pain. Again, an ultrasound performed in the emergency department showed gallstones. The next afternoon, an open cholecystectomy was performed. This patient received nothing by mouth for 2 days postoperatively. On POD 3, the doctor wrote orders for a clear liquid diet. On POD 4, the patient was allowed to advance his diet as tolerated. He tolerated a full liquid diet at lunch and a soft diet for dinner. His bowels were functioning, he was ambulating in the hallway, and he was taking oral pain medications. The following day, POD 5, the physician discharged the patient—on hospital day 7.

These two disparities are not uncommon. Both hospitals received the same DRG reimbursement. Studies have shown that case management has made a difference in cases such as these. Hospitals can no longer afford not to manage their resources wisely, and case managers are proving to be one of the best resources for this. They follow up on care progression and manage the LOS on the basis of the patient's condition and required services.

In October 2007, the CMS overhauled the DRG system with the development of "severity-adjusted DRGs." Specifically, the CMS replaced DRGs with "Medicare-severity

DRGs," referred to as MS-DRGs. The CMS phased-in this revised system over a 3-year period during which the payment was blended under the old DRG and the new MS-DRG systems. Today the MS-DRG system is in effect. While there are similarities between these two systems such as the existence or absence of complications or comorbidities, the MS-DRG system adds a third category: major complications and/or comorbidities. Under the revised system, patient cases are classified into MS-DRGs for payment on the basis of the principal diagnosis, up to eight additional diagnoses, and up to six procedures performed during the patient's hospital stay. In a number of MS-DRGs, classification is also based on the age, sex, and discharge status of the patient. The diagnosis and discharge information is reported by the hospital using codes from the *International Classification of Diseases*, 9th Revision, Clinical Modification (*ICD-9*-CM) which today has been replaced with the *ICD-10*-CM version, the 10th Revision.

LENGTH OF STAY

Some insurance companies allow the hospital a standard number of days for a patient's condition. A laparoscopic cholecystectomy may be given a 1-day LOS. An uncomplicated appendectomy may be given a 2-day LOS. Books of LOS are broken down by regions in the country and by diagnosis. They are further delineated by age and other factors such as surgical procedures. The estimated LOS for each category is given in percentiles—10%, 25%, 50%, 75%, 90%, 95%, and 99%. For example, a patient 65 years of age or older with paroxysmal supraventricular tachycardia may be given an LOS of 1 day (10th percentile) to 7 days (99th percentile). Most insurance companies use the 10% to 50% range for assignment of LOS.

A landmark legal case developed around an assignment of an LOS in *Wickline v. State of California* in the late 1980s (Saue, 1988). This case involved a Medi-Cal (California's Medicaid plan) patient, Mrs Wickline, with peripheral vascular disease and occlusion of the abdominal aorta. Mrs Wickline was admitted to a California hospital, where an artery was removed and replaced with a synthetic graft. The postoperative course was described as "stormy" with several complications, so the attending physician asked the state agency for 8 additional days after the LOS was established. The LOS was extended for only 4 more days, at which time the patient was discharged in stable condition. Home health nursing was provided, but within days after discharge, the patient's leg became more painful and started to change color. At about 9 days after discharge, the leg pain became unbearable. It was determined that at some point Mrs Wickline developed a clot in her leg and a graft infection. Antibiotics, anticoagulants, and bed rest failed to save the leg, and a below-knee amputation was deemed necessary and performed. Nine days later, the patient needed an additional above-knee amputation.

Subsequently, Mrs Wickline filed a multimillion dollar lawsuit against the state of California, stating that Medi-Cal forced her out of the hospital prematurely and that the physician was intimidated by the Medi-Cal program and complied with their LOS. This case went to the California Supreme Court, which ruled in favor of the state. In its judgment, the Court stated that the attending physician—not Medi-Cal—was ultimately responsible for treatment decisions concerning the care of patients and that the physician cannot abdicate that responsibility for any reason. It is important then for case managers to know that physicians are legally responsible for the treatment plan. As the court warned in the Wickline Case, "A physician could not shift legal responsibility for his patient's welfare to a third party by complying with a cost containment program" (Saue, 1988, p. 83).

At the time of this case, Medi-Cal did not have an appeals process; it is now law that beneficiaries must be provided with an appeals process. Physicians, case managers, and the treatment team must put patient welfare above payment. Appeals are frequently won on the side of the hospital and in the patient's best interests.

Insurance companies frequently give short LOS—24 to 48 hours—for admission diagnoses that are more symptomatic than diagnostics such as chest pain or abdominal pain. As the case develops, additional LOS days can usually be negotiated. If a patient is stable after several days and care can be given at a less cost-intensive setting (a lesser level of care), the company may not extend the LOS further but may agree to pay for an alternate plan. (More on LOS can be found in "Utilization Management Modalities" in Chapter 5.)

PER DIEM REIMBURSEMENT

Per diem reimbursement is based on a fixed dollar amount per day for services provided to a patient regardless of actual costs, rather than on charges or patient acuity. Cost-based reimbursement is based on the actual costs of a patient's care. Many insurance companies favor the per diem method of payment. They often pay for the day of admission, but not for the day of discharge. Occasionally, certain expensive items can be billed separately. Per diem reimbursement may be a different dollar amount for different service lines. Intensive care services have a higher per diem rate than surgical service lines; a medical patient may be reimbursed more than a behavioral health patient in a per diem system.

CAPITATION

Capitation is a type of reimbursement or payment method that is primarily used in a managed care context where a fixed monthly payment to a provider is paid in advance of services and regardless of whether services were needed and provided. In reality, however, a full range of medical services may be expected for each member of a capitated health insurance plan (Kongstvedt, 2003). The amount paid to a provider is based on a per member per month negotiated rate. Capitation started out as a popular method for reimbursing primary care physicians (PCPs)/gatekeepers and became more common with increased use of managed care health plans. Now capitated contracts can be seen in every area of healthcare.

Here is a simplified fictitious example of how capitation works for a PCP. Dr. Jones has 100 members from Managed Care Insurance Company A. The capitated rate is $15 per member per month, so Dr. Jones will receive $1,500 per month from Insurance Company A to manage all its members.

Capitation rates vary widely across the country and even among counties in one given state. Also variable is what the PCP, hospital, or other capitated facility/agency includes in the capitation rate. For example, a capitation for office visits would be less costly than a capitation that includes office visits and all laboratory tests. The capitation rate will be higher still if the PCP agrees to see these members in the event that they are hospitalized. From the managed care standpoint, capitation allows a health plan to budget for medical costs. For years, capitation was used essentially as a budget tool for outpatient services such as physician office visits. Now that capitation has moved into all managed care settings, case managers will need to manage the use of all resources.

Capitation provides a powerful incentive to contain costs, but balances in this system are delicate; underutilization of services can have far-reaching consequences through compromised quality of care. Some feel that the capitation system is unfair to those PCPs with sicker patients who require more office visits per month; conversely, a healthy member is a profitable member. The thought, however, is that the mix of sicker and healthier patients an individual healthcare provider is responsible for on the basis of the capitated plan agreement will balance out the expenses and revenues, perhaps resulting in a positive bottom line. One hopes that this is the usual case. The reality remains, however, that the provider faces the financial risk in such arrangements. Physician incentives to not refer to specialists or provide various procedures have visited the legal arena in the past several years; in response, many laws and accreditation organizations require that financial "incentives" be provided openly.

FEE-FOR-SERVICE

Fee-for-service is the old method of reimbursement, in which a healthcare provider sends a bill (referred to as a claim) to the health insurance company and then the insurance company pays it. The bill is determined on the basis of the services provided and is reflective of the actual costs incurred. With this form of reimbursement, healthcare costs go up as more services are provided. Some feel that fee-for-service was a major reason for the healthcare crisis, and at this time most insurance companies are agreeing to pay only "reasonable" charges. PPOs use a variation of fee-for-service: the physician gets paid each time the member requires services (in contrast to capitated physicians) but at contracted rates agreed on in advance. High-level specialists may be paid fee-for-service by some insurance plans.

There is an interesting dilemma that occurs when, for example, a hospital is paid by an HMO using the capitated method, and yet the physicians in the network are reimbursed on a fee-for-service basis. The hospital case manager may have his or her hands full with these cases; the hospital is at financial risk, but the physicians are "encouraged" to provide more services. Add to the equation that the physician incentives/actions also strengthen the patient's resolve to demand more resources. Patient benefit books prescribing what is allowed are vague at best and therefore are of little assistance in this scenario. The good news is that phrases like "appropriate utilization of services" and "medical necessity" are becoming more concrete with the evolution of resource utilization protocols, medical guidelines and pathways, and more precisely written benefit designs.

DISCOUNTED FEE-FOR-SERVICES

In the discounted fee-for-services reimbursement schedule, healthcare providers are reimbursed similar to the fee-for-service method; however, the reimbursements are discounted. The percentage discount is usually agreed upon between the insurance company and the healthcare provider in advance of the provision of services.

PAY-FOR-PERFORMANCE AND VALUE-BASED PURCHASING

Pay-for-performance (P4P) structures have been implemented recently as incentive structures by some commercial insurance companies, and over the past few years have infiltrated the governmental health benefit programs, including Medicare and Medicaid. In the commercial insurance arena, P4P is being paid in the form of incentives for healthcare providers and organizations who meet certain predetermined outcomes criteria such as reduction in the need for acute care admissions, emergency department visits, or other clinical outcomes that are disease specific in nature. Examples of clinical outcomes are patient's knowledge of medication (including compliance with use), and mortality and morbidity rates.

Governmental health benefit programs are currently moving away from the incentive approach of P4P and are implementing reimbursement approaches that are based on performance. Examples of the measures used to assess performance and determine reimbursement include mortality rates, morbidity rates, medical errors, nosocomial infections, pressure ulcers, and patient satisfaction with the care experience.

Over the past several years, the CMS has transitioned to the value-based purchasing system of reimbursement where hospitals and other providers are incentivized on the basis of the quality of care they provide to the

Medicare fee-for-service beneficiaries. How hospitals perform on quality and resource use measures is linked to the inpatient PPS. This system rewards acute care hospitals and providers with incentive payments for the quality rather than the volume of services they provide. Congress authorized this type of reimbursement in Section 3001(a) of the Patient Protection and Affordable Care Act of 2010. Quality in this case is defined on the basis of clinical care (process and outcome indicators/measures), patient- and caregiver-centered experience of care including care coordination, safety and serious events, and efficiency including cost of care. When this approach was first initiated, the patient and caregiver experience of care measure was allocated a lower percentage weight in the calculation of the incentive or financial risk; today it has reached higher than the other measures.

BUNDLING AND UNBUNDLING

Bundling case rates indicate that the facility charges and the physician charges are all bundled together and reimbursed on the basis of one bill/claim. This is also known as package pricing or global payment. For example, a plan may negotiate a rate of $30,000 for a cardiac bypass. This would include everything from the surgeon and anesthesiologist to postoperative hospital-based care (Kongstvedt, 2003). Usually use of the terms bundling and unbundling refers to the inclusion or exclusion of professional fees in the hospital-based charges and therefore the claim provided to the insurance plan for reimbursement of services rendered to a patient/member.

Unbundling is a term that explains the practice of billing separately for items that were once bundled together in a single bill (Kongstvedt, 2003). For example, a minor surgical procedure was once a single charge. When unbundled, it may include fees for the procedure, physician services, instruments, hospital room, and dressings.

▶ Enrollment Terms and Qualification for Special Insurance

ENROLLEE

An enrollee, also known as a beneficiary, member, or participant, is an individual eligible for health benefits under a health insurance plan/contract. HMO beneficiaries are usually referred to as members, whereas PPOs may refer to these individuals as enrollees. A member of a government-based health insurance program is referred to as a beneficiary.

ENROLLMENT

Enrollment in a health plan may require specific qualifications. Medicaid, for example, requires the patient to be financially impoverished; Medicare Part A requires a specified number of work hours into which Social Security is paid and may stipulate age restrictions or a disabled health condition. Private insurance plans may (although rare today) refuse enrollment for persons with preexisting medical conditions or accept a chronically ill member for a high monthly premium. The following three definitions explain aspects of a member's enrollment.

OPEN ENROLLMENT PERIOD Open enrollment is a time period, usually during a specified month of the year, when a member may change health insurance plans (Kongstvedt, 2003). As a rule, most managed care plans (specifically HMOs) have their open enrollment period in the fall; the changes become effective from January 1 of the following year. Government-based health insurance plans may not necessarily follow such a timeline. In Arizona, for example, open enrollment for the state's Medicaid plan is in August and goes into effect from October 1. For members unhappy with their health insurance plan, it is important to know when open enrollment periods come around, because it is the one time of year when a plan change can be made without having the need to pay any financial penalty, regardless of health status.

DISENROLLMENT Disenrollment is the process of terminating insurance coverage (Kongstvedt, 2003). Voluntary termination involves a member quitting simply out of personal desire. Involuntary termination can include reasons such as losing or changing jobs (see "Consolidated Omnibus Budget Reconciliation Act" [COBRA] in the following paragraphs). A serious form of involuntary disenrollment can be for reasons such as fraud, abuse, nonpayment of agreed-on copayments or premiums, or a demonstrated inability to comply with recommended treatment plans. Disenrollment for some of these reasons may be very difficult to prove and is therefore rare.

SPEND DOWN Spend down is the process by which a patient or a family can financially qualify for welfare medicine, most commonly known as Medicaid. In essence, the patient must impoverish him- or herself with medical bills. These medical expenses are subtracted from the patient's annual income until the income eligibility limits for Medicaid benefits are met. This yearly financial income allotted depends on such factors as family size and personal property ownership.

Following is a simplified example with no extra variables of a spend down in a patient. Mrs Barrett receives an annual income of $12,000. To qualify for Medicaid, it was assessed that she must not earn over $5,000 per year. Therefore, she must incur $7,000 in medical expenses or, in other words, spend down $7,000 to qualify for Medicaid benefits. Mrs Barrett was in the hospital in February this year and was billed $4,500. She spent $1,000 in medications and outpatient doctor bills. In May, she was in the hospital again as an inpatient. Her hospital bill had exceeded the remaining $1,500 charge, so she had met her spend down amount. Mrs Barrett became eligible for Medicaid coverage.

CONSOLIDATED OMNIBUS BUDGET RECONCILIATION ACT

Under the COBRA, employers with 20 or more employees are required to offer terminated employees an opportunity to continue the same health insurance coverage under an existing medical plan in exchange for a monthly premium. This is why COBRA is sometimes referred to as "continuation coverage." This premium may cost up to 102% of the actual cost of the premium, with 2% being administrative expenses (Williams & Torrens, 1993). The former employee has 60 days to decide if he or she desires to purchase an insurance under COBRA. If a COBRA policy is desired and the person is eligible, the employee can pay for it for 18 to 36 months. The length of time a person is allowed to maintain COBRA insurance depends on several variables, ranging from reason for eligibility (e.g., termination versus disability) to whether the person is the primary beneficiary or a family member.

▶ TYPES OF INSURANCE MODELS/ SYSTEMS

The following section discusses various types of insurance strategies. Matching needed services for patients with available resources is a primary case management responsibility. Few people can afford medical services without the benefit of some form of health insurance. A basic understanding of insurance types is essential for the case manager: what the benefits are, what is covered, how the services are reimbursed, what the patient's fiscal responsibility is, what the care provider's responsibility is, with whom the patient is allowed to follow up, where the patient must fill prescriptions—these and many other questions must be assessed with the insurance company for effective care planning and reimbursement.

It is a well-known fact that managing healthcare came about because of the tremendous price tag of this care; the price is still escalating. Managed care can be defined as an organization that provides and/or finances medical care using provider payment mechanisms that encourage cost containment, involves selective contracting with networks of healthcare providers (individuals and organizations), and imposes controls on the utilization of healthcare services and resources. More than 130 million Americans are enrolled in managed care, and it is the predominant mode of healthcare delivery and financing for privately insured populations in the United States. In addition, many states have shifted their Medicaid and Medicare beneficiaries into managed care programs, and some states have chosen managed care as the mode for the state children's health insurance program, which was included in the Balanced Budget Act of 1997 (BBA) as well as that for the Medicaid beneficiaries in the form of Managed Medicaid plans.

Managed care has infiltrated nearly every health insurance strategy: even the last great indemnity plan—traditional Medicare. Although Medicare is separated into the "traditional" (fee-for-service) track and the managed Medicare track (advantage plans) for the purposes of clarification in this textbook, the extensive changes in Medicare reimbursement today have most definitely changed the definition of Medicare forever. Both traditional Medicare and managed Medicare are now intensely "managed."

▶ Coordination of Benefits

Many families possess health benefit plans from more than one health insurance company. Multiple coverage can occur in such instances when both parents (spouses) are working and each has insurance as an employee benefit, when a child has a catastrophic condition or is developmentally disabled, or when automobile insurance or workers' compensation is involved. State laws have been written to deter fraud by standardizing coordination of benefits (COB) for the holders of multiple health insurance plans.

When a patient has more than one insurance plan, it is important to first determine who is the primary payor; that is, which one is the primary health insurance plan. If the case manager is working on a case with health plans from two or more insurance companies, then the tertiary payor must also be determined. The "rules" can be quite interesting. One group we worked with uses the birthdays of the married couple as the gauge; the health plan of the person with the first birthday in the year becomes the primary plan. In general, however, if there is a private health insurance plan and Medicaid coverage, Medicaid is usually the payor of last resort. However, because there are no absolutes in healthcare, the case manager must determine the rank order on a case-by-case basis. Plans covered under the rules of the Employee Retirement Income Security Act, for example, are exempt from traditional COB regulation.

To ensure healthcare coverage for dependent children, special rules apply when parents are divorced or separated. Divorced parents and their dependent children may follow a sequence such as the following:

1. The plan of the parent in custody of the child(ren).
2. The plan of the spouse of the parent in custody of the child(ren).
3. The plan of the parent without custody of the child(ren).
4. The plan of the spouse without custody of the child(ren).

▶ Medicare

Perhaps the most well known of all health insurance plans in the United States, Medicare is a federally funded program under Title XIX of the Social Security Act, enacted in 1964. Medical services are provided to US citizens older than 65 years of age who have worked at least 10 years (40 quarters, considered work credits), to those who qualify for SSD for at least 24 months, to those under 65 and with certain disabilities, and to persons with permanent kidney failure/end-stage renal disease and requiring either dialysis or kidney transplant. This federal health insurance program is overseen by the CMS.

Not all citizens automatically receive Medicare in their 65th birthday month. They often need to file an application. For a patient who is 65 years old or older with a reliable work history and who does not show coverage under Medicare, social services may be able to help get the person on Medicare; the case manager and/or social worker could be of value in this case, especially in guiding the person through the application process. Persons with renal failure may also apply (CMS, 2017). Renal patients are eligible for Medicare after 3 months of hemodialysis; if private group health insurance is in effect, that policy must cover hemodialysis for 30 months before Medicare takes over. No age limits are imposed in this case. Benefits will continue until 1 year after hemodialysis stops or a kidney transplantation is performed.

The care of Medicare patients is monitored by quality improvement organizations (QIOs) in each state. These are independent groups of physicians and other healthcare professionals, including nurses and social workers, hired by the federal government to assess whether the care Medicare beneficiaries receive meets standards of quality, is reasonable and necessary, and is provided at the most appropriate level. They also review any complaints from Medicare members; these range from poor care to premature discharge. Additionally, QIOs are involved in auditing care rendered by healthcare organizations and individual providers not only for the purpose of reviewing the quality of care, but also for identifying any acts of fraud, waste, and abuse. QIOs provide quality improvement consultation through state projects. Display 3-1 lists three important websites for government benefit programs.

MEDICARE PART A

Medicare is divided into two distinct and separately financed parts. Part A is known as hospital insurance and includes coverage for hospital care, including critical access hospitals, inpatient rehabilitation facilities, inpatient stays at an SNF, home healthcare, hospice care, and inpatient care in a religious nonmedical healthcare institution. Part A is usually premium free and is earned on the basis of a person's or a spouse's employment credits. It is financed through a portion of the Social Security tax that all employees and employers pay.

Part A may be purchased by those who are 65 years of age or older and who are not eligible for premium-free benefits. Examples include those who did not work or did not pay enough Medicare taxes while working, and those who are disabled and have returned to work. In most cases

display 3-1

IMPORTANT GOVERNMENT-RELATED WEBSITES

Three important pieces of website information about the government-based health insurance benefit programs:

1. www.cms.hhs.gov: the official Centers for Medicare & Medicaid Services (CMS) website. The CMS address is:
   Centers for Medicare & Medicaid Services
   6325 Security Boulevard
   Baltimore, MD 21207-5187
   Telephone: (410) 786-3000
2. www.medicare.gov: a website that offers useful information to Medicare beneficiaries and case managers working with this population. Among other important information, this site includes the *Medicare and You Handbook* (online) and has a section entitled *Medicare Compare*, which displays comparisons of various Medicare health plans.
3. www.medicaid.gov: a website that offers important information about the Medicaid benefits with special description of offerings by state, eligibility criteria, and application process. It has special sections about drug benefits, long-term care benefits, improvement initiatives, Managed Medicaid, among many others.

those who buy Part A must also have or purchase Part B benefits. If a person has limited income or resources, the state government may be able to help.

Medicare benefit periods are also known as "spells of illness." They measure the beneficiary's use of Part A or inpatient care. The dollar amounts change yearly for Medicare. The following is based on the year 2017 (CMS, 2017).

- ▶ Most people don't pay a monthly premium for Part A. If you buy Part A, you'll pay up to $413 each month. If you have paid Medicare taxes for less than 30 quarters, the standard Part A premium is $413. If you have paid Medicare taxes for 30 to 39 quarters, the standard Part A premium is $227.
- ▶ A benefit period begins on admission to an inpatient facility.
- ▶ A benefit period ends when the member has been out of a hospital, an SNF, or a rehabilitation facility for 60 consecutive days (including the day of discharge).
- ▶ There is no limit to the number of benefit periods the member can have for hospital and other SNF care.
- ▶ Each time a benefit period is begun, a $1,316 hospital deductible charge is incurred. There is no coinsurance for days 1 to 60 for each benefit period.
- ▶ Medicare will pay for 100% of the beneficiary's hospitalization (minus the above deductible) for the first 60 days of any benefit period.

▶ From the 61st day until the 90th day in the hospital, the Medicare beneficiary is responsible for $329 per day. This charge is referred to as coinsurance.

▶ If more than 90 inpatient days are needed in a benefit period, lifetime reserve days help offset medical expenses. In this case, for days 91 and beyond, the coinsurance increases to $658 per each "lifetime reserve day" for each benefit period.

▶ Only 60 lifetime reserve days are given per beneficiary. These may be used up in one, two, or any number of benefit periods. If 10 reserve days are used up in 1 year, the member has 50 left to use any time that a benefit period exceeds 90 days. They are not renewable.

▶ Beyond lifetime reserve days, the beneficiary is responsible for all costs.

▶ Inpatient psychiatric care in a freestanding psychiatric hospital is limited to 190 days in a lifetime.

▶ Members can opt out of using the reserve days by informing the hospital in writing of their wishes.

Long or frequent inpatient admissions can cause eventual loss of Part A benefits. To lose these benefits, the patient would have to be in the hospital or in the SNF for 150 days (using up 90 days plus the 60 lifetime reserve days), without a reprieve of 60 consecutive days out of the hospital or the SNF. Although this rarely happens, case managers need to be aware of this possibility. Medigap plans cover an additional 365 hospital days after the lifetime reserve is used up. If the patient does not have a Medigap plan, he or she will most likely have to spend down to become eligible for a Medicaid plan.

Medicare Part A also pays for some posthospital SNF care. The beneficiary must have been in the hospital under an acute admit (not observation status) for 3 nights at the minimum. The patient may be discharged directly into a Medicare-certified SNF or can go home and, if a skilled SNF need is discovered, can be admitted to an SNF within 30 days of the hospital discharge date.

Medicare Part A helps pay for a maximum of 100 days in each benefit period for skilled care in an SNF (Display 3-2). The member pays nothing for the first 20 days; Medicare pays 100%. If the patient still needs additional skilled care at an SNF level, 80 additional days will be paid for, but the coinsurance to the member is $164.50 per day (CMS, 2017). After 100 days in each benefit period, Medicare will not be financially responsible.

Medicare Part A also pays for home healthcare provided in lieu of hospitalization if certain criteria are met. Essentially, the member must be homebound, have a physician-ordered home healthcare treatment plan, and must require intermittent (rather than intensive) skilled nursing or skilled rehabilitation services. As long as the abovementioned criteria are met, the Catastrophic Coverage Act of 1988 ensures that home health services can be covered for a maximum of 38 consecutive days. If the services are deemed appropriate, they will be reimbursed at 100%. However, dramatic changes are shifting the provision of home health services to Medicare beneficiaries in the reimbursement of Medicare home health services.

Durable medical equipment (DME) has a coinsurance payment of 20%; Medicare will pay for 80% of covered DME. Hospice care is also covered under certain conditions. Inpatient psychiatric care is reimbursed for up to 190 days, if needed and offered in a freestanding psychiatric facility.

MEDICARE PART B

Part B is also known as medical insurance and includes coverage for medically necessary services including physician's services, outpatient hospital services, DME, other miscellaneous services, or those not covered by Part A. The monthly premium for Part B in 2017 for a single individual started at $134 or higher depending on the beneficiary's income. Those who already receive Social Security benefits pay about $109 on average.

display 3-2

PAYMENT ACCORDING TO LEVEL OF CARE IN EACH BENEFIT PERIOD (2017)

	Member Pays	Medicare Pays
Hospital		
Day 1–60	Deductible $1,316	All other qualified expenses
Day 61–90	$329/day coinsurance	All other qualified expenses
Day 91–150	$658/day	All other qualified expenses
Lifetime reserve days[a]		
Skilled Nursing Facility		
Day 1–20	$0	All qualified expenses
Day 21–100	$164.50/day	All other qualified expenses
Day 101 and over	All costs	$0
Home Healthcare		
Home care services	$0	All qualified expenses
Durable medical equipment	20% of Medicare-approved amount	80% of approved amount

NOTE: Medicare Advantage Plans cover these services. However, costs vary by plan and may be higher or lower than those stated above.
[a]Unlike other benefit periods, lifetime reserve days are not renewable and can be used only once in a member's lifetime. These are up to 60 days over the lifetime. However for inpatient psychiatric care in a freestanding psychiatric facility, the reserve days are 190 in a lifetime.
From the Centers for Medicare & Medicaid Services. *Medicare and you, 2017.* Retrieved from www.medicare.gov

Medicare Part B can be purchased even if Part A requirements have not been met. Some Medicaid plans purchase Medicare Part B for their ineligible (Part A) members as a cost-saving method. Part B has an annual deductible of $183, and any Part B service can be used to fulfill that deductible. The member also owes a 20% coinsurance payment for many Part B services, especially after the deductible has been satisfied. In general, Part B helps cover physician services, outpatient hospital care, diagnostic tests, radiology and pathology services (inpatient or outpatient), DME, home health services, physical/occupational/speech therapies, and limited chiropractic, podiatry, dentistry, and optometry services.

Like Medicare Part A, Part B will pay for 100% of approved home health services and 80% of DME, but not until after the $183 annual deductible is met. Kidney dialysis and kidney, liver, and heart transplantations may be partially covered under Part B when strict criteria are met.

Both Part A and Part B cover blood components such as red blood cells, platelets, and fresh-frozen plasma. Both sections of Medicare require the recipient to pay for any replacement costs on the first three units. This replacement fee is the amount charged for blood that is not replaced. The replacement fee criteria can be satisfied with the use of either the Part A or Part B side. Part A pays all costs from the fourth pint each calendar year. Part B pays for 80% starting with the fourth pint. The annual Part B deductible must also be met.

Displays 3-3 and 3-4 summarize the detailed list of insurance-covered services in both Part A and Part B. The Medicare system is not only complicated, but also subject to changes in any year. Case managers may benefit from the most recent CMS publications accessible on their website at www.cms.hhs.gov.

Medicare also has recently supported payment for *Chronic Care Management Services*. This applies to those beneficiaries with two or more chronic conditions that are expected to last for at least 1 year. A chronic condition could be arthritis, asthma, diabetes, hypertension, heart disease, osteoporosis, and others. This benefit is voluntary and the beneficiary must consent to it for the primary care provider to be able to bill Medicare for it. If effective, the beneficiary assumes responsibility for a copayment and coinsurance similar to those in other outpatient visits and services as well as the annual deductible based on Medicare Part B benefit.

The services offered under this arrangement consist of a comprehensive care plan that lists the beneficiary's health problems and goals, need for other healthcare providers, medications, community services, and other information about the person's health. The plan also explains the care the beneficiary needs and how this care will be coordinated. The healthcare provider expects the beneficiary to sign an agreement for this service after which the provider prepares the care plan, including medications management, provides 24/7 access for urgent care needs, supports the beneficiary during the transition from one healthcare setting to another, reviews the medications prescribed, and assists in coordinating the beneficiary's chronic care needs.

MEDICATIONS AND HOME INFUSION PUMPS

Under certain circumstances, Medicare Part B pays for or helps to pay for the following:

▶ Antigens if they are ordered by a physician and administered by a properly instructed person (who could be the patient/family) under the supervision of a physician;
▶ Erythropoietin if the patient has end-stage renal disease and is on dialysis, and requires it for treatment of anemia;
▶ Hemophilia clotting factors;
▶ Hepatitis B vaccine;
▶ Immunosuppressive drugs within 1 year of organ transplantations;
▶ Flu and pneumococcal pneumonia vaccines;
▶ Oral chemotherapy for cancer, if the same drug is available in injectable form.

In the 1990s, traditional Medicare approved a limited number of IV medications to be administered in the home setting, where previously no such medications were covered in the home. Because the cost of the medications was very high, many, otherwise independent, patients had to be transferred to nursing homes, where IV medications are covered for long-term IV antibiotic regimens.

According to the Medicare Durable Medical Equipment Regional Center (DMERC) Guide, the criteria for home IV medications include use of an infusion pump and a prolonged infusion of at least 8 hours or infusion of the drug at a controlled rate to avoid toxicity. Another means of accomplishing the infusion is not acceptable or safe. The DME portion of the home health benefit covers approved supplies, drugs, and biologicals. These claims are subject to review on a case-by-case basis.

External infusion pumps are covered for the following indications:

▶ Deferoxamine for the treatment of chronic iron overload;
▶ When treating primary hepatocellular carcinoma or colorectal cancer in cases in which this disease is unresectable or in which the patient refuses surgical excision of the tumor;
▶ For morphine when used in the treatment of intractable pain caused by cancer.

Some approved medications (with the abovementioned criteria) include the following:

▶ Administration of fluorouracil, cytarabine, bleomycin, doxorubicin, vincristine, or vinblastine by continuous infusion over at least 24 hours when

display 3-3

MEDICARE (PART A): HOSPITAL INSURANCE-COVERED SERVICES FOR 2017

Services	Benefit	Medicare Pays	Member Pays
Hospitalization			
Semiprivate room and board, general nursing, medications, and other hospital services and supplies	First 60 days	All but $1,316/benefit period	$1,316
	Day 61 to 90	All but $329/day	$329/day
	Day 91 to 150[a]	All but $658/day	$658/day
	Beyond 150 days	Nothing	All costs
Skilled Nursing Facility Care			
Semiprivate room and board, general nursing, skilled nursing and rehabilitative services, and other services and supplies[b]	First 20 days	100% of approved amount	Nothing
	21–100 days	All but $164.50/day	Up to $164.50/day
	Beyond 100 days	Nothing	All costs
Home Health Care			
Part-time or intermittent skilled care, home health aid services, durable medical equipment, and supplies and other services	Unlimited as long as Medicare conditions are met	100% of approved amount; 80% of approved amount for durable medical equipment	Nothing for 20% of approved amount for durable medical equipment
Hospice Care			
Pain relief, symptom management, and services for the terminally ill	For as long as physician certifies need	All but limited costs for outpatient drugs and inpatient respite care Doesn't cover room and board if hospice care is offered in the beneficiary's home or another facility where the beneficiary resides if other than home such as an SNF	$5 copay per prescription for outpatient drugs and 5% of approved amount for inpatient respite care
Blood	Unlimited if medically necessary	80% of all but first three pints per calendar year	First three pints and 20% of all other pints[c] starting with the fourth

NOTE: Medicare Advantage Plans cover these services. However, costs vary by plan and may be higher or lower than those stated above.

Most people do not pay Part A monthly premiums because they paid Medicare taxes while working. If not eligible for premium-free Medicare Part A hospital insurance, premium is $423/month, or more for those who must pay a surcharge for late enrollment.

[a]This 60-reserve-days benefit may be used only once in a lifetime.

[b]Neither Medicare nor private Medigap insurance will pay for most custodial care.

[c]Blood paid for or replaced under Part B of Medicare during the calendar year does not have to be paid for or replaced under Part A.

From the Centers for Medicare & Medicaid Services. *Medicare and you, 2017.* [Online]. Retrieved from www.medicare.gov.

display 3-4

MEDICARE (PART B): MEDICAL INSURANCE-COVERED SERVICES FOR 2017

Services	Benefit	Medicare Pays	Member Pays
Medical Expenses			
Doctors' services, inpatient and outpatient medical and surgical services and supplies, physical and speech therapy, diagnostic tests, durable medical equipment, and other services	Unlimited if medically necessary	All expenses for most preventive services if provided by a qualified provider 80% of approved amount for other services (after $183 deductible); 50% of approved charges for most outpatient mental health services	$183 deductible,[a] plus 20% of approved amount and limited charges above approved amount

display 3-4

Chronic Care Management Services	If two or more conditions are present and are expected to last for at least 1 year	Expenses covered depending on the services provided and after the $183 normal deductible	A monthly fee and coinsurance applies if the beneficiary agrees to the services including the normal $183 deductible
Clinical Laboratory Services			
Blood tests, urinalyses, and more	Unlimited if medically necessary	Generally 100% of approved amount	Nothing for services
Home Healthcare			
Part-time or intermittent skilled care, home health aide services, durable medical equipment, and supplies and other services	Unlimited as long as you meet Medicare conditions	100% of approved amount; 80% of approved amount for durable medical equipment	Nothing for services; 20% of approved amount for durable medical equipment
Outpatient Hospital Treatment			
Services for the diagnosis or treatment of illness or injury	Unlimited if medically necessary	Medicare payment to hospital based on hospital cost	Copayment or coinsurance that varies by service (after $183 deductible)[a]
Ambulatory surgery	Unlimited if approved	100% of approved amount after deductible	Coinsurance applies as well as $183 deductible if it was not yet satisfied
Blood	Unlimited if medically necessary	80% of approved amount (after $135 deductible and amount starting with the fourth pint)	First three pints plus 20% of amount approved for additional pints (after $183 deductible[b]) No cost if the provider obtained the blood from a blood bank at no cost, except for the fees of handling the blood
Mental health	Unlimited if medically necessary	Medicare Part A coverage applies All costs for an annual depression screening 80% of approved amount (after $183 deductible[b])	Based on Medicare Part A coverage 20% of approved amount (after $183 deductible[b])
Clinical research	Unlimited if medically necessary and for qualifying studies	80% of the Medicare approved amount, including coverage for services that otherwise would be covered regardless of research protocol	20% of approved amount
Ambulance services	If medically necessary and depends on the seriousness of the condition	Approved amounts after $183 deductible	Coinsurance and $183 deductible apply
Tele Health			
Office visits, psychotherapy, consultations, and certain other medical or health services	If services provided using an interactive, two-way telecommunications system (like real-time audio and video) by an eligible provider	80% of costs of approved services after $183 deductible	20% of the Medicare-approved amount, and the Part B deductible of $183 applies

NOTE: Medicare Advantage Plans cover these services. However, costs vary by plan and may be higher or lower than those stated above.

In 2017, there were limits on physical therapy, occupational therapy, and speech-language pathology services. There were also exceptions to these limits.

2017 Part B monthly premium for a single individual starts at $109 (premium might be higher if one is a late enrollee and is not already a recipient of Social Security benefit).

[a]Once $183 of expenses for covered services in 2017 is spent, the Part B deductible does not apply to any further covered services received for the rest of the year.

[b]Blood paid for or replaced under Part A of Medicare during the calendar year does not have to be paid for or replaced under Part B.

From the Centers for Medicare & Medicaid Services. *Medicare and you, 2017.* [Online]. Retrieved from www.medicare.gov.

the regimen is proven or generally accepted to have significant advantages over intermittent administration regimens.

▶ Administration of selected narcotic analgesics (in addition to morphine) for intractable pain not responding to, or if the patient cannot tolerate, other forms of pain control.

▶ The following antibiotics/antivirals: acyclovir, foscarnet, amphotericin B, vancomycin, and ganciclovir.

▶ Dobutamine if the individual meets *all* the following criteria:

1. The individual is an accepted cardiac transplant candidate on an active status;

2. Even with treatment of maximum doses of diuretics and angiotensin-converting enzyme inhibitor, along with a simultaneous administration of a vasodilator, the individual remains dyspneic on minimal exertion or at rest;

3. Physiologic response readings demonstrate an increase in cardiac output, an increase in left ventricular ejection fraction, and a decrease in the pulmonary wedge pressure;

4. The documentation supports the deterioration in the client's condition when dobutamine is discontinued under observation in the hospital; *and*

5. There is no need for intensive electrocardiograph monitoring in the patient's home, and any life-threatening arrhythmia is controlled.

Note: The aforementioned information was obtained from the *Federal Medicare Intermediary* in Oxnard, California.

The home health agency called in to care for the patient can help the case manager in assessing which home IV medications are covered under Medicare. Most prescription medications are not covered under either part of Medicare. This causes a real hardship for chronically ill persons on fixed incomes. Frequent readmissions should be assessed for "noncompliant patients" who are not taking their prescribed medications. The following reasons for noncompliance should be assessed:

▶ Can the patient afford the prescribed medications?
▶ Is the patient carefully doling out the medications, cutting the dose so the bottle will last longer?
▶ Some patients hoard old prescriptions for "emergency" use; the medications may be expired or the dosage may be too low or too high.

People with no pharmacologic insurance coverage should be assessed and possibly helped to acquire needed medicines.

MEDICARE ADVANTAGE PLANS (PART C)/ MEDICARE HEALTH PLAN CHOICES— TRADITIONAL AND MEDICARE MANAGED CARE

Medicare Advantage Plans (MAPs or MAs) are health plan options (like HMOs and PPOs) approved by Medicare and run by private companies. MAPs are not supplemental insurance and must follow rules set by Medicare. For several years Medicare risk contracts have offered prepaid, comprehensive health coverage to Medicare beneficiaries. Instead of paying hospitals the traditional DRG payment, these risk contracts are actually commercial, private, or managed care plans that contract with the CMS to provide services to Medicare beneficiaries for a fixed monthly payment paid by Medicare on behalf of the beneficiaries who opt to enroll in a MAP. The plan is "at risk" if the needed services are more costly than the fixed payment. From a member perspective, the out-of-pocket costs (coinsurance, copayment, and deductibles) may be different than those in traditional Medicare.

Services provided to beneficiaries include all of those offered under Medicare Part A and Part B; however, MAPs may offer additional services such as preventive and wellness care, dental care, hearing aids, and eyeglasses. They also include Medicare prescription drug coverage, usually for an extra cost. As in all managed care plans, MAPs have provider networks, services must be preapproved, and authorized care providers (individuals and facilities), which may include a referral from a primary care physician/provider (PCP) to a specialist, must be used. If urgent care is required, it can be provided outside the plan's service area. Gatekeeper-style PCPs are generally required.

Case managers often have to coordinate care with the Medicare plan's case manager to manage and facilitate necessary services and discharge planning including posthospital services. These plans offer less freedom of choice in that the case manager must match the home health agency or the SNF (for example) to the Medicare-contracted networks. Some advantages include more home IV medication coverage and added pharmacy and ancillary coverage for the patient.

The BBA required many stipulations that protect Medicare beneficiaries and changed Medicare forever. MAPs are intended to provide Medicare beneficiaries with a range of options for the financing and delivery of their healthcare. Under the MAP choices, beneficiaries may be able to choose from one of the following:

▶ Managed care plan, specifically an HMO, with or without a point-of-service (POS) option
▶ PPO
▶ Provider-sponsored organization (PSO)
▶ Medical savings account (MSA)
▶ Private fee-for-service (PFFS) insurance plan
▶ Original "traditional" Medicare.

Generally and as a rule of thumb, the case manager must remember that under the MAP arrangement, beneficiaries are expected to receive at a minimum the same services they would otherwise have received under the original Medicare benefits program; they also have the same rights. The main case management/patient advocate role will be to assure the Medicare beneficiaries that the

CMS will work with them; the traditional fee-for-service plan is always an option, so they will not be left without healthcare services.

The BBA also provides Medicare beneficiaries with other benefits, including screening mammograms, screening Pap smears and pelvic examinations, colorectal cancer screening tests, prostate cancer screening tests, coverage for diabetic supplies and diabetic education (whether the beneficiary is insulin dependent or not), and procedures to identify bone mass/density or bone quality in certain at-risk patients. Flu and pneumococcal vaccine benefits will continue to be covered as well.

Emergency department care has come under scrutiny because many insurance plans have denied payment for emergency care when the medical problem turned out to be nonemergent. The BBA stipulates that under any chosen plan, coverage for care that a "prudent lay person" would consider to be an emergency must be considered and paid. In other words, if a patient was admitted to the emergency department with complaints of chest pain and it turned out to be a hiatal hernia (nonemergent), a prudent lay person would not have known that—the emergency department claim must be paid.

Medicare has paid managed care companies a fixed monthly amount per beneficiary, adjusted only by geographical area. To "level the playing field" for those health plans that care for frail and elderly Medicare beneficiaries, the CMS has implemented a new payment method. Known as risk adjustment, this method reflects the health status of Medicare beneficiaries. It is hoped that this will lessen the incentive to enroll only the healthiest of the Medicare population. Risk adjustment looks at a person's diagnosis in 1 year and predicts how much, if any, additional cost there will be for that person the next year. If a Medicare beneficiary has an appendectomy for 1 year, that may not increase costs; however, if the person has a major stroke, the plan would receive a larger payment-per-month to cover expected expenses. These risk-adjusted payments began in January 2000 with a 10% incremental increase; they came into full effect in 2004. There are rules for this method of payment. For example, the CMS is excluding hospital admission diagnoses that are rarely the principal reason for inpatient hospital care or that are vague or ambiguous; 1-day hospitalizations are also excluded to reduce the incentive to increase marginal admissions.

MEDICARE PART D

Medicare offers prescription drug coverage for everyone with Medicare. This coverage is called Medicare Part D. A beneficiary is eligible to receive this benefit after joining a Medicare drug plan; such plans are usually run by insurance companies approved by Medicare. Plans vary in cost on the basis of options and drugs covered. If one does not take a lot of prescription drugs and opts not to join this benefit, he or she can join later on when drug expenses have increased and pay a required late-enrollment penalty fee.

There are two ways for a Medicare beneficiary to join a prescription drug plan: (1) join a Medicare Prescription Drug Plan, known as MPDP, or (2) Medicare Advantage Prescription Drug Plan known as MAPDP. Everyone with Medicare benefits is eligible to join any of these Medicare drug plan options. When a beneficiary joins a plan, he or she pays a separate monthly premium in addition to the original Medicare fees. Monthly premiums vary by plan; on average the 2017 premium is $42.17 per month which is 9% higher than that of 2016. This is in addition to the monthly premium spent on the original Medicare Part B plan and do not include any copays that may be expected upon filling a prescription. Depending on the beneficiary's annual income, the premium may be higher. For example, on the basis of the 2015 income tax returns, an individual with an annual income above $85,000 and less than $107,000 was expected to pay in 2017 the premium plus and additional $13.30 per month for the prescription drug plan. Late penalty fees are also charged if one does not join the drug plan during the annual enrollment period. However, if a person's needs change after joining a plan, one can switch to another plan that better meets his or her needs. MAPs that offer prescription drug coverage do not require additional monthly premiums for prescription drugs.

Medicare drug plans have a list of drugs covered by the plan, known as a "formulary." Plans by law are standardized to cover the most common medications. At a minimum, a plan must cover the following:

▶ At least two different drugs for each of the medications categories and
▶ At the least the majority of drugs for the categories of cancer, immunosuppressants, antidepressants, antipsychotics, and HIV/AIDS.

To access these drugs, the patient's condition and need must always meet Medicare's requirements. There may be special rules for filling a prescription even if a drug is included in the formulary. The list of drugs may change at any time because of changes in therapies, the addition of new drugs, and the removal of others. If the formulary stops including a drug a person is taking, the drug plan must notify the individual at least 60 days in advance. In this case the individual may either change the drug to another on the list or may be required to pay more into the plan to continue taking the same drug.

Those who join Medicare drug plans are also responsible for a deductible and coinsurance or a copayment. These amounts are determined on the basis of the plan a beneficiary chooses to enroll in. An example of a plan's tiers is available in Display 3-5. After a person spends a certain amount of money for covered drugs (called the limit), he or she will have to pay all costs out of pocket. This situation is called "coverage gap." The beneficiary will continue to pay the monthly premium even during the coverage gap. Each state offers at least one plan with

TIERS OR CATEGORIES ON A MEDICARE DRUG PLAN/FORMULARY

Tier (Formulary)	Beneficiary Pays/Copayment	What Is Covered?
1	Lowest Copayment	Most Generic Prescription Drugs
2	Medium Copayment	Preferred,[a] Brand-name Prescription Drugs
3	Higher Copayment	Nonpreferred, Brand-name Prescription Drugs
Specialty Tier	Highest Co-payment or Coinsurance	Unique, Very High Costs

NOTE: Medicare drug plans place drugs into different tiers called formularies. Drugs in each tier have different costs. Some plans may have more tiers, whereas some may have fewer.

[a]Preferred brand-name prescription drug is a drug that has been determined by the plan to be less costly, but is as effective as other more costly drugs.

From the Centers for Medicare & Medicaid Services. *Medicare and you, 2008.* [Online]. Retrieved from www.medicare.gov.

some type of coverage during the gap. Plans with gap coverage may charge a higher monthly premium. Some may cover brand-name drugs only and may offer generic drug coverage during the gap. Some, even when they offer gap coverage, may not cover all the drugs a beneficiary may need.

Medicare Part D plans (Display 3-6) generally pay around 60% of brand-name and 49% of generic prescription drug costs. Once the plan pays for a total of $3,700 in costs for the year, the coverage drops to 50% for brand-name and 14% for generic drugs. However, once the Medicare beneficiary has spent a total of $4,950 out of his or her pocket for the year (that is has reached the limit set by the plan for the year), catastrophic coverage begins.

Catastrophic drug coverage benefits beneficiaries with extremely high drug costs. Under such arrangements, the individual pays a coinsurance or copayment after spending no more than $4,950 for drugs covered. The plan thereafter will pay for nearly all the prescription drug costs. By 2020, Medicare Part D plans will pay for 75% of all prescription drug costs. Because case managers will potentially incur such a high deductible for drugs, it is important for them to advice their patients when shopping for a Medicare plan to check if the prescription drugs the patients are currently taking or those they think

PRESCRIPTION DRUG COVERAGE MEDICARE PLAN D (2017)

	Medicare Pays	Beneficiary Pays
Initial deductible	All costs after the initial deductibles of $400 per coverage year and up to the initial coverage limit	$400 per coverage year and any costs that exceed the initial coverage limit
Initial coverage limit	$3,700 per coverage year after initial deductibles	All costs after the initial coverage limit of $3,700 per coverage year
Coverage gap	Begins upon reaching the initial coverage limit and ends when the out-of-pocket reaches $4,950 per coverage year	Copays and deductibles up to the initial coverage limit and costs that are not covered during the coverage gap range
Cost sharing in catastrophic coverage	The greater of 5% or $3.30 for a generic or preferred drug that is a multisource one and the greater of 5% or $8.25 for all other drugs	
Generic prescription drugs	49% of the price during the coverage gap	51% of the price. This amount is expected to decrease each year until it reaches 25% by year 2020
Brand-name prescription drugs[a]	60% of the price during the coverage gap Excludes manufacturer discount if one is in effect	Up to 40% of the plan's cost for covered brand-name prescription drug Manufacturer discount may be up to 50%

NOTE: Medicare drug plans place drugs into different tiers called formularies. Drugs in each tier have different costs. Some plans may have more tiers, whereas some may have fewer.

[a]Preferred brand-name prescription drug is a drug that has been determined by the plan to be less costly, but is as effective as other drugs.

From the Centers for Medicare & Medicaid Services. *Medicare and you, 2017.* [Online]. Retrieved from www.medicare.gov.

may be needed at some point are covered as part of the plan. This is important as each plan may have a different list of covered drugs (formulary) despite those that are considered standard across plans. If a drug is not on the list, then the beneficiary will generally be responsible to pay the full price.

MEDIGAP PLANS

In July 1992, the federal government approved standardized insurance policies designed to supplement, or fill in the gaps of, original Medicare coverage. Today, there are 10 Medigap plans in use nationally compared with 12 plans in 2008. These supplemental health insurance plans help pay for Medicare Part A and B deductibles, copayments, coinsurance, and other out-of-pocket expenses for healthcare services and supplies not covered by Medicare. Some policies also include coverage for certain health services not covered by Medicare. Some Medigap policies cover extra benefits for an additional cost. Before these plans were standardized, Medicare beneficiaries had to choose among so many vague Medicare supplemental policies that often case managers would find that their patients had supplements that were both inadequate and duplicative; in some instances, patients were unaware that they had supplements. Although the federal government does not offer these policies (because they are private insurance policies), it does require strict adherence to guidelines.

Both federal and state laws govern the sales of Medigap insurance. Insurers may not sell a policy that duplicates the member's existing health plan or one that is not one of the approved standard policies. The premiums for these policies have increased tremendously over the past several years. This has put the beneficiaries with fixed incomes under much difficulty, and the consequence is that they are enrolling in the managed Medicare plans.

The 10 standardized plans available in 2017 are identified by specific letters A through N (Display 3-7). In most states, all 10 standardized plan options are accessible. Plan F is the most popular option and is the only one that includes all nine Medigap benefits. In Massachusetts,

display 3-7

STANDARD MEDIGAP SUPPLEMENT INSURANCE POLICIES—MEDIGAP PLANS (2017)

Benefits	Plans									
	A	B	C	D	F[a]	G	K[b]	L[c]	M	N
Core benefit (Basic)	100%	100%	100%	100%	100%	100%	100%	100%	100%	100%
Medicare Part A coinsurance and hospital costs (up to an additional 365 days after Medicare benefits are used)	100%	100%	100%	100%	100%	100%	100%	100%	100%	100%
Medicare Part B coinsurance or copayment	100%	100%	100%	100%	100%	100%	50%	75%	100%	100%[d]
Skilled nursing facility coinsurance			100%	100%	100%	100%	50%	75%	100%	100%
Part A hospice care	100%	100%	100%	100%	100%	100%	50%	75%	100%	100%
Blood (first 3 pints)	100%	100%	100%	100%	100%	100%	50%	75%	100%	100%
Part A Deductible		100%	100%	100%	100%	100%	50%	75%	50%	100%
Part B Deductible			100%		100%					
Part B Excess charges					100%	100%				
Foreign travel emergency (up to plan limits)			80%	80%	80%	80%			80%	80%
Preventive care coinsurance (included in Part B)	100%	100%	100%	100%	100%	100%	100%	100%	100%	100%

[a]Medigap Plan F also offers a high-deductible plan in some states. If a beneficiary chooses this option, it means the beneficiary will be responsible for Medicare-covered costs (coinsurance, copayments, and deductibles) up to the deductible amount of $2,200 in 2017 before the policy pays anything.

[b]Medigap plan K also requires an out-of-pocket of $5,120 annually according to 2017 plans.

[c]Medigap plan L also requires an out-of-pocket of $2,560 annually according to 2017 plans.

[d]Medigap Plan N pays 100% of the Part B coinsurance, except for a copayment of up to $20 for some office visits and up to a $50 copayment for emergency room visits that don't result in an inpatient admission.

From the Centers for Medicare & Medicaid Services. (2017). *2008 Choosing a Medigap policy: a guide to health insurance for people with Medicare.* Baltimore, MD: Author.

Minnesota, and Wisconsin, they are standardized in a different way. Each plan must include a core package of benefits. All plans cover an additional 365 days of approved inpatient hospitalization after the long-term reserve days have been used (see "Medicare" section). These plans only work with the original Medicare plan and cannot be used to pay the copayments or deductibles for MAPs. In addition, all must be clearly identified as Medicare Supplemental Insurance.

The nine core benefits of the Medigap plans include the following:

❱ Part A hospital coinsurance or copayment
❱ Part B coinsurance or copayment
❱ Part A hospice coinsurance or copayment
❱ Blood first three pints
❱ SNF care coinsurance
❱ Part A deductible
❱ Part B deductible
❱ Part B excess charges
❱ Foreign travel emergency

The monthly premium for Medigap plans is set or rated in one of three ways:

1. *Community-rated (also called no-age rated)*: The same monthly premium is charged to everyone who has the Medigap policy regardless of age. Premiums may go up because of inflation and other factors.
2. *Issue-age-rated*: The monthly premium is set on the basis of the age the beneficiary is at the time a policy is purchased. Premiums are lower for people who buy a policy at a younger age, and will not change as the person gets older. However, premiums may go up because of inflation and other factors.
3. *Attained-age-rated*: The monthly premium is set on the basis of the beneficiary's age at the time the policy is purchased; however, the premium increases as the person gets older. Premiums are low for younger buyers. This policy type may be least expensive at first, but may become the most expensive in later years. The premiums may also go up because of inflation and other factors.

In most cases, a beneficiary may not have the right under federal law to switch Medigap policies unless he or she is within the 6-month open enrollment period. Beneficiaries may switch between policies for reasons that include the following:

❱ You are paying for benefits you do not need.
❱ You need more benefits compared to your needs at the time you signed up.
❱ Your current Medigap policy has the right benefits, but you are unhappy with the insurance company.
❱ Your current Medigap policy has the right benefits, but you would like to find one that is less expensive.

The Medicare beneficiary does not have to wait for open enrollment to buy a Medigap policy. The best time to buy is in the first 6 months after the person turns 65 years of age and has already enrolled in Medicare Parts A and B.

MEDICARE SELECT

In some states, one may be able to buy another type of Medigap plan called Medicare SELECT. Medicare SELECT is a plan that supplements traditional Medicare; it allows the same choice of the 10 plans as any Medigap insurance supplement does. The only difference is that Medicare SELECT requires the use of specific providers (hospitals and, in some cases, specific doctors) to receive full benefits. Emergent care may be out-of-network. The premiums are generally lower than those of the standard Medigap policies.

❱ Medicaid

Medicaid, like Medicare, is a federally funded healthcare program under Title XIX of the Social Security Act. Medicaid was enacted into law on July 20, 1964 and is part of the federal and state welfare systems. Before 1965, physicians and hospitals often gave out charity care or billed on a sliding-scale basis. Eligibility for Medicaid is based on income and/or various welfare categories such as AFDC. Generally speaking, Medicaid provides medical benefits to groups of low-income people and some who may have no or inadequate medical insurance. Although the federal government establishes the general guidelines for the program, Medicaid requirements are actually established by each state. Whether a person is eligible for Medicaid depends on the state where he or she lives. Some states may include people in the Medicaid program other than those specified in the federal guidelines.

Many Medicare recipients also financially qualify for Medicaid. If a patient has both Medicare and Medicaid, a supplemental policy may be redundant. The Medicaid portion will cover all Medicare deductibles, coinsurance, medically necessary care, and prescription medications. Home IV medications may also be covered under this insurance arrangement.

The member with only Medicaid generally has no premiums, deductibles, or coinsurance costs. Prescription drugs are paid for, although some states have a "negative formulary list," which excludes some medications and substitutes others. Some states may also require a small out-of-pocket charge for doctor visits or prescriptions; this is rarely enforced.

Medicaid programs are subject to state regulatory agencies; therefore, wide variations in coverage and eligibility exist among the different states. Title XIX of the Social Security Act mandates certain basic health services. Each state, however, may determine the scope of services offered or may offer optional services such as clinic services and dental or optometry services.

MEDICAID ELIGIBILITY

The following are some of the categories that allow Medicaid eligibility. To be categorically eligible, individuals must fit into a category that makes them eligible according to Title XIX (Medicaid) of the Social Security Act. Recipients of SSI and those who qualify for AFDC are automatically eligible for Medicaid.

- *Medical assistance only (MAO):* A special category of Medicaid recipients under AFDC or SSI who receive only Medicaid benefits and not financial assistance.
- *Medically needy/medically indigent (MN/MI):* A category of Medicaid recipients in which Medicaid receives funds only from country and state treasuries. Other categories may also receive matching federal funds.
- *Sixth Omnibus Budget Reconciliation Act (SOBRA):* One of Medicaid's maternal and child health reforms that was passed by Congress and became effective in 1987. Pregnant women and children with family incomes at or below the poverty level become eligible for Medicaid.
- *Persons with specific medical conditions that states may include under Medicaid plans:* One is a time-limited eligibility group for women who have breast or cervical cancer; the other is for people with tuberculosis (TB) who are uninsured. The first group receives all services; TB patients receive only services related to the treatment of TB.

Blind and disabled persons who also receive SSI, and persons in certain other specifically defined categories, are also eligible for Medicaid. If a case manager has a patient who may qualify for Medicaid, he or she will work with the patient to complete a Medicaid application and coordinate the process for seeking eligibility for Medicaid benefits. Most large hospitals and Department of Economic Security (DES) or Social Security Administration offices have eligibility workers who assist in the processing and review of such applications. These are employees of a county, DES, or Social Security, whose job is to determine eligibility for Medicaid through interviews and assessment of medical and financial data. Social workers are another valuable source with whom case managers can work closely to coordinate the application process.

Some core Medicaid benefits, which are considered mandatory and which states are required to offer by law, include the following:

- Hospital inpatient care.
- Hospital outpatient services.
- Pregnancy-related services including prenatal care and services for other conditions that might complicate pregnancy. This also includes 60 days of postpartum pregnancy-related services.
- Laboratory and radiography services.
- SNF care for persons 21 years of age and older.
- Home health services for those who meet home care criteria. This includes home health aides, medical supplies, and appliances for use in the home.
- Physician services.
- Family planning services and supplies.
- Certified pediatric and family nurse practitioners (when licensed to practice under state law).
- Rural health clinic services.
- Medical and surgical services of a dentist.
- Early and periodic screening, diagnosis, and treatment for persons younger than 21 years of age.
- Nurse-midwife services.
- Certain federally qualified ambulatory and health center services.
- Transportation to medical care.
- Tobacco cessation for pregnant women.

Some of the Medicaid benefits that are considered optional and states have the choice to offer, include the following:

- Prescription drugs
- Case management
- Therapy services: physical, occupational, respiratory, and speech, hearing and language
- Hospice
- Dental and denture services
- Optometry
- Aids: hearing, glasses
- Personal care
- Services for individuals aged 65 or older in an institution for mental disease
- Services in intermediate care facility for individuals with intellectual disabilities
- Self-directed personal assistance services
- TB-related services
- Inpatient psychiatric services for individuals under 21 years of age
- Health homes for enrollees with chronic conditions

The vagueness of some covered Medicaid services means that the case manager may be able to negotiate resources for the patient. If services requested are in lieu of hospitalization or an SNF placement or are necessary for patient safety, the Medicaid plan may choose to accommodate the request. Because of budget cuts, however, fewer nonemergent services are being provided. This makes the patient advocacy role of the case manager even more critical when it comes to planning safe and adequate discharges.

Some Medicaid plans do not cover services such as inpatient drug or alcohol programs. The case manager and the social worker may be limited to community programs, which might be free or may charge on a sliding-fee scale.

A baseline knowledge of what your state's Medicaid coverage includes can save the case manager from assessment of time-consuming plans that will not be approved.

Medicaid began as a fee-for-service program in the 1960s. Currently, all states have changed to some form of Medicaid managed care, using capitated payments or per diem rates as a primary method of reimbursement. In Arizona, for example, the AHCCCS pays hospitals on a per diem basis. As an example, the medical patient receives approximately $750 per day for care in the hospital. Magnetic resonance imaging uses up most of that, but also included in the per diem rate is all care from laboratory tests to radiology to nurses. Because hospital patients are very ill, it is easy to see that for many multisystem-failure patients who need resource-intensive care, this rate will be inadequate. Tight utilization of resources is important. The challenge is providing medically necessary care to ill patients while striving for a fiscally healthy institution—all within the confines of a Medicaid per diem rate.

▶ Tricare

Tricare, formerly known as the Civilian Health and Medical Program of the Uniformed Services, is a program of medical benefits for all covered military personnel and eligible family members or survivors. These include the Army, Navy, Marine Coprs, Airforce, Coast Guards, Public Health Services, and the National Oceanic and Atmospheric Administration. By strict definition, Tricare is not an insurance program. It does not involve a contract guaranteeing medical coverage in exchange for a premium, and it is not subject to the state regulatory agencies that cover most insurance plans. Tricare is provided for by US governmental funds, which are appropriated through Congress. Medically necessary and certain psychologically necessary services are covered and are detailed in the U.S. Department of Defense directive (Kongstvedt, 2003). Benefits under Tricare are equivalent to high-option plans of the public sector.

Because of Tricare's historical generosity to its members, expenditures and claims have doubled since 1985. Reform initiatives are changing the face of Tricare, and now some Tricare programs strongly resemble HMOs and PPOs; like Medicare, they reimburse hospitals at a DRG rate. Tricare reform has created two major channels:

1. *The indemnity option*: TRICARE standard is most expensive to the beneficiary but provides the most freedom.
2. *The managed care options*: TRICARE Extra (the PPO option) and TRICARE Prime (the HMO option).

▶ Workers' Compensation

Workers' compensation laws began in 1908 by federal statute. The first state to enact the law was New York in 1914, in response to a factory fire in which 146 women died. Mississippi was the last state to enact the law, doing so in 1950. Workers' compensation is compulsory in most states and is designed to provide compensation and medical benefits if an employee is hurt or becomes disabled while on the job. Workers' compensation laws and programs have been implemented not only in all states, but in US territories as well.

Three types of benefits are provided, although the scope is mandated by individual states.

1. Indemnity cash benefits in lieu of lost wages
2. Reimbursement for necessary medical and vocational rehabilitation expenses
3. Survivors' death benefits.

Workers' compensation, like all facets of the healthcare industry, is a victim of a system out of control. In 1992, workers' compensation claims reached an estimated $70 billion people, which is triple the benefit figure of 1980 (InterQual Inc., 1993). In 2000, compensation programs incurred costs in claims for 126.5 million workers (National Academy of Social Insurance, 2002). It is reported that, on average, each claim costs about $19,000. To offset the spiraling costs, recent changes have been implemented, including adaptations of PPOs, HMOs, hospital utilization review, and case management. These types of managed care modalities are growing rapidly; they have already proven effective in reducing LOS and even avoiding medically unnecessary acute care admissions.

Workers' compensation claims frequently involve trauma, repetitive motion, or neuromuscular impairment. There is a growing trend toward alleged soft tissue claims with nonspecific diagnoses. These claims pose a challenge from the utilization review perspective because they often lack objective physical findings. From a patient advocate perspective, an admitting diagnosis of severe back pain (especially without positive test results) often opens up these patients to denials of insurance-covered hospitalizations and even judgmental attitudes among hospital staff. Yet, as healthcare providers such as nurses (who are especially prone to back injuries) know, the most painful sprains, muscle spasms, and pinched nerves do not show up on scans, but can lead to inability to work and frequent reinjuries. Often the patient needs reassurance that care is necessary and that it can be provided for at a different level of care (i.e., it does not always need to be done in the hospital). The primary goal of workers' compensation is for the patient to return to work.

▶ Indemnity Plans

Indemnity plans are the traditional plans used before the days of managed care. Although they now use some managed care concepts such as prehospital certification and catastrophic case management, indemnity plans still offer the most flexibility (Kongstvedt, 2003); virtually any hospital or doctor can be chosen by the member. Monthly premiums are generally higher for this freedom, and other out-of-pocket expenses may include deductibles and a percentage of the bills (usually 20%) up to a ceiling of $500 to $5,000 per year. As with all insurance companies, the case manager needs to know the specific types of allowable coverage and possible patient costs to formulate a workable discharge plan. Indemnity plans often cover behavioral health and alcohol and drug detoxification treatment, both inpatient and outpatient, within certain limited time frames and dollar amounts. Indemnity plans, by their very nature, do not require tight control of utilization. In fact, the incentive may be to use up services and resources; it is this type of insurance planning that has been blamed for the necessity for managed care.

▶ Managed Indemnity Plans

As an evolution of the old indemnity plans, managed indemnity plans use utilization management strategies such as hospital preadmission screening, authorization for services to be rendered, concurrent review, second surgical opinions, outpatient procedure services review, and case management. They keep the traditional indemnity approach of members' freedom of choice of physicians/providers and fee-for-service payment to these providers.

▶ Managed Care Organization

Managed care organization (MCO) is a generic term that applies to managed care health plans. These plans have programs that include utilization management modalities: authorization for services, preadmission, concurrent and retrospective review programs, case management, referral management, utilization reporting and evaluation programs, and provider incentive programs. MCOs also focus on quality assurance activities, such as credentialing, quality assessment studies, and peer review. The evolution of healthcare is toward some variation of MCO, such as HMOs, PPOs, and POS plans (Kongstvedt, 2003).

▶ Health Maintenance Organizations

In its purest form, an HMO is nearly synonymous with managed care; a member must go through the chosen PCP who acts as a gatekeeper for any needed services (Kongstvedt, 2003). Only HMO-contracted facilities and physicians are allowed. Members who use unauthorized physicians or facilities are usually placing themselves at risk for being required to pay for services rendered. Limited psychiatric and dental care and limited coverage when traveling are other disadvantages.

HMOs have potentially the least expensive premiums, often with no or low deductibles, coinsurance, or claim forms. Some copayments at the time of service may be expected. Physicians and other healthcare professionals are paid for through capitation, thereby sharing the risk of financing the healthcare services for the enrolled population. If the provider incurs expenses exceeding budgeted cost, they would be required to absorb those excesses and not the member.

HEALTH MAINTENANCE ORGANIZATION MODELS

There are five models of HMOs: staff model, group model, independent practice association (IPA), network model, and the direct contract model. The relationship between the HMO and the physicians distinguishes the various models.

1. *Staff model*: In this model, the HMO employs the physicians who work in HMO clinic-type settings (exclusively) for salaries. This model is considered the most cost-effective but also the most restrictive.
2. *Group model*: Here, the HMO contracts with multispecialty physician groups. These groups provide all services to the HMO's members. The members' choice of providers is wider in this model.
3. *IPA*: IPA model HMOs recruit physicians from the various specialties to care for their HMO members. These physicians are contracted by the IPA and are also free to service non-HMO patients, if desired. The IPA is paid on a capitation (per member per month) basis by the HMO, and the physicians are in turn paid in either a fee-for-service or capitated manner.
4. *Network model*: This model combines elements of the staff, group, and IPA styles. The HMO contracts with more than one group practice. The group practices tend to be located in various locations to allow access to services in the various regions where the members reside.
5. *Direct contract model*: In this model, the HMO contracts directly with the physician, rather than through an intermediary such as an IPA. The gatekeeper approach is common in this model. Fee-for-service or capitation is the reimbursement method, although capitation is the preferred method because it limits financial risk for the HMO and places it on the care provider side. The physicians are free to care for other non-HMO individuals.

PRIMARY CARE PROVIDER/PHYSICIAN

The PCP is the main physician assigned to a member of a healthcare insurance plan. This physician tends to be a generalist, a family practitioner, or a pediatrician. HMO-style insurance companies use PCPs in a gatekeeper role (see in the following paragraphs). Members of these types of health plans are expected to go through the PCP before accessing other providers of care such as specialists; that is, require a referral from the PCP.

SPECIALIST CARE PROVIDER

The specialist care provider (SCP) is a physician specializing in a particular area of healthcare such as cardiology, digestive diseases, infectious diseases, or neurology. Health insurance plan members may not be able to access the SCP without a referral from the PCP.

GATEKEEPER

The gatekeeper concept is an important one in the world of managed care. *Gatekeeper* is an informal term used to define the role of the PCP. Essentially, the PCP stands at the gate of available medical services and decides which services each member requires. The gatekeeper is responsible for the basic medical care of the patient and also determines when that member needs laboratory tests, radiographs, a specialist, or virtually anything medicine has to offer, including referral to an SCP. True emergencies are excluded when members may be served in emergency departments. The gatekeeper concept is a predominant characteristic of HMOs.

Although the gatekeeper concept can be an excellent method to manage escalating healthcare costs, it can also become a barrier to access of specialty services. Depending on a physician's practice pattern and financial incentives, the PCP may under-refer or over-refer to various specialists or services.

▶ Preferred Provider Organizations/ Preferred Provider Arrangements

The PPO/Preferred Provider Arrangement (PPA) model falls somewhere between an HMO and an indemnity insurance plan. PPOs use a preferred panel of physicians who have been selected because of their cost-efficient and quality care (Kongstvedt, 2003). The member has a monthly premium, a deductible, and often a 10% to 20% coinsurance up to a specific ceiling of about $500 to $2,000 per year. The premium is higher than that in HMO arrangements. A major advantage for some members is the ability to use physicians who are not in the plan (referred to as out-of-network), but reimbursement is at a lower rate (i.e., more out-of-pocket for the member). This is important to some people who hesitate to choose an HMO because HMOs do not pay at all if outside facilities or physicians are used. In many PPOs, members are encouraged, but not obligated, to use the gatekeeper PCP concept. Medicare beneficiaries are being offered HMO and PPO options. Medicare pays more for contracted providers; however, noncontracted providers may be used, although a higher out-of-pocket expense is incurred.

▶ Point-of-Service

POS plans combine elements of an HMO model and an indemnity insurance plan. The member does not have to choose how to receive services up front; when a service is needed, the member may choose to stay in the plan or use outside providers (Kongstvedt, 2003). Significant differences in out-of-pocket expenses for the member may apply (e.g., 100% compared with 60%). The physicians may be reimbursed through capitation or performance-based methods and may act as gatekeepers. POS plans were hybrids of HMOs mainly in response to a market that clearly wanted freedom of choice to pick a well-known specialist if the need should arise.

▶ Provider-Sponsored Organizations

PSOs are a form of managed care and are similar to HMOs. The difference is that PSOs are formed by a group of hospitals and physicians who directly take on the financial risk of providing comprehensive health benefits for Medicare (and other) beneficiaries. These types of arrangements are less common today than in the 1990s.

▶ Private Fee-for-Service (PFFS)

PFFS is an option for Medicare beneficiaries established in 1999. Beneficiaries may elect a private indemnity-type insurance plan. The insurance plan, rather than the Medicare program, decides how much to reimburse for services provided. Medicare pays the private plan a premium to cover traditional Medicare benefits. Providers are allowed to bill beyond what the plan pays (up to a limit), and the beneficiary is responsible for paying whatever the plan does not cover. The beneficiary may also be responsible for additional premiums.

▶ Physician Hospital Organizations

The Physician Hospital Organization (PHO) model bonds a hospital with the attending physician staff for the purpose of linking with a managed care plan (Kongstvedt, 2003). Like IPAs, PHOs have their own internal political structure and therefore can define on their own terms what is high quality or cost-effective. Some PHOs use outside utilization review firms; such arrangements allow some degree of objectivity. Like PSOs, PHOs were more popular in the 1990s.

▶ Medical Savings Accounts

In the late 1990s, the U.S. Congress authorized up to 390,000 Medicare beneficiaries to participate in an MSA demonstration project. This option is not as popular today. The plan works in the following manner: The beneficiary chooses a Medicare MSA plan—a health insurance policy with a high deductible. Medicare pays the premium for the MSA plan and makes a deposit into the Medicare MSA that is established by the beneficiary. The beneficiary uses the money in the Medicare MSA to pay for services provided before the deductible is met and for other services not covered by the MSA plan. Unlike other Medicare plans, there are no limits on what providers can charge above the amount paid by the Medicare MSA plan. In addition, individuals who enroll in MSAs are locked in for the entire year.

Long-Term Care

In some ways, LTC has become one of the biggest challenges for the case manager. Although an increasing number of people are buying private LTC insurance policies, and most states have coverage for poor, chronically ill patients, there are often waiting periods of up to 3 months for all the paperwork to be approved and placement of an individual in LTC facilities to commence. Sometimes families can manage in the interim. Often, this is a time of frequent readmissions into the acute care setting. Medicare, Medicaid, and most private health insurance plans will pay for short stays in a nursing home for skilled care. A case manager can assess patients for a possible need of greater than 3 weeks of nursing home care or for a probable deterioration of the patient's condition with little chance of recovery. It is vital to start LTC paperwork quickly; early, careful assessment of postdischarge needs (sometimes with a "plan B" in mind) is also essential. Custodial care needs, as well as skilled needs, are assessed. Many LTC programs have home-based and SNF-based support. Family support and available respite can be assessed for possible home-based LTC placement. A case manager who is familiar with the eligibility requirements and enrollment process of their state's LTC program will be better prepared to meet such challenging situations. Display 3-8 lists two helpful resources for the patient and the family.

Some types of private LTC insurance policies are referred to as "tax qualified long-term care insurance contracts." They provide federal income tax advantages. Patients should contact their state insurance counseling office and tax advisor if considering one of these policies. Another consideration is that not all nursing facilities accept all types of contracts. The contract must be matched to the desired placement.

SUGGESTED RESOURCES FOR LONG-TERM CARE AND NURSING HOME PLACEMENTS

display 3-8

Two good resources for long-term care and nursing home placement are
A Shopper's Guide to Long-Term Care Insurance
National Association of Insurance Commissioners (NAIC)
120 W. 12th Street, Suite 1100
Kansas City, MO 64105-1925

Guide to Choosing a Nursing Home
Centers for Medicare & Medicaid Services
Medicare Hotline: (800) 638-6833

Other Weird Arrangement

The acronym OWA (for other weird arrangement) applies to any new, nonconforming, or hybrid managed care plan that provides a new twist (Kongstvedt, 2003).

Self-Funded Employer Health Insurance Plans

In 1974, the Employee Retirement Income Security Act (ERISA) created laws that govern the health insurance plans of employees. The intent was that when a large employer or union group crossed state lines, they would not have to comply with conflicting individual state laws; rather, ERISA laws would apply. For example, ERISA plans cannot be forced to comply with various state rules that cover COB; they must comply with federal regulations instead.

In self-funded plans, the organization often hires a third-party administrator to handle claims, utilization management, and case management activities. Claims are often handled by a separate company than the one handling utilization of services and case management. This lends an extra level of protection to the employees, with the independent opinion of the utilization and case managers. These independent utilization/case management firms hire and train expert personnel and retain large panels of specialists for second opinions, determinations of medical necessity in tough circumstances, and during the appeals process. Case managers may also be internally hired by the self-funded plan; however, if the employee is well known to the company, the element of objectivity may be threatened. Self-funded plans usually have stop loss carriers that protect the fund in catastrophic cases. These stop loss amounts can range from $25,000 to $100,000 or more depending on the fund amount, number of employers, past claims, and other factors.

Viatical Settlements

Viatical settlements, or living benefits, are not classified as health insurance products. Rather, they involve selling one's life insurance policy to a third party before one's death. The funds can then be used to improve the quality of the last weeks, months, or even years of the individual's life. This process can be better explained by an example.

Mr A had a rare type of aggressive cancer and a rare type of health insurance coverage, whereby he must work at least 30 hours per week or lose his benefits. Another option would be to pay approximately $370 per month for continued coverage. His financial situation did not allow Mr A the luxury of quitting work; his basic food and rent needs would not be met, and he certainly did not have an extra $370 per month. But in hospice care, he continued to go to work and put in 30 hours per week. There came a time when he was so weak and exhausted that family and friends had to drive him to and from his job. His last days were being spent working to pay bills and continue to qualify for health insurance coverage. He had a small life insurance policy that was sold as a viatical settlement; that act helped him to die with dignity.

Viatical settlements allow the policy holder, rather than the beneficiary(ies), to benefit from life insurance policies. The term comes from the Latin word, *viaticum*, which means "provisions for a journey." To *viaticate* means to sell a life insurance policy; the *viator* is the seller of the policy. There are some serious considerations that case managers should be aware of if viatical settlements are a potential option for a patient.

- ▶ When the seller of the policy accepts an offer, all persons listed as beneficiaries must sign a release to waive any current and future rights to the policy. In reality, there are obvious reasons that this may be a touchy subject, ranging from greed to need.
- ▶ Viatical settlements take at least 4 to 6 weeks for completion. There must be time or the effort will be wasted.
- ▶ There may be tax ramifications. The Health Insurance Portability and Accountability Act (HIPAA) of 1996 allows that individuals with a life expectancy of 24 months or less can sell their life insurance policy tax free if the viatical settlement company complies with specific licensing and regulatory requirements; however, the settlement may be subject to state and local taxes.
- ▶ Additional funds can sometimes jeopardize the patient's current assistance, such as Medicaid or other public assistance programs. The settlement may cause the patient to lose important benefits.
- ▶ The policy is usually sold for between 40% and 90% of the face value, depending on several circumstances. Life expectancy is the main issue; if a patient is expected to live for less than 6 months, the settlement will be closer to the 90% range.
- ▶ The case manager should suggest a financial planner for assistance. There are often other options such as accelerated death benefits on selected plans.
- ▶ Not all states have licensing requirements at this time for viatical settlement companies. The case manager should call the Viatical Association of America or the National Viatical Association for licensed companies (Display 3-9).
- ▶ Some policies contain a rescission clause of 15 to 30 days, to allow for a change of mind.

▶ INSURANCE PLAYERS

▶ Third-Party Payor

Third-party payor is any organization, public or private, that pays or insures health or medical expenses on behalf of beneficiaries or recipients of such services. This is usually

---

display 3-9

VIATICAL SETTLEMENT RESOURCES

Viatical Association of America
1200 19th Street, NW—Suite 300
Washington, DC 20036
Telephone: (800) 842-9811 or (202) 429-5129
Web site: www.viatical.org\viatical

National Viatical Association
1200 G Street, NW—Suite 760
Washington, DC 20005
Telephone: (800) 741-9465
Fax: (202) 393-0336
Web site: www.nationalviatical.org

---

a private insurance carrier, prepayment plan, employer, or government agency, for example, commercial health insurance companies, Medicare, and Medicaid.

A person generally pays a premium to the insurance company (the payor) for coverage; the company then pays the claims (bills) on the insured's behalf. These payments are called third-party payments; they separate the individual receiving the service (the first party) from the individual or institution providing it (the provider of care, the second party) and the organization paying for it (the third party).

In this arrangement, the two primary parties are the patient/recipient of care and the provider. The third party is the payor of the medical care that is provided to the patient.

▶ Claims Administrators

This group reviews insurance claims to determine whether to pay claims to enrollees, physicians, hospitals, or others on behalf of the health benefit plan. Many case managers must work with claims personnel to determine what benefits a patient is allowed and how much of the benefit the patient has used. However, claims data are usually not current, so the case manager may get only a general idea of how much of the benefit has been exhausted.

▶ Reinsurance/Stop-Loss Personnel

Case managers may work with carriers for reinsurance (previously discussed in this chapter). Experience has determined that once a patient reaches stop loss, some companies want the stop-loss carrier case manager to take over the case. However, this is not always the situation, especially if the current case manager has a good relationship with the patient/family and especially if there may be legal ramifications in the case. Understanding of the procedures of stop-loss insurance by the case manager is essential for effective management of benefits and coordination of care and services.

▶ Employer Groups

When an employer group self-funds its insurance benefits, the case manager may be working with a benefits specialist in the group. This contact is crucial for the case manager, as everything from authorization for case management services to special benefits may be obtained through this person. One other "level" of contact may be the health-care consultant that the employer group uses to develop the self-funded plan. For very tough situations, the case manager may have to go "all the way up" to the consultant for answers. These people may, in turn, have to consult the company's board for the answer.

▶ BILLING-RELATED TERMS

▶ Current Procedural Terminology

CPT codes list procedures and services and differentiate them with a five-digit number. These codes function as a record of physician utilization practices by HMOs (and other insurance companies/benefit programs) and are useful for billing purposes. The American Medical Association revises and publishes CPT annually.

▶ International Classification of Diseases

International Classification of Diseases, 9th Revision—*Clinical Modifications* (*ICD-9*) (formerly called *ICD-9-CM*) and *ICD-10* (10th Revision) are the most widely used classifications of diseases in the world. These alphanumeric codes are used by hospitals and other providers when reporting diagnostic and treatment information about members of federally funded programs such as Medicare, Medicaid, and Maternal and Child Health. All third-party payors are required to submit ICD codes for billing purposes. When a claim is submitted, it usually includes primary and secondary *ICD-10* codes reflective of diagnostic and treatment categories/procedures.

▶ Fee Schedule

A fee schedule consists of a listing of fee allowances for specific procedures or services that a health insurance plan will reimburse.

▶ Global Fee

Global fee is a predetermined all-inclusive fee for a specific set of related services, treated as a single unit for billing or reimbursement purposes.

▶ Withhold

Withhold is a portion of payments to a provider held by the managed care company until year end. This amount is not returned to the provider unless certain targets are achieved. Typically, withhold is used by managed care companies to curtail costs such as utilization of services rates including referrals to SCPs, use of ancillary services (e.g., lab and radiology expenses), and emergency department visits.

▶ IMPORTANT MISCELLANEOUS ORGANIZATIONS AND TERMS

▶ The Joint Commission

The Joint Commission (TJC), formerly known as the Joint Commission on Accreditation of Healthcare Organizations, is a private organization founded in 1951. It establishes quality standards and surveys healthcare organizations of various types, including hospitals, nursing homes, home care agencies, and other outpatient facilities to accredit the facilities. Accredited facilities are deemed to meet the U.S. Department of Health and Human Services certification requirements. It is hoped that the accreditation process encourages the facility to maintain the highest quality, safety, and performance levels. TJC accreditation is necessary for hospitals and other facilities to be eligible to receive reimbursement from Medicare and other health insurance plans.

▶ Grievance

Grievance is a term that refers to the complaint process that can occur when an adverse action, outcome, decision, or health insurance policy is challenged. A member can file a grievance for any number of reasons, such as a physician complaint, denial of a medical claim or service, denial of a piece of equipment, or a poor hospital outcome. A hospital or other facility may file a grievance for a denial of a claim it felt was medically justified.

▶ Management Information System

Management information system is the computer term for hardware and software that provides support for managing health insurance plans, including case management.

▶ Office of Prepaid Health Care Operations and Oversight

The Office of Prepaid Health Care Operations and Oversight, a federal agency that is part of the CMS, oversees eligibility and compliance of HMOs and competitive medical plans.

▶ Clinical Data Abstraction Centers

Clinical data abstraction centers are data collection firms contracted by the CMS. These centers are expected to collect clinical data from medical record reviews of a large national sample of patients' records; millions of records are reviewed. The data gathered are then analyzed by the Medicare QIOs to identify areas of care for quality improvement projects.

▶ Notch Group

The term *notch group* refers to the portion of the US population whose annual income is too low to afford medical insurance premiums but too high to be eligible for Medicaid programs. This concept seems innocuous enough, but a staggering statistic is attached to it: according to the Census Bureau in 2007, more than 45 million Americans are uninsured. This number has decreased by half because of the Patient Protection and Affordable Care Act of 2010.

▶ Days per Thousand

Days per thousand is a measurement that states the average number of hospital days used per year by 1,000 members each (Kongstvedt, 2003). This is commonly used by health insurance companies. This is a measure of healthcare utilization that MCOs tend to track over time. Other measures include average cost per case and average number of visits to the emergency department per 1,000 members.

▶ MANAGED CARE CONTRACTS

Healthcare providers (individuals and organizations) have been engaging in MCCs since the inception of MCOs. The impetus for establishing a MCC may originate from either the MCO or the provider. Such arrangements assist the MCO in reducing the costs of healthcare services and the provider in securing new or maintaining old business. Issues that are negotiated in an MCC are numerous. Display 3-10 lists the major issues that are discussed and agreed upon in the contract. Some of these issues have a direct impact on the provider's case management program, including the role of the case manager; others impact the MCO's case management program, including utilization management, and the payor-based case manager.

The team involved in negotiating an MCC consists of representatives from both sides: the provider and the MCO. These include senior administrators/executives, finance, case management, quality, accounts payable, marketing, and legal counsel. Some organizations include clinicians on an ad hoc basis; others may exclude case management. In any case, consulting with clinicians and including case management as a permanent member of the negotiation team is essential, especially because most of the procedures to be agreed upon impact the role of the case manager. Examples are utilization review and management procedures, notification of services, and denials and appeals management processes. Clinicians' feedback on the scope of services being agreed upon in the MCC

---

display 3-10

GENERAL ISSUES FOR NEGOTIATION IN A MANAGED CARE CONTRACT

1. Scope of services to be provided to the covered population/enrollees
2. Services to be excluded or carved out from the contract
3. Agreements with other providers, especially those across the continuum of care and settings
4. Payment methodology (e.g., capitation, case rate, discounted rate) and reimbursement rates including withhold and incentives
5. Administrative procedures such as notification of admission to the hospital, submission of reports
6. Claims filing and management process
7. Marketing arrangements
8. Legal issues such as settlement of disputes
9. Denials and appeal rights and procedures for handling these
10. Utilization review and management procedures including referrals and areas of noncoverage
11. Quality management and reporting procedures
12. Incentives, if any and criteria for such.

---

is also important to make sure that the provider will be able to meet the scope of service expectations and that what is agreed upon does not place the provider at risk for noncompliance or any cost inefficiencies. Examples of issues that impact the practice of clinicians are the pattern of referrals by primary care providers to SCPs and noncoverage of certain treatments or procedures. A rule of thumb for the effective management of MCCs is "approach the negotiation as a system; that is, include representatives from administration, finance, patient financial services, quality, and clinicians."

During the negotiation period (usually occurring over a series of meetings) both parties share important information about themselves. This exchange of information tends to be covered under HIPAA agreements. Privacy and confidentiality are maintained and an HIPAA agreement is executed before such exchange takes place. Information the provider of care shares includes a general description of the organization, availability and type of services, costs of care, discharge planning, utilization review and case management procedures, staffing, and quality of care and patient safety programs.

Information shared by the MCO also includes a description of the organization, the number of the enrollees or covered lives (the population being contracted), demographics of the population and its historical healthcare utilization data, costs of care, desired goals of the MCC, utilization review procedures including denials and appeals processes, reimbursement arrangement, and measures of quality of care. Once the exchange of information has occurred, negotiation commences. During the negotiation process, issues are identified, prioritized, and discussed, and resolutions are achieved.

▶ Implications for Case Management Practice

There are certain areas in the MCC that have a direct impact on the case management department or program, case management staff, and the role of the case manager. These include the scope of services to be provided to the population, agreements with other providers across the continuum of care and settings, utilization review procedures including denials and appeals, compensation for case management services, and quality/outcomes measurement and reporting. These issues have a great impact on the daily operations of case managers. For example, knowing the services to be furnished to the covered lives informs the case manager whether outpatient and ancillary services are included and allows him or her to manage the follow-up visits and cost of services more effectively.

Arrangements with other providers across the continuum of care provides the case manager with information about how to manage referrals between one provider and another and how to arrange for posthospital discharge services (e.g., home care, rehabilitation, and transportation services). Lack of such arrangements may impact negatively on the provider's performance; that is, the provider may incur increased costs because of prolonged length of hospital stay and overutilization of acute care services.

Information about the utilization review procedures allows the case manager to better meet the MCO's expectations in the areas of preadmission reviews, authorization of services, concurrent and care progress reviews, and the appeal process in case of denial of services. Compensation for case management services, if offered, helps the provider to offset the expense needed to enhance its case management program to meet the demands of the negotiated MCC. Not every MCO or MCC offers compensation for case management services. If offered, it is usually a specific amount per month, calculated on the basis of the size of the population.

In the area of quality and outcomes measurement, knowledge of the metrics the MCO uses to measure the provider's performance is important for proactive management of these outcomes. Some of these metrics may directly impact the role of the case manager. For example, timeliness of preadmission reviews, authorization of services, referral patterns, and members' experience of care are measures the case managers can impact greatly and influence not only adherence to procedures, but achievement of desired performance as well.

Every MCC includes provisions and stipulations that impact the role of the case manager, including decision making (whether clinical or operations in nature) and daily case management activities (whether utilization review or resource allocation related). Involving the case management department in contract negotiation allows a provider to negotiate a more desirable contract, reduce risk, and increase its chances to meet the demands of the contract successfully. After all, the case manager is the key member in an organization that will allow the provider organization to meet the demands of the negotiated contract.

▶ THE FUTURE

Future changes to the face of healthcare leave the possibility of wide revisions on many types of medical insurance. Even Medicare—almost a part of American tradition —is dramatically changing in an effort to lower its budget and expenses. Many visions of future healthcare have been proposed. Although the first major attempt at national health reform in the 1990s was unsuccessful, one thing is certain: the cost of healthcare is high and rising rapidly, and change is still sorely needed to cover the needs of millions of uninsured Americans. Although certain improvements such as reduction of the uninsured by over 20 million individuals have been achieved since the enactment of the Patient Protection and Affordable Care Act (PPACA) in 2010, the future of this act is uncertain. Repealing this act has been in progress at the time this textbook was being revised. The question remains, what will exactly happen to the PPACA? The crystal ball has not revealed the final answer, but one probability looms large: that case managers, in grassroots fashion and on a case-by-case basis, will continue to make an impact on the high cost of health services and to help ensure quality, cost-effective care in the bargain.

DISCUSSION QUESTIONS

1. What health insurance plan do you personally have? What type is it? How does it compare to those cited in this chapter?

2. How do Medicare and Medicaid benefits compare and contrast?

3. How many reimbursement structures for healthcare services are there? What are they? Are they available in every state? Which one presents more risk for the payor? For the provider? For the patient?

4. Is a Medicare beneficiary better off enrolling in a MAP or in a Medigap plan? What are some of the reasons for your decision?

5. Under what circumstances should someone be advised to switch his or her Medigap policy?

6. What do you think of the withhold concept? Who benefits the most from it? How does it affect the consumer of healthcare services?

7. What can a case manager do to assist a patient in understanding his or her health benefits?

8. What role can a case manager play in effectively implementing the MCC in which the healthcare institution is participating? What is the rationale of each of these activities?

▶ **REFERENCES**

Centers for Medicare & Medicaid Services. (2017). *Medicare and you 2017.* Baltimore, MD: Author.

InterQual Inc. (1993). *Utilization review and management training manual.* North Hampton, NH: Author.

Kongstvedt, P. R. (2003). *Essentials of managed health care* (4th ed.) Gaithersburg, MD: Aspen Publishers.

National Academy of Social Insurance. (2002). *Workers' compensation benefits, costs, and coverage, 2000 new estimates.* Retrieved from, www.nasi.org.

Saue, J. M. (1988, August). Legal issues related to case management. *Quality Review Bulletin, 14*(8), 239–244.

Williams, S., & Torrens, P. R. (1993). *Introduction to health services.* New York, NY: Delmar.

PART 2

The Case Management Process and Related Activities

"You ought not attempt to cure the eyes without the head, or the head without body; so you should not treat body without soul."

SOCRATES

CHAPTER 4

The Case Management Process

"Don't prepare patients for discharge; prepare patients for self-management success."

LEARNING OBJECTIVES

Upon completion of this chapter, the reader will be able to:

1. Describe each stage of the case management process.
2. List five criteria that qualify a patient for case management services.
3. Determine the essential components of a case management assessment.
4. Develop a case management plan of care, including establishing goals and prioritizing needs.
5. Describe four strategies that ensure effective implementation of the case management plan of care.
6. Recognize the importance of ongoing monitoring and evaluation of the case management plan of care.
7. Identify three strategies for effective closure of case management services.
8. Describe how the Medicare Conditions of Participation (CoP) infuse every stage of the case management process.

ESSENTIAL TERMS

Alternative Therapies • Assessment • Care Planning • Case Closure • Case Evaluation • Case Management Assessment • Case Management Outcomes • Case Management Process • Case Plan Goals • Case Screening • Case Selection • Continuous Monitoring • Criteria for Case Management Services • Cultural Diversity • Current Medical Status • External Case Management • Financial Assessment • Functional Assessment • Home Environment Assessment • Implementation • Internal Case Management • Medicare Conditions of Participation (CoP) • Medication Assessment • Nutrition Assessment • Potential Problems • Psychosocial Assessment • Reassessment • Screening • Service Planning • Socioeconomic Indicators

▶ INTRODUCTION TO THE CASE MANAGEMENT PROCESS

This chapter discusses the direction and activities needed to guide a patient and family through the complex healthcare maze. Nurses will find the process familiar, because it uses some of the same components as those of the nursing process: assessment, planning, implementation, monitoring, and evaluation. The focus, however, is much broader in case management. In the nursing process, the nurse assesses a patient for changing physical, medical, psychosocial, and safety needs on a shift-by-shift basis as compared with the plan of care. In case management, however, the case manager must also assess the patient's condition before the current illness or event, determine whether his or her environment (physical and social network) will continue to meet present needs, investigate how the needs will be met financially, and then plan future care. Additionally,

during this process the case manager also considers the patient's health insurance plan and benefits and contrasts them with the needed plan of care. Therefore, the steps may be slightly reordered, new ones added, and the emphasis and purposes altered.

This reordering and altering may also apply when considering different types of case management programs and care settings. Case selection is often based on facility or Medicare and other health insurance–related data, and newer techniques have been evolving in the past 10 years, such as "predictive modeling." Case selection for a hospital case manager may be filtered through the institution's admissions and utilization management and/or denial management processes. An independent case manager may receive referrals from a variety of sources such as physicians, insurance companies, employers, and private citizens. Other case managers may select cases according to a predetermined specialty or condition such as spinal cord injuries, asthma, heart failure, AIDS, or cerebral palsy. The monitoring component may be done less frequently for a case manager with patients in private homes or in sheltered care than for a hospital case manager, who may have to monitor patients more frequently.

Follow-up and termination of case management services will depend, in part, on the type of case management work or practice setting. Some hospital case managers are finished with a case at the time of a patient's discharge. Others perform posthospital follow-up for a brief time. Hospice case managers may assess their patients in the home or hospital, but they do not actively take on the case until patients are formally "admitted" to hospice care; this may occur when the patient arrives home or at a skilled facility after discharge or if the patient becomes a hospice candidate while using home health services. Hospice case managers may follow up on the patient until death. Still other case managers follow up on their patients in whatever care and service setting the patients' health conditions warrant.

Responsibilities are also different in various case management positions. Independent case managers and case managers who work outside institutional settings (referred to as outside-the-walls case management) must often obtain signed consents for case management services from the payors or for release of information or medical records. Negotiation and cost-benefit evaluation are daily activities. Reports to consultants and health insurance claims managers are different from the facility-based documentation that internal case managers (referred to as within-the-walls case management) must provide. Health insurance case managers may have varied duties, also depending on where the patient or member is located. For example, Medicaid case managers rely on hospital personnel and other sources for much of the assessment information, especially for medical and psychosocial aspects. They often work closely with hospital or skilled nursing facility (SNF) transitional planners, case managers, and social workers to fulfill a safe and timely discharge or transfer.

Generally speaking, the stages of the case management process are the same regardless of the healthcare provision setting (e.g., outpatient, acute, or rehabilitation), case manager's practice setting (hospital, disease management, health insurance), or type of professional who assumes the case manager's role (e.g., nurse, social worker, rehabilitation counselor).

▶ STAGES OF THE CASE MANAGEMENT PROCESS

Each patient is unique and case management styles are individual; therefore, case management is a personalized process in every case. However, it must be noted that the

case management process is carried out within the ethical and legal realms of a case manager's scope of practice, using critical thinking and evidence-based knowledge. "Note that the case management process is cyclical and recurrent, rather than linear and unidirectional. For example, key functions of the professional case manager, such as communication, facilitation, coordination, collaboration, and advocacy, occur throughout all the steps of the case management process and in constant contact with the client [/patient], client's family or family caregiver, and other members of the inter-professional health care team" (Case Management Society of America [CMSA], 2017, p. 18).

Taking this into consideration, the process discussed in this chapter should be used as a guideline: the skills and creativity of each case manager are still the essential ingredients. In general, the case management process involves the following stages:

1. Case/patient identification, selection, and engagement in case management
2. Assessment and identification of potential issues
3. Development and coordination of the plan of care
4. Implementation and coordination of the plan of care
5. Evaluation and follow-up
6. Continuous monitoring, reassessment, and reevaluation
7. Case closure and termination of case management services
8. Communication with the patient/family postclosure of the process.

As mentioned earlier, different styles and settings of case management lend themselves to different processes. As a rule of thumb, the stages of Assessment/Problem Identification, Development and Coordination of the Care Plan, and Continuous Monitoring, Reassessment, and Reevaluation have many universal principles that may apply to several types of case management. However, other stages may vary significantly in different case management settings. Case Selection is different for a medical case manager in an acute care setting than for a disease-specific case manager. A disease-specific case manager may provide services only to a patient population centered around one diagnosis; within that diagnosis, the case manager must prioritize those who need more or less intense case management services. In other words, the amount of case management service is dependent on the risk category the patient falls under, such as low, moderate, or high risk, which means simple/limited intensity, moderate intensity, or complex/high intensity case management services. Case managers who work in a provider setting may have functions that are different from those of their counterparts who work in a payor setting. For example, a payor-based case manager may engage in more telephonic triage and utilization management activities, whereas the provider-based case manager may spend more time on activities such as facilitation and coordination of clinical care including treatments, tests, and procedures. This is illustrated in Stage IV: Implementation and coordination of the plan of care. The stage of evaluation and follow-up is also very specific to the type of case management. The rest of this chapter will attempt to consider case management from many perspectives. However, refer to recent journals and magazine articles for information on how other case managers are coping with problems specific to your type of case management.

One issue that will come up with new names and differing opinions is about what and who make up an interdisciplinary care team. In fact, articles and entire chapters have been written about the nuances of definition, and we encourage the reader to review those pages (Treiger & Fink-Samnick, 2016). The bottom line is this: case management practice and the entire case management process depend on knowledge from multiple professionals on each patient situation or case. Patients are becoming more complex as we enter into a bold, new technological age; the brainpower of everyone involved is needed, as are patient care rounds (in whatever terminology you use). They are critical to the best outcome for patients.

▶ STAGE I: CASE IDENTIFICATION, SELECTION, AND PATIENT ENGAGEMENT

Case selection is the "first cut" in the process. Basically, this step weeds out patients who probably will not need case management services; put differently, it means selecting those patients who would benefit most from case management services. Occasionally, one of the patients placed on the "probably not" list will actually need services. A patient's condition can deteriorate or the needs change drastically to the point of needing SNF or acute rehabilitation placement, or, more simply, a piece of durable medical equipment (DME) may become necessary. But don't let the seemingly simplistic need lull you, because regulations, insurance benefits, and high deductibles make even obtaining a humble piece of DME a time-consuming endeavor. Sometimes a quirky hitch arises such as a patient losing a lease or being evicted from an apartment by a roommate during the time of hospitalization. On the other hand, not all those who are put on the "probably" list (i.e., needing case management) will need the same degree of case management services; some may need only a bit of education or a walker for safety purposes. Regardless, all patients need screening for case management services; those patients who are selected need a basic assessment, at the minimum, to determine the type and intensity of the required services.

Universal case management is not necessary. Some patients neither require case management nor benefit from it. Previously healthy people who are admitted for uncomplicated procedures such as hysterectomies,

cholecystectomies, transurethral resection of the prostate (TURP), or an occasional exacerbation of asthma or chronic obstructive pulmonary disease, and who have some social support, usually require little or no posthospital support. In these cases, a mere requirement of short-term home care services postdischarge from the episode of care does not directly amount to a need for case management.

However, a simple ailment in combination with a poor social environment may signal the need for further assessment. Diagnosis or chief complaint alone does not determine whether a patient/family would benefit from case management services. Screening a patient by focusing on the patient/family's total situation (i.e., health condition, financial and insurance status, psychosocial network, availability of community resources, literacy and knowledge, ability for self-care and self-management, and so on) is the best strategy for deciding whether to weed a patient out or to place the patient on the probable or definite list. It is necessary for a case manager to complete such screening as early as possible during a patient's encounter with health care services; indeed, it is a regulatory requirement in some levels of care (for example, upon admission to the hospital) to be screened within 24 hours of admission.

These regulations are spelled out in Medicare's Conditions of Participation (CoP). The CoPs are a set of stringent measures designed to regulate how hospitals and other medical establishments use Medicare aid. Every healthcare facility that receives reimbursement for Medicare-related costs must adhere to the guidelines specified by the Centers for Medicare & Medicaid Services. These rules are published in the Federal Register and stipulate regular inspections of hospitals to ensure that all healthcare facilities follow the guidelines consistently. These regulations also make sure that all patients receive a minimum standard of health service, which is the right of every Medicare Beneficiary (American Case Management Association, 2016).

In general, if a patient meets intensity of services (degree and amount of resources/services required for safe care) and severity of illness (acuity and acuteness of health condition) criteria, but if no major discharge barriers are identified, readmission is not a problem, and there are no financial or psychosocial concerns, then case management may be required only minimally. A case manager may be required only for those patients with moderate-to-complex problems: (1) moderate-to-complex medical conditions and comorbidities, (2) moderate-to-complex transitional care needs, or (3) moderate-to-complex social and financial issues. Other criteria may include risk for deterioration in health condition, experience of untoward events, or presence of ethical and/or legal issues/concerns. Although a comprehensive assessment of the patient is considered Stage II, a cursory assessment must be conducted during case selection to make an accurate "cut" about who may require, and be expected to benefit from, the services of a case manager. Several indicators are commonly used to flag situations that may require case management services. Some indicators, although useful to trigger a case management investigation, warrant careful use. By their very nature, they are intrinsically flawed and may defeat some of the goals of case management, such as early intervention and cost containment. Consider the following common indicators:

▶ Length of stay longer than 5 days (or another arbitrary number)
▶ Charges greater than $50,000 (or another dollar amount).

Both indicators exclude the possibility of early case management. Perhaps with early use of case management services, a patient who is now on hospital day 4 could have been discharged by hospital day 2 or 3. In addition, if this patient requires intensive care needs and resources after discharge, such as a transfer to an extended care facility, it may take an extra day (or more) to plan and implement the discharge or transfer. Such delay could have been prevented if screening had been done early on during the hospital stay. Such delay may also result in a denial to the patient by the health insurance plan of a day or two, with the rationale being unnecessary prolonged length of stay in the acute care setting.

The second indicator (even if the dollar amount is considerably less, such as $10,000) may still pose barriers to the case management process. Again, early case management is precluded. Chances are lost to effect improved utilization and allocation of resources, to establish a productive and beneficial relationship with the patient and family early on during the illness and care encounter, and to steer any variances back on track. There are situations when a patient does not have health insurance and cannot afford self-pay; in such cases, focusing on cost alone without consideration of reimbursement issues may result in a hospital not getting paid at all for services rendered. Perhaps such a patient would meet the criteria for emergency Medicaid. If case management had not been involved from the time of admission to the hospital, it is likely that this patient would have been discharged without having undergone this process at all, hence losing the opportunity to apply for Medicaid benefits and ultimately resulting in "no reimbursement."

Other commonly used indicators are too general to be used on their own merit and warrant secondary screening for possible case management needs. However, to a new case manager, this list of issues could signal a red flag, until he or she develops a good case management knowledge base and acquires the required skills and competencies.

▶ *The patient lives alone (or with someone with a disability)*: A psychosocial assessment would be useful in such a case. If the patient lives alone, is there an informal support system strong enough to match his or her needs? If the patient lives with a disabled or debilitated roommate or family member, can that roommate or family member meet the patient's needs at discharge? Often the patient has been the primary caregiver in the relationship. If so, who is caring for the person left at home?

▶ *The patient is older than 65 years*: People of all ages may need case management services. (Some facilities use age indicators of 70 or 75 years.) Most case managers have discharged "spunky" patients in their 90s. The opposite is also true case managers have cared for fairly young patients being discharged with complex health conditions, needs, and services. On the other hand, as the treatment options for patients with AIDS have advanced, more young men and women are living longer with the disease and need supportive care.

▶ *Payor source*: Some types of health insurance may be clues to possible medical or psychosocial needs such as Medicare disability. Also, patients without any (or with limited) insurance resources may need creative case management for safe transitional planning.

▶ *Readmission within 15 days (or 30 days) for the same problem(s)*: This may be a quality issue or a sign of an inadequate/early or unsafe discharge plan during the previous admission. It could also signal patient nonadherence, such as a patient with congestive heart failure who loves pretzels and pizza or the patient with diabetes who does not check blood sugar levels, take insulin as directed, or follow a diabetic diet.

▶ *Physicians*: Some physicians' practices, such as those of trauma surgeons or geriatric specialists, signal a possible need for case management. Other physicians request the services of case management because of its efficacy and patient satisfaction. Another red-flag indicator may be a patient being cared for by multiple physicians in consultation or in an extensive multidisciplinary team. Here, the case manager can serve as the conductor, ensuring that all the disciplines are involved in time and playing the same song, ultimately integrating the plan of care, ensuring the patient is safe and care is progressing appropriately.

▶ *First-time mothers*: Giving birth to a first child does not automatically mean a need for case management services. An abundance of family support may limit the degree of case management services needed. Ultimately, a quick assessment (screening) of the mother's knowledge, needs, and availability of social support may place the mother and baby on the "weed out" list. In the case of a premature newborn, the story may be very different. Coping with a premature newborn alone or a stillbirth may result in the need for case management services.

▶ *Diagnosis-related group (DRG)*: Not all people with a specific diagnosis require case management services, especially in the early stages of a disease process; educational activities or counseling services may be all that are needed. A medical record review and possibly a patient/family interview or assessment will show the level of independence and severity of illness. All complex medical conditions or psychosocial/financial problems will require some degree of case management intervention.

▶ Psychological Indicators

Certain mental health, behavioral, and substance use conditions warrant, at the very least, a psychosocial assessment. Often, a psychiatric evaluation is also required. The specific case details will guide the case manager to the appropriate referrals. The following are some red-flag indicators.

▶ *Overdose (unintentional)*: Unintentional overdoses of prescription medications can result from a lack of knowledge about correct dosages or inability to properly self-medicate, or as a result of confusion or poor eyesight. Unintentional overdoses can also be of the illegal, polydrug variety.

▶ *Overdose (intentional)*: Suicide gestures always need careful assessment and initiation of proper referrals.

▶ *Alcohol and drug use*: This may present as a primary or secondary cause of admission.

▶ *Eating disorders (e.g., bulimia, anorexia nervosa, "failure to thrive")*: Psychological causes may warrant psychiatric assessments. Conditions such as anorexia and failure to thrive may also have medical causes. Assessment will determine the extent of case management that may be needed.

▶ *Chronic mental illness*: This may include various psychoses, schizophrenia, neurotic disorders, depression, bipolar disorder, and severe anxiety. Is the mental or emotional condition stable enough for the patient to return to previous living arrangements, or is the condition unstable and the patient a danger to self or others?

▶ *Alzheimer's/dementia*: This may include any form of confusion or disorientation, especially if it is a new change.

▶ *Nonadherence*: Frequent readmissions may be an indicator.

▶ *Uncooperative/manipulative/aggressive behaviors*: The perpetrator may be the patient, a family member, a friend, a personal caregiver, or any combination of these. Often, these people create havoc in a case by refusing tests and procedures (delay of diagnosis), "firing" physicians, or making outrageous demands for unnecessary and costly tests (overutilization of resources). Early recognition of potential manipulative behavior and identification of ways to limit these behaviors are necessary.

▶ *Miscellaneous conditions such as Münchhausen syndrome or Münchhausen syndrome by proxy*: The very definition of Münchhausen syndrome lends itself to overutilization of resources because those suffering from this condition intentionally produce symptoms of illness to assume the role of sick people. Münchhausen syndrome by proxy is a form of child abuse in which, for example, the parent (usually the mother) produces illness in the child. This, as in all forms of child abuse, is a reportable event. The extent to which one with Münchhausen syndrome will go to receive medical care can be dramatic and often requires investigative work to make a diagnosis of this syndrome.

▶ Socioeconomic Indicators

Some socioeconomic factors alert the case manager that further screening for case management services is required. High-risk situations, such as reportable events, need immediate and close assessment. The occurrences may include the following:

▶ Suspected child abuse or neglect
▶ Suspected elder abuse or neglect
▶ Violent crime
▶ Domestic violence

Other socioeconomic red flags include:

▶ Homelessness
▶ Poor living environment such as inadequate housing; poor sanitary conditions; and lack of water, electricity, or heat
▶ No known social or familial support systems
▶ Admission from an extended care facility or other sheltered living arrangement
▶ Need for transitional care in an extended care facility or sheltered living arrangement
▶ Out-of-state or out-of-country residence
▶ Residence in rural community where services are poor or nonexistent, thus limiting posthospital follow-up
▶ Limited or no financial resources
▶ No health insurance or inadequate amount of health insurance
▶ Single parent (assessment of care of minors left at home)
▶ Dependent on others for activities of daily living (ADLs).
▶ Repeated admissions to acute care
▶ Frequent visits to the emergency department, family physician, or clinic
▶ Disruptive or obstructive family member or significant other.

Some general clues may reveal possible future problems. Appropriate case management, referrals, and support may make a tremendous difference to the patient's quality of life. Be alert to situations such as the following:

- ▶ Any condition that will necessitate a major life change or a major quality of life change. Will the patient no longer be able to carry out his or her previous type of employment? Can the patient no longer live in his or her home of 40 years? Life changes may also include smaller behavioral changes such as quitting smoking, refraining from drinking alcoholic beverages, or following a strict diet or exercise regimen.
- ▶ Any condition that may negatively affect physical or sexual function or self-image
- ▶ Unrealistic expectations about the prognosis, treatment, or ability to go back home.

With the exception of reportable events, no single condition or diagnosis is automatically a problem that necessitates full case management services. Certainly, those with obvious home health needs or hospitalizations that include any quality or risk management issues need careful attention. The examples that have been provided here serve as guidelines, and many patients meeting these guidelines will need some discharge or transition services. The next step is a thorough assessment.

▶ Patient/Family Engagement in Case Management Services

Case management is implemented differently in different healthcare organizations. When selection criteria are used—and these may range from data-driven predictive modeling techniques to the number of readmissions within a specified time frame—an organization must prospectively determine these criteria and communicate them clearly to all healthcare providers to encourage their use. Case managers must also become familiar with these criteria, apply them when screening patients, and help educate and support fellow members of the healthcare team on their use. Allowing staff to deviate from the use of criteria exclusively for screening and case finding is also important. Sometimes a case manager knows intuitively the importance of providing case management services for certain patients, even though those patients do not meet the selection criteria. Personal judgment is necessary in such situations. Follow-up assessment and monitoring may best determine whether to continue the services.

On completion of the screening and determination that a patient/family would benefit from case management services, it is important for the case manager to inform the patient/family about such a decision. At this time, the case manager explains to the patient/family "what case management is; how it will benefit the patient/family; and what are the expectations." The case manager also describes her/his role in the provision of care and answers questions, if any, from the patient/family. During this exchange, the case manager ensures that the patient and family understand what is expected and verbalize agreement with or declination of provision of case management services. It is important for the case manager to obtain and document such consent, which essentially provides the case manager with the right or duty to advocate on behalf of the patient and family and for what is in their best interest. This will lead to the initiation of a trusting, respectful, and therapeutic patient/family–case manager relationship.

▶ STAGE II: ASSESSMENT AND IDENTIFICATION OF POTENTIAL ISSUES

After the selection process has red flagged a case and the patient/family has consented to case management services, Stage II—Assessment and Identification of Potential Issues—follows. It involves data gathering, analysis, and synthesis of information for the purpose of developing a patient-centric case management plan of care. Unless it is obvious that at this time the patient needs little or no case management services, a thorough and accurate assessment is performed. Assessment determines patient needs and establishes plans that will overcome problems (actual or potential) and move the patient forward. Data collection and analysis focus and direct the case manager to the treatment, interventions, resource utilization, care coordination activities, and transitional plans needed for that individual patient. Potential or actual problems are exposed; goals start taking shape. In this stage, the case manager finds out what gaps need filling, what services are necessary, and what quality of life issues require special focus. All anticipated needs are considered for a transitional plan that will allow the optimal quality of life for that patient.

A lengthy discourse on assessment is contained in this section. The reason a lot of attention is given to it is that assessment is the pivot around which the case management process revolves. Comprehensive assessment of the patient condition and family situation is essential for the planning of quality, safe, and appropriate care. If one misses a sufficiently important condition, event, or circumstance, the whole plan of care, including the transitional plan, becomes unstable. In addition, the allocation of resources may be inappropriate, which ultimately affects the utilization management activities. At best, much confusion results and last-minute changes may be needed, sometimes delaying discharge for 1 or 2 days. A case manager once worked hard to set up a complex discharge, complete with high-tech equipment, only to discover at the last minute that the patient's house had no electricity. This was a troublesome situation and was caused by inattention to details. At worst, an inaccurate or poor assessment can lead to an unsafe discharge plan or follow-up care and a possible lawsuit. A complete and concise evaluation of all data is key to holistic, comprehensive, and individualized management of the patient. Time spent performing a careful in-depth assessment may be time and money saved later. Backtracking and changing plans can be confusing and frustrating for the patient and/or family, leaving them perhaps less than confident with the idea of case management.

There are several sources of assessment information. The patient is the primary contributor of data, which include medical, social, functional, financial, historical, personal preferences, and other types. If the patient is incapable of giving an interview, secondary sources can be used, starting with the patient's closest support system: parents and/or foster parents (especially if the patient is a minor), spouse, significant other, adult children, other family members, close friends, personal caregiver(s), and neighbors. When using surrogate sources for information, it is important to ensure that the plan will incorporate what the patient might desire. For example, case managers and other healthcare providers must incorporate in the plan the wishes and interests the patient and/or family have communicated previously to a healthcare proxy or in an advance directive.

Sources of medical information include the family physician and related office records, hospital and ancillary medical staff, and hospital records (both past and present), any supervisory care staff and related medical records, and home health personnel and related records. Dental, hearing, and vision records may also be helpful. Other types of important data can be gathered from physical, occupational, and speech therapists; social workers and transitional planners; and psychiatric nurses.

The patient's home environment is a crucial place to evaluate for safe transitional planning. Sometimes the insurance company social worker or case manager has visited the patient's home for evaluation purposes and can be asked to share the findings from that review. Other important people who make home visits are therapists, home health nurses, social workers, and psychiatric nurses. They may contribute data needed for a safe discharge plan and follow-up services.

The patient's employer can often be helpful in evaluating the patient's functional capacity before the current illness or event. Care must be taken not to violate confidentialities.

Sometimes in the course of gathering information, conflicting stories are revealed. These contradictions can show up in medical records in which several different physicians are recording medical, social, and functional data. Inconsistencies need further probing. The nature of the incongruity determines the route to clarification. Some contradictions clarify themselves; for example, a patient whose clinical picture is consistent with an alcohol consumption problem may deny such a problem and then experience delirium tremens. In other cases, interviewing the sources of the conflicting

data may be necessary. Care must be taken to avoid adopting an accusatory or confrontational tone during the interview because such an approach makes people defensive and may compromise the quality of the patient/family–case manager relationship. The reason for a contradiction may be a seemingly insignificant typographic or dictating error. If resolution of the conflict is vital to the treatment plan (grandma wants full resuscitation measures, not merely comfort care), a family or even multidisciplinary team conference may be required to sort it out.

A discussion of several assessment categories follows.
Patient's History and Demographics

▶ Note the patient's name, age, ethnic group, address, marital status, children (with ages), employment, languages spoken, educational level, and religion.

▶ Note all medical history, past and present. Most hospital medical records contain a "History and Physical" section. This may or may not be comprehensive. A thorough medical history may include all previous diagnoses, diseases, childhood diseases, serious/chronic illnesses, accidents, injuries, hospitalizations, surgeries, obstetric procedures, and mental illnesses.

▶ Look for complicating factors, chronicity, and comorbidities.

▶ Look at nonadherence issues. They can often be uncovered in the history. Reasons for nonadherence can be explored and hopefully altered. Nonadherence has many causes, some of which can be resolved, such as lack of money for medications and lack of understanding or knowledge about the disease process. Other reasons for nonadherence make behavioral changes more difficult. These reasons can range from burnout caused by the chronicity of a disease to an "I don't care" attitude (sometimes so severe that it appears to be a form of passive suicide).

▶ Note all medications the patient is taking, including over-the-counter drugs, illicit drugs, alcohol, and herbal preparations.

▶ Look at family histories for possible diabetes, cancer, Alzheimer's disease, heart disease, hypertension, epilepsy, sickle cell disease, renal disease, alcoholism, mental illness, and others.

▶ Be aware of allergies: food, drug, and environmental.

▶ Evaluate how your patient uses care facilities. Is he or she inconsistent in the use of medical resources? For example, does your patient rush to the emergency department when the clinical condition could be taken care of at a lesser level, such as in the physician's office?

▶ Be familiar with the use of nontraditional or holistic modalities. People are increasingly using alternative healing methods, especially patients with incurable diseases or chronic conditions not helped by traditional medicine.

▶ Examine the patient/family self-management behavior, knowledge, and skills. These can reveal a lot about the patient's condition, disease progression, and utilization of resources. If found inadequate, the case manager is then clear that health education, counseling regarding care expectations, and motivational interviewing for healthy lifestyle behavior change are warranted.

Although many give no credence to alternative healing methods, the National Institutes of Health in Washington, DC, has a designated budget for the study of "unconventional" methods of healing. Several medical schools, including Harvard University and the University of Arizona, also offer courses on alternative medicine. Some of the alternative therapies are thousands of years old, and new forms and variations of them are cropping up. It is recommended that case managers have knowledge of some of these modalities, because more patients are using them. Many outcomes studies are taking place to find exactly why millions of patients are willing to spend billions of out-of-pocket dollars on nontraditional healing. Some forms of alternative therapies, although very limited, are being reimbursed by insurance companies, and case managers should be aware of them and their impact on patients' choices of therapy. Examples include chiropractic care and acupuncture.

▶ Current Medical Status

If the patient is at home, interviewing home health professionals can be useful to assess a patient's medical status. Such professionals include physical, occupational, and speech therapists as well as home health nurses, social workers, aides, and homemakers. The family physician may also be able to provide helpful information. If a physical appraisal is part of your job responsibilities, a head-to-toe assessment can be done.

If the patient is in the hospital or in a SNF, all available data can be used: medical and health records including laboratory results; special test results; radiographs; MRI and CT scans; vital signs; progress notes; nurse notes; physical, occupational, and speech therapist notes; consultations; respiratory therapist notes; surgical reports; allergies; medications, and your personal observations. The following steps should also be taken:

▶ Assess utilization review modalities: The use of intensity of service/severity of illness criteria, whether InterQual, Milliman Care Guidelines, other health guidelines, or critical pathways, should be reviewed. This careful review alerts the case manager to a possible need for changing the patient's level of care, and it may also be necessary for the authorization of insurance resources.

▶ Find out the patient's health goals, interests, and major health concerns.

▶ Check assessments of direct care nurses and other care providers.

▶ Evaluate diets: Does the patient follow a special diet for health conditions, religious purposes, or personal preference? Is the diet adequate or is a dietary consultation needed?

▶ Evaluate all skin conditions.

▶ If the patient is in acute care, determine what tubes, catheters, and equipment should be continued at discharge. Are urinary catheters, tracheostomies, and suction machines and supplies, jejunostomy (J-tube) and gastrostomy tube care, drains, feeding tubes, IV or feeding tube pumps, medication pumps (e.g., insulin), oxygen, and miscellaneous ostomy supplies required? Is any wound care needed?

▶ Review medications: Is the medicine regimen complicated enough to require a consult with a pharmacist or a visiting nurse to help coordinate and educate about proper intake? Do medications such as anticoagulants and isoniazid require laboratory studies on an ongoing basis? Assess any over-the-counter drugs or therapies for possible problems. Assess patient compliance knowledge about, and adherence to, the use of medications. Can the patient afford the medications? Is there a problem getting transportation to the pharmacy?

▶ Assess bowel and bladder incontinence.

▶ Analyze patient understanding of conditions and educational needs pertaining to diagnosis/illness.

▶ Assess the patient's views and interests pertaining to advance directives. Does the patient have a designated healthcare proxy? Has the patient made his wishes known regarding end-of-life care, do-not-resuscitate status, and withdrawal of life and/or nutritional support?

▶ Nutritional Assessment

Proper nutrition is an important factor in a person's health status; it contributes to positive health outcomes and saves healthcare dollars if managed carefully. It is common knowledge that proper nutrition can delay the onset of many health conditions from heart attacks to osteoporosis; early nutritional assessment and intervention is the key to prevention of many complications once a patient is ill. Long-term marginal nutritional status may be the cause of many (or most) of the problems in healthcare today and certainly contributes to functional and cognitive decline.

Nutritional assessments are required by accreditation organizations in most levels of care. Research indicates that malnutrition is a serious problem. Annually, almost 17 million patients are treated for conditions that place them in a high-risk category for malnutrition. Outcome research indicates that personalized nutrition therapy can reduce healthcare costs. Of the 10 leading causes of disease, 8 are related to nutrition. Studies document that poorly nourished patients require care for longer periods, have higher complication rates, have higher mortality rates, and require more frequent readmissions and emergency care.

Case managers must identify various nutritional needs such as home delivery of meals (e.g., Meals on Wheels, Gods Love We Deliver), assistance with shopping or cooking, or nutritional education. Case managers must also be able to assess risk factors for malnutrition. Collaborative work with registered dietitians is worth the effort. Registered dietitians are usually on the staff of major hospitals or can also be accessed through the American Dietetic Association.

The following represent some nutritional risk factors. Much of the information can be found in the patient's medical records.

▶ *Inadequate or inappropriate food intake*: Each diagnosis requires its own variation of foods that can or cannot be tolerated. Compliance with the proper diet is a common problem. Case managers can examine the frequency, amount, and quality of choices for food intake. Is it too little or too much? Is the food of the wrong type (pretzels and fast-food pizza in congestive heart failure patients)? Assess for other issues such as excessive alcohol use.

▶ *Financial issues*: Quality food costs money. Vitamins, minerals, and herbs often touted as helpful are not covered under health insurance plans. Some impoverished people will pay rent and utilities and have little money left for food. Stories are common about elderly people living on cat/dog food or spending the little money they have on food for their pets, thus leaving themselves to starve or eat poorly; unfortunately, these stories are often true.

▶ *Social isolation*: This can cause a decreased desire to eat; some people hate to eat alone. It can also cause depression, which often results in low appetite levels.

▶ *Dental/oral assessment*: If eating is a major source of aggravation or pain due to lack of teeth, poorly fitting dentures, or other mouth and gum problems, the end result could be decreased nutritional levels.

▶ *Ability and disability*: Can the patient shop for food? Is the patient able to prepare food and clean up after the meal? Does the patient have any help or active support system?

▶ *Weight loss and gain*: Has the patient gained or lost 10 lb recently? A recent and sudden change in body weight of 10 lb is strongly associated with functional and instrumental ADLs; it is also associated with increased healthcare costs. Assess the adequacy of food intake, new prescription or over-the-counter medications, and changed mental or functional status. Certain medications cause nutritional deficiencies and should be assessed carefully. Did the patient have a recent trauma, infection, or surgery that required an additional load of calories? Were the additional needed calories supplied?

▶ *Acute and chronic diseases*: Examine the patient's history and present health condition for clues. Look for major diagnoses and assess whether patient is over- or underweight or has mental health issues and dental and mouth problems.

▶ Medication Assessment

Medication assessment is a part of nearly all other types of assessments in this chapter. Its contribution to health or morbidity cannot be overemphasized. At every level of care, pharmaceuticals must be examined, and this responsibility belongs to many professionals, including physicians, nurses, case managers, pharmacists, and even dietitians. The Institute of Medicine reports that more than 100,000 Americans die in hospitals annually in the United States from adverse medication reactions, both prescription and over-the-counter. In addition, 2.1 million people suffer from serious medication-related complications such as gastric bleeding, cardiac irregularities, and allergies.

Case managers should review medications—prescriptive, herbal, and over-the-counter—and carefully assess if a physician or pharmacist should be consulted. Some medication issues to consider include:

▶ Review all allergies—whether associated with medications or with herbal products.

▶ Review for polypharmacy and consult the physician and/or pharmacist to ascertain if there is a potential problem .

▶ Assess the patient/family self-management skills as they pertain to medication intake. Check if the patient is taking medications according to the physician's orders. Assess for general compliance and safe storage.

▶ Assess lack of transportation as a cause of not obtaining ordered medications.

▶ Assess financial problems as a cause of not obtaining ordered medications. Are generic equivalents a possibility? Would a change to generic make it more feasible for the patient to buy the medication?

▶ Assess insurance for pharmacy benefits.

▶ Assess for adverse interactions and contraindications.

▶ Assess for adverse reactions to common food. Is the patient aware of the potential for an adverse reaction? For example, one common medication was determined to be unsafe when taken with grapefruit juice. Several people became ill before this was discovered.

▶ Because many medications such as anticoagulants require ongoing laboratory monitoring, check whether scheduled appointments to monitor serum levels or other pertinent blood work are attended.

▶ Assess whether the medications are prescribed at the lowest effective dose and for appropriate duration.

▶ Assess whether the supplied medications use the simplest dosing regimen. Sometimes a medication has been taken for many years; meanwhile, advancements that would allow simplified dosing have occurred.

▶ Assess whether the most effective routes have been prescribed for the medications.

▶ Assess whether the medication containers are accessible (e.g., not all arthritic patients can open child-proof containers).

▶ Assess patients with renal or hepatic problems to see if they are taking medications that do not get cleared through those vital organs.

▶ Carefully assess for any knowledge deficit about medications. Does the patient know:
  1. The name of the medication.
  2. The purpose of the medication.
  3. The dosage of the medication.
  4. The frequency/timing of administration of the medication.
  5. The relationship between taking the medication and taking meals.
  6. Red flags or adverse side effects that require a call to the doctor.
  7. The method of administration of the medication: chewed, sublingual, swallowed, swish-and-swallow, crushed, through the feeding tube, etc.

Provide simple explanatory handouts about the medications when necessary. Medication calendars or prepackaging in "Medi-set" containers is often the answer.

▶ Financial Assessment

▶ Does the patient have inadequate insurance coverage or no coverage? What health benefits does the insurance plan include? Does the insurance plan have any restrictions, limitations, or carve-outs?

▶ Have you checked for any governmental entitlements (Medicare, Medicaid, Supplemental Security Income, Social Security Disability)?

▶ Can the patient/family meet copayments and deductible demands?

▶ Can the patient/family pay for necessary supplies, medications, and miscellaneous items not covered by insurance?

▶ If necessary, can the family contribute toward a SNF placement or supplemental home help?

▶ Can the patient meet basic financial obligations (rent, utilities, food) during this episode of illness?

▶ If the patient must be discharged with high-tech equipment, can he or she afford the additional utilities? For example, some air-flow beds may increase electric bills up to $200 per month. Patients on fixed incomes cannot usually afford this monthly increase.

▶ Functional Assessment: Environmental Factors

It is important to assess for patient safety in transitional planning. Was the patient safe and at an adequate level of care before this event? Many elderly patients fall in the home and are admitted to hospitals. If hospitalization has been caused by an unsafe home environment, can it be modified for safety or is a more supervised setting needed?

It is also vital to look at the patient's level of independence. How well did the patient perform functional tasks before this event? Was he or she independent in all ADLs and ambulatory, or was there a prior psychomotor deficit?

THE HOME ENVIRONMENT ASSESSMENT

The home environment assessment is a key activity for safe transitional planning. The following should be checked:

▶ *Stairs*: Can the patient get into and out of the house or apartment safely? Are there stairs inside that the patient needs to negotiate?

▶ *Telephone (landline or cell)*: Telephone communication is especially important to consider if the patient lives alone or is alone for several hours at a time. Can the patient see and hear adequately to use the telephone? If not, can adaptations be readily made?

▶ *Toilet, tub, and shower*: Check for conditions and safe access. Does the patient require the use of an elevated toilet seat or bars in the shower and tub for assistance in mobilization? Is the floor condition unsafe? Does it place the patient at risk for slipping, falling, or tripping?

▶ *Utilities*: Check electricity, heat, fans, and air conditioning to ensure that they are in working order. Many older people are admitted to hospitals with dehydration or heat stroke in the summer and with pneumonia in winter, both caused by poor environmental conditions. Gas heaters and heat from gas stoves are often major fire hazards. Is the electrical wiring safe for DME use?

▶ *Sanitation*: Are running water, working toilets, and clean conditions available? Are rodents or roaches a problem? We have seen more than one patient readmitted with maggots invading postsurgical wounds, caused by poor sanitary conditions.

▶ *Equipment needs*: Does the patient have a bed? Does he or she require a special hospital bed, other DME, a Hoyer lift, or portable ramps?

ADLs ASSESSMENT

Both prior and present self-care deficits and present learning capabilities are to be noted. If the patient is currently less independent in daily activities than at a prior time, transition planning compensations may be needed. The discharge disposition must match and compensate for the patient's deficits. The following questions about the patient's capability for self-care must be addressed:

- Can the patient dress and undress?
- Can the patient put on vision and hearing aids and stump prosthesis?
- Does the patient have the ability to perform the following hygiene tasks:
  - Bathing
  - Shaving
  - Brushing teeth or dentures
  - Testing temperature of bath or shower water
  - Entering and exiting the tub/shower safely
  - Lowering and raising self from toilet
  - Cleaning self after elimination
- Can the patient handle nutritional needs: shopping for and preparing food, using utensils, chewing, and swallowing? Is extra help needed, such as for shopping and food preparation or perhaps Meals on Wheels?
- Is the patient able to perform housekeeping and yard work?
- Can the patient take prescription medications as ordered, or is the task too complicated, requiring home health nurse supervision? Are wrong doses, expired medications, or discontinued medications still in the patient's possession?
- Can the patient handle transportation needs to get to the store, pharmacy, place of worship, or health clinic for follow-up care?
- Does the patient have balance and coordination problems? Does he or she tend to fall or have difficulty with motor skills? Does the patient hold onto home furniture to manage getting around?
- What is the patient's ability to see, hear, speak, read, and write? Is his or her native tongue English? Are translators or bilingual nurses and support care providers needed?
- If the patient uses a wheelchair, is this a new development? Is the previous dwelling accessible to the wheelchair? If not, can modifications be made, or does the patient need to change living arrangements? Is the wheelchair the correct size and type, with properly fitting cushions and trays?
- Does the patient know how to telephone for emergency services? This is especially important in areas without 911 capabilities. Does the patient have the telephone numbers of utility companies and medical equipment supply companies in case of equipment malfunction or a need for medical supplies?
- Now the big question—is safe home care a possibility for this patient? (The psychosocial assessment is the other major factor that affects the patient's ability to be discharged home safely.)

▶ Psychosocial Assessment

In the psychosocial part of the assessment process, the case manager treats the whole family unit as the patient. The family, significant other, personal caregiver, and close friends are an extension of the patient, and all needs and desires should be heard. The family's effect on the patient is too important to overlook. In some social cultures, the extended family is a primary social unit; the parents are the decision makers and not the patient.

A relationship does not necessarily exist between the severity of the illness and psychological functioning; therefore, the patient's response to the illness or event must be assessed along with the family's adjustment to it. This is most important in the case of a chronic illness that is life altering in nature, especially when it is a new diagnosis.

- What other stresses are taking a toll on the patient's family life at the time of the illness? These possibilities include divorce, moving, a death in the family, job change/loss, or a new baby. What family dynamics are revealed? How do the patient and family usually cope with stress? These methods can include religious activities, meditation, sports, talking with friends or a professional counselor, anger, physical violence, and the use of alcohol and drugs. Even if the family dynamics were functional and safe before this event, will they continue to be so now?
- Who is at home? If the patient is a single mother, are the children safe? If the patient is a casualty of the "sandwich generation" and is responsible for caring for an ill parent, who is caring for that parent now? If the patient is elderly, is there a spouse (or other relative) at home who is unable to care for his or her own needs without the patient's assistance? Are there pets at home that need attention?
- Assess the family for exhaustion and burnout. Can respite care be provided to help ease the burden?
- Ask about hobbies and recreational activities. One case manager once shared with us that she had a chronically ill patient who loved to sew as a diversion, but she lost an arm. With her primary form of entertainment made so much more difficult, the case manager needed to find another way for her to relax. For this type of situation, it is necessary to explore other relaxation outlets.
- Assess the formal support system. Is it adequate, inadequate, lacking, or dysfunctional?
- Assess the patient's informal resources such as neighbors, church or synagogue groups, friends, and relatives. Can these be expanded if more help at home is needed?
- School or employment records may be assessed as appropriate or if job placement is a part of your

particular case management responsibilities. Patient or family-signed release forms may be required. School records may be necessary if you are dealing with a pediatric patient.

▶ Assess the patient's level of care prior to the current illness. Can the patient return to the same environment, or is short- or long-term SNF or acute/subacute rehabilitation care needed? Do the people associated with the previous living arrangement agree to have the patient discharged back into their care? Sometimes, the decision to send the patient to a SNF is a challenging one, especially when the patient is fairly lucid and wants to go home. Early intervention with family or team conferences should begin.

▶ Secondary gains to illness often serve conscious or unconscious needs. Some patients do not want to get well. They like the special attention from family and medical staff. Some feel it is a way to gain power over others. For others, dependency needs are met while ill. For still others, a hospital stay represents a warm or cool place to sleep and eat. Occasionally, the hospital is a refuge—a safe place—where a parent or spouse cannot abuse them. Patients such as these are often the "frequent fliers," who are admitted regularly for exacerbations of their basic problem (often rotating from hospital to hospital). A depression screening and psychiatric consultation with possible referrals to outpatient support groups may assist such persons. Depending on the problem, an Adult Protective/Child Protective Services referral may be needed. If the patient is homeless, referrals to shelters may help or, preferably, a social service plan can provide a more permanent solution.

▶ Cognitive or mental status assessment may be needed. Not infrequently, a patient at home or in a hospital desires an unsafe or detrimental disposition (in the medical team's professional judgment). If that person is otherwise alert and oriented, ancillary assistance may be all you can provide. If the person's mental capacity is in question, the next step would be a psychiatric referral to evaluate the patient's judgment, competence, and orientation. If the psychologist or psychiatrist feels this person is incompetent, legal action may be necessary, especially in the case of a patient without a healthcare proxy or one who has no family members or other relatives. Mental incompetence sometimes must be verified in a court of law.

▶ The brick wall syndrome: Occasionally, a psychosocial situation occurs in which a very ill patient requires intensive care, 24 hours a day. Family members insist that they can handle the patient at home. Your instincts as the case manager are that it will not work, that the family will not be able to get enough rest, or that the patient may not be cared for adequately. Families have the right to try to care for their loved ones, and all necessary equipment and available help can be provided. Many times, after this plan has been implemented, reality sets in. The family members "hit the brick wall" and realize that they are unable to handle the care of the patient alone and therefore request SNF placement. If there is a considerable chance that the home placement will not succeed, making necessary copies of the medical record for a SNF placement before the record goes to the hospital's health information management (previously medical records) department may ease and speed up a transfer request by the family. Suggestions for supervisory homes may also be given to the family if need be.

▶ Cultural and Religious Diversity

To provide appropriate case management services, the case manager must be aware of cultural and religious preferences and differences; this is both confusing and gratifying. Fortunately, diversity is now front and center in the media and in healthcare. It is important to evaluate patients according to their cultural beliefs, value systems, and traditions.

▶ *Gestures*: Nonverbal body language is an important communication method. However, this is not always clear when caring for individuals from different cultures. The same gesture may mean "goodbye" in one culture and "come here" in another. A smile and a "yes" nod may not indicate agreement, but rather the wish to be polite and respectful.

▶ *Language barriers*: These go beyond simply not speaking the same language. Misunderstood basic language concepts can hinder the case manager–patient/family relationship. Ruth Beebe Hill (1979) writes in her introduction to *Hanta Yo*:

Admit, assume, because, believe, could, doubt, end, effect, faith, forget, forgive, guilt, how, it, mercy, pest, promise, should, sorry, storm, them, us, waste, we, weed—neither these words nor the conceptions for which they stand appear in this book; they are the Whiteman's import to the New World, the newcomer's contribution to the vocabulary of the man he called Indian. Truly, the parent Indian families possessed neither these terms nor their equivalents.

The word "maybe" is another concept not readily understood by some Native American tribes, and the use of this word may produce lack of trust in a relationship.

▶ *Cultural traditions, differences, and taboos*: Some people do not approve of eye contact, either feeling that it is impolite or believing that it robs them of their spirit. Others do not like casual touching. Silence is essential in some cultures and uncomfortable in others.

Some ethnic groups are uncomfortable discussing topics that medical professionals and case managers may consider necessary. In some cultures, healthcare decisions are the responsibility of the elder family members (parents/grandparents) rather than of the patient. Expressions of pain, from stoic to expressive, vary among different cultures. Knowledge that the patient may be acting stoically can help you to determine how to offer optimum comfort.

▶ *Religious and spiritual beliefs*: For some, the spiritual belief system is a major source of strength. Assess the feasibility of pastoral/rabbinical visits or tapes and reading materials for spiritual nourishment. If daily prayer or meditation was previously an important part of the patient's life, some time could be set apart without any interruption for this purpose.

Some religious practices may affect healthcare subtly, such as dietary practices or beliefs that illness is a punishment from God. Overt practices, such as the Jehovah's Witness's rejection of blood transfusions, can affect the treatment plan and have far-reaching consequences. Consideration should be given to all spiritual and cultural differences because they can affect the patient–case manager relationship.

▶ *Cultural and religious conflicts within the individual*: Humanity is now in the global information age. Cultures are merging, and information on anything is at one's "beck and call." This can create conflicts within people. An example of such a conflict is in Display 4-1.

At times, providing culturally relevant care may be better left outside the realm of case management services. The conflict shared in Display 4-1 was solved among the members of a large family in their own unique way. However, case managers must be aware of such conflicts, be prepared to not fully understand, and yet be nonjudgmental and supportive when such issues arise. If, by chance, you have a personal cultural knowledge to assist more fully, then your patients are indeed fortunate.

In your role as a case manager, it is important to recognize that the comprehensive and individualized assessment of your patient and family may be an overwhelming and time-consuming undertaking. The diverse aspects of the assessment described in this stage of the case management process may not all apply to every individual patient situation. Here is some advice:

▶ Be thoughtful in determining what is most relevant and informative for the development of an effective plan of care for each patient.

▶ Remember that you may not need to conduct every aspect of the assessment personally yourself. Take the time to review the assessment findings of other members of the healthcare team (e.g., physician; nurse; social worker; physical, occupational and speech therapists; nutritionist).

▶ Your skills in drawing meaningful conclusions from these assessments, identifying areas requiring further clarification from the patient/family or the healthcare team, and determining your very next step to begin to map out the important focus areas of your case management plan are key success factors for both the patient/family and yourself in your case management practice.

---

display 4-1

EXAMPLE OF A CULTURAL AND RELIGIOUS CONFLICT

A large Navajo tribe lives in Arizona. A Navajo newspaper reporter once wrote about this conflict when her father died.

Like most Navajos, she follows the Earth-based traditional faith of Hozho—a concept about beauty, stability, and order—yet traditional Christianity also plays a strong role in her life and the lives of many of her extended Navajo family. It took her 4 years to write about the conflict. During her father's illness and struggle with Parkinson's disease, she prayed to and cursed two gods—the Christian God and the Holy People, who show themselves as lightning, dawn, rain, wind, snow, water, and fog.

She asked much of her Christian God during the difficult college years; *maybe she asked too much and used up her quota of assistance. Maybe she was being punished for holding on to her Navajo beliefs.* Among taboos of the Navajos are contact with dead bodies, staring straight into a person's eye, driving away from a coyote that crosses your path without sprinkling corn pollen in his tracks, and saying harsh words, because they have the power to kill. *Maybe the Holy People were punishing her for not covering her eyes quickly enough during a bloody scene she had to witness for her newspaper job. Maybe the power of words (which she uses to craft her work) has caused harm to Navajos or others.*

During the burial process, many other conflicts arose. Her father was a traditional Navajo who never saw the inside of a Christian church; he followed the way of the Holy People. Traditional ceremonies for the dead do not mesh well with hermetically sealed coffins that preserve dead bodies for many years. The Christian and traditional factions of the family had differing needs.

▶ STAGE III: DEVELOPMENT AND COORDINATION OF THE PLAN OF CARE

If assessment aids the case manager in deciding where to go with a particular case, or patient situation, then Stage III helps the case manager to choose the best way to get there. In this stage, the needs and services are matched into a seamless plan based on the assessment data and the desires of the patient and family/caregiver.

According to the CMSA Standards of Practice for Case Management, the "case management plan of care is a structured, dynamic tool used to document the opportunities, interventions, and expected goals, the professional case manager applies during the client's engagement in case management services" (CMSA, 2017, p. 18). The case management plan is necessary to establish goals of the treatment, prioritize the patient's needs (actual and potential), and determine the services required to attain the established goals and desired outcomes. It helps reduce the risk of inappropriate, unnecessary, or incomplete care CMSA, 2017).

Creativity is the keynote at this point; often there is more than one "best" way to do something. Maintaining a patient/family-centered approach to care coordination and management is essential to choose what is best for the case (patient and family). Flexibility is another important factor; the patient and family may desire changes, or the patient's condition may change. Amending the plan in the light of these changes is necessary to meet the goals designed for the case. It is also essential for maintaining a plan of care that is relevant to the current and changing condition of the patient. Here is where the role of patient advocate becomes most evident. Creatively finding ways to meet the basic needs of your patient is reflected in quality treatments, interventions, and transition plans. The "gift" a patient advocate gives to the patient is a plan of care that promotes the patient's optimal level of self-care, self-management, and control over his or her life.

The case manager has just spent many hours putting together a thorough clinical, financial, and psychosocial assessment. The patient's individual strengths, weaknesses, resources, and lack of resources have been identified. Now the multidisciplinary team, which can include several professionals such as the case manager, social worker, physical or occupational therapist, pharmacist, patient, family/caregiver, physician, payor, and others in the patient's case, must decide the following:

- ▶ What needs to be done
- ▶ How best to do it
- ▶ How does what is needed meet the patient/family interests and preferences
- ▶ Who will provide necessary services
- ▶ When each need will be met

- ▶ Where and when the next level of care will be provided
- ▶ How the patient/family can best manage after discharge (after this episode of care).

For this planning stage to be successful, the patient and family must actively participate in all decisions, including any changes in the plan of care. If the patient or family is not in agreement with the plan, it most likely will fail in addressing the identified needs or meeting the care goals. The family can add to a successful plan by identifying any informal resources that may be needed to fill in the gaps. These informal resources may be friends, neighbors, or volunteers from religious organizations or community agencies.

▶ Establishing Care Goals

The first step in this stage of coordinating and developing treatment and transitional plans is establishing care goals. What must be accomplished by whom and by when? Most goals are composed of many smaller goals or tasks that must be met for successful completion of the main goal. Missed details can delay or hinder the smooth sequence and progression of the plan. Objectives such as home safety at discharge or the promotion of an optimal level of independence for the patient may require two, three, a dozen, or more modifications in the home setting to make the goal of home safety a reality. A grandmother's transfer to the SNF may consist of several tasks, such as finding an appropriate SNF, finding a physician who will follow up at the SNF, setting up appropriate transportation and DME, copying/faxing/securing electronic software transfers of all the necessary medical records, notifying the family of transfer time, obtaining physician's orders for her care at the SNF, coordinating transportation to the SNF, and obtaining reports from the multidisciplinary team. The ultimate goals of case management are quality of care, safety, and efficient use of resources. This entire textbook is dedicated to the smaller tasks needed to ensure that these three major goals are met.

Long- and short-term goals may also need to be established. Consider short-term goals for a previously independent, elderly gentleman who recently had total hip replacement surgery. These goals may include the removal of all tubes and drains, stable blood tests, transfer from bed to a chair with assistance, and walking a few steps with assistance. This man's long-term goals—possibly in a SNF or acute rehabilitation—may be walking 300 feet or more with a walker or cane, ultimately walking without assistive devices, and achieving independence in ADLs, which would allow the patient to return home safely.

▶ Prioritizing Needs and Goals

The second step in the planning stage is to prioritize the needs and care goals that were assessed. Again, the patient's and family's input is insightful here. What is their idea of the most pressing problem? Each person views life and adversity from his or her own perspective and value system. A "can't live without" for one person might be a minor irritation to someone else.

There may be times when the patient's or family's idea of a priority problem does not match the professional staff member's idea of a priority. One case manager had a case that involved an elderly lady who was in the terminal stage of cancer. Whereas the case manager, physicians, and social worker repeatedly tried to speak to her daughter about hospice care, the daughter focused on her mother's dental cavity. The prospect of hospice was too much for the daughter, so she narrowed down the problem into something she could handle. Sometimes hard reality is just too overwhelming. Starting to work with the patient and family at their stage of acceptance of a health condition, diagnosis of a terminal illness, or prognosis is necessary to get to the most important discussions or decisions regarding the plan of care. Neglecting this makes it too much of a challenge to address the important issues. This strategy allows the patient and family to be more involved in the care and the related decisions.

At other times, families or patients may adamantly disagree with the assessed priority needs. An alert and oriented elderly lady may insist on going home alone, when a short-term SNF placement is the obvious safe choice. Perhaps a patient is readmitted to the acute care level within 1 week of discharge. During the first admission, the family and patient refused services that the case manager deemed a priority and an immediate need. Through education and negotiation, a revised plan may be successful the second time around.

Some limiting factors often narrow the choices, which may make prioritization of treatments and activities easier but the treatment and transition plans less than optimal. Consider financial and health insurance resource allocation and its limitations. The limitation may be as simple as the fact that the health insurance company will not pay for both a front-wheeled walker and a wheelchair, which both the patient and case manager feel are needed. On the other hand, the limitation may be as critical as a need for bone marrow transplantation with no payor source. Therefore, concentrating on conditions that can be improved is one way to prioritize. Because not all circumstances can be "fixed," the focus should be on attaining the best quality of life possible for the patient.

▶ Service Planning and Resource Allocation

After priority goals have been ascertained, the case manager compensates for assessed deficits, fills in healthcare gaps, and reduces duplication through thoughtful coordination of services and resources. This third step, service planning and resource allocation, requires knowledge of public and private organizations that may be helpful. Medical insurance

companies are often the first place to try for funding needed services, and they usually consent to medically necessary requests. If your idea of medical necessity does not coincide with the health insurance company's idea of medical necessity, you have the options of negotiating, speaking to the company's medical director for clarification, or finding other resources such as charitable and community support agencies.

Resource allocation for a patient with no or inadequate health insurance is a challenge and requires creative case management. The second place to look is "informal" resources such as the patient's family, friends, neighbors, community-based agencies, and religious groups. Matching the patient with government entitlements such as Medicare, SSD, or Medicaid may be helpful but may sometimes require long waiting periods. Geographically convenient resource books are a funnel of information for local social services. Often you may find information about such resources available online. Make use of social service personnel, who sometimes can provide invaluable help.

The unique features of each case will determine the service planning and coordination details. If a patient can be independent with intensive education and a few follow-up home health visits for education and review of the skills taught, then education and home health are provided. If long-term placement is needed, a facility is matched with the patient's skill needs, health insurance benefits, and available resources. If the family and multidisciplinary team agree that hospice and a duplication of the hospital room at home are required, the case manager will coordinate these services. Transitional planning can be simple or multifaceted and complex, but these activities are always personalized to meet the needs and interests of the patient and family.

Even with the best intentions and the most careful planning, changes, interruptions, and detours are common. During busy winter seasons, many SNFs and shelters may be full, with waiting lists of several days to several weeks. If one SNF gives you a "definite maybe" for a day or two hence, it may be good assurance to place the patient on a second waiting list that also meets with the patient's/family's approval. An unexpected deterioration (or improvement) in the patient's medical status may necessitate an entirely new service and transitional plan. A change of heart/mind of the family members may upset the plan. Sometimes families, overcome by guilt, refuse SNF placement at the last minute or, overcome by exhaustion, feel incapable of taking the patient home again. Family and team conferences should be convened as soon as possible to prevent additional unnecessary/avoidable hospital days. New goals and new plans may have to be considered and evaluated.

For some patients who undergo planned, elective surgeries, transitional planning may be done before surgery. If complications occur and are serious enough, those plans may need reassessing. Anything can happen, so a "plan B" or an alternate plan is always a good idea. A "plan B" strategy keeps the case manager ahead of the game and proactive in meeting the care needs of the patient and family.

Coordinating treatments and services during a hospitalization is another important function of the case manager. Efficiency saves not only valuable resources but also entire hospital days. This may be accomplished in several ways. Clinical pathways are a chosen tool for decreasing lengths of stay. Observation for correct sequencing of tests can also prevent unnecessary additional hospital days.

Several consultants treating one patient often make their own individual plans. The case manager can bring those plans into alignment to cause the least trauma to the patient. For example, if a patient needs a major debridement for osteomyelitis and requires 6 weeks of intravenous (IV) antibiotics, the case manager can coordinate a long-term venous access placement to be done concurrently with the debridement. Perhaps a patient requires a TURP (genitourinary surgeon) and a hernia repair (general surgeon). If the patient and physicians are in agreement, a single coordinated surgery saves the patient from receiving general anesthesia for two procedures at two different times. Such a surgery also saves operating room and postoperative hospital time, and cuts down on the use of miscellaneous resources. However, good clinical judgment is necessary when suggesting a "better way"; poor or unsafe suggestions, at the very least, diminish the case manager's credibility and effectiveness.

The team has assessed the problems, ascertained what needs to be done, orchestrated a time frame (pending medical stability of the patient), and determined the contributions and limitations of the health insurance company. Informal supports are verified and available. Referrals are in for SNFs, rehabilitation facilities, mental health facilities, home health agencies, community-based resources such as Meals on Wheels, and whatever else the patient needs. Transportation needs are assessed. DME is approved. Educational factors—what needs to be taught to whom—have been evaluated. This stage culminates when assessed needs are linked with chosen interventions and desired outcomes. Most importantly, however, a plan of care meets the patient's/family's needs, desires, care goals, and preferences, not only those of the healthcare team.

▶ STAGE IV: IMPLEMENTATION AND COORDINATION OF THE PLAN OF CARE

Implementation is the process of putting the plan of care into action. In the implementation of the plan, the patient's assessed needs have been linked with private and community services. The gaps are filled, there is no duplication of services, and the patient and support systems have expressed agreement with the plan. The goal of this stage is to maximize the safety and well-being of the patient, using the most independent and necessary level of care. A cost-effective setting must match the patient's health condition, needs, capabilities, desires, and financial abilities. This is where the case manager shows a talent for coordination, facilitation, negotiation, and brokerage. The patient is now discharged home, transferred to a supervised setting, or remains in the same setting but with a more appropriate service and treatment plan because of case management.

By Stage IV in the case management process, the case manager has accurately assessed the patient's and family's needs. Weaknesses and opportunities have been delineated and problems solved. The treatment plan may have made a few detours from the expected clinical path, but variances have been expediently identified and promptly brought back in line. The total case has been assessed, reassessed, negotiated, and coordinated. The treatment and transitional plans are realistic and workable and have been approved by the multidisciplinary team, patient, family, and third-party payor.

The case manager has the service vendors and facilities chosen and the patient/family, team, and payor have approved the choices. All informal supports are in place. The case manager is comfortable that this plan will work, but still is flexible and has a pretty good idea what "plan B" might entail if needed. The team, patient, and family are depending on the case manager to take care of all the details and to get them right.

There are as many types of implementation of a case management plan of care as there are types of case management programs. For the purposes of simplification, this section will separate essential issues by differentiating between internal and external case managers.

▶ *Internal case managers* are those within a facility or agency, such as a hospital, acute rehabilitation facility, SNF, home health agency, or hospice; some refer to this as "within-the-walls" case management. Internal case managers are employed by the providers of care. They are on-site case managers and assume responsibility for the creation and coordination of the patient's plan of care in a way that meets the patient's needs and the payor's demands.

▶ *External case managers* are those who work outside facilities, such as insurance/third-party payor case managers, health maintenance organization (HMO)/preferred provider organization (PPO) case managers, disability management and life care planning agencies, or those private/independent or contracted with self-insured plans or union groups. External case managers essentially work for payors of care. They often work telephonically and may also function on-site according to contracts. Most often, however, they practice "outside-the-walls" case management.

▶ Case Managers Within Facilities (Internal)

There are no distinct lines that can be drawn in the separation of duties of the various case managers who practice in a specific care setting. All case managers may be responsible for any of the tasks described in Displays 4-2 and 4-3. Knowing what is expected of you by your employer, the clients who refer the patients, and by state and federal laws is essential for effective case management services. Often, your responsibilities span the development and implementation of the plan of care, including the discharge or transitional plan, among numerous other activities. These, however, are physically limited to the confines of the healthcare

organization in which you are employed. These also extend in focus on what is beyond your physical practice setting as you coordinate your patient's plan of care across care settings, care providers, and in collaboration with external case managers.

It may be useful for your healthcare organization to assess the issues described in Displays 4-2 and 4-3. Make a permanent check sheet for your charts with these points; brainstorm pertinent job responsibilities necessary for your organization. A check sheet can help to ensure that no important information or steps will be missed. When there are perhaps innumerable details to take care of in each case together with the possibility of human error, even the most basic of responsibilities may be overlooked.

---

display 4-2

EXAMPLE OF KEY CASE MANAGEMENT ACTIVITIES FOR A PATIENT'S DISCHARGE— DAY BEFORE DISCHARGE

▶ Medical stability and discharge screens are monitored.

▶ Patient education continues, and return demonstrations identify any misinformation or incomplete learning processes. Teaching is stepped up for the patient's discharge the following day. If home health is required, home health professional staff is notified of learning weaknesses and continued learning opportunities.

▶ Evaluate pain control and attempt to change to oral pain management, if possible.

▶ Anticipated tests (hemoglobin and hematocrit, room air oxygen, arterial blood gases for supplemental oxygen, prothrombin time/partial thromboplastin time, and so on) are ordered. Results are reported to attending physicians and healthcare team.

▶ Transportation needs are evaluated. If the patient is from out of state or county (or even out of the country), transportation plans need clarification as early as possible. If the patient requires a ground or air ambulance or stretcher van, calls should be made 24 hours in advance; cancellation may sometimes be necessary but is preferable to holding up a discharge because an appropriate transport vehicle is not available. Wheelchair vans may also require 24-hour notice. Families can confirm approximate pickup times on this day if they can transport the patient home.

▶ Find out when the attending physician and consultants need to see the patient after discharge and, if necessary, help the patient make follow-up appointments.

▶ Confirm outpatient physical therapy, occupational therapy, and speech therapy appointments and give the patient the times, days, and a contact telephone number.

▶ Any needed outpatient IV therapy (such as antibiotics and chemotherapy), wound care, and scheduled tests and procedures need orders and appointments. This is often needed for patients who are not homebound and therefore do not qualify for home health services.

▶ Coordinate the DME. Delivery of all large equipment that must be brought to the home or the apartment needs to be timed appropriately so that someone is there to accept it at the door. Smaller DME (e.g., small volume nebulizer [SVN] machines, portable oxygen tanks) can be sent to the hospital. Often, a patient cannot go home without continuous oxygen; a smaller oxygen tank must be taken to the hospital before discharge and the larger unit needs to be coordinated for

house delivery. When assessing equipment needs, ask about room sizes and space availability. This should be done as soon as DME need is assessed. Many patients require a hospital bed but must move home furniture around to make it fit into the room. Even three-in-one toilets do not always fit if the patient lives in a small trailer. Shower equipment also needs to fit in the type of bathroom facilities the patient has (full-size bathtub, smaller trailer-size tubs, or shower stall).

▶ Get all supplies ready for wound care, tracheostomy, ostomy, or other procedures. Some home health agencies want the patient to go home with a few days' worth of supplies for the purpose of continuity of care. This is especially important on weekends.

▶ Confirm hemodialysis days and times with the accepting facility. Confirm transportation needs.

▶ Call the home health agency and/or IV infusion therapy company to confirm impending discharge, and update the company on the social and medical status of the patient. Discuss any change of instructions.

▶ For discharge to the home setting, verify the patient's need for transportation services, including type (e.g., stretcher-ready transportation). Confirm that transportation has been arranged.

▶ For transfers to a SNF, call for validation that the patient's bed is still available. Update the SNF on the social and medical status of the patient. Ask whether the SNF supplies transportation from the hospital to the facility or you set it up. Confirm that there is a physician to follow up; if not, find one. If possible, get transfer orders written, get reports from the multidisciplinary staff, and copy pertinent parts of the medical record.

▶ Get confirmation from the patient, the family, and the attending physician that they still agree with the discharge plans (whether home or SNF transfer).

▶ Make a list of all pertinent agencies, companies, and community referrals and their telephone numbers. Give this to the patient and the family.

▶ Call the insurance company with up-to-date medical and discharge data; obtain authorization for the final hospital day (many insurance companies pay for the day of admission but not for the day of discharge), and obtain authorization for any discharge disposition services.

▶ Gather any other details specific to a particular case.

EXAMPLES OF KEY CASE MANAGEMENT ACTIVITIES FOR A PATIENT'S DISCHARGE—THE DAY OF DISCHARGE

- ▸ Monitor medical stability and discharge screens.
- ▸ Give written discharge instructions. Work on fine-tuning any assessed educational insufficiencies.
- ▸ All test results have been reported to the physician and healthcare team. Those that are not normalizing have been discussed, and documentation verifies the physician's notification and permission to continue with discharge as planned.
- ▸ Transportation to home or another facility is set up and confirmed. The patient/family, nurses, and physician are notified of final times for pickup.
- ▸ The patient and family are given written instructions for follow-up with physician(s).
- ▸ The patient and family are given written dates, times, and addresses for any outpatient needs (physical therapy, occupational therapy, speech therapy, IV therapy, tests, hemodialysis, etc.), including appointments already confirmed.

- ▸ DME is delivered to the home or the hospital.
- ▸ Supplies are delivered to the home or the hospital.
- ▸ Home health agencies are called for medical updates and for confirmation of time and day when a first visit will commence. Often, a home health agency will not begin servicing a patient until the day after discharge if the care can be completed in the hospital on the day of discharge. If a patient needs a twice daily treatment or IV antibiotics, the home healthcare worker will come on the day of discharge. Communicate these arrangements to the patient and the family.
- ▸ For SNF transfers, calls are placed with medical updates and to confirm transfer on that day. Final validation is obtained that physicians/family/patient all agree with the transfer; transportation is set up, a physician will follow up, the chart is copied, orders are complete and correct, and all reports are included.
- ▸ Gather any other details specific to a particular case.

▸ Case Managers of Outside Facilities (External)

Case managers working within acute and postacute facilities can benefit from the support of external case managers. The external case managers are knowledgeable about patients' benefits and about which agencies and facilities are contracted with the patient's health insurance plan. This information is valuable and can save time when seeking follow-up care.

The aforementioned internal case management responsibilities may also be required of external case managers. Because of the different healthcare relationships in these two types of case management practices, additional responsibilities often are incurred with external case management. Many of the tasks are more aligned with business, rather than clinical job descriptions. External case managers are frequently required to document and report differently than those in hospitals or SNFs. Proof of negotiation and pricing agreements must be in writing, confidentiality and release of information forms may be required, and often even agreement and consent for case management services may need to be obtained. Reports to consultants and claims to payors demonstrating improvement in quality of life and cost-benefit savings because of case management services are required on a regular basis. Return-to-work plans and life-care planning documentation are required for some external case managers. In addition, careful documentation and recording of activities, decisions, and observations are required on a day-to-day basis for both external and internal case management.

▸ STAGE V: EVALUATION AND FOLLOW-UP

The stage of evaluation and follow-up is an important one; it ensures case continuity and sends the patient and family a message of caring. The job responsibilities of your particular type of case management determine what you do in Stage V and how you do it. Episodic case management is provided for a specified encounter of care in a patient's life. Some hospital case managers follow a patient in the hospital during an illness, but do little follow-up after the patient's discharge or transition to another care setting or level of care. Other case managers start their responsibilities after the patient is discharged. Home health case managers follow up on the patient/family in the home setting; extended care facility case managers follow up patients while they reside in that facility; hospice case managers follow up their patients from admission into hospice until death (unless the patient or family opts otherwise); other case managers manage their patients throughout all levels of care until the latter's independence, formal release of the case, or death.

▸ Familial Needs

Several research studies have been conducted to find what families with chronically ill family members need to help them cope with illness and hospitalization. The original landmark study was conducted by Molter in the late 1970s. The universal need identified as extremely important was the need for hope (Molter, 1979). Another study distilled the responses of seventeen previous studies and revealed that fourteen of the top twenty-one needs were concerned with obtaining information about family members (Hickey, 1990; Kleinpell, 1990). Case managers are often the disseminators of the information that the family needs to cope. Families are an integrated system in which a change in one member's normal condition, (e.g., the ill patient) directly affects all other members (the family), often disrupting the equilibrium of the whole system (Kupferschmid, 1987). The sharing of accurate information by the case manager with the family empowers the family to make informed decisions; in this way, the case manager helps the family to gain understanding and a feeling of control over a difficult situation (Bouley, Von Hofe, & Blatt, 1994). Although studies such as these belong to an older period, human needs rarely change quickly, remaining more or less the same throughout.

Fifteen of the most important family needs are discussed in this chapter. The needs may have been ranked differently, depending on the study performed, and the year in which a study that was performed influenced its findings. Earlier studies show comfortable furniture in the waiting room of a care setting as well as waiting room and bathroom locations ranking higher in importance than do later studies. A reason for this may be that many hospitals have addressed these issues, and they no longer loom as major concerns today.

It is interesting how often a case manager can make an impact on the fifteen most important needs. When appraising the final evaluation of a case, assess the success and impact that case management services have had in meeting these needs.

1. *To feel there is hope*: Hope helps people to cope with a current life crisis by helping them to believe that the future holds promise; it is the universal need expressed. There is a delicate balance that case managers must achieve between giving too much hope or too little. We must often talk about the gravity or difficulty of a situation. It is not always easy to do this without destroying hope. Assess how well this was done in some of your most challenging cases.

2. *To have questions answered honestly*: People respond positively to honesty and expect it. In 10 studies, 100% of the respondents rated this need as extremely important (Hickey, 1990). Even grave news has the benefit of preparing family members for the worst. Less than honest answers—or providing false hope—can leave a family member in shock and disbelief if they were not told of the possibility of a poor outcome before its occurrence. This is especially difficult if the physician or family member wants information kept away from the patient or another family member. Assess how well this was done in a difficult situation.

3. *To be assured that the hospital personnel care about the patient and that the best possible care is being provided to the patient*: Families want to be assured that their ill relatives and loved ones are important to the staff and are treated kindly, respectfully, and with total honesty. They also need to know that the care provided is appropriate for the illness. Clinical pathways, especially those prepared for the consumption of patients, when shared with patients and families, have been noted to ease their worries. If the patient is moving along the pathway fairly steadily, the family can see that the care is standard protocol and that the patient is responding as expected. Using patient- and family-focused clinical pathways enhances patient and family control over the situation, alleviates their anxiety concerning the type of care/treatments to be provided, and allows them to anticipate their role in the treatments to be provided and understand their responsibilities.

4. *To know the prognosis*: Often after the family is briefed about the prognosis by the attending physician, it has many questions that do not surface immediately. The case manager can act as a safety net, being there to allow the family to vent, grieve, or ask questions as they come up and perhaps to make one of the most difficult decisions—whether to sign a do-not-resuscitate (DNR) order or to withdraw life and/or nutritional support.

5. *To know specific facts about the patient's progress on a daily basis*: This knowledge was also an extremely important need for 100% of the respondents in 10 studies (Hickey, 1990). Some of the angriest family and patient complaints have resulted from their feeling that they were not updated regularly about the patient's progress and could not get the information they needed. Frequent visits by case managers to answer questions and clarify any misconceptions can prevent unnecessary anger and anxiety. Assess the patient's/family's satisfaction on this point.

6. *To have explanations given in understandable terms*: Explaining complicated concepts in an easy-to-understand language is an art. Some physicians are excellent at doing this; other times it may be necessary for the case manager to assess for gaps and misunderstandings in the patient or the family. When a patient is in pain or a family is in crisis because of the acute, severe nature of the illness or injury, even clear and simple explanations may be more than a person can process. The explanations at such times must be simple, concrete, and clear, conveying only the most immediately necessary facts. Speaking slowly and calmly and making eye contact aid this process. Assess whether the family/patient received this kind of attention.

7. *To see the patient frequently*: This is more difficult in some areas of case management than in others,

such as when the patient is in an intensive care unit (ICU). The inability of a family to see, touch, and assess how their loved one is doing is a constant reminder of the threat of permanent loss of that person. This is especially true in sudden, acute situations such as traumas. One case manager remembers when, as a fairly new bride in the late 1970s, she was called at work with information that her husband had been involved in a motorcycle accident. She arrived at the scene and stayed with him for 45 minutes until the ambulance came. During that time, he was in and out of consciousness, his pupils were dilated, and it was obvious that several bones were broken, including his clavicle, which was protruding through the skin. In the 7 hours that followed—during which he was in the emergency department—the only information volunteered to her was the name of the ward to which he was being transferred. The only time she saw him was when she sneaked into his room in the emergency department and was then promptly ushered out. The anxiety she felt was intense; it could have been eased greatly by regular updates and closer physical proximity.

Perhaps because of that experience, that case manager now uses more cots on her unit—and has been known to run out of them—than are used on other units. Both patients and families usually respond with decreased anxiety when they can be near each other. Case managers who work in ICUs or emergency departments can plan times that are acceptable to the area and the family for visitation. Keeping the patients and families informed of what is going on is essential to reducing their anxiety and ultimately increasing their cooperation and involvement in care and decision making. Assess family satisfaction on this point as part of the final evaluation.

8. *To know exactly what is being done for the patient and why it is being done*: This is important in helping patients and families to make informed decisions. The case manager aids the family by sharing accurate and consistent information. This is a shared responsibility with the physician and has legal ramifications when this information is used for the purpose of signing an informed consent. As in all informational needs, assess how well this was covered in the case plan.

9. *To talk to the physician every day*: Usually a patient, if alert and oriented, speaks daily to the physician. But issues arise when family members and significant others are unable to make contact with busy physicians. After a couple of days pass with no word from the patient's doctors, family members are likely to become upset, displaying attitudes that lead the staff to label them as "difficult," "manipulative," or "interfering." Again, anxiety is often the cause of this behavior, and it can be diminished by a physician telephoning the family, sometimes supplemented with information offered by the case manager.

One communication disaster paired a physician with a less-than-empathetic bedside manner with an angry man whose grandfather—his only living relative—was in the hospital. As the patient's hospitalization stretched longer and longer, the worried grandson threatened to file lawsuit after lawsuit, fired multiple physicians, and became tangential in his conversations. The physician withdrew, doing his best to avoid communication. The situation was reaching a dangerous point, because staff nurses were becoming frightened of the grandson. When the case was transferred to another unit, the case manager there made a deal with the physician that if he would speak daily—at least briefly—to the grandson, she would fill in the gaps. The grandson agreed to this arrangement, after she assured him that she was available for further informational needs. Working on the tangential nature of his personality was a little more challenging, however. She limited the number of main points for each conversation (frequent reorientations to those main points were necessary), and the main points were written down for the grandson to hold onto. At first, the grandson asked the same questions over and over without seeming to hear the answers. Within 3 days, he was much less hostile, and the frequency of repeated questions was dramatically reduced. Finally, the patient was transferred to an extended care facility with the same physician following up, and the grandson was in agreement with the plan.

In the final evaluation, assess whether the family and patient were comfortable with the one-on-one attention from the attending physician and other staff involved in care.

10. *To be called at home when the patient's condition changes*: Because case managers are not present 24 hours a day, the responsibility of calling to update families may fall on the staff nurses, physicians, or some other designated health professionals. Many nurses are very conscientious about this. If the family is upset over poor communication, staff guidance and support may be needed.

11. *To have a specific person to call if the family cannot make it to the facility*: The three-shift structure of facilities that give 24-hour care translates into many caregivers for each patient. Families often feel more comfortable if they have a single contact person whom they can ask for by name. The case

manager is a reasonable choice that benefits everyone. The family has a knowledgeable contact, and the case manager often picks up important information about transitional planning from these conversations. Information appears to be a vital need for families, and the case manager can be a primary link between that information and the family. If too many people are calling from one family unit, it helps to have the family appoint a spokesperson to call the case manager. The other family members can then call this designated person. In the final case evaluation, assess your role in this pivotal communication position.

12. *To be told about transfer plans*: When a patient is being transferred to another unit within the hospital, let the family know. Family members get frightened when they visit and find an empty bed, especially if the patient is critically ill. When the transfer is to another facility, the plans should be agreed to by the family and coordinated with them. One uncomfortable type of situation occurs when a family approves of the hospital where the patient is, but the health insurance company wants the patient transferred to one of their contracted hospitals. The present hospital could suffer financially if the transfer is not made, and few families can afford to pay for a hospitalization. In the final evaluation, assess transfer coordination with the family.

13. *To feel accepted by the hospital staff or those of the care setting where the patient is receiving healthcare services*: Family members often feel like "strangers in a strange land" and need to feel supported if they are to be a support for their ill family member. A case manager remembers a very difficult case involving a husband and wife. The wife was a heavily built woman who was essentially a quadriplegic as a result of multiple sclerosis. She had many chronic conditions, including infections that frequently necessitated IV antibiotics. Although she required 24-hour care, her husband adamantly refused nursing home placement. He was a challenging person, and many home health agencies could no longer deal with his demands. Therefore, this case manager's challenge became finding a home health agency that would accept the wife each time she was discharged. The staff always groaned when this patient was admitted; although she was extremely pleasant, her husband's demands could not be satisfied. One afternoon, while making rounds with the nurse manager of the unit, the husband went into his usual tirade of complaints and demands. The nurse manager approached him in a way no one else had. She touched his arm and gently asked how long he had been caring for his wife in this condition. He looked surprised but answered, "Seventeen

years." "And who," she asked, "takes care of you?" Breaking into tears, the man said quietly, "No one." Suddenly someone had accepted him. This nurse manager's compassion opened a door, and the man responded with a remarkable mellowing.

Some patients and family members are also apprehensive that if the staff disapproves of them, they will not receive good care. This fear is not uncommon. If the case manager or the staff cannot connect with the family, perhaps a minister, rabbi, or psychologist may be able to do so. In the final evaluation, assess whether the case manager was instrumental in helping the family to feel accepted and welcome.

14. *To have directions about what to do at the bedside*: Families are often afraid to touch their ill family member, especially if there are many tubes and machines in use. Neonatal intensive care nurses routinely show parents how to handle the "preemies" and sick newborns. Parents of older pediatric patients are also routinely given directions for safe handling of the child. Many family members, especially spouses, would like to do more for the patient but are not sure what they are allowed to do. The staff nurse and case manager can explain any invasive lines, assess the extent to which the family member would like to help with basic care, and help dispel any fears. Assess family satisfaction in this area.

15. *To talk about the possibility of the patient's death*: Some people have a great need to talk about their loved one's possible death; it is almost as if, by rehearsing it, they might be better prepared when it happens. Others will not verbalize the possibility as if afraid that by talking about it, they might bring it on. Sensitivity to the family's needs on this point is critical, and some families prefer to speak to a member of the clergy. In the final evaluation (if this is applicable), assess whether the family's needs were met.

▶ Case Evaluation

In general, families want reassurance that their loved one is well cared for, that they have access to the patient and the healthcare team, and that they have all the information they can handle. If these points are addressed, the family is usually satisfied. Overall, how well did the patient/family unit respond to the plan of care? The following are some general questions to ask in case evaluation and follow-up.

1. Were the care goals and objectives met? Essentially, there are only three possibilities: the goals were met, partially met, or not met at all. Any shade of gray must be addressed. Determine why the goals were partially (or not) met:

- Were the goals realistic?
- Were appropriate treatment, resources, procedures, or case management interventions selected? Were all the essential needs of the patient and family identified and addressed? Did other issues come to light after the initial interventions that demonstrated a new strategy might be more successful or necessary?
- Was the patient or family motivated and fully engaged?
2. Were all services delivered as planned?
3. Were there any problems with the agencies or companies that were set up for certain services and resources?
4. Are new needs surfacing that are serious enough to destabilize the whole plan of care?
5. Were any patient or family needs missed?

Some cases do not go smoothly, and the case manager is not surprised. Perhaps the patient wanted more than the health insurance agency would pay for and refused other options. Perhaps the patient's needs and the available resources were a poor match. What if the case management interventions appeared to go fairly routinely, yet later the patient or family expressed disappointment or resentment? The following are some possible questions to ask.

- Did the patient and family truly agree to the plan, were they pressured or coerced, or did they simply lack understanding?
- Was the family or patient unrealistic, or in denial, about the options?
- Did the patient's medical status change, necessitating revisions to the plan of care, transitional plan, and/or care goals?
- Was poor or inadequate planning responsible for patient/family disappointment?
- Was the suboptimal intervention due to the fact that the patient had virtually no resources (socially or financially/insurance) and refused other available assistance (shelters, community assistance)?
- Was the follow-up agency/facility less than adequate, or was poor "chemistry" with the staff to blame? Case managers are responsible for using credible resources; however, sometimes even reliable agencies and facilities have intermittent problems.

There are as many reasons for case management interventions and plans to falter (in whole or in part) as there are details to a particular case. If improperly evaluated and executed, any detail can destabilize the whole plan.

▶ Case Management Outcomes

Outcomes evaluation is not precisely a step in the case management process but is essential for case management to continue to grow and be recognized as a value-added

part of the healthcare system. In discussing the Standards of Practice for Case Management, the Case Management Society of America (CMSA, 2016) focuses on the following standards of care:

1. Assessment/case identification and selection
2. Problem identification
3. Planning
4. Monitoring
5. Evaluation
6. Outcomes

The final standard of care, outcomes, is important because case management is a goal-directed process. Case managers collaboratively determine care goals with the patient/family unit, the physician, and the multidisciplinary team. Next, case management interventions are set in motion that will have the greatest likelihood of achieving those goals. Then, case managers identify what the outcomes, or results, of those case management interventions will be. For a patient suffering a new onset of stroke with left hemiplegia, for example, the goal may be ambulating 50 feet with a walker. The time frame may be in weeks or months, depending on the severity of the paralysis, and the general health condition of the patient, and the involvement of the family in care. Both the goal in feet and the goal in a specified time frame are measurable. That is the key—any outcome must be the result of a measurable goal.

On a more global level, case management outcomes may not necessarily be patient related from a quality of life or clinical point of view. Rather, outcomes in case management can also be measured in terms of cost-effectiveness because of a given case management intervention. Does case management presurgical teaching shorten lengths of stay? Does diabetic education reduce the frequency of hospitalizations because of diabetic ketoacidosis or uncontrolled diabetes? Does close monitoring of pharmaceuticals in a congestive heart failure patient lessen the number of avoidable readmissions to the hospital or emergency department visits?

Proof of good case management outcomes, for both cost and quality, is expected in today's healthcare environment. The key purpose of measuring case management outcomes is to quantify and qualify the impact of case management services. In fact, the role of an outcomes manager is becoming one of the hybrid case management roles in many care settings today. Hands-on case managers are being asked, at the very least, to collect the information used for outcomes analysis. Administrative case managers may be required to develop quality improvement projects.

Outcomes management is, at times, a frustrating and complex activity requiring knowledge about topics such as how to develop and improve outcomes; how to identify and develop quality indicators that are measurable, reliable, and valid; and how to interpret the data. It is not, however, an activity that will disappear anytime soon. Accreditation standards are written with outcomes in mind, and accreditation status depends on them. The healthcare industry is demanding evidence of quality care, customer/patient satisfaction with the care experience, and efficiency of care delivery. These expectations are embedded in today's healthcare-related regulations and pay-for-performance standards. Case managers no doubt are able to contribute to adherence to these expectations and to ensure that the patient/family has an optimal, quality, and safe care experience.

▶ STAGE VI: CONTINUOUS MONITORING, REASSESSING, AND REEVALUATING

Case management monitoring, reassessing, and reevaluating continue until the patient's case management services are officially concluded. Therefore, it is not really a stage, but rather an ongoing review process. Ongoing activities include (CMSA, 2016):

- ▶ Follow-up with the client, family, and/or family caregiver and evaluation of the client's status, goals, and outcomes.
- ▶ Monitoring activities include assessing client's progress with planned interventions.
- ▶ Evaluating whether care goals and interventions remain appropriate, relevant, and realistic.
- ▶ Determining whether any revisions or modifications are needed to the care needs, goals, or interventions specified in the client's case management plan of care.

Rarely does the case management process proceed directly from Stage I to Stage VI, in which the patient is miraculously being fully and perfectly cared for! More often, this continuous process of reassessment and monitoring reveals changes in the patient's medical condition or hidden social circumstances hitherto unknown, necessitating changes in the plan of care and services. Through the activities of Stage VI, the service plan is revised, refined, and fine-tuned. This iterative, back-and-forth flow may occur several times before implementation of the final plan becomes a reality.

The stability and the type of the case determine the frequency of the monitoring and reevaluating. Some patients in hospital need more than daily attention, whereas a stable patient residing in a long-term facility may need only weekly visits (although the patient would be monitored daily at the facility). Disease-state case management monitoring depends on the issues of the particular disease. Other types of case management require specific care plans and have policies about exactly when these care plans must be reviewed. Reassessment may also be required at specific intervals by state laws in long-term care and other programs. Each case management model has its own challenges and unique clientele, requiring customized monitoring and reevaluation of standards and procedures.

For some types of case management (mostly external case managers), the payor of case management services must also be monitored. There are times when details of a patient's case change, so the payor may no longer desire to continue providing case management services. Some patients may eventually qualify for Medicare or another insurance as a primary payor; most payors do not want to continue to pay for case management services because they are not financially liable, but some (a few) continue because case management can benefit the patient and ultimately reduce unnecessary costs in the long run. The details of the patient's condition may change, so the payor of case management services may decide on a new goal for case management. Perhaps initially, case management was called on to find a perfect placement for a hard-to-place patient, complete with reasonable per diem negotiations. That was all the case manager was hired to do. However, once in the facility, problems may develop with the family and care, so case management may be asked to stay on for a longer time.

The process of case selection eliminates patients who are essentially stable. The remaining cases, by their very nature of severity and instability, require continuous monitoring. Akin to a domino effect, a change in the patient's medical status could affect the entire continuum from the treatment plan to the final disposition. As the case manager monitors the medical and psychosocial stability of the patient, a moderate-to-severe change could necessitate the reassessment of the total balance of services planned for in previous stages. The change may be minor, such as a new need for home oxygen, which would be added to any other home health needs that were previously evaluated. Perhaps a major reevaluation of the whole service, treatment, care plan, or transfer plan may be needed. Most case managers have at some time needed to upgrade a discharge disposition from home-based services to admission at a SNF because of medical deterioration; the reverse may also take place. The following is an example of the importance of continuous case management.

Mrs. Bolton was 97 years old and lived with her 79-year-old daughter. Mrs. Bolton had a medical history that included hypertension, osteoarthritis, congestive heart failure, and colon cancer, necessitating J-tube feedings for nutrition. She was admitted to the hospital in a cachectic condition with hypotension, dehydration, acute renal failure (creatinine, 4.3 mg/dL), and pneumonia.

Within 48 hours of admission, Mrs. Bolton became unresponsive, with a temperature of 34°C. A DNR order was signed, and comfort care and gentle IV hydration were provided. It was also decided that IV antibiotics would be continued for the pneumonia. The next day, her stools became grossly heme-positive, and her hemoglobin and hematocrit levels dropped significantly. The daughter and physicians decided to transfuse one unit of red blood cells and monitor her hematocrit and hemoglobin daily. The family did not wish the patient to undergo a colonoscopy. By the week's end, the doctors assessed the prognosis as "grim."

The following Monday morning, the case manager noted that Mrs. Bolton's name was still on the census board. She checked with the unit secretary and was told that she was indeed still on the unit. Imagine the case manager's surprise when, in the morning report, the night charge nurse mentioned that Mrs. Bolton was ambulating with assistance through the hallways! While the family and medical team were making "final disposition" plans, Mrs. Bolton had other ideas. She remained in the hospital for additional (somewhat rocky) days, during which time her pneumonia and gastrointestinal bleeding both cleared. Her creatinine decreased to a reasonable level, and physical therapy helped with strengthening. Once her J-tube feedings were tolerated at the prescribed rate, she was discharged home with her daughter.

It is said that the only thing constant is change; this is certainly true in case management. Constant change is the prime reason why this stage of continuous monitoring and reevaluating is so essential. Each case has unique features and important aspects that need monitoring. The following represent some basics that need to be monitored.

❱ Changes in Medical Status (Improvement or Deterioration)

Change in medical status (improvement) is the desired outcome when a patient enters the hospital. When a patient comes in sick, it is hoped that the illness can be changed to a more homeostatic condition. If the lungs are wheezy, physicians try for clear lungs and to achieve acceptable arterial blood gases. If bowels are obstructed, the medical team attempts to clear the obstruction with conservative or surgical methods. A multisystem failure patient or a level I trauma victim may deteriorate further or may stabilize at a level of health that is lower than the previous baseline. All body systems, laboratory results, and vital signs must be monitored. Patient changes may signal the need for change in the treatment plan. Anything that varies from the patient's baseline may indicate a need for compensations in the transitions plan.

Medical status changes often must be monitored for utilization and insurance authorization purposes. Clinical pathways, intensity of service, severity of illness, and other utilization modalities may demonstrate a need for a change in the level of care and the case plan. A patient who is not in an appropriate level of care may be at risk medically if a more acute level of care is needed; he or she may be overutilizing resources if a less acute level of care is available to treat the medical condition.

❱ Changes in the Social Stability of the Patient

Life changes that occur while a patient is in the hospital or in the convalescent phase of an illness can sometimes be more trying than the illness itself. A lost lease or apartment may leave a patient homeless and worried about his or her possessions. If pets or family members also live there, the emotional trauma is multiplied. During hospitalizations and convalescent periods, patients can lose roommates, significant others may depart, parents may die, spouses may also need to be hospitalized, pets may be left uncared for, bills pile up, utilities are turned off, and employment is terminated—all these may have a significant effect on the total psychosocial picture and often cause stress-related exacerbations of illnesses. Prompt attention from social services and modifications of the transition plan may be needed.

❱ Quality of Care

Acceptable standards of care and careful, ethical treatment of patients and their medical conditions are the minimal expected norms. Unfortunately, accidents and oversights take place. A clinically astute case manager can often prevent or impede an adverse outcome. Ideally, a maloccurrence can be averted. If that is not possible, quick action may minimize the negative consequences. If an undesirable outcome takes place, it may be wise to call the risk management department and follow the facility's protocol.

❱ Changes in Functional Capability and Mobility

Functional changes are especially important for older adults who may have been independent prior to the current ailment. Some conditions, such as recent surgery, profound weakness, deep vein thrombosis, and hemiparesis, preclude early mobilization. An aggressive approach to early mobilization is essential to prevent further weakness and decline. Patients often feel that illness and bed rest are a natural marriage, whereas nurses know that bed rest may lead to a host of possible comorbidities. Sometimes, the physician's order for restorative nursing, physical therapy, or ambulation is missing and therefore not considered until late in the admission. Patients who may be restrained for safety purposes often are capable of walking with assistance. Case managers should guard against extra lengths of stay because of minimal mobilization until late in the hospitalization. It jeopardizes the independence of some patients and may cause insurance denials at the acute care level.

❱ Evolving Health Education Needs

As the patient or family is ready, knowledge deficits about the disease process, its course, and treatment should be identified and educational sessions can be added. Opportunities for teaching seem endless. Health education by staff nurses or other healthcare professionals concerning the disease process, dressing changes and wound care, medical equipment, nutrition and dietary plan, rehabilitation activities and exercise, tube care, medication usage, medication interactions and side effects, suctioning, and many other techniques and informational aspects of care is essential. Case managers should note that the health teaching aspect expands into areas such as explanations about the individual's health insurance benefits and coverage, deductibles, copay plans, DRGs, prescription costs, and location of contracted pharmacies and hospitals. Patients are often uncertain who their primary care physicians are or how to access the medical system. Overuse of emergency departments is often a clue to the latter knowledge deficit. Community resources and how to access these may be important to many individuals.

Patients retain only approximately 10% of the information given to them in teaching sessions. Visual demonstrations, books, and audiovisual handouts are helpful. As the patient's and the family's readiness and receptivity increases, they can review the education materials as needed. Studies have shown that informational materials are best understood when written at the sixth grade reading level or lower, in large print, and including several illustrations. Tapes should be interesting but concise, because people who are ill often have short attention spans. If headphones are available, they can be used to block out distractions.

Physical and psychosocial influences must be taken into consideration when assessing a patient's readiness to learn. Pain, weakness, nausea, and drowsiness from medications weigh heavily on a person's ability to learn. A person who is still in shock over a new diagnosis may be too depressed or in the denial stage and therefore unreceptive to learning. Body image is another powerful factor. Occasionally, a previously independent patient who lives alone may need to go to an extended care facility after a colostomy or tracheostomy because of refusal to accept—and subsequently care for—the tracheostomy or colostomy. Some people simply need more time. Learning cannot be forced; the information must be accepted and absorbed in cooperation with the free will of the patient.

▶ Pain Management

Pain management is one aspect of care that often brings out the "judge" in the medical staff. Perhaps it is because pain is a subjective experience that often does not correlate with objective criteria. This is further complicated by an individual's tolerance to pain and psychological, sociologic, and cultural elements. Studies have shown that although pain is cited as the most common reason why people seek medical attention, the management of pain is often inadequate. Early and adequate pain management is part of the case manager's obligation to relieve suffering as much as possible. It also produces earlier mobilization of patients, shortened hospital stays, and reduced costs.

The psychosocial aspect of pain control is important for the case manager to consider, and some comprehensive pain management clinics include psychosocial care and alternate methods in their programs. Pain management programs at numerous institutions teach relaxation, stress reduction, and meditation as a pain reduction plan. The perception of pain is perhaps the most important component in pain control. Humans have a unique way of experiencing pain, one that is mixed with fear; when the fear component is missing, the experience is very different from what is typically witnessed in adults after a stay in the hospital. The Beth Israel Deaconess pain clinic found that if patients could modify the way they perceived pain, the pain often lessened.

▶ Care Goals

It is important to assess and reassess whether all the identified and agreed upon care goals in the case management plan that were determined to be essential to a case continue to be realistic and appropriate, as the case evolves and unfolds. Priorities change as patients either improve or become more accepting of their current situations. Life care plans must be modified when patient/family goals are changed or the patient's condition changes. Perhaps the major goal was to keep the patient at home; after major mental deterioration, the burden may become so huge that a residential placement is in order. The case manager's role may shift to assisting the family to find a place where they feel the care will be good for their loved one; grief counseling for the family may also be needed, because this is a major life shift.

▶ STAGE VII: CASE CLOSURE AND TERMINATION OF CASE MANAGEMENT SERVICES

Closure of case management services is about bringing mutually agreed upon closure to the patient–case manager relationship and engagement in case management. Case closure focuses on discontinuing the case management services when the patient has attained the highest level of functioning and recovery, the best possible outcomes, or when the needs and desires of the patient have changed (CMSA, 2016).

And sometimes, saying goodbye is one of the most challenging tasks a case manager must complete. Case managers who follow patients throughout the continuum of healthcare and human services have been invited to birthday parties, retirement parties, and even funerals. Obviously, a patient's death terminates case management services, but other reasons for termination are also notable:

- ▶ The patient, provider, or payor requests termination.
- ▶ The patient is no longer eligible for the insurance that covers case management services.
- ▶ Changes in the medical condition that warrant concluding the case management services: a healthy baby is born, the medical condition is stabilized, or disease-specific education and monitoring have been maximized.

▶ The patient/case management goals have been achieved.

▶ The patient and/or family opt for a change in the case manager or the private case management company.

▶ The patient died.

▶ The case manager is no longer available for any of several reasons, such as relocation, change in job, change in organization/employer.

▶ The case management company closed or relocated.

▶ The case management program was discontinued.

Case closure or termination of case management services requires special skills and talents. Terminating services is as challenging as building a trusting relationship between the case manager and the patient/family. Case managers should exercise caution in how they go about closing a case or terminating a relationship with a patient and/or family. They are advised to:

▶ Educate the patient and family about the need for case closure.

▶ Share the expectation of case closure with the patient and family at case selection and intake time.

▶ Transition the case to the next case manager or provider to maintain continuity of care if closure is done because of relocation or change in insurance company or provider.

▶ Answer patient and family questions.

▶ Alleviate patient and family anxiety.

▶ Reintroduce the need for case closure a few days prior to the last date of involvement in the case.

▶ STAGE VIII: COMMUNICATION WITH THE PATIENT AND FAMILY AFTER CLOSURE OF THE PROCESS

Communication and follow-up with the patient and family after closure of the case management process and services have recently become popular and integral to ensuring safe patient discharge from an episode of care or transition to another level of care or provider for continued care and services. The purpose of such communication is patient centered—that is, checking if the patient is safe, the services needed after the care encounter have been secured and commenced as planned, and continuity of care has not been compromised.

Communication after the patient's discharge or transition from a setting such as a hospital, rehabilitation center, or SNF may be done by telephone or occasionally in person. The follow-up may be helpful in ensuring that postdischarge or transition services are supporting the patient— whether these services are minimal, such as a few home care visits by a healthcare professional (e.g., registered nurse, physical therapist), or as significant as an extensive rehabilitation transitional period. This follow-up is usually appreciated, and often needed, by the patient and family.

Many times after discharge, unexpected events occur, questions surface, ordered services fall through the cracks or do not meet expectations, or durable medical equipment does not arrive or is different from the type that the family was taught how to use in the facility. Perhaps the patient/family expected more hours of help or had a different idea of needed help from that of the home health agency or that approved by the health insurance plan. Caring for the patient may present more challenges than the family had anticipated; perhaps proper encouragement and a couple of added services would be all that are needed to turn the situation from one of panic to one of success. In addition, a family may be having a difficult time securing a medication. The family may not know which pharmacy is contracted with the patient's health insurance plan, or the medication is not covered and is found to be unaffordable. A patient may feel that a physician is not responsive to telephone calls; on the other hand, some patients and families would rather direct their enquiries to a case manager than "bother" their physician. Any number of unanticipated situations may arise.

This follow-up contact, as it occurs by phone, may act as a vehicle to answer questions, discuss possible solutions, reassure the patient/family, and often prevent complications or even readmissions and trips to the emergency department. Multiple telephone calls may be needed in some instances; it is important for the case manager not to give up after one or two calls when still unable to connect with the patient/family. Telephone calls to the physician, the home health agency, the DME company, social service agencies, or any other part of the plan of care and the postdischarge services may be required.

Other important benefits of communicating with the patient/family after discharge or transition include inquiring with the patient/family about their experience with care provision, their level of satisfaction with the services, and their recommendations, if any, for improvement. Additionally, case managers may explore the patient's (or the family's) knowledge of red flags and degree of comfort with self-management and ability to maintain adherence to the plan of care including healthy lifestyle behaviors. Accordingly, case managers are then able to institute action to enhance self-care management and prevent avoidable return to the acute care setting or emergency department.

The case management process is not an easy one, but a skilled and experienced case manager can usually overcome obstacles, regardless of what they are or when they occur. Most patients and families are very appreciative of the case management process and the guidance and support extended to them. The final question, the answer to which will test the efficacy of the whole case management process, is, Did case management efforts improve or at least optimize the quality of life for this person and this family unit? Within this question lies the heart of case management.

DISCUSSION QUESTIONS

1. Cite an example of a case that was not selected for case management but should have been. How did this case fall through the cracks? What did you do to prevent such mistakes from happening in the future?

2. Discuss the importance of a thorough assessment. What are some barriers to a thorough assessment?

3. Discuss the steps needed to coordinate and develop a treatment or discharge plan. What are some barriers to this stage of the case management process?

4. How would you go about developing a list of community resources and agencies in your area?

5. Discuss changes that must be monitored in the case management stage of continuous assessment and monitoring. Evaluate how one change can affect the structure of the whole case plan.

6. Cite a case example in which a discharge was held up because all services were not evaluated and set up by the day that the patient was ready for discharge. What could have been set up the day before discharge? Would this have allowed the discharge to go on as scheduled?

7. Discuss the important issues cited by families. How can a case manager help meet those needs?

8. Consider a case that you managed. Did you include all the steps and stages? What would you do differently?

9. Discuss a case where closure was challenging. What were the issues? What strategies were effective? What activities were ineffective?

▶ REFERENCES

American Case Management Association. (2016). *Compass: Directional training for case managers. Version 3.0.* Little Rock, AR: Author.

Bouley, G., Von Hofe, K., & Blatt, L. (1994). Holistic are of the critically ill: meeting both patient and family needs. *Dimensions of Critical Care Nursing, 13*(4), 218–223.

Case Management Society of America. (2016). *Standards of practice for case management.* Little Rock: Author.

Case Management Society of America. (2017). *Core curriculum for case management* (3rd ed.). Philadelphia, PA: Author.

Hickey, M. (1990). What are the needs of families of critically ill patients? A review of the literature since 1979. *Heart & Lung, 19*(4), 401–415.

Hill, R. B. (1979). *Hanta Yo: An American Saga.* Garden City, NY: Doubleday Publishers.

Kleinpell, R. M. (1990). Needs of families of critically ill patients: a literature review. *Critical Care Nurse, 11*(8), 34–40.

Kupferschmid, B. (1987). Families of critically ill patients. *Critical Care Nursing Currents, 5*(2), 7–12.

Molter, N. (1979). Needs of relatives of critically ill patients: a descriptive study. *Heart & Lung, 8*(2), 332–339.

Treiger, T., & Fink-Samnick, E. (2016). *Collaborate for professional case management: A universal competency based paradigm.* Philadelphia, PA: Wolter Kluwer.

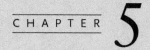

CHAPTER 5

Utilization Management

Management of the allocation and utilization of resources is not a guessing game or streamlining workloads of professionals. It is about being timely, fair, and equitable in the access and distribution of resources to various individuals while making decisions that are based on standards, rules, policies, evidence-based criteria, and care guidelines. It also is about meeting the care needs of individuals while assuring that services provided enhance quality and safety, facilitate reimbursement, and avoid financial risks for all involved.

LEARNING OBJECTIVES

Upon completion of this chapter, the reader will be able to:

1. Define terms and key activities of utilization management.
2. Describe the use of criteria and guidelines in the utilization management process.
3. Differentiate between the various types of reviews.
4. Differentiate between various admission statuses.
5. Determine the role of the case manager in utilization management.
6. Recognize the impact of documentation on avoiding denial of services.
7. Implement a Medicare discharge appeal.

ESSENTIAL TERMS

Admission Review • Appropriate Level of Care • Authorization of Services • Avoidable Delays or Days • Case Management Plans (CMPs) • Certification of Services • Clinical Document Specialist • Clinical Pathways/Critical Pathways • Concurrent Authorization • Concurrent Review • Condition Code 44 • Continued Stay Review • Criteria—evidence-based • Denial • Discharge Appeals • Discharge Reviews • Discharge Screens • Intensity of Service (IS) • InterQual • Length of Stay (LOS) • MCG Health • Medical Necessity • Observation Status • Patient Advocacy • Pending Review • Physician Advisor • Preadmission Review • Precertification • Present on Admission (POA) • Prospective Authorization • Prospective Review • Quality Improvement Organization (QIO) • Recovery Audit Contractors (RACs) • Resource Management • Retrospective Authorization • Retrospective Review • Severity of Illness (SI) • Subauthorization • Subsequent Reviews • Telephonics • Two-Midnight Rule • Utilization Management (UM)

▶ INTRODUCTION

Case managers who came from the ranks of the utilization review (UR) nurses feel at home with the utilization management (UM) role. However, many case managers who came straight in through the clinical doorway (intensive care unit [ICU] nurses, staff nurses) find UM overwhelming and challenging. This chapter breaks down the concepts into clear and usable pieces. It is not difficult, so relax and take a deep breath! However, it is sometimes frustrating. Not all patients fit neatly into the allotted categories, and the UR/UM criteria

are constantly changing, getting stricter, and becoming more demanding every year.

Good UM practices include the use of medical instincts or nursing intuition. Often a patient does not meet official criteria to be hospitalized, but the case manager senses something unstable about the patient. Within 24 hours, the patient "crashes" and is admitted to an ICU. Perhaps the case manager spoke to the health insurance plan's UM department earlier and received a denial notice; a second telephone call would rescind the denial and substantiate why the case manager was hesitant to push for a discharge or transfer to a lesser level of care or setting. Occasionally, an insurance reviewer is very set on using the company's chosen UM modality as though it were law. Cookbook UM is frustrating and probably accounts for the primary reason why many case managers prefer "root canals" to UM responsibilities.

Today's healthcare pressures to provide safer and cost-conscious care with less resources have placed case management in a unique position as a connector between the revenue cycle and UM. As resource stewards, also known as "resource management," case managers apply evidence-based guidelines and practices when recommending resource allocation and utilization options to promote the most effective and efficient use of healthcare services and financial resources (Case Management Society of America [CMSA], 2016).

Although some still use the term "utilization review," this indicates the review, or monitoring, of resource utilization. There is so much more to do and therefore, the term "utilization management" better defines the role. UM evaluates the appropriateness, medical necessity, and efficiency of healthcare services and procedures according to evidence-base criteria. It is intended to help control costs while ensuring that quality of care is delivered and not compromised. UM requires that the payor receives timely clinical reviews of inpatient care and that the reviews contain sufficient information for the payor to make a determination of medical necessity and consequently approve the inpatient stay for payment. In cases where there may be disagreement about medical necessity, effective case managers will facilitate discussion between the physicians caring for the patient and the payor's medical director. In addition, case managers can help identify patients classified incorrectly as observation or inpatient status and collaborate with physicians to rectify the status according to hospital and regulatory policies. This larger role translates into opportunities for case management departments to demonstrate their value within the revenue cycle process (Miodonski, 2012).

▶ HISTORICAL BACKGROUND

UM is not new to the healthcare industry; it has been in existence since the 1970s. It began with the professional standards review organizations, previously known as peer review organizations (PROs), and known today as quality improvement organizations (QIOs). These review organizations were created to evaluate the healthcare services rendered to Medicare and Medicaid beneficiaries. Initially, the main focus of UM entailed the review of hospital-based services provided to Medicare and Medicaid beneficiaries. This UR necessitated matching patients' needs to necessary care interventions with the goal of reducing waste and overutilization of services. Such review was coordinated through independent but state-related agencies (e.g., QIOs).

To maintain compliance with resource utilization standards, hospitals employed nurses to assume UR functions. The UR nurse reviewed the patients' record, and if a patient did not meet acute care criteria, the nurse rectified the situation with the physician and instituted appropriate action. Gradually these functions expanded to outpatient services and by the mid-1980s to commercial health insurance companies. As a result of this expansion, UR shifted from being merely a review function to UM activities that impacted not only quality of care and resource utilization, but reimbursement as well. Today UM is an integral aspect of case management and is applied to the care of every patient regardless of the type of health insurance plan (private or governmental) he or she carries.

Health maintenance organizations, preferred provider organizations, workers' compensation, and virtually all payors at every level of care use a form of UM today. This has resulted in the evolution of case management programs employed by a healthcare organization from being focused on nursing/clinical care management to having clinical care, transitional planning, and UM functions all integrated into one program; often these functions are also integrated into the role of one key healthcare professional—the case manager. This evolution increased the complexity of the case manager's role and, at the same time, raised its importance for the organization. More recently, the regulatory changes have been coming rapidly and this task often goes to the Case/Care Management Department or Program.

UM allows an organization to review its compliance with healthcare-related laws and regulations (e.g., provision of care at the appropriate level of care/setting) and managed care organizations' (MCOs) utilization procedures and practices (e.g., authorizations for care and services). UM functions have direct impact on reimbursement for care rendered. The case manager ensures that patients meet preestablished criteria to support the level of care being delivered, including the setting where patients are cared for. Therefore, reimbursement is dependent on a match between the patient's health/clinical condition (acuity or severity), the treatment plan and options (intensity of resources), and the level of service (care setting/physical location across the healthcare continuum).

▶ THE UTILIZATION/CASE MANAGEMENT TEAM

UM has evolved in the past several years to become more regulation-driven and more precise. It is no longer the case that the nurse case manager, the practice, and the physician advisor constitute the inner UM circle. The evolutionary changes in case management have seen many models come and go, and, it seems, everything old is new again. Today, like in the 1990s and early 2000s, larger healthcare enterprises are separating the UM work from the transitional planning activities. But that does not mean UM nurses are in a silo (as may have been the case in the past). Today's team includes several members, including (but not always limited to):

▶ Nurse Case Manager (NCM)
▶ Social Worker (SW)
▶ Physician Advisor (PA)
▶ Clinical Documentation Specialist
▶ Denial and Appeals Manager
▶ Care Management Assistant (CMA)
▶ Physician Practices/Attending Physicians

The team cannot happen in isolation of the contribution of other healthcare professionals; the practice of case management *is* a team approach (CMSA, 2017). Sometimes the topics get passionate; see Display 5-1 for some tips.

▶ Nurse Case Manager

Interestingly, the role of the NCM may be separated into one that promotes transitional planning and necessarily works closely with patients and families. The NCM in the UM role will likely have less contact with the patients and families, but must huddle regularly with the rest of the healthcare team, who need all the critical information to

---

display 5-1

PRACTICAL TACTICS FOR EFFECTIVE TEAM COMMUNICATION

▶ Be aware of the purpose of the conversation and the most important information or issues to convey before you engage in the conversation with the other party.
▶ Focus on the patient. The patient-centered approach diffuses suspicion and allows everyone to focus on the same goal.
▶ Be colloquial and not adversarial in your approach. Gain a reputation for solving problems, not for creating problems.
▶ Be succinct and to the point about your needs and concerns. Everyone is busy and often may have a low tolerance for rambling conversations.
▶ Make sure you have an accurate and thorough clinical assessment of the situation before you begin your conversation.
▶ When discussing discharge or transfer plans, make sure you have the patient's/family's cooperation in a plan before you discuss it with the physician; this saves wasted steps. On the other hand, some physicians would have known their patients and families for many years and can provide preliminary information that will be very helpful when assessing the plan.
▶ Be assertive, not aggressive.
▶ Keep lines of communication open and follow through on what is discussed. You will gain more trust because of a good follow-through than any other approach you may use.

---

advocate for the best interests of the patient and family. Many companies and third-party administrators provide both UM and case management services. The UM division often detects and substantiates patient triggers that require a referral to case management. Such cases are complex and require more than what UM services typically provide. The patient must be looked at from a broader perspective.

UM is important. It allows services to be authorized by insurance companies; simply put, providers must get paid for the services they provide to survive. Utilization modalities also encourage fiscally responsible length of stay (LOS) and offer the case manager an efficient template for determining medical necessity as the patient moves through the healthcare maze and across the continuum of health and human services. However, in a real sense, simply UR is reactive to medical criteria, whereas nursing case management is proactive. Cookbook UR (i.e., poor or suboptimal UR) has the goal of removing the patient from cost-intensive settings as quickly as possible. Good or optimal case management may have the same end point, but it uses patient advocacy and an interdisciplinary team approach to planning and implementing care to achieve that end point.

▶ Social Worker

Social work is a practice-based profession and an academic discipline that promotes social change and development, social cohesion, and the empowerment of self-choice. SWs collaborate with case managers and other members of the interdisciplinary healthcare team to assist in the coordination of needed community resources (CMSA, 2017). SWs are instrumental in assessing the patient's psychosocial needs, coping with complex and chronic illness, including behavioral and grief modalities and support.

▶ Physician Advisor

The PA is not only a critical role in the team, it is one that has regulatory components and therefore must be accessible. PAs must be a part of some of Medicare's regulations such as ensuring compliance with the Medicare Conditions of Participation (CoP), discharge appeals, and Condition Code 44 (CC44) activities. There are several major advantages to having dedicated PAs. Typically (in addition to regulatory duties), these include:

▶ Improved clinical documentation.
▶ Assistance in reducing avoidable delays/hospital or acute care days.
▶ When a denial occurs, PAs are a resource to help get it overturned. Payor medical directors may deny authorization with an option sometimes given for peer-to-peer discussion; that is, a physician-to-physician communication. A facility may escalate cases to PAs before, during, or after the authorization/denial process.

- Acting as liaisons and educators between case management and practice partners; this is not only about medical necessity, but also about education on laws, rules, regulations, and accreditation standards especially those that pertain to UM and discharge/transitional planning.
- Supporting case managers in addressing patient flow and throughput issues in the acute care setting when the physician caring for a patient declines to cooperate or respond to case management recommendations. For example, a patient may no longer meet criteria for an intensive-care setting and the physician does not transfer the patient to a lesser level of care.
- Serving as a resource for case management in many ways! This partnership is key to our success.
- Facilitating or chairing UM committees.

▶ Clinical Documentation Specialists

Clinical Documentation Specialists, sometimes referred to as Clinical Documentation Improvement Specialists, are often nurses who demonstrate a high level of critical thinking and a strong clinical background. In many ways, they are a link between the coding department and the medical staff, as they strive to garner the most accurate and thorough medical record documentation for coding. This entails a comprehensive review of a medical record, and looking for what is, and what is *not*, in that record. Incomplete, ambiguous, or conflicting information must be rectified. It is the role of the clinical documentation specialist to make sure the medical record captures the patient's condition, comorbidities, risk of mortality, and the SI; if not documented precisely, the clinical documentation specialist will seek clarification from the medical practice professionals.

With the advent of the International Classification of Diseases and Related Health problems—Clinical Modification 10 (*ICD-10 CM*) coding, these professionals fiscally assist organizations by reviewing patient medical records for areas where greater specificity is needed to ensure the most accurate coding. In addition, these experts are the ones to call upon when the case manager cannot get a firm answer from the medical record (or the practice) about a diagnosis, yet must target something less vague (more specific) for both UM functions and in support of the quality core measures.

▶ Denials and Appeals Manager

Many larger healthcare facilities or systems have a department entitled "Denial Management" or "Denials and Appeals Management." Usually, this includes a clinically astute registered nurse (RN) with the strong presence of physicians, including the PAs. This RN understands UR and UM criteria and procedures, especially those required by health insurance plans, whether governmental or private. This RN is the point-person for denials and appeals. Trending of denials and missed opportunities is critical and can be used as a tool to change practices and processes, with the intent to garner less denials. In the section (in this chapter) that discusses the most common reasons for denials, trending can assess if there are people problems, documentation issues, and systems or processes in need of improvement. Denial management takes a lot of human resources; if the number of denials can be reduced due to improved processes, the precious manpower thus saved can be used for more constructive purposes.

▶ Care Management Assistant

Case management assistants, also known as case management aides (CMAs) or case management support associates, play a pivotal role in the success of case management departments. The main function of a CMA is to provide administrative support to case managers (both nurse and SW); however, the responsibilities differ considerably, depending on the type of case management and the care or practice setting. CMAs work under the direction of a professional, usually a licensed person, and their work helps maintain a high level of efficiency and output by the professional team.

Responsibilities are different in various settings. In hospitals, CMAs may send clinical information to insurance companies, information that was previously gathered by the RN or the SW. They may assist with obtaining signatures on regulatory letters, such as the Medicare Outpatient Observation Notice (MOON) or IM (see MOON and IM in this chapter). They may assist with transitioning patients to the next level of care, through collating important records and finding an appropriate service or bed in a skilled care facility. CMAs in the human services sector perform a vital function and may have responsibilities such as data entry and maintaining case files by updating referral information and verifying various kinds of information; some CMAs interact with clients and their families; they may formulate treatment plans under the guidance of case managers or SWs; and CMAs may help review treatment progress.

▶ UTILIZATION MANAGEMENT DOCUMENTATION

As in all aspects of medical care, documentation for UM activity is vitally important. If, for example, you are working with a physician who is a poor documenter (yes, even in the electronic age, they still exist), your documented conversations with the physician(s) and insurance reviewer may make the difference between an insurance authorization or a denial of inpatient days, services, or reimbursement.

Insurance companies today demand that physician documentation be evident in the patients' charts, so the case manager's responsibility will be to attempt to obtain that documentation or make sure that it is completed if it is found to be lacking.

UM documentation does not have to be lengthy, but proper documentation of facts is necessary to validate the patient's diagnosis and support the necessity of the treatment plan. Most insurance plans will not pay for services if a doctor's order is missing or if they could not find documentation that the service was necessary and, in fact, performed.

The use of evidence-based utilization criteria is not a substitute for thorough and accurate documentation. For example, if in a court of law, a healthcare provider claims to have followed a clinical pathway, the documentation must support that declaration. When documenting from a UM perspective, the case manager should perform the following functions:

▶ Record all clinically pertinent data. Objective data should be exact. For example, record a patient's temperature as 39.2°C, rather than "high temp." Other clinical data may include results of laboratory work, radiographs, scans, vital signs, biopsies, cultures, and so on. Avoid saying that a test result or a physiologic parameter is abnormal without including the actual value or what is exactly the abnormality. Subjective data may support the facts. All data should validate the diagnosis, appropriateness of the level of care, and necessity of the treatment plan.

▶ Document any time a patient deviates from the evidence-based utilization criteria or critical pathway implemented. It is not enough to show that a patient deviated from the critical pathway; document how and why the patient went "off the path" and what was done to address any problems.

▶ Record the patient's response or lack of response to the treatments, interventions, and services.

▶ As stated earlier, accurately document conversations with physicians, insurance reviewers, and all other people pertinent to the services needed and treatment plans. We all can remember situations where documentation could not support the plan because it was lacking and the patient was at risk for denial of treatment or continued hospital stay. For example, one novice insurance nurse denied the continued hospital stay when a patient with a persistent high fever had all IV antibiotics discontinued (this patient had been given three antibiotics). What was lacking in this patient's medical record was the plan to discontinue the antibiotics and pan-culture the patient in the hopes of "catching" the offending bug. The reviewer missed the order to pan-culture, and the documentation lacked a clear picture and a black-and-white plan. After the reviewer was explained that this was an approved standard of treatment for a fever of unknown origin, she rescinded the denial, but she required physician documentation of the medical plan to back her decision.

▶ Include times and dates of conversations: Many insurance companies (not all) give the facility 24 hours to supply requested data before the denial goes into effect. Other companies simply end the LOS. If the case manager or the physician can provide pertinent data, the insurance companies will also approve the day of the conversation (usually until midnight).

▶ Demonstrate the patient's status at any given point in time. If another reviewer picks up the case, no backtracking should be needed.

▶ Document accurate and thorough discharge, transition, or transfer plans: If a discharge or transfer plan needs to be changed, include the reasons for the changes in the report. Also include the level of care that is planned, home health nursing services, durable medical equipment needed, transportation and all other arrangements made, and the reasons for medical necessity. It is also important to reveal the name and title of the insurance company representative who approved payment of these discharge services.

▶ Document outcomes of care, especially those that are tied to the goals of care, the treatment plan, or the critical pathway if one is in use. Documenting progression, or lack of it, allows a better concurrent review process between the hospital-based case manager (or those in other inpatient facilities) and those in the health insurance company. Lack of progression, when well-documented, enhances the argument a case manager makes to obtain approval for continued/extended hospital stay.

▶ Document authorization or certification numbers as you obtain them: All insurance companies provide certification (also referred to as authorization) numbers for services that are approved for a particular patient. Documenting the number is important for reimbursement or for following up with the insurance company in certain situations such as the case of retrospective claim denial. The case manager or UM nurse can use the certification number when attempting an appeal.

The Centers for Medicare & Medicaid Services (CMS) requires specific documentation to ensure Medicare reimbursement for care rendered. See section on "Status" in this chapter for more descriptions of the nuances of CMS documentation. These requirements pertain to patients and care providers in the acute care setting.

1. Physician orders that clearly designate admission status (inpatient, outpatient, or observation), including date and time.
2. History and physical (H & P) that justifies the admission and course of treatment. This must be performed within 30 days prior to or within 24 hours of the admission. The H & P must include the patient's chief complaint, history of present illness, past medical history, allergies, medication intake, family and social history, and complete systems exam, with special focus on the reason for a procedure if applicable.
3. Daily progress notes that should include the patient's current health condition and progress; any revisions made to the diagnostic impressions, especially in the case of new evidence/findings; conditions or possible diagnoses that have been ruled out; conditions that verify or support the reason for admission to an inpatient setting; reasons for the patient's need to stay hospitalized, and rationale for change in admission status (e.g., change from inpatient to observation status).
4. Discharge summary that includes the principal and secondary diagnoses as well as the principal and secondary procedures; a brief description of the hospitalization, disposition, and follow-up care arrangements; and the results of diagnostic findings, especially those that confirm the principal diagnosis. If any surgical procedures were performed, these must be included as well. Secondary diagnoses are as important as the primary diagnosis because they provide evidence of comorbidities at the time of admission to the hospital.
5. Discharge summary addendum if any. This may consist of clarifications requested by medical record personnel after the patient's discharge concerning the principal or secondary diagnoses and procedures. This may also include the addition of test results or other information obtained post discharge.
6. Documentation of communications with the patient about the plan of care and discharge plan including postdischarge services; also documentation reflective of the patient's involvement in decision making about and agreement with the plan.

▶ Telephonic Review

Telephonic review is UM that is performed via telephone, usually concurrently while the patient is still receiving care. Telephone triage and telephonic UM continue to grow in use because an increasing number of health insurance companies use demand management strategies and 24-hour coverage. Telephonic reviews are a less expensive way for insurance companies to perform UM, but the reviews are only as good as the information elicited. Poor or inadequate information can result from the reviewer's lack of knowledge to ask medically important questions for a particular admitting diagnosis. The information must be elicited systematically; the reviewer must ask the questions that will efficiently demonstrate whether the patient needs continued stay at the present level of care. The staff nurses should know what IV medications the patient is receiving, some laboratory test results, and the patient's response to treatment.

Telephonic review, without a good UM nurse or case manager on the patient end, is the least effective means of UM; further, it can result in case management actions fraught with liability. Many companies have a mechanism to tape reviews for evidence that one was done and what was included in the review.

Your voice is your tool and it can relay a message that can cause cooperation or a problem. Display 5-2 describes some telephone tips for those engaged in telephonic UM reviews.

▶ STAGES OF REVIEW

The following are the main types of UM services. Each one reflects management of the utilization of resources in various stages of the delivery of healthcare services. Essentially, there are five stages within the UM process:

---

display 5-2

TIPS FOR TELEPHONIC UTILIZATION MANAGEMENT AND REVIEW

▶ Always begin by introducing yourself. Do not assume that the person on the other side of the phone will recognize your voice just because you frequently communicate with this person.
▶ Take the time to establish rapport; frequent conversations with the same person may facilitate building rapport and respect.
▶ Listen to your tone of voice. The voice is your connection to the patient or insurance company representative; sincerity, frustration, hurriedness, or kindness does come through.
▶ Be clear on your reasons for the call. Your words can give you away if you are not clear on the reason for the call. Take a minute before reaching for the telephone to gather your thoughts and objectives for the call.
▶ Name-drop. Use the name of the person you are talking to; make it a point to at least use the name while saying goodbye. However, using a person's name too often has become a wornout tactic in the sales industry, so do not overdo it.
▶ Demonstrate credibility. Keep your promises and complete the follow-ups you commit to.
▶ Use active listening. No one can hear you nod your head, so use verbal forms of active listening.
▶ Be focused and answer the necessary questions. If you have additional important information, volunteer that information as long as you think it will enhance a positive/affirmative decision.

1. Preadmission/Precertification Stage
2. Admission Stage
3. Concurrent/Continued Stay Stage
4. Discharge Stage
5. Postdischarge Stage/Retrospective

Each activity can impact the revenue of the organization, especially for "authorizations/certifications" or "denials." Most health insurance plans require preauthorizations (certifications) of planned procedures and elective acute care admissions. Emergent admissions may not require an authorization; however, that does not preclude the services from being denied. In such cases, it is important to notify the health insurance plan of the patient's emergent admission within the required time frame on the basis of the plan's UM requirements and procedures. The following describes UM activities in each stage.

▶ Preadmission/Precertification Stage

Precertification, prospective review, or preadmission review is often completed by a representative from the healthcare provider agency to ensure that the decision to admit a patient to an inpatient facility is appropriate or justified and that an authorization for the provision of specific aspects of care will be obtained from the insurer. This review takes place before ("pre") services are rendered. Here the reviewer determines whether admission to the facility (i.e., hospital, rehabilitation unit, surgical center, skilled nursing facility [SNF]) is reasonable and medically necessary. Because the attending physician has the ultimate responsibility for the patient, this physician will determine admitting status, regardless of authorization. A compromise may be a 24-hour authorization to see whether the patient needs that particular level of care or a pending review status.

Most MCOs require this type of review and preauthorization for nonemergent/elective procedures. The advantage to such a review is that utilization of resources or quality issues can often be found before the delivery of patient care; the major disadvantage is that necessary services may be delayed or denied.

Prospective review addresses the following:

▶ Insurance coverage and benefits are verified.
▶ Managed care program requirements/procedures are met.
▶ Quality of care issues are identified, addressed, and resolved when possible.
▶ Alternatives to care are identified before admission.
▶ Care is medically necessary.
▶ Healthcare services are rendered at the most appropriate level of care and setting.
▶ Selection of the provider is appropriate and within the preferred network if possible. If going outside-of-network is justified and the health insurance

plan has authorized such services, documentation of the authorization prevents the insurance plan from issuing a denial at a later date. This assists in the continued stay review.
▶ Assessment of needs/discharge planning is initiated.
▶ Initial LOS is determined if the patient is an inpatient.

For emergent care, it is within the role of the case manager or utilization manager to work with physicians to assess if those patients who come in through the emergency department (ED) should be admitted, placed in observation, sent to another lower level of care, or discharged home with or without postdischarge services.

▶ Admission Stage

The hospital admission UM stage is familiar to most UM nurses. The critical case management functions during the admission phase include admission review for medical necessity using evidence-based guidelines or criteria, and assisting the practices to choose the appropriate statuses. This is a prime function in case managers' scope of practice. The American Case Management Association (ACMA) *Scope of Services & Standards of Practice for Hospital/Health System Case Management* states that case management, with respect to payor requirements, will ensure timely notification and communication of pertinent clinical data to support admission, clinical condition, continued stay, and authorization of postacute services (ACMA, 2016c).

These UM activities play a crucial role in alignment with the revenue cycle. Examples of how this role is imperative to the facility's bottom line include (Miodonski, 2012):

▶ *Providing clinical reviews to payors for urgent/emergent admissions*: Provide the health insurance plans with clinical admission reviews required (according to payor contracts) and the clinical reviews at the time of admission for the inpatient stay.
▶ *Admission review of elective admissions*: Even if the elective surgical procedure has been precertified by the payor, changes in patient condition following surgery or procedures will necessitate the case manager to review and follow up with the health insurance plan. It is also important to compare what was authorized with the actual surgery or treatment; often, more was done than originally planned, making a new authorization necessary. Sometimes a "worst case scenario" may have been anticipated; however, it was determined during the surgery that the less intensive-care approach is appropriate. Therefore, following up with the insurance plan after surgery keeps everyone on the same page.
▶ *Early identification of discharge needs*: The saying that "discharge planning begins at admission"

assumes importance when there is visualization of the connection between the revenue cycle and case management. Here, the UM case manager may realize that this patient has undergone multiple readmissions and therefore requires a root cause analysis on "why" this is occurring. Can another readmission be prevented?

Although each case is unique, some of the issues that need to be addressed in the admission review include:

▶ What is the admitting diagnosis? What was the patient's past medical history?
▶ What is the expected LOS?
▶ What were the signs and symptoms of the patient upon admission and what are the current ones?
▶ What was the patient's functional level prior to admission?
▶ What intensity of the services is needed for a safe hospitalization: are the services appropriate? Is there overutilization, underutilization, polypharmacy?
▶ What quality initiatives must be triggered for this patient?
▶ What is the medical plan, both current and future?
▶ What may be the discharge plan, and is this your role or do you need to huddle with others in the organization?
▶ Are there delays in care (see section on avoidable delays/avoidable days)?
▶ When and how often must the payor be notified?
▶ Is there a request for additional information that may require you to follow up at a later stage, and when should that take place?

▶ Concurrent/Continued Stay Stage

Although the admission phase sets the stage for the concurrent stage, the concurrent stage is often the busiest time for case managers/UM nurses as there is a continuous evaluation of the patients' clinical condition and plan of care. A concurrent review is performed while the patient is in the healthcare facility and being cared for. Here, the UM case manager must validate the patients' ongoing stay for medical necessity, and the appropriateness of the status and level of care (such as ICU, step down, telemetry, floor care, extended care, rehabilitation care, or home with home health). Medical appropriateness is gauged by monitoring and evaluating the medical condition of the patient against the services performed. Finally, all must be communicated with the health insurance company. Where there is no obligation to send information to some payors, such as fee-for-service Medicare, the continued stay review serves as the vehicle for case managers to act as a patient and organizational advocate to manage the utilization of resources.

Concurrent review often includes two parameters:

1. Admission review—performed within 24 hours of admission to a facility.
2. Continued stay review—performed at specific points during the patient's stay to determine that each day of a hospital stay is necessary and that care is rendered at the appropriate level, by the right providers, and in the right setting. If the patient is critical, a review every 2 to 3 days may be an acceptable time frame. If the patient is nearing a change in the level of care, daily reviews are necessary. Continued stay reviews focus on monitoring the patient's health condition and healthcare resources utilized during the inpatient stay.

Examples of how concurrent activities are imperative to the facility's bottom line include the following alignment with the revenue cycle (Miodonski, 2012):

▶ Application of UM criteria such as InterQual, Milliman Care Guidelines (MCG), today referred to as MCG Health, or other proprietary clinical decision support tools to all patients. This includes all commercial and governmental payors, including international payors.
▶ Provision of timely concurrent continued stay reviews for payors and taking appropriate action when the criteria are not met. Missed reviews prolong the revenue cycle, and passive case managers result in extended LOS and increase the probability of denials.

During the concurrent phase of hospitalization, the UM case managers are conduits of communication with physicians, the hospital healthcare team, the patient and family members, the health insurance plan CM, and sometimes the postacute providers and community resources. Concurrent review is intended to ensure that:

▶ The patient information is captured in a timely fashion and reviews of the patient's clinical status and progress are accurate.
▶ Healthcare services continue to be provided at an appropriate level of care and setting, and with the appropriate utilization of resources (avoiding over- or underutilization).
▶ Care is coordinated and no delays occur.
▶ Complex clinical and psychosocial situations are referred to the interdisciplinary team.
▶ Insurance coverage and benefits still match the patient's requirements (includes communication with the payors).
▶ Quality issues are monitored and, if triggered, appropriate notification is made.
▶ Barriers are identified to advance the medical treatment plan and discharge plan, and a plan of action is implemented to address these barriers.
▶ Case management plans (CMPs) and interventions are documented.

▶ Patient/family involvement in decision making regarding care options is documented.

The concurrent stage often requires significant physician communication (both with the physician practices and with the PA). Questions to get answered and issues to address include the following:

▶ In fee-for-service Medicare cases that are inpatient for one midnight, changing the status back to observation (CC44) requires discussion with both the physician practices and the PA, or a representative physician from the Utilization Management Committee at the hospital; it is regulation.

▶ In commercial cases where the patient does not meet continued stay criteria, the UM case manager should discuss the case with the attending physician and, if necessary, forward for a second-level review by the PA.

▶ The UM case manager will often need for input on clinical issues at the physician level. The documentation may not be clear or thorough, or does not give a picture of the plan of care or the progression with the medical plan. Some issues include:

▶ Is medical necessity met and are the care and/or the discharge plan on track? If not, what is the revised plan and why? What may be issues around procedure timing or appropriateness? (Do delays in care need to be documented?)

▶ If there are inconsistencies in the documentation, what is the correct diagnosis/treatment plan/other inconsistency?

▶ In some cases, reviews will prompt PAs and case managers to advocate for appropriate services and plans for patients. Frequently, the UM case manager will communicate with the payor, though some payors will work with PAs on cases. Often, the payor will only budge on the status or days authorized after a peer-to-peer review (meaning the attending/PA with their health insurance plan's physician or medical director).

▶ Discharge Stage

The discharge stage is when all the loose ends are wrapped up and patient safety issues must be addressed. If a patient does not meet criteria for continued stay, it becomes necessary for UM case managers to evaluate the patient's readiness for discharge or the potential safety of the discharge and appropriateness of the postdischarge services.

This phase of hospitalization has been the focus of many transitions of care projects for decades. National Transitions of Care Coalition, The Joint Commission, and legislation mandating healthcare reform have highlighted the need for clinicians across the continuum of care to communicate with each other as handoffs occur. Improving care transitions has an obvious effect on the quality of care

and now, with the advent of the value-based purchasing initiative, quality measures will have a financial component as well, especially in preventing financial risk because of repeated avoidable admissions to the hospital or another facility. An assertive UM case management program assists both patients and organizational financing in several ways:

▶ Longer-than-necessary hospital stays have nosocomial consequences; this is well-documented. Patient safety and patient satisfaction with the care experience are at stake with long hospitalizations. Additionally, incidence of healthcare-associated conditions or infections presents a financial risk for the healthcare provider and is part of value-based purchasing initiative.

▶ The final review of authorized days and an assurance that all days are authorized for medical necessity are imperative for making payment. Delays in payment, denials, and denial appeals will cost the hospital heavily in terms of both financial and staff resources.

▶ Executing the discharge plan may not be the role of the UM case manager; however, coordination with the interdisciplinary team is imperative. Discharge plans that are not comprehensive and do not incorporate best practices may result in readmissions. Patients readmitted with diagnoses targeted by value-based purchasing and/or quality initiatives may have a negative effect on revenue.

▶ Postdischarge Stage/Retrospective Review

Retrospective authorization is approved after services have been performed. Often the patient would have already been discharged from the hospital. The insurance company may authorize the whole hospital or SNF admission or deny payment in whole or in part. Although concurrent review seems to be more honest and up front, retrospective review is a reality that case managers need to be aware of. Retrospective review is less common than in the past, because more payors require precertification for most services or real-time authorization.

During this stage, paying prompt attention to payor requests for retrospective reviews, providing discharge reviews and any additional clinical information required for authorizing inpatient days, and following up on postbilling denials have a direct impact on the revenue cycle. Case management follow-up with targeted patient populations (for example those with readmissions and frequent ED visits or those with chronic diseases) may help reduce readmissions and improve patient and physician satisfaction. Although these tasks may, or may not, be within the role of the UM case manager, essential case management activities in the postdischarge period that impact the revenue cycle include:

▶ Timely response to denials and outstanding reviews are necessary. While the goals of any case management program include *prevention* of denials, postbilling denials for medical necessity cannot be entirely eliminated. A successful appeals program will reduce writeoffs and enhance your company's revenue.

▶ Follow-up contact for patients with complex discharge needs is an established best practice and may reduce readmissions—and readmissions may impact the fiscal health of the organization.

Retrospective review is a useful tool for looking at quality control. Monday morning quarterbacking can often prevent similar quality issues from repeating themselves if a preventive plan is assessed and implemented. However, a major disadvantage is that when the review is done after the fact, it does not allow intervention to change and improve a course of events that have already happened.

▶ DENIAL MANAGEMENT

Denial of payment to facilities and organizations is a common, and often frustrating, message. Denials can occur at any phase of the healthcare process: preadmission, admission, continued stay, or retrospectively. More frequently, denials can be carved out, meaning specific days or procedures may be denied. There are level-of-care denials where the health insurance plan will pay for medical-surgical level of care, but not for intermediate level of care, and status denials, where the plan will approve the observation level of care, but not the inpatient level of care. With Medicare denying more cases, especially one-midnight stays, (see section Recovery Audit Contractors), there is no stone to hide under.

ACMA Standards of Practice and Scope of Services states that case management will proactively prevent medical necessity denials by providing education to physicians, staff and patients, and interface with payors by documenting relevant information (ACMA, 2016c). The CMSA, in its Standards of Practice for Case Management, advocates for resource management and stewardship where the case manager is expected to demonstrate "evidence of promoting the most effective and efficient use of health care services and financial resources" (CMSA, 2016, p. 29). Additionally, the case manager should complete "documentation which reflects that the intensity of case management services rendered corresponds with the needs of the client" (CMSA, 2016, p. 30). Such expectations promote successful UM activities and assist in the prevention of denials.

It is critical for the UM case manager to recognize the impact that documentation has on avoiding denials. If documentation is inconsistent or ambiguous, the UM case manager should contact the physician and ask for clarity. Sometimes the denial would be valid, where the services would have been out of the scope of the benefits, or the patient could have been treated at a lower level of care. It may be that the contract personnel should reexamine the contracts if the denial is without merit or is not within standards of medical practice.

The following are some of the most common reasons for denials. Sometimes, a denial is a call to investigate or to change a process.

▶ Lack of prior authorization or notification of admission is often a large source of denials. Some health insurance plans will accept case manager communication as notification, whereas other plans will not. It is important for case managers to know the requirements of their payors; if these types of denials occur regularly, the process of obtaining prior authorization may need tightening up.

▶ The patient has no benefit for the service performed. UM case managers should ensure that the services being appealed are not excluded from the patient's health insurance benefits plan and that documentation supports the medical necessity of the services provided.

▶ Medical necessity is not met for the level of care that the patient is assigned. The payor may pay for a lesser level of care, as long as medical necessity meets that level.

▶ Billed services do not match the authorization: Investigate why this has happened and change processes as needed.

▶ Incomplete clinical reviews were provided or no review was provided: if this is a trend, workflow processes may not be optimal, or staff may completely overlooked performing a review.

▶ Information was not shared within reasonable or requested time frames: The care management department may need to change or adjust processes if this is a trend.

▶ A valid order for a particular treatment or procedure is missing from the patient's medical record: This may be an unfortunate oversight, but again, processes should be investigated: How did this occur? How can the organization stop it from occurring in the future?

▶ Weekend-related services (and days) were denied due to lack of services during weekends, resulting in additional hospital days: Some facilities have rectified this with adding services on the weekend, especially radiologic services.

▶ APPEALING A DENIAL

An appeal, also known as a reconsideration or grievance, is a formal process or request to reconsider a decision made not to approve an admission or a specific aspect of care and services. Often, appeals are managed by the UM case manager on behalf of the care provider (e.g., hospital) and/or the patient.

An appeal should be filed on the basis of the contractual agreement between the care provider or agency and the health insurance company. It also should comply with insurance and public health laws. The denial letter usually gives the time frame allowed to file an appeal and the insurance company is obligated to review the appeal and respond within 30 to 60 days of the date it is filed. When the review is completed, it may result in the appeal being upheld in its entirety, the denial being amended to a portion of the care/services, or a complete reversal.

Grievances may be won, especially with good physician and UM case management documentation. When writing an appeal letter, it is best to involve the attending physician of record. It is also important to reference any authorization numbers obtained during UM interactions with the representative of the insurance company. In addition, it is advisable to reference in the appeal letter the UM criteria/guidelines used by the insurance company such as InterQual or MCG (described in this chapter). The appeal letter must reflect how the criteria match the patient's condition, including the interventions applied and the outcomes achieved.

Case managers need to be aware that, if they think the care was reasonable, the appeal process should not stop with discussions between hospital (or facility)-based case managers and payor case managers. Case managers have the option of peer-to-peer physician discussions, which occur between the health plan medical director and the attending physician; this is especially key when there is strong supporting clinical information that the health insurance plan denied payment inappropriately or refused authorization to transition the patient to the next level of care (ACMA, 2016a).

On the basis of their knowledge and expertise, PAs can make a significant contribution in denial management. They conduct verbal and written reviews and appeals of denials or downgraded coverage determinations made by MCOs. As governmental requirements become more prevalent, PAs help manage the governmental appeals process for inappropriate denials on behalf of the hospital, including representing the hospital during Administrative Law Judge hearings. The partnership between case managers and PAs is critical for success. Both groups need to remain up-to-date on ongoing regulatory guidance changes, managed care/hospital contract updates, and the latest evidence-based care guidelines and outcomes as they exercise their role in financial stewardship and delivery of quality care.

When working with managed care payors, it is also important to realize that an authorization is not a *guarantee* of payment. Upon review by the managed care payor, if it is determined that the care rendered was not medically necessary, was clinically in appropriate, or

was rendered in the "wrong" setting, payment can still be denied. Moreover, just because a patient is an inpatient at a sending facility it does not necessarily translate to an inpatient hospitalization at the receiving facility.

▶ QUALITY IMPROVEMENT ORGANIZATIONS

QIO programs have been around since the 1970s and have gone through many name changes. In general, QIOs hire health quality experts, clinicians, and consumers to improve the care delivered to people with Medicare. QIOs are chosen via a request-for-proposal process and work under the direction of the CMS to assist with quality improvements, beneficiary protection, and the protection of the Medicare Trust Fund. They ensure payment for appropriate goods and services in the correct setting and address consumer complaints related to provider appeals and violations of the *Emergency Medical* Treatment *and Labor Act*. The CMS is required to publish a Report to Congress every fiscal year that outlines the administration, cost, and impact of the QIO Program (ACMA, 2016a).

In 1972, Medicare Professional Standards Review Organizations began to oversee quality of care at the local level and, in 1982, became PROs with new authority to protect Medicare beneficiaries from underuse of necessary health services. In 1996, the QIO program expanded in scope and PROs could systematically collect data, measure progress, and identify areas for improvement. This allowed PROs to shift their focus from auditing of charts and following up on complaints to more targeted efforts. PROs began to focus on specific diseases and improving the management of common *chronic condition*s such as diabetes and cardiovascular disease (QIO, 2016).

By 2002, PROs had been renamed *QIOs* to reflect the multidisciplinary approach of all team members—physicians, nurses, and administration—working together to improve the quality of care. QIOs became the boots on the ground in communities, helping patients, families, and providers carry out local activities that rolled up into national progress. More recently, QIOs have established strong partnerships and collaboration with *stakeholder*s and patients, as well as each other. *Learning and Action Network*s were developed in 2011 in an effort to bring together like-minded individuals around the achievement of a common goal. Around that time, the program also began to align its efforts with other healthcare agencies like the Agency for Healthcare Research and Quality and the Centers for Disease Control and Prevention, as well as the private sector, to improve the healthcare system (QIO, 2016).

Today, the QIO Program is one of the largest federal programs dedicated to improving health quality at the community level. In August 2014, the CMS established a new functional structure for the program. There are much fewer QIOs than decades ago and their responsibilities are separated into two primary roles:

1. *Beneficiary and Family Centered Care (BFCC-QIO):* Currently there are two BFCC-QIOs in the United States: Kepro BFCC-QIO and Livanta BFCC-QIO. These BFCC-QIOs are tasked with improving healthcare services and protecting Medicare beneficiaries through expeditious statutory review functions, including complaints and quality of care reviews for people with Medicare. These BFCC-QIOs are where case managers will interact if a Medicare Beneficiary submits a discharge appeal (see section on Medicare Discharge Appeals in this chapter). These are also the QIOs that will monitor the short (1-day) hospital stays for Medicare patients (see sections on one-day stays, two-midnight rule).

2. *Quality Innovation Network QIN-QIOs:* QIN-QIOs improve healthcare services through education, outreach, and sharing practices that have been successful in other areas, using data to measure improvement and convening community partners (including hospitals, home health agencies, SNFs, governmental agencies, etc.) for communication and collaboration. QIN-QIOs work to improve the quality of healthcare for targeted health conditions and priority populations and to reduce the incidence of healthcare-acquired conditions to meet national and local priorities (ACMA, 2016a).

▶ MEDICARE DISCHARGE APPEALS

In general, an appeal is a process that seeks to overturn a denial; it is often a part of the role of the "denial manager" (see section on "denial manager" under "The Utilization Management Team"). This section will include a variation on the appeals types, entitled the Medicare Discharge Appeal. However, more on Appeals, in general, is included in Chapter 8, Legal Considerations in Case Management Practice.

Now, a little history on the Medicare discharge appeal. On November 27, 2006, the CMS published a final rule, CMS-4105-F: Notification of Hospital Discharge Appeal Rights. Hospitals are mandated to deliver the "Important Message from Medicare (IM)" to inform Medicare beneficiaries who are hospital inpatients about their hospital discharge appeal rights. Notice is required both for Original Medicare beneficiaries (fee-for-service) and for those enrolled in Medicare health plans. The IM must be provided when a patient is admitted with an inpatient status and again within 48 hours of discharge. Beneficiaries who choose to appeal a discharge decision will receive a more detailed notice ("Detailed Notice of Discharge"). Refer to Display 5-3 for details on who can appeal the discharge.

Medicare beneficiaries are getting more savvy about their patient rights, including the right to appeal a hospital discharge if they feel they are being discharged too early. The anatomy of a discharge appeal may go like this:

1. A patient wishes to appeal his or her discharge usually after receiving the second IM. The second IM must be given to the patient/representative no more than two calendar days before discharge, but at least 4 hours before discharge.

2. The case management department will get a notice from the BFCC-QIO stating that a patient is appealing his or her hospital discharge.

3. The next step for the case manager to do, immediately, is to check if an active discharge order has been written. If no discharge has been written, the appeal is not valid. The care manager should notify the BFCC-QIO. This is also a good time to recheck whether a discharge plan that meets the patient's identified discharge needs is in place. The patient does not have to be agreeable to the discharge plan, but there needs to be an acceptable plan in place along with the discharge orders, that is, an accepting SNF or home health agency.

4. You should also direct the patient (or the person appealing the discharge) to call the BFCC-QIO once an actual discharge plan is written, if he or she still feels that the discharge is too early. The patient has time until midnight on the last covered day (the day when the discharge plan was written) in order to request an appeal for discharge. The case manager should explain (as does the IM) that the patient will not incur any extra financial responsibility while the review process is underway.

---

display 5-3	WHO CAN/CANNOT APPEAL A MEDICARE HOSPITAL DISCHARGE

Who *can* appeal a Medicare discharge:	Who <u>cannot</u> appeal a Medicare discharge:
▶ Any patient with Medicare of any type: fee-for-service, Medicare Advantage Plans (MAPs), Medicare Part A only, Medicare Part B only, Medicare as a second insurance ▶ Any patient with the above-mentioned insurance who is in an *inpatient* status	▶ Any patient in an *outpatient* status: observation, outpatient in a bed ▶ Any patient who is planned to transition to a lateral level of care (e.g., acute hospital to acute long-term care hospital)

5. Once a valid discharge appeal is called in and the department has been notified of the appeal by the BFCC-QIO, instructions will also be sent as to what the BFCC-QIO needs from the hospital to determine the outcome of the appeal. Minimal information that should be provided in the fax include:

   ▶ First/second IM—signed or notated that the patient/representative refused to sign
   ▶ Detailed notice of discharge or detailed explanation of noncoverage
   ▶ Face Sheet/admission order/ED notes, if applicable
   ▶ Admission history and physical/discharge summary
   ▶ Consultations and final operative/test results, radiology/procedure notes
   ▶ Physician orders and physician progress notes—past 2 weeks or less.
   ▶ Case management/discharge planning/SW notes—past 2 weeks including current notes. MUST contain a current, viable plan (not a "possible" plan initiated on the day of discharge)
   ▶ Wound care notes (as indicated)
   ▶ Up to last 7 days of the following:
   • Nurse's notes, vital signs, flow sheets
   • Laboratory test results
   • Medication Administration Records
   • Ancillary notes: physical therapy, occupational therapy, speech and language therapy, and respiratory therapy evaluations, goals, and progress notes (as indicated), dietary, etc.

6. The BFCC-QIO will notify the case management contact as to whether the decision to discharge the patient was upheld within one calendar day after receiving all necessary information. Refer to Display 5-4 for tips on maximizing success in upholding the discharge decision.

   ▶ If the BFCC-QIO decides that the patient is not medically ready for discharge or that the discharge plan is not appropriate, the hospital will be informed, along with the reason(s) for their decision. The patient is not financially responsible if the BFCC-QIO disagrees with the discharge plan (agrees with the discharge appeal).
   ▶ If however, the BFCC-QIO agrees with the discharge plan, the patient must leave the facility (or incur fiscal responsibility) by noon on the day after the BFCC-QIO determination is made, or on the last covered day (whichever is later).

▶ AVOIDABLE DAYS/DELAYS

"The avoidable day is the most expensive item commonly provided by a hospital."

ELGIN KENNEDY, MD (MAGE CORPORATION)

display 5-4

TIPS FOR GETTING THE BEST OUTCOME OF A MEDICARE DISCHARGE APPEALS REVIEW

▶ Make every attempt to keep the faxed record to 50 pages maximum.
▶ The case managers will be viewed as "advocates" for the patient with the appeal process; this is the patients' right under Medicare. The case managers will assist patients and families through this process.
▶ It is imperative to demonstrate that a safe, thorough, and accurate discharge plan has been offered. It is imperative that documentation is consistent. For example, the final plan should not state that the patient plan was for an SNF level of care in one note and a long-term acute care level of care in another note. If it does state two plans, modify a final note to explain the true level of care.
▶ It is imperative to demonstrate that the patient is stable for discharge. If this cannot be provided, speak to Leadership and/or the PA, as the discharge may be inappropriate. It is imperative that documentation is consistent. For example, it must not state that the patient is medically stable on one note and not medically stable in another.
▶ Prior to faxing the information to the BFCC-QIO, a social worker, nurse case manager, or team lead should look over the documentation.
▶ Prior to faxing, it is good practice to call the BFCC-QIO and notify it of the incoming fax.

An *avoidable day* is defined as a patient day in the hospital during which acute hospital services were not rendered or could have been safely and appropriately performed in an alternate setting or less acute level of care. Avoidable days may occur at the beginning of a hospital stay (on admission), during the stay, or at the end of a hospitalization when a patient could have been discharged or transferred sooner than was actually done. Such days are considered nonacute by health insurance companies; here overutilization of resources becomes apparent. It is not uncommon for insurance companies to deny portions of a hospitalization (on admission, during, or at the end of a stay) if they feel these portions were due to avoidable delays. In fact, there is a growing correlation between avoidable days and insurance denials. *Avoidable delays* may be defined in a similar way as an avoidable day, but the time parameters are less: typically 4 hours or one-half day of delay (ACMA, 2016b).

Good case management can minimize these avoidable days and delays, and hospitals are witnessing an encouraging impact in this area. At times, the avoidable day may be "unavoidable"; when this happens, the case manager should help get the case back on track as quickly as possible.

Given all the people involved and factors that make up each patient's case, it is not surprising that avoidable days occur with monotonous consistency. The reasons for avoidable days are varied, and closely related to these nonacute days is the issue of unjustified variation of practice. Avoidable days are deviations from normal, quality care. Unexpected or worrisome occurrences that affect the course of illness can be identified through analysis of avoidable days data. These data, in turn, can identify possible opportunities for performance improvement. In fact, one of the primary goals of tracking and analyzing avoidable days data through the use of CMPs, clinical pathways, or other UM tools is to aid in early identification and resolution of healthcare issues. In continuous quality improvement circles, avoidable days, or variations, are considered a basic cause of instability in a process. Stability in a process depicts a process that is well-defined and consistent in methods used and application. Variability in a process is just the opposite; variable processes are inconsistent and changeable. It is difficult to attribute outcomes to processes that are unstable. Case managers who perform outcomes studies on the basis of such tools as clinical pathways often use avoidable days data to draw conclusions and improve care processes.

Sources for avoidable days identification used by case managers include nurse and physician documentation, verbal communication with the interdisciplinary healthcare team, and avoidable days found on clinical pathways. The patient or family members are another source (and sometimes a cause) of avoidable days.

The causes of avoidable days, which may lead to avoidable days and undesired outcomes, are generally assigned to four categories as follows:

1. Patient/family reasons,
2. Practitioner reasons,
3. Institution/systems reasons, and
4. Community reasons.

Avoidable days can be caused by social factors, financial factors, environmental factors, patient or family responses or lack of responses, physician-induced reasons, or hospital (institution) responsibilities. Display 5-5 lists some examples of avoidable days. The list is by no means complete, as creative and interesting circumstances can (and do) pop up unexpectedly!

The causes of avoidable days are seemingly endless. The more complicated the discharge, the more opportunities for avoidable days to occur and the more a detailed social evaluation is needed. We heard of one case in which the case manager worked very hard putting together a complicated discharge with various pieces of durable medical equipment. On the day of discharge, someone in the family happened to mention that there was no electricity at home. Assessment had missed this crucial fact. This, of course, delayed the patient's discharge. Therefore, the case manager should always be alert to possible changes and be prepared with a "plan B."

---

display 5-5

EXAMPLES OF AVOIDABLE DAYS

Characteristics of Avoidable days/delays

▶ Occurs when what is supposed to happen does not take place or is delayed
▶ Deviates from a standard, norm, goal/target, or threshold
▶ Omits an activity
▶ Does not meet expectations or expectations are met too soon.

Patient/Family Avoidable days/delays

▶ Unsafe home environment
▶ Refusal to leave the hospital
▶ Lack of family support (i.e., no caregiver at home)
▶ Refusal of procedure and/or treatment regimen as prescribed by physician
▶ Indecision regarding treatment or discharge plan
▶ Indecision about a test, procedure, or surgery
▶ Insistence that the patient is too ill to be discharged
▶ No family shows up to pick up the patient after arrangements were made.
▶ Inability of family member responsible for at-home care to arrive from out of state on the day the patient is ready for discharge
▶ Lack of patient cooperation with the medical program, causing delayed diagnosis and treatment.
▶ The patient suffering from an intraoperative myocardial infarction or from other medical complications (e.g.,

hemorrhage, shock, ileus, postoperative infection, or pneumonia)
▶ Although educational needs were attended to early in the admission, significant knowledge deficit exists, and additional teaching needed for patient or family.
▶ Delayed transfer or discharge because of inadequate discharge planning details
▶ Family members changing their minds about the discharge plan at the last minute (e.g., the case manager's suggestion that an extended-care facility may be appropriate suddenly sounds good!)
▶ Chronically ill patient with inadequate (or no) insurance support and poor social support, causing a difficult discharge dilemma (if available, charity care may be needed)
▶ Inability to reach family members
▶ Pressure ulcer present on admission that requires treatment
▶ No clothes or key to apartment; therefore cannot be discharged yet
▶ Inability to self-care or administer insulin injections
▶ Poor historian or withholding important information.

Practitioner Avoidable days/delays

▶ Physician is late in providing service, scheduling procedures, writing prescriptions, and/or ordering laboratory tests.
▶ Discharge order is not written by the physician in a timely manner.

display 5-5

EXAMPLES OF AVOIDABLE DAYS *(continued)*

▶ Primary physician is inaccessible.

▶ Specialist is inaccessible.

▶ Physician insists on an inappropriate level of care.

▶ All SNFs in which the patient's physician will follow are full; the physician will not go to other suggested SNFs; or the patient refuses care by a "strange" physician. This avoidable days can be attributed to the patient/family or physician, depending on how one looks at it.

▶ The doctor writes the discharge order at 10:00 pm, when visiting hours are over and patients and their families are usually asleep!

▶ The physician comes in early—before the day's laboratory test results are back and before the patient's progress for the day can be assessed—and writes "will discharge tomorrow if the patient is stable today."

▶ The patient was admitted for a problem outside the expertise of the attending physician. Delays occurred getting specialist consultations.

▶ The physician's practice pattern is such that only one test is ordered at a time, and the results must be back before any other diagnostic action is taken.

▶ Tests are ordered in poor sequence, causing delays because of extensive preparation.

▶ Poor practitioner's techniques cause complications.

▶ There are delays in ordering needed services (i.e., social service, physical therapy, rehabilitation consultation).

▶ There is a failure to conduct proper financial screening.

▶ There is inappropriate use of medical equipment.

▶ Miscommunication occurs among healthcare team members or with patient/family.

▶ There is a delay in checking results of tests and therefore there is delay in progressing the treatment plan.

▶ There is a failure to obtain certifications for services.

Institution/Systems Avoidable days/delays

▶ Orders are not transcribed in a timely manner.

▶ Equipment malfunctions or breakdowns.

▶ Delay occurs in services, tests, and/or procedures.

▶ No beds are available (all levels of care).

▶ There is refusal to accept patient in the next level of care.

▶ There are transportation problems.

▶ Scheduling delay for tests, procedures, or surgery may be the result of full operating rooms or tests that are run only on specific days.

▶ Test or biopsy results are delayed, which postpones further procedures or discharge.

▶ A lower level of care would have adequately met the needs of the patient, but traditional Medicare requires 72 hours in acute care before transfer to an SNF level.

▶ The institution does not have the necessary equipment, so that transfer to another hospital is necessary for a test or procedure.

▶ Beds are unavailable for new admissions.

▶ Weekend coverage is lacking in certain services.

Community Avoidable days/delays

▶ Private insurance causes delay (authorization, transfer problems, finding contracted providers).

▶ Durable medical equipment is unavailable or is delivered late.

▶ SNF is unavailable (reason: no beds) or refuses patient at the last minute.

According to the ACMA Standards of Practice and Scope of Service, "Case management will utilize a validated system/defined methodology for tracking avoidable days/delays and use this information to identify and communicate opportunities for improvement. Case management will participate in the development of performance improvement activities relevant to identified opportunities" (ACMA, 2016a, p. 239). One methodology approach worth looking at is the ACMA's "Compare AD: Avoidable Delay and Utilization Management (UM)" system (ACMA, 2016b).

This system uses five categories. Each category contains subcategories with codes to track and trend avoidable delays/days. The overarching categories are:

1. *Financial/Payer caused delays*: This category codifies and tracks delays caused by payors because of funding issues, lack of prior authorization, or lack of funding source (no insurance).

2. *Care Transitions*: This category codifies and tracks delays caused by the family/patient or community service. Examples in this category include Medicare discharge appeals, psychosocial issues, and bed not available at the designated level of care (hospice, rehabilitation, inpatient psych, etc.). This category may demonstrate areas outside of the organization that may need better relationships and transition processes.

3. *Care Progression*: This category codifies and tracks delays in the progression of care or the plan of care. Examples in this category may be physician-driven, nursing-driven, case management-driven, or therapy-driven. This category may demonstrate areas within the organization that may need process changes.

4. *System Services*: This category codifies and tracks delays caused by services within the organization, such as in the operating room, admission/registration, and procedures/tests. This category may demonstrate areas within the organization that may need process changes.

5. *UM*: This category codifies and tracks delays caused by barriers where the patient spent time in the incorrect level of care. This category is coded by timing: (a) beginning of stay or (b) during the stay. Note that after discharge, delays are not coded.

Avoidable delays are bad for everyone. Yet, case managers, as resource stewards and facilitators of patient care services, are in the best position to identify potentially avoidable days/delays. They may directly affect quality of care (potential hospital-acquired infections or falls), increase costs (overuse of bed days), and ultimately have a negative impact on patient satisfaction.

▶ MEDICAL NECESSITY CRITERIA/USE OF EVIDENCE-BASED CARE AND PATHWAYS

The out-of-control economics of healthcare have been apparent since the 1980s. Various ways and modalities of managing the utilization of healthcare resources have come and gone; more will likely emerge. The staggering dollar amounts being spent for healthcare are forcing this search for better management of resources. Some UM tools have changed and become more efficient. Still others are in their adolescence—raw, but with good potential. There are many UM tools. The four modalities discussed here are the most commonly used UM tools at this time: LOS, InterQual, clinical pathways, and MCG Health. Application of approved medical necessity criteria will assist in determining the appropriateness and accuracy of levels of care.

When using UM tools, it should be kept in mind that they are just that—tools. They are not mandatory. More importantly, they are only a part of total case management. They do, however, speak a language that insurance companies understand, and insurance companies pay the bills.

Sometimes merging the roles of UM and patient advocacy seems to cause conflict. This conflict may signal the need for discussion between a physician and a case manager, or even a full conference with the multidisciplinary team on the case. There have been times when case managers have felt sandwiched between an insurance company's threat to deny payment unless the physician moves the patient to a lesser level of care and a physician angry over the insurance company's decision. During such times it helps to get everyone's focus back on the patient and what that patient needs to receive proper and safe care. At other times, the physician is grateful for the added "support" of an insurance denial if the patient or family is adept at manipulating or malingering. In either case, knowledge of utilization modalities will aid the case manager; impending insurance denials will not be a surprise because the case manager would have already predicted the possibility and therefore the discharge plan would have already been in place well into the case management process.

▶ Length of Stay

LOS is perhaps the most fundamental attempt at controlling costs of healthcare. An LOS is a term to describe the duration of a single episode of hospitalization. Inpatient days are calculated by subtracting the day of admission from the day of discharge for a specific diagnosis or procedure (Display 5-6).

Do you remember when was a total knee or hip replacement a week-long LOS? Many factors have affected LOS over the past three decades, including:

▶ Case managers;
▶ New regulations, such as the two-midnight rule;
▶ The Prospective Payment System (PPS), especially the inpatient PPS;
▶ The type and prevalence of managed care strategies in different geographical regions;
▶ New technology that allows less invasiveness and earlier recovery;
▶ More postacute capabilities at all levels of care;
▶ Community resources;
▶ Accreditation agencies and new standards requiring closer attention to patient safety and patient flow;
▶ Focus of inpatient facilities (e.g., hospitals) on efficiency and patient flow;
▶ Attention given to outpatient and observation statuses versus inpatient status;
▶ Case management's skillful coordination of complex and catastrophic cases.

There are many venues to get LOS data. LOS is embedded in evidence-based criteria sets, and healthcare organizations subscribe to regional and/or national databases to which they contribute their own organization-based data. In return, they are given the opportunity to benchmark against the performance of other organizations. An organization has the choice to benchmark against the other organizations in its region or in the nation, or against a select group of organizations that shares the

---

display 5-6 | LENGTH-OF-STAY TERMS

A *LOS* is a term to describe the duration of a single episode of hospitalization. Inpatient days are calculated by subtracting the day of admission from the day of discharge.

An *average length of stay* (ALOS) is calculated by dividing the sum of inpatient days by the number of patients admitted with the same diagnosis-related group (DRG) and it is often used as an indicator of efficiency. If all factors are equal, a shorter LOS will reduce the cost per discharge.

Patients admitted and discharged on the same day have an LOS of less than one day.

A geometric mean length of stay (GMLOS) is used to compute reimbursement and removes extreme outlier cases and focuses on the frequency of each los occurrence. Medicare uses the GMLOS to minimize the impact of those outliers. If the number of patients is relatively low, one patient with an uncharacteristically long or short los can significantly increase or decrease the ALOS respectively. The goal is to get to a number that can be utilized fairly in the DRG payment formula.

same database. The benchmark data usually are reported in averages, with the opportunity for an organization to see its variance from the average and the percentile in which it falls. The benchmark data include other metrics besides the LOS, such as volume, demographics (gender, age, socioeconomic class), case mix index, health plan distribution (Medicare, Medicaid, commercial insurance), distribution by diagnosis and procedure, and others. Data are calculated on the basis of reviews of millions of actual patient discharge records from the hospitals that are included in the database. When healthcare organizations compare their performance with those in these national databases, they report excess days and ratio of observed to expected LOS.

Healthcare professionals use the databases to generate LOS guidelines that can be reported as national data or broken down by region/state in the United States. Custom reports can also be generated, such as choosing a select group of hospitals for benchmarking purposes; in this latter case data are reported on the basis of the medical records submitted from the select set of hospitals. But benchmark data used by an organization should be updated annually, so that the most recent benchmarks are used to maintain current, logical, and meaningful comparisons, good reputation, competitiveness, and efficiency. Although benchmarking data are rarely used by health insurance companies as the sole consideration for authorization of hospital stays, they are a useful tool for case managers to grasp an average length of time a patient should stay in the hospital for a specific diagnosis or procedure. If a patient is admitted, and the case manager is not familiar with the illness or procedure, knowing the usual LOS (average based on national or regional benchmark data) may be a comforting place to start. One idea is that case managers make a cheat sheet of 10%, 25%, and 50% for common problems encountered on the service they are mostly involved in. For case managers who perform case management duties telephonically in different geographical areas of the country, it is a helpful guide because there is a difference in LOSs in various regions.

The bottom line is that the case manager's role in managing LOS is to avoid a negative financial impact by appropriately progressing the patient through the system, facilitating appropriate patient discharge, and/or coordinating care throughout the continuum of care. It is the responsibility of each case manager to know the targeted LOS for the facility overall, the targeted LOS for the unit(s) on which they work, and the targeted LOS for specific diagnosis-related groups (DRGs) in order to better balance cost and outcomes (ACMA, 2016a).

▶ InterQual Criteria

InterQual was first introduced in 1978 in printed form and, not only has it experienced many revisions and additions

with each annual release, but each revision has changed significantly over the years. It is currently in its 2016 edition and is one of the most widely used evidence-based UR and management criteria for use by hospitals, health plans, government agencies, and other care/case management providers. InterQual is designed to serve as a "common language" between payers and providers on the basis of a synthesis of current evidence and best practices. It is accessible in a variety of different technology solutions, including software applications, online access, and even on mobile devices, with the book format retiring in 2017. Healthcare is changing at a breakneck speed, and the use of electronic-only form allows more "real-time" updates than print does.

The InterQual portfolio consists of four content suites:

▶ Level of Care
▶ Care Planning
▶ Behavioral Health
▶ Complex Care Management

1. InterQual's *Level of Care Criteria* assist healthcare organizations assess the clinical appropriateness of patient services across the continuum of care, prospectively, concurrently, or retrospectively. Robust clinical detail allows organizations to consider the patient's SI, comorbidities, and complications, as well as the ISs being delivered. In addition, it contains objective endpoints for service, allowing healthcare professionals to perform reviews of discharge or transfer readiness on the basis of the individual's clinical needs. The clinical review process guides the reviewer toward the safest and most efficient level of care. It also assists the care manager in discharge planning and transitioning care across the continuum. The Level-of-Care suite includes the following criteria sets:
   a. Acute Adult (see Display 5-7)
   b. Acute Pediatric (see Display 5-8)
   c. Long-Term Acute Care
   d. Acute Rehabilitation
   e. Subacute and SNF
   f. Home Care
   g. Outpatient Rehabilitation and Chiropractic

Since 2012, the acute adult and pediatric criteria have been structured into a condition-specific format, which presents evidence-based interventions that are specific to the condition selected. The specific conditions are then laddered into an "Episode-Day" structure, which assists the reviewer further to evaluate if the patient is responding as expected. Another method InterQual used to further delineate the detailed specifics of the patient's case is through the use of "responder" criteria or "non-responders" criteria. Depending on the clinical indications, there are notes and recommendations for interventions in the event of complications or a slower-than-expected response to treatment; the criteria then incorporates clinical measures,

INTERQUAL: ACUTE ADULT

Acute adult example:

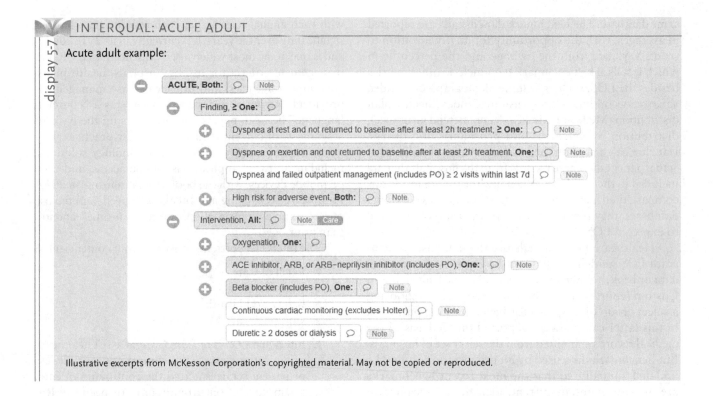

Illustrative excerpts from McKesson Corporation's copyrighted material. May not be copied or reproduced.

comorbidities, and complications to support the most appropriate care and best outcomes for patients. All this assists the case manager in moving patients through the care continuum, with the ultimate intent to reduce inappropriate admissions, avoidable days, and readmissions.

Only the acute care criteria (both adult and pediatric) use the episode-day structure. Just a few of the over three dozen adult topics include (McKesson, 2016b):

▶ Acetaminophen Overdose
▶ Acute Coronary Syndrome

INTERQUAL: ACUTE PEDIATRIC

Acute Pediatric example:

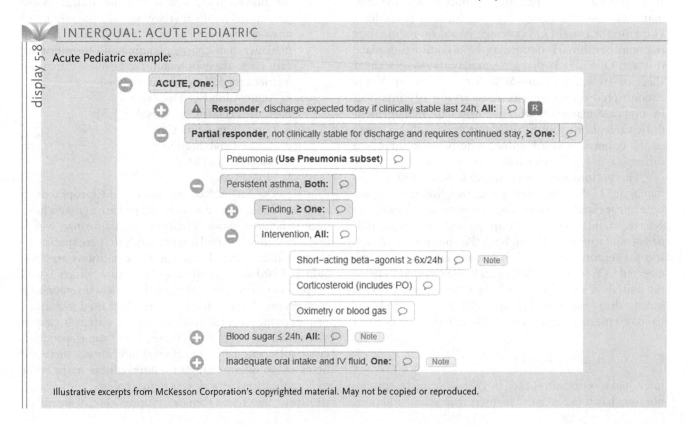

Illustrative excerpts from McKesson Corporation's copyrighted material. May not be copied or reproduced.

◗ Anemia/Bleeding
◗ Arrhythmia
◗ Heart Failure
◗ Inflammatory Bowel Disease
◗ Pancreatitis
◗ Pulmonary Embolism
◗ Stroke/TIA

Just a few of the over 30 pediatric topics include (McKesson, 2016b):

◗ Acetaminophen Overdose
◗ Anemia/Bleeding
◗ Antepartum
◗ Asthma
◗ Bronchiolitis
◗ Diabetes Mellitus
◗ Failure to Thrive
◗ Hyperbilirubinemia
◗ Meningitis

If you are one of the more seasoned case managers, who are used to thinking in terms of Intensity of Service (IS) and Severity of Illness (SI) descriptions, this thinking is still utilized today, as stated in a 2016 brochure: "InterQual's novel approach, evaluating Severity of Illness along with Intensity of Service, provides a clinically-specific approach to stay determinations" (McKesson, 2016a, p. 3). Consideration of comorbid conditions is a welcome addition because those "seasoned" case managers of earlier versions often had to choose one condition over another; this is more streamlined.

InterQual made two additional enhancements to the criteria in 2016. It has added Proactive Care Management Guidance in the form of content to assist the care manager in understanding the evidence surrounding what the trajectory of care should be for the condition so that they may add value to the care management process by making suggestions that can help improve the response of the patient to treatment. Also, alternate level of care recommendations are made to assist in moving the patient across the continuum. LOS targets have been added to specific conditions derived from vast claims data sources, representing millions of patient discharges. These targets create guidance to facilitate efficient management of the patient to that target.

1. InterQual's *Care Planning Criteria* assist healthcare organizations to determine when imaging studies, procedures, molecular diagnostics, durable medical equipment, specialty referral consultations, and specialty pharmaceuticals are medically appropriate, on the basis of the evidence, and are typically used prospectively to manage resource utilization, or retrospectively as a quality management tool. They can also serve as an educational tool to help promote efficient use of resources, as well as foster communications between physicians and health plans. The Care Planning suite includes the following criteria sets:
   a. Durable Medical Equipment
   b. Imaging
   c. Molecular Diagnostics
   d. Procedures
   e. Specialty Referral
   f. Specialty RX Non-Oncology
   g. Specialty RX Oncology
   h. SIM plus Retrospective Monitoring
2. InterQual's *Behavioral Health Criteria* assist in making initial and continued stay level-of-care decisions on the basis of each patient's presentation and allow for movement up and down the continuum of care. Content addresses the unique needs of geriatric, adult, adolescent, and child patients with psychiatric and substance use disorders. The depth of criteria allows care managers to consider symptoms, functional status and quality of support system as determinants for the most appropriate level of care. The Behavioral Health suite includes the following criteria sets:
   a. Adult and Geriatric Psychiatry
   b. Child and Adolescent Psychiatry
   c. Substance Use Disorders
   d. Behavioral Health Procedures
3. InterQual's *Complex Care Management* suite supports the management of complex, high-risk patients. This suite includes the InterQual Coordinated Care Content that includes a patented assessment that blends multiple conditions or disease states and generates a unique, patient-specific care plan. There is also a separate readmission reduction assessment to aid in mitigating avoidable readmissions within 30 days of hospital discharge, as well as a palliative care assessment to help address end-of-life concerns.

◗ Clinical Pathways and Case Management Plans

Of all utilization modalities, clinical pathways and CMPs most completely take into account the total multidisciplinary aspects of the patient's care. Various names and formats for these pathways have been used: clinical pathways, critical pathways, practice parameters, integrated care pathways, clinical protocols/guidelines, Care Medicare Advantage Plans (MAP) (Zander, 1992), progress pathway, progress maps, treatment pathways, patient pathways, or, simply, pathways. Although we look at pathways as a medical tool, the methodologies have been around for decades in the construction and engineering fields; they were not invented for healthcare. They were used as early as the 1950s in industry (aviation and construction work). In industry Critical Path Methods and Program Evaluation and Review Techniques were used to control and manage complex processes.

display 5-9

NOTE ABOUT INTERQUAL

InterQual
Address: McKesson Health Solutions
275 Grove Street,
Newton, MA 02466
Telephone: 800-522-6780
Web site: www.mckesson.com/interqual

In the mid-1980s, Karen Zander and Kathleen Bower, working at the New England Medical Center (Boston, MA), translated the standard operating procedures (in the Industry field, were called Critical Path Methods and Program Evaluation and Review Techniques) into Case Management Plans (CMPs), and later into clinical pathways. Coincidentally, or not, the DRG system was introduced in US hospitals in 1983, suggesting a high financial incentive. Zander and Bower used clinical pathways as plans to help nurses and case managers codify or formalize patterns of care (Chawla, Westrich, Matter, Kaltenboeck, Dubois, 2016; Vanhaecht, Massimiliano, van Zelm, Sermeus, 2016). Clinical pathways have become popular standard tools in case management programs, and case managers use them to monitor a patient's care progression. Generally, these tools have come to be known as case management plans.

Clinical pathways are an interdisciplinary management tool that proactively depicts important events that should take place in a day-by-day sequence. Throughout the entire episode of illness, the key events change daily and move the patient and the healthcare team toward discharge. The overall goal is to achieve optimal quality of care while minimizing delays and unnecessary resource utilization; they are also written to stay within the DRG-allotted LOS. Pathways can be used by all team members to coordinate, plan, deliver, and monitor care, and document and perform UM activities concurrently.

Clinical pathways have been written for various patient populations. Some are based on DRG-related diagnoses such as pneumonia or acute coronary syndrome. Other pathways have been written for patient conditions such as ventilator dependency weaning. Surgical procedures such as total knee replacements or lumbar laminectomies comprise many pathways. Some pathways are used for more chronic conditions. Patients with end-stage renal disease, chronic obstructive pulmonary disease, benign prostatic hypertrophy, or Crohn's disease could benefit from these pathways in the ambulatory setting. Clinical pathways can also be written for various timelines of care. The first and most common scope of care was the inpatient hospital pathway; however, pathways can now be found in use across care settings such as from SNFs to home health agencies, and connecting through the continuum.

Pathways are characterized as a method for managing patient care on the basis of clinical practice guidelines.

They are said to improve care, reduce variation, and increase the efficient use of healthcare resources. However, pathways vary in content, implementation, and place of service. Currently, there is a lack of standardization or policy on best practices in either the development or the implementation of pathways (Chawla et al., 2016).

Visually, many pathway formats are set up similarly. An inpatient clinical pathway will be used as an example. In chart form, the patient days stretch across horizontally, and the key categories align vertically (Display 5-10). The medical events are cross-referenced by category and hospital day; these events may differ (e.g., a clinical path for a total hip replacement alters from that for congestive heart failure). Generally, clinical pathways have four basic components:

1. *Aspects of care*, such as assessment, monitoring, treatments, medications, activity, diet, patient teaching, discharge planning, or outcomes evaluation.
2. *Phases of care* or the time intervals for the treatments or care.
3. *Clinical pathway functions*, such as the activities, processes, or interventions implemented by the interdisciplinary staff. The functions section also includes case management activities such as coordination of care, referrals to specialty care providers, and brokerage for postacute services.

Note: Here is where a disclaimer is important: no clinical guideline must preempt the medical judgment of a professional. Consider how the pathway will be used in areas such as documentation and

display 5-10

CRITICAL PATHWAY CHART

	Day 1	Day 2	Day 3	Day 4	Day 5
Diagnostic tests					
Treatments					
Consults/ referrals					
Medications					
Activities/ safety- mobility					
Diet/ nutrition					
Transitional/ discharge planning					
Health teaching/ education					
Outcomes					

communication. Also consider if it is a permanent part of the medical record; take into consideration the legal aspects of a clinical pathway. Determine all the disciplines that must use the pathway. Is it adequate to meet their documentation requirements or is it just another piece of paper?)

4. *Outcomes*: Clinical pathways must be updated as and when best practices change and new evidence is discovered; they must also be updated when the outcomes determine that there is a better method or time frame to address a clinical issue. Both cost and quality issues must be measured and evaluated.

Clinical pathways leave unanswered questions and signal limitations. They are not ideally suited to patients with multiple concurrent medical problems, although many healthcare professionals are working on solutions to this problem. In general, it is recommended that the staff use the clinical pathway matching the most immediate problem the patient presents with, which is usually the primary driver for care decisions. For example, if a postoperative patient is having a difficult time weaning from mechanical ventilator assistance, change the pathway to a ventilator pathway until the patient can get back on the original path. In less extreme circumstances, the patient may deviate from the pathway and smaller adjustments may need to be made; pathways are an outline and a tool, and it may not always be possible to follow them exactly. Other problems may arise if one patient has multiple physicians with multiple practice patterns. If an agreement cannot be reached, the pathway may cause additional stress and defeat its purpose.

Although not a limitation per se, the event changes are not standing orders; rather, these are clinical protocols as defined earlier. If an attending physician has already visited the patient that day, and the nurse has been prompted by the clinical pathway that a change to oral (from IV) medication may be recommended, the nurse can call the physician for clarification. Perhaps the physician had a reason to continue the IV medication (e.g., the patient is nothing by mouth [NPO]); perhaps it was an oversight and the telephone call could save resources and possibly an extra day in the hospital. More facilities are writing concurrent standing orders that coincide with each day's events.

Many organizations and professionals have created clinical pathways for patients using lay, rather than technical, terminology. Popular patient-focused pathways are those that include pictures and graphics, engage the patient in tracking progress toward discharge, and encourage the patient to speak up about any concerns or ask for clarifications if confusion exists. Clinical pathways have proved to be a support to both patients/families and medical staff. Patients who can "see" that what they are experiencing is common are not as anxious as those who do not understand what is happening to them. Many physicians appreciate the at-a-glance interdisciplinary charting. They have also received positive feedback from their patients. Patient-focused pathways are an important tool for patient teaching and for encouraging a patient to assume an active role in his or her care.

Over the years, reactions to clinical pathways have been mixed, especially from physicians. Although physicians have been essential to their development, underlying fears include increased liability and loss of autonomy, especially in the area of decision making and judgment about a patient's treatment plan. Some physicians believe that clinical pathways are a road map for a plaintiff's attorney; certainly they are sometimes used as a sword—and sometimes used as a shield—in court. Physicians also state that pathways represent a loss of their own autonomy, usually referred to as cookbook medicine. Legal recommendations in the literature state that a disclaimer should be on the clinical pathway, because it is a guideline and does not preempt the clinical judgment of a physician. A disclaimer should include that the pathway is only a representation of a common pattern of treatment and that all patients are different; acceptable medical practice includes a variety of responses to a particular clinical problem.

In the near future, with the advent of more bundled or episode-based payments, pathways should have even more influence. For example, currently, the CMS is launching the oncology care bundle and pathways are expected to play a major role; accountable care organizations and integrated delivery systems are expected to do likewise (Chawla et al., 2016). These tools can certainly create greater standardization of treatment regimens and sequencing, as well as improved outcomes, from both a quality-of-life and a clinical outcomes perspective.

Today, there are clinical pathways that are integrated into computerized provider order entry and electronic documentation systems. This is a result of the recent advancement in health and clinical information systems. Special features of these pathways include the availability of clinical/medical order sets, integration with electronic documentation, and embedding care recommendations on the basis of current evidence and best practices.

DEVELOPMENT OF A CLINICAL PATHWAY

Crozer-Keystone Health System in Pennsylvania introduced a process for the development of extended-care clinical pathways used in disease management programs in 1997 (Anonymous, 1997); refinement came in the 2000s (Panella, 2003). If your organization is inclined to develop or improve your pathways, the following steps may assist:

1. *Select a target population.* This is based on the individual organizational needs. You may choose an area with a selection matrix, including diagnoses, with higher costs, higher volumes, higher

mortality, higher LOS, or a greater number of outcome variations.

2. *Build the interdisciplinary work-team.* This is a task of prime importance. Most teams involve physicians (from family practitioners to specialists), nurses, therapists, SWs, and administrators providing care in the selected area. One of the most important success factors, before undertaking a change such as use of clinical pathways, is the choice of a "physician champion." A respected physician at the beginning will lessen physician resistance at the implementation stage. The rest of the work group can consist of adjunctive specialists who have knowledge of the disease state and comorbidities, case managers who understand UM and discharge planning strategies, computer systems personnel if the pathway is going to be computerized, and any other pertinent persons with knowledge of the process.

   Another important factor is the support from finance and decision support/data analytics. Finance and decision support share key information about the target diagnosis with the team including LOS, excess days, resource utilization and practice patterns (e.g., use of radiology tests, laboratory tests, devices or prosthesis, medications), and cost per case. It is helpful for the team to see such information analyzed by provider/physician and service. Such analysis allows the team to determine the practice pattern of the provider with optimal performance and others who may be lagging behind.

3. *Define the diagnosis and/or the patient population,* and assess the care and service needs of the chosen population. Match existing services to the population's needs. Fill in gaps through creative approaches. If additional knowledge is required at this stage, bring other experts into the working group.

4. *Review practice and literature.* Analyze the care processes and research the best evidence for the patients. Research the literature for various pathway formats and come to a consensus on one that will work for your culture and organization.

5. *Develop the clinical path.* Define appropriate goals to satisfy the multidimensional needs of the patients. Translate the results from the review phase into elements of care detailed in protocols and documentation, including the sequence of events and expected progress of the patients over time. You may choose to develop high-level flowcharts that define the process flow for all steps in the delivery of care. When developing a clinical pathway, consider how it will flow to all parts of the continuum and with all members of the interdisciplinary team.

6. *Develop quality improvement feedback loops to track and report the selected indicators.* Reporting of outcomes is expected. Developing quality indicators and using them to target areas of improvement is one excellent use of clinical pathways. This step may necessitate inclusion in the planning team of information systems and quality management experts.

7. *Pilot test and implement the pathway.* Make this a test drive, rather than the long haul. If something in the pathway causes problems, the small-scale effort may involve tweaking rather than a full-blown organizational change.

8. *Establish benchmarks.* A benchmark is essentially a goal to be achieved and is derived from the best in the field. When a facility implements a change in a process, it wants to know if that change has caused a good result or a negative situation (unintended consequences). Benchmarks are one method to measure the effect of the process; they demonstrate if goals have been met.

9. *Regularly monitor (every 3 months), evaluate, and update (yearly) the pathway.* This is a basic tenet of quality improvement; anything that can be done can be done better. You may want to investigate if/why there were any deviations from the pathways and measure patients' outcomes.

10. In Display 5-10, the following may be filled in applying a specific time frame (e.g., day 1 or day 2):
    ▶ Diagnostic tests include measurable data, such as radiology, radiography, laboratory tests, ECG, urine or stool studies, and blood sugar monitoring.
    ▶ Treatments include interventions that must be performed by the healthcare team, such as tube/catheter and site care, telemetry, daily weights, Foley catheter care, vital and neurological sign checks, suture removal, IV site changes, and small-volume nebulizer treatments.
    ▶ Consults/referrals bring in other members of the healthcare team, such as those in ostomy care, social service, diabetic education, rehabilitation, physical therapy, or dietary services.
    ▶ Medications include the drugs ordered with dosage, times, and route. IV antibiotics may be ordered on days 1 and 2, whereas oral antibiotics may be charted for the following hospital days. Medications may include anything from anticoagulants to stool softeners. Pain control is also documented, along with route of medications (oral, intramuscular, IV, or epidural).
    ▶ Activities/mobility outlines the patient's allowable activities. Across the days, this may progress from bed rest to chair to ambulation, or sitting up in a chair or head-of-bed elevations. The length of time that the patient sat in the chair or how far he or she ambulated should be documented.

▶ Diet/nutrition defines the patient's dietary needs and may advance from NPO to a regular or specialty diet, depending on the patient's requirements. The percentage of diet taken and how well the patient tolerated it must be charted. Discharge planning optimally starts before admission. Because this is not always possible, a social service referral may be charted for day 1 or 2. Insurance eligibility or SNF placement referrals may be recommended.

▶ Transitional/discharge planning defines the activities that will need to take place to move a patient from one level of care to another, less intense level, in preparation for discharge to home or another less acute facility. These may include UM review and other activities that focus on ensuring a safe discharge plan and coordination of services.

▶ Health teaching/education interactions are necessary to help the patient/family become more independent and self-sufficient. Teaching may include physical therapy safety modalities, proper administration of medications (with possible side effects), insurance explanations, tube-feeding administration, diet, exercise, posttransplantation necessary lifestyle modifications, or disease process. All events are tailored to the needs of the diagnosis and hospital day. A special focus here is the patient's self-management knowledge, skills, and abilities.

▶ Outcomes define the intermediate and discharge outcomes. Intermediate outcomes are the milestones that will need to be achieved to ensure that a patient is progressing well toward discharge to a lesser acute setting (home or SNF), which is indicative of improvement in the patient's condition.

▶ MCG Health

In 2012 MCG Health joined Hearst Health, a provider of care guidance solutions with practice-proven content. The software product makes the current evidence readily available, allowing the documentation of care management decisions, consistent and coordinated care plans, identification of gaps in care, all with an intent to enhance care management operational efficiency.

MCG Health's editors develop the care guidelines in strict accordance with the principles of evidence-based medicine. The staff that produces MCG content uses the hierarchy of evidence-grading that ranges from randomized controlled trials at the top, through other published sources, and finally including appropriate unpublished data. All content is reviewed annually and updated as necessary. Epidemiologists then examine extensive population databases to validate that published research results are achievable in real-life situations.

MCG offers content solutions that span the entire healthcare continuum. Each content solution addresses both adult and pediatric guidelines.

INPATIENT CARE RESOURCES

MCG has four content solutions that address care in the inpatient setting. Case managers use these solutions to assess, plan, and implement care during the inpatient stay. The inpatient content includes decision-making tools and supports transitioning the patient to the next most appropriate level of care. Finally, the inpatient content supports the case manager in collaborative discussions between all members of the healthcare delivery team. The four content areas are:

1. *Inpatient and Surgical Care* includes evidence-based diagnosis or procedure-specific and level-of-care (NICU, ICU, telemetry, etc.) guidelines. Inpatient and Surgical Care includes admission criteria, goals, care pathways, readmission risk assessments, goal LOS data, discharge planning, and patient education resources.

2. *General Recovery Care* provides guidelines that address more complex patient scenarios or cases where a single condition-specific guideline could not be easily applied.

3. *Multiple Condition Management* addresses the challenges of patients who present with more than one clinically active condition. These evidence-based guidelines provide direction on many common pairs of diagnoses, such as a single guideline addressing patients with heart failure and diabetes. This guideline solution provides the same resources as those of Inpatient & Surgical Care, but streamlines the workflow and provides a more holistic view of care options on the basis of the combined diagnoses. (See Displays 5-13 through 5-15 for example.)

4. *Patient Information* includes preoperative information, inpatient care plans, and discharge instructions written at a fourth to sixth grade reading level. These tools are written and formatted to be distributed to the patient and their care givers. (See Displays 5-11 through 5-15 for examples of MCG Guidelines and Optimal Recovery Courses).

POSTACUTE CARE RESOURCES

MCG has two primary solutions that address postacute care. Case managers can use these to assess, plan, and implement care in the postacute and home care settings. The tools within the postacute resources support collaborative discussions between all members of the healthcare delivery team. The two content areas are:

1. *Recovery Facility Care* provides diagnosis or procedure-specific evidence-based guidelines that

GUIDELINE FOR SEPSIS, NEONATAL

Inpatient & Surgical Care > Optimal Recovery Guideline > Neonatology and Pediatrics

Sepsis, Neonatal, Confirmed

ORG: P-425 (ISC)
Link to Codes

Print View

- Care Planning—Inpatient Admission and Alternatives
  - Clinical Indications for Admission to Inpatient Care
  - Alternatives to Admission
- Hospitalization
  - Optimal Recovery Course
  - Goal Length of Stay—**4 days**
  - Extended Stay
  - Hospital Care Planning
- Discharge
  - Discharge Planning
  - Discharge Destination
- Evidence Summary
  - Hospitalization
  - Length of Stay
- References
- Footnotes
- Codes

© 2016 MCG. All Rights Reserved. Confidential, Do Not Distribute.

Guideline: Sepsis, Neonatal, Confirmed

support transitioning patients from the hospital to the most appropriate recovery care setting. These address care at the skilled nursing, subacute, and inpatient rehabilitation (acute rehabilitation) levels of care. Recovery Facility Care includes LOS data (both Medicare and commercial), treatment courses, patient education, and discharge planning content.

2. *Home Care* includes evidence-based guidelines that support the multidisciplinary healthcare team as they deliver or manage care in the home setting. This content solution includes decision support criteria, data (both Medicare and commercial) for nursing and other rehabilitation services, treatment courses, patient education, and discharge planning.

▶ Ambulatory Care (Test and Treatments)

Ambulatory Care focuses primarily on authorization of tests, treatments, procedures, injectables, and high-cost pharmacologic agents and durable medical equipment. Included in Ambulatory Care are extensive evidence-based genetic medicine authorization guidelines and referral management guidelines. Ambulatory care includes rehabilitation data to help organizations determine goals and benchmarks

for rehab service visits. Case managers use Ambulatory Care to assess, plan, and implement care primarily in the outpatient setting.

▶ Behavioral Health

The Behavior Health evidence-based care helps case managers manage psychological, behavioral, and pharmacologic therapies for health challenges at five levels of care and across 15 diagnostic groups. Behavioral Health Care provides level-of-care and diagnosis-specific criteria, care plans, treatment options, discharge planning, therapeutic treatment options, and LOS for healthcare providers.

▶ Disease and Case/Care Management

The two content solutions to address the overall care needs of complex, chronic, or diseased-managed patients are:

1. *Chronic Care*: This addresses complex case management and chronic outpatient conditions. The evidence-based guidelines include patient assessment tools, care plans, care management tools, and patient education details. Case managers can use these tools to provide case and ongoing or long-term disease management.

CLINICAL INDICATIONS FOR HOSPITALIZATION FOR SEPSIS, NEONATAL

Guideline Clinical Indications for Admission

Clinical Indications for Admission to Inpatient Care

Return to top of *Sepsis, Neonatal, Confirmed—ISC*

- Admission to Level II or Level III nursery is indicated for **1 or more** of the following(1)(2)(3)(4)(5)(6)(7):
  - Suspected or proven sepsis

© 2016 MCG. All Rights Reserved. Confidential, Do Not Distribute.

Hospitalization
Return to top of *Sepsis, Neonatal, Confirmed—ISC*

Optimal Recovery Course
Return to top of *Sepsis, Neonatal, Confirmed—ISC*

Day	Level of Care	Clinical Status	Activity	Routes	Interventions	Medications
1	• Level II or Level III nursery[A] • Discharge planning	• **Clinical Indications met[B]**	• As tolerated	• IV fluids, medications • Oral feedings as tolerated	• Temperature support[C] • Cardiorespiratory monitor • Pulse oximetry • Lumbar puncture, CSF culture and analysis • CBC, renal and liver function tests • Glucose monitoring • Aggressive fluid resuscitation • Blood cultures • Possible C-reactive protein and other inflammatory markers • Possible CXR	• Parenteral antibiotics • Possible red cell transfusion
2	• Level II or Level III nursery	• **CSF analysis not indicative of meningitis** • **Temperature normal, stable, or improving**	• As tolerated	• IV fluids, medications • Oral feedings as tolerated	• WBC • Glucose monitoring • Pulse oximetry	• Parenteral antibiotics
3	• Level II nursery	• **Temperature normal or improving** • **Hemodynamic stability, neonatal** • **Respiratory status acceptable, neonatal** • **CSF cultures negative** • **WBC stable or improved**	• As tolerated	• Nipple feeding tolerated • IV fluids, medications	• Wean to open crib • If necessary, establish long-term access for antibiotics	• Parenteral antibiotics
4	• Level IIc nursery	• **Fever absent** • **Need for temperature support absent** • **Toxic appearance absent**	• Routine	• **Oral hydration, medications[D]** • Nipple feeding advancing	• **Open crib**	• Parenteral antibiotics
5	• Level IIc nursery to discharge[E] • Complete discharge planning	• **Hemodynamic stability, neonatal[F]** • **Respiratory status acceptable, neonatal** • **Alert** • **Fever absent** • **Need for temperature support absent** • **Toxic appearance absent** • **WBC normal or improved** • **Antibiotic regimen for next level of care arranged** • **Discharge plans and education understood**	• Routine	• **Oral hydration, medications** • **Adequate nipple feeding**	• **Open crib**	• Parenteral antibiotics

(1)(2)(4)(7)(9)(11)(12)⒩ © 2016 MCG. All Rights Reserved. Confidential, Do Not Distribute.

Guideline: Optimal Recovery Course

GUIDELINE FOR HEART FAILURE WITH CLINICALLY ACTIVE DIABETES

Inpatient & Surgical Care—Multiple Condition Management > Optimal Recovery Guideline

Heart Failure with Clinically Active Diabetes MCM

ORG: M-190-DM (MCM)
Link to Codes

Print View

- Care Planning—Inpatient Admission and Alternatives
  - Clinical Indications for Admission to Inpatient Care
  - Alternatives to Admission
  - Alternative Care Planning
- Hospitalization
  - Optimal Recovery Course
  - Multiple Condition Benchmark Length of Stay—**Ambulatory or 2 days**
  - Extended Stay
  - Hospital Care Planning
- Discharge
  - Discharge Planning
  - Discharge Destination
- Evidence Summary
  - Criteria
  - Alternatives
  - Hospitalization
  - Length of Stay
- References
- Footnotes
- Codes

© 2016 MCG. All Rights Reserved. Confidential, Do Not Distribute.

Guideline: Heart Failure with Clinically Active Diabetes

---

2. *Transitions of Care*: This is designed to assess a patient's transition-of-care needs, provide evidence-based care planning, and promote patient condition self-management for those with postacute care needs. These guidelines are disease specific or condition -specific and are for situations in which patients are likely to benefit from case management to ensure they understand their care needs and that these needs are met appropriately.

▶ OVERVIEW OF STATUSES AND THEIR IMPORTANCE

Physician documentation is always the basis for determining the status for hospital admissions. Placing the patient in the correct status is both a function of critical decisions and seeking a crystal ball; in other words, especially in the first several hours, you may not have enough clinical data or know the plan of care to determine the correct status. What follows in this section on 'Status' are levels of status and some case studies to demonstrate nuances—taking into consideration the condition of the patient, governmental regulations, and commercial health insurance benefits and authorizations. Put all this together accurately (with the assistance of evidence-based clinical decision tools) and your healthcare facility will get paid/reimbursed for the services provided; get it wrong and denials may result, posing financial risk to your facility.

Choosing the correct status is critical and often takes the clinical minds of the case manager, the PA, the practitioner, and others who may be on the patient's team. Still, with all that brainpower, the patient's condition may suddenly improve or deteriorate—and consequently, it may turn out that the wrong status has been chosen. The topics in the section on "Status Determinations" will necessarily include the following:

CLINICAL INDICATIONS OF ADMISSION FOR HEART FAILURE WITH CLINICALLY ACTIVE DIABETES

Clinical Indications for Admission to Inpatient Care

Return to top of *Heart Failure with Clinically Active Diabetes MCM—MCM*

*Note: For patients who do **not** have clinically active diabetes, **see** Heart Failure* ⬀ ISC.

[Expand All / Collapse All]

- Admission is indicated by **1 or more** of the following(1)(2)(3)(4)(5)(6)(7):◼
  - ◦ Hemodynamic instability
  - ◦ Severe electrolyte abnormalities requiring inpatient care
  - ◦ Cardiac arrhythmias of immediate concern
  - ◦ Precipitating cause for acute decompensation (e.g., pneumonia, pulmonary embolism) requires inpatient care
  - ◦ Acute cardiac ischemia causing or associated with failure. See Angina ⬀ ISC or Myocardial Infarction ⬀ ISC as appropriate
  - ◦ Pulmonary edema that is very severe (e.g., mechanical ventilation needed, imminent or likely, need for 100% oxygen to keep oxygen saturation above 90%)
  - ◦ Massive skin edema (anasarca) with complications (e.g., tissue breakdown with infection, inability to void because of edema)[A](14)
  - ◦ Inpatient admission required[B] rather than observation care (see <u>Heart Failure: Observation Care</u> ⬀ ISC guideline as appropriate) because of **one or more** of the following:
    - ⊞ Pulmonary edema that is persistent
    - ▪ Altered mental status that is severe or persistent
    - ▪ Increased creatinine (new on laboratory test) with reduction of more than 50% in estimated glomerular filtration rate from baseline ▦ GFR—Adult Calculator
    - ▪ Progressively (ongoing) rising creatinine (known from past laboratory test) with reduction of more than 25% in estimated glomerular filtration rate from baseline ▦ GFR—Adult Calculator
    - ▪ Acute renal failure
    - ▪ Acute peripheral ischemia (e.g., examination shows pulseless, cool, mottled, or cyanotic extremity)
    - ▪ Oxygen administration or respiratory treatments have been needed for over 24 hours that are performable only in acute inpatient setting

e.g.,
    - ▪ Pulmonary artery catheter monitoring needed
    - ▪ Other condition, treatment, or monitoring requiring inpatient admission.

Guideline Clinical Indications for Admission

- ▶ Outpatient Status and Inpatient Only (IPO)
- ▶ Observation Status
  - ▶ Medicare Observation Guidelines
  - ▶ Commercial Insurance Observation Guidelines
- ▶ Inpatient Status
  - ▶ Two-Midnight Rule
  - ▶ Physician certification/recertification
- ▶ Changing Statuses
  - ▶ Commercial Insurance
  - ▶ Medicare Regulations
    - • CC44
    - • MOON

Determining the correct status (Display 5-16) was never to be a black-and-white. But in the past few years, the number and types of regulatory changes that have been finalized has made these decisions even more difficult. The medical practices often do not have the most up-to-date knowledge on these regulations and, therefore, depend on the case manager to keep them current and guide them through the ever-changing regulatory terrain.

▶ Outpatient Status and Inpatient Only (IPO)

Determining Medicare beneficiaries' status after surgery poses multi-level challenges. If the patient has an outpatient procedure without complications, he or she would be designated an outpatient status. If the patient has an inpatient-only procedure, he or she gets an inpatient status. It is everywhere in between these two scenarios that the case manager must be alert, aware of regulations, and clinically astute. It is also necessary that the case manager makes the correct decision on the basis of the evidence as document in the patient's medical record to avoid a denial and ensure no financial risk for the healthcare organization or medical practice.

EXTENDED RECOVERY/OUTPATIENT

Typically, Medicare does not cover observation services under the following circumstances and should not be billed as such. The following instances should alert the case manager to keep the patient in an extended recovery/outpatient status and *not* change to observation:

- ▶ Services were provided for the convenience of a patient, the patient's family, or the physician.

▶ The services provided were standard for diagnostic, surgical, or therapeutic procedures.

▶ The services were part of the standard preparation or recovery period for diagnostic, surgical, or therapeutic care.

▶ The monitoring was incidental to other diagnostic, surgical, or therapeutic services.

Observation must be medically necessary, and that it is rarely appropriate for a postsurgical procedure. Payment for the standard recovery period following surgery is built into the outpatient Ambulatory Payment Classification payment structure. However, to every Medicare rule, there are exceptions. An observation order should be obtained by the provider and entered into the electronic medical record (EMR) when a Medicare patient completes the 4- to 6-hour extended recovery period, but has experienced a complication. The following criteria *may* signal observation status following the 4- to 6-hour time frame post procedure:

▶ pain management,
▶ oxygen requirements,
▶ nausea,
▶ hyper/hypotension,
▶ arrhythmias,
▶ abnormal laboratory values, or
▶ failure to void.

Should any of these criteria be met, observation could be the appropriate postoperative status. The patient will then be transferred to a hospital unit bed for an overnight admission. It must be noted that Medicare permits observation status to continue for up to two midnights if inpatient criteria are not met. When this issue occurs, the surgical practice and/or the hospital PA should be consulted for plan-of-care considerations.

Let's look at two case examples (Coulter & VanGelder, 2014):

CASE STUDIES

CASE STUDY 1:

A patient is admitted for a scheduled thyroidectomy (CPT code 60240). Post procedure, the patient is taken to the postacute anesthesia unit (PACU), orders are written, and the patient is placed in extended recovery. The case manager reviews the patient's progress 4 hours later. Hypertension and nausea are noted and documented by the PACU nurse. The patient has received three doses of an intravenous beta-blocker, two doses of intravenous ondansetron (Zofran), and oxygen at 3 L/minute with continuous pulse oximetry. Following this review, the case manager determines that observation status is appropriate. The provider is contacted and an observation order is obtained and entered in the EMR.

CASE STUDIES

CASE STUDY 2:

In this example, the reason for a decision to change a patient's status is not always obvious. The patient

---

display 5-15

OPTIMAL RECOVERY COURSE FOR HEART FAILURE WITH CLINICALLY ACTIVE DIABETES

Optimal Recovery Course

Return to top of *Heart Failure with Clinically Active Diabetes MCM—MCM*

Day	Level of Care	Clinical Status	Activity	Routes	Interventions	Medications
1	• ICU[D] or intermediate care [E] after emergency treatment • Readmission risk assessment • Discharge planning	• **Clinical Indications met**[F] • Tachypnea, edema, and dyspnea • Possible hypoxia and hypotension • Hyperglycemic and possibly acidotic	• Initial bed rest	• Parenteral medications • Oral hydration • Low-salt diabetic diet	• ECG, CXR, ABG • Cardiac biomarkers, BNP • Possible pulmonary artery catheter[G] • Oxygen • Echocardiogram • Digoxin level if previously prescribed • Weigh • Possible fluid restriction • Serum glucose, serum ketones, electrolytes, bicarbonate, ABGs or venous pH measurements, urinalysis • Bedside glucose monitoring	• IV diuretics • ACE inhibitor or ARB • Beta-blocker[H] • Possible aldosterone antagonist • Possible IV vasodilator (e.g., nitrates, hydralazine) • Glucose control with insulin • Potassium, phosphorus, and magnesium replacement as indicated

OPTIMAL RECOVERY COURSE FOR HEART FAILURE WITH CLINICALLY ACTIVE DIABETES (*continued*)

2	• Intermediate care or floor	• Hemodynamic stability • **Mental status at baseline** • **MI excluded** • **Oxygenation at baseline or improved** • **Pulmonary edema absent or improved** • **Electrolytes normal or improved** • **Dehydration absent** • **Metabolic acidosis absent** • **Glucose control acceptable for next level of care or improved**	• Advance activity as tolerated	• **Oral hydration, medications, and diet** • Low-salt diabetic diet • Adjust fluid restriction	• **Pulmonary catheter absent** • Weigh • Possible CXR, ECG, BNP • Oxygen • Serum glucose, electrolytes, and bicarbonate • Bedside glucose monitoring • Diabetic education	• **Outpatient diabetic medication regimen initiated** • Taper parenteral medication and optimize oral medication • Diuretics • ACE inhibitor or ARB • Beta-blocker • Possible aldosterone antagonist • Possible nitrates, digoxin, hydralazine • Electrolyte supplementation as needed
3	• Floor to discharge • Complete discharge planning	• Hemodynamic stability • **Tachypnea absent** • **Oxygenation at baseline or acceptable for next level of care** • **Cardiac rate and rhythm acceptable** • **Pulmonary edema absent or acceptable for next level of care** • **Peripheral or sacral edema absent or improved** • **Volume status acceptable on oral medication** • **Mental status at baseline** • **Acceptable acid-base balance** • **Blood glucose under acceptable control** • **Electrolytes acceptable** • **Diet tolerated** • **Discharge plans and education understood**	• **Ambulatory**	• **Oral hydration, medications, and diet** • Low-salt diabetic diet	• **Oxygen absent** • **Diabetic education complete** • Weight	• **Outpatient diabetic medication regimen established** • Diuretics • ACE inhibitor or ARB • Beta-blocker • Possible aldosterone antagonist • Possible nitrates, digoxin, hydralazine

(1)(13)(32)(33)Ⓝ

Guideline Optimal Recovery Course

may meet criteria for an inpatient stay; however, the question may arise as to whether the patient will require a hospital stay longer than one to two midnights. This decision must involve critical thinking and astute nursing and case management assessment skills as the following case illustrates.

Scenario: A patient was admitted to the Cardiac Catheterization Laboratory for a left-sided heart catheterization. The CPT code 93452 is an outpatient procedure. Before the procedure, an arterial catheter was inserted because of a history of uncontrolled hypertension. During the procedure, two drug-eluding stents were placed. Admission to the

STATUS TERMS AND DEFINITIONS (BASED ON TRADITIONAL MEDICARE/ FEE-FOR-SERVICE)

Ambulatory: Anticipate discharge from the postacute anesthesia unit (PACU) postsurgical procedure.

Extended recovery: A 4- to 6-hour time frame in PACU post procedure that is billed as recovery room services.

Outpatient in a bed: A status that is used following extended recovery when criteria for observation are not met.

Observation: A status that is used following extended recovery on the basis of medical criteria.

Inpatient: A status that is determined by being on the inpatient-only list or by complex medical factors that necessitate an inpatient stay.

Condition Code 44: A code used on outpatient claims when a Medicare inpatient admission has been changed (in status) to observation prior to discharge.

PACU was accompanied with an extended recovery order. Throughout the next 4 to 6 hours, elevated systolic blood pressures remained uncontrolled, and a nitroglycerin drip with titration was initiated. When the patient was stable, an order for transfer to the intermediate/step-down unit was entered for close monitoring. At this juncture, the inpatient criteria were met; however, the discharge plan had not been determined. A call was placed to the intermediate/ step-down RN caring for the patient, and several inquiries were made concerning the condition of the patient, recovery time, and intended care plan. The unit RN had spoken to the provider and understood the care plan of the patient; the PACU case manager asked specific questions:

Question: How long do you anticipate that the intravenous nitroglycerin drip will continue?

Answer: The patient is scheduled to go to dialysis this afternoon and following his dialysis treatment, the drip will be discontinued.

Question: How long do you anticipate keeping the arterial catheter in?

Answer: The arterial catheter will also be discontinued following dialysis treatment.

Question: Do you think the patient will be discharged home tomorrow?

Answer: Yes, the patient's attending physician has indicated that the patient will be discharged tomorrow if he remains medically stable.

On the basis of the information given by the unit RN, an order for observation was obtained from the provider and entered in the EMR. The care plan as stated by the intermediate/step-down unit RN was executed; the patient went for dialysis treatment later in the day. Both the nitroglycerin drip and arterial catheter were discontinued that evening, and the patient was discharged home the

next morning. The total hospital stay, from admission to discharge, was only one midnight. Observation was the correct status for this Medicare patient.

MEDICARE INPATIENT-ONLY (IPO) LIST

Note: This section pertains to Medicare fee-for-service beneficiaries who have had a surgical procedure. Commercial beneficiaries are usually preauthorized for surgeries on the basis of their health insurance benefits.

The Medicare Inpatient-Only list (IPO) is composed of a number of surgical procedures which the CMS deems to be inpatient-only encounters. Each procedure has an attached CPT code. The CPT codes are published and are updated annually by the American Medical Association. The list is organized by physiologic systems that are generally grouped in numerical order. Any Medicare patient who has a procedure on this list must be admitted as an inpatient to the hospital following the procedure. The CMS has stipulated that services appearing on the IPO list and supporting an inpatient admission may be appropriately billed under Part A payment, regardless of the expected LOS. To comply with this directive, a surgical procedure on the IPO list must have a written physician preprocedure inpatient order before the patient is taken to the operating room (Coulter & VanGelder, 2014).

Status is critical: there is a delicate balance between the "revenue cycle and case management" that benefits acute care facilities. A surgical procedure on the Medicare IPO list that is not ordered in the correct status prior to the commencement of surgery will not be able to be billed to Medicare and will represent a revenue loss to the hospital. Conversely, if the proper orders are written and certified by the attending physician, the hospital will be able to obtain inpatient funds from the CMS.

The following cases illustrate how focused attention to correct status and orders result in substantial cost savings. Reviewing and updating the Medicare IPO list annually cannot be overlooked. Knowing the nuances of regulations (a prime case management role), especially when it comes to Medicare surgeries, is critically important to the fiscal health of the organization. These three cases underscore the importance of an astute case manager in the PACU, who is well versed in both inpatient-only surgeries and their contiguous regulations (VanGelder & Coulter, 2013).

CASE STUDIES

CASE STUDY 1:

A Medicare patient is admitted to the PACU following a cervical fusion with instrumentation. The CPT code for this procedure is 22845 and is on the Medicare IPO list. The preprocedure order for inpatient was entered correctly; however, the neurosurgeon elected to enter a discharge order to home with self-care directly from the PACU. The case manager in the PACU questioned the discharge order since a Medicare patient must be admitted to the floor in an inpatient status before being discharged home to receive appropriate reimbursement from the CMS. The neurosurgeon was contacted and educated on the reimbursement consequences regarding the current discharge plan from the PACU. The order for the inpatient was reinstated, the patient was transferred to the floor, and a discharge order was written later in the day. The net savings for this case was $13,212.

CASE STUDIES

CASE STUDY 2:

This case demonstrates the importance of the preadmit procedure order prior to the commencement of surgery. A Medicare patient was scheduled for aortic and mitral valve replacements. The case manager in the PACU, reviewing the day of surgery schedule, noted the lack of a preprocedure admit order. The attending physician was contacted and a preprocedure admit order was obtained and entered. Had this omission not been found, the entire case that includes the charges of the surgery and postoperative care in the ICU and the telemetry unit of approximately $75,000 could have been lost.

CASE STUDIES

CASE STUDY 3:

A scheduled Medicare procedure had a CPT code that was not on the Medicare IPO list. The preprocedure admit order was correctly entered as Extended Recovery; however, the surgery was more extensive than planned. The updated procedure was found on the Medicare IPO list. An order was obtained for a status change to inpatient and the facility received the appropriate reimbursement.

▶ Observation Status

HISTORY AND OVERVIEW OF OBSERVATION

The history of observation status goes back many decades—at a time when healthcare was dramatically different than today. In 1983, Medicare was reimbursing hospitals according to their costs on a fee-for-service basis. However, it was felt that providers were not motivated to keep their costs low, as that only served to reduce their own reimbursement. There was little regulatory oversight during the pre-1980 years, and efficiency and effectiveness were not monitored. Then, the DRGs were born, and this pay structure to prospectively set rates for certain diagnoses changed everything; for example, hospitals were keen to reduce LOSs and the rising costs of healthcare began to slow down and NCMs were embedded in hospitals to look more closely at clinical issues (Powell, 2013).

At first, observation status had no written regulations and, therefore, provided relief from the constraints of the DRGs' payment methodology and the regulatory oversight. Then, in 1994, the Prospective Payment Assessment Commission identified observation stays as problematic because many of the observational stays should have been coded as "inpatient admissions." So after this investigation, the Health Care Financing Administration—now the Centers for Medicare & Medicaid Services—published the rules for appropriate use of observation status in the September 1996 Medicare Hospital Manual, Publication 10. And, the current problems began (Powell, 2013).

Fast forward to November 3, 2011: a lawsuit was filed by the Center for Medicare Advocacy and cocounsel National Senior Citizens Law Center seeking to end the use of hospital "Observation Status" (*Bagnall v. Sebelius* [*No. 3:11-cv-01703, D. Conn*]). The suit was filed on behalf of seven individual plaintiffs from Connecticut, Massachusetts, and Texas who represent a nationwide class of people harmed by the illegal "observation status" policy and practice. *Bagnall v. Sebelius* stated that the use of observation status violates the Medicare Act, the Freedom of Information Act, the Administrative Procedure Act, and the Due Process Clause of the Fifth Amendment to the Constitution. It stated that Medicare is using observation status to deny reimbursement to beneficiaries for hospital services and nursing home stays. If a Medicare beneficiary cannot safely go home and requires physical, occupational, or speech therapy (for example), Medicare does not have to pay for an SNF—the beneficiary pays for it. Is this not a form of cost shifting (Powell, 2013)?

Other lawsuits have also challenged the observation regulations. Most simplified, some merely want observation days to contribute to the 3-day qualifying SNF stay. In the Outpatient Prospective Payment System (OPPS) 2010 guidelines, the CMS clarified expectations about the use of observation services, physician interventions, and documentation.

But the real challenge came in 2013 with the advent of Medicare's two-midnight rule. The CMS dealt with the growth in long-stay observation cases (those greater than 48 hours), which increased from 3% of all observation cases in 2006 to 8% in 2011 (ACMA, 2016a). The two-midnight rule redefined what inpatient versus observation status is all about. Evidenced-based criteria, such as InterQual or MCG, have attempted to keep up with the changes. However, the patient often falls into a gray area, where just crossing two midnights is not enough clinical reason to make the status "inpatient." Medical necessity plays a significant role. Note that, in this new world, observation days still do not "count" toward the 3-day qualifying SNF stays in Medicare fee-for-service beneficiaries (commercial health insurance and some MAP may not be this strict). However, if beneficiaries receive outpatient services in the ED, in observation status, or in the operating rooms, they can count those midnights

INPATIENT VERSUS OUTPATIENT OBSERVATION STATUS

Inpatient vs. Outpatient Observation—*8 Key Questions for Physicians to Ask*

1. In what condition will the patient most likely be tomorrow?
2. "Better"=Consider observation
3. Is it risky to send the patient home today?
4. "Yes"=Consider observation
5. Is it likely I will know whether to admit or send the patient home by tomorrow?
6. "Yes"=Consider observation
7. Are vital signs stable?
8. "Yes"=Consider observation
9. Will a diagnosis likely be made in 24 hours?
10. "Yes"=Consider observation
11. Will treatment, such as IV fluids, require standard monitoring and be completed within 24 hours?
12. "Yes"=Consider observation
13. Is the patient being admitted with symptom(s) (e.g., chest pain, abdominal pain, TIA)?
14. "Yes"=Consider observation
15. Is the patient having an unusually long recovery period following an outpatient procedure (e.g., pain management issues, cardiopulmonary concerns, urinary retention)?
16. "Yes"=Consider observation

Reprinted from Richards, F., Pitluk, H., Collier, P., Powell, S., Dion, C., Struchen-Shellhorn, W., & Plunkett, M. (2008). Reducing Unnecessary Medicare Hospital Admissions for Chest Pain in Arizona and Florida. *Professional Case Management, 13*(2), 74–84, with permission.

toward the 2-day inpatient status. And new legislation includes a proposal to the OPPS 2016 regulations that will require the bundling of services into observation services. This will further complicate the effectiveness with which hospitals can manage this service (ACMA, 2016a).

Commercial payors and several Medicare Managed Care Plans can have different expectations about what constitutes an observation versus an inpatient status. The case manager must know the patient's insurance benefits, and apply their rules, authorizations, and regulations to each case. Constant vigilance is necessary, along with a strong knowledge of guidelines when discussing observation cases with the PAs. Because observation stays incur greater out-of-pocket expenses for the beneficiaries and do not contribute to a qualifying 3-day SNF stay, case managers must don their advocacy role to manage any difficult scenarios.

OBSERVATION GUIDELINES

Observation status is an administrative classification of patients, seen in hospital emergency rooms or outpatient clinics, who have uncertain conditions that are potentially serious enough to warrant close observation, but usually not so serious to warrant admission to the hospital. Healthcare providers and hospitals tend to place these patients in beds, usually for less than 24 hours, without formal admissions to the hospital as inpatients. During this time frame, the patient is monitored and frequently assessed until a final determination is reached whether to admit or discharge.

The CMS defines observation services as those that are furnished by a hospital on its premises, including the use of a bed; at the least, they include periodic monitoring by a hospital's nursing or other staff. These services must be reasonable and necessary to evaluate an outpatient's condition or determine the need for a possible inpatient admission. The purpose of observation status is to evaluate and treat a patient's medical condition to determine if there is a need for further treatment in an inpatient setting or stability for discharge. Figure 5-1 includes a decision tree hospitals may implement as part of their observation status guidelines. Display 5-17 is another helpful tool that can aid case managers and physicians in effectively determining if a patient's condition warrants an inpatient admission or observation status.

There are as many points of entry as there are places where a patient may enter into the hospital as an observation patient: ED, PACU, direct admission from a physician's office or clinic, or a change from another status to observation status. Generally, patients who have a *symptom*, rather than an admitting diagnosis, are appropriate for observation status: during the next 24 hours, monitoring and observing the clinical symptoms to assess if a diagnosis presents (or the patient improves) is appropriately observation. Usually within 24 hours, or 48 at the latest, the improvement or diagnosis will show itself. (Also see section, this chapter, on Outpatient scenarios, for other observation nuances.)

Documentation by the physician practice is key to demonstrating correct status. When a patient is in observation status, documentation of progress must include the need to continue observation. The patient's medical record must include documentation at certain intervals during the 24 hours. If documentation of progress includes the conversion in status to an inpatient admission, the record must reflect the presence of evidence that the patient's condition meets admission and medical necessity criteria. If documentation of progress indicates the decision to discharge the patient, the record must reflect evidence of medical stability and a plan for follow-up care as needed. As in all cases, documentation indicating that the physician assessed risk to the patient as a rationale why the patient remains in the hospital (and in the chosen status) is key to reimbursement.

Another important point for case managers to know is that when a Medicare beneficiary is under observation status, he or she is categorized as "outpatient services" and

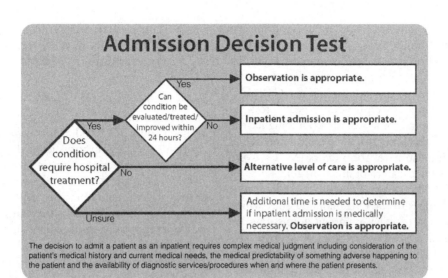

Admission Decision Test

Does condition require hospital treatment?

- Yes → **Can condition be evaluated/treated/improved within 24 hours?**
  - Yes → Observation is appropriate.
  - No → Inpatient admission is appropriate.
- No → Alternative level of care is appropriate.
- Unsure → Additional time is needed to determine if inpatient admission is medically necessary. **Observation is appropriate.**

The decision to admit a patient as an inpatient requires complex medical judgment including consideration of the patient's medical history and current medical needs, the medical predictability of something adverse happening to the patient and the availability of diagnostic services/procedures when and where the patient presents.

Figure 5-1 Deciding on a patient's admission status. (Courtesy of Health Services Advisory Group, Phoenix, AZ.)

must be billed as such. The other impact to the patient is that they have no Medicare rights to appeal a discharge (see section this chapter on Medicare Discharge Appeals) because they are not considered an inpatient.

A physician's order must specify "admit to observation" and must be signed and dated. When a change in status occurs, physician notes and orders must also specify such change. Changing statuses in Medicare beneficiaries is another area where regulations play a critical role. (See the section on "Changing Status" in this chapter.)

▶ Inpatient Status

Like the observation status, inpatient status can occur in any level of care: ICU, medical-surgical, intermediate, step down, and other unique levels of care. It is obvious that many patients meet the criteria for inpatient status; however, there are red flags that case management should be aware of, especially given regulations such as the two-midnight rule and IPO surgeries. Case studies in this chapter on "Outpatient and Inpatient Only" discuss close calls, where a wrong order, or an incorrect discharge from the PACU, could have caused significant loss of revenue for the hospital.

In the past few years, there has been more scrutiny on short, inpatient admissions. In part, this is due to the advent of the two-midnight rule. All one-day inpatient stays should be investigated carefully, as they are the subject of audits. Commercial insurance looks at these and may deny the admission, or give the facility the opportunity to change the status to observation. For Medicare beneficiaries, one-day stay audits have been done by both the Recovery Audit Contractors (RACs) or the two BFCC-QIOs (Livanta and KEPRO). Their charge is to evaluate the appropriateness of short-stay inpatient admissions that extend over less than two midnights.

Of course, the reason for this focus on auditing one-day admissions is directly related to reimbursement issues. Hospitals are paid by DRG; therefore, if the patient is an inpatient for just one day, Medicare still pays the hospital the entire DRG amount. This makes Medicare look twice to see if these patients could have been managed as outpatients. As stated earlier, hospitals are also receiving increased attention from commercial payors. Case managers should be aware of the percentage of one-day stay cases attributed to their facility (ACMA, 2016a).

Case managers need to examine why a patient has a one-day inpatient admission. There may be completely appropriate reasons (see exceptions to the two-midnight rule). However, they should be sure that this was a medically necessary inpatient admission and that there was no hint of a social admission or gaming the system. And case managers must make sure there is accurate and thorough documentation in the medical record of the clinical picture of the patient at the time of admission, what treatments were done, and what the risk of discharge to the patient may be.

TWO-MIDNIGHT RULE

The CMS has been looking for processes to address some of the disagreements around observation versus inpatient hospital admissions. On the one hand, it wanted to reduce long observation stays, a prime complaint of Medicare beneficiaries. On the other hand, RACs found high numbers of admissions they felt should have been outpatient observation (rather than inpatient) status. These conflicting findings, and hospitals and other stakeholders, mandated that the CMS come up with more clarity on what constitutes an inpatient admission that will be paid for under Medicare Part A.

The original two-midnight rule, released in August 2013, stated that a hospital inpatient admission was considered reasonable and necessary if the physician (or other qualified practitioner) ordered the admission on the basis of the expectation that the patient would require at least two midnights of medically necessary hospital services (or if the patient required a procedure on the CMS IPO list). However, if the physician/provider expected to keep the patient in the hospital for less than two midnights, the services would be billable for outpatient payment only. RACs and Medicare Administrative Contractors (MACs) were responsible for reviewing claims for inpatient admissions. In October 2015, the CMS released the OPPS 2016 final rule, which finalized changes to the two-midnight rule, which addresses the question of when inpatient admissions are appropriate for Medicare Part A payment (Ollapally, 2016).

The significant change to the 2015 ruling was that, under certain circumstances, hospital admission stays of less than two midnights may be allowed to remain inpatient. Another modification will transition review of claims for inpatient admissions from RACs and MACs to QIOs. By 2016, after much feedback by the healthcare community, the CMS had allowed more weight to be given to the physician's medical judgment in meeting the needs of Medicare patients. If the attending physician anticipates that the patient will need fewer than two midnights of hospital care (and the procedure is not on the IPO list or otherwise specifically listed by the CMS as an exception), the inpatient admission may be payable under Medicare Part A on a case-by-case basis. Medical record documentation must support that an inpatient admission is appropriate (Ollapally, 2016).

Another change was the mandate for certification of the attending physician's signature on the admission order. After much scrambling by hospitals, and many resources utilized, this was softened. Effective January 1, 2015, the certification requirement of the two-midnight rule is no longer required. However, if a patient remains in the hospital for 20 days or more, a certification requirement is needed and should include the rationale and medical necessity documentation of why the patient remains hospitalized.

EXCEPTIONS TO THE TWO-MIDNIGHT RULE

If a Medicare patient is discharged after one midnight, do not change from inpatient status if the patient had a surgery performed that is on the IPO list; the two-midnight rule does not apply to these surgeries. Other exceptions to the two-midnight rule in Medicare patients that should be applied include:

▶ The patient leaves against medical advice.
▶ The patient is transferred to hospice care (and not previously in hospice).
▶ The patient was unexpectedly placed on a mechanical ventilator after a procedure (and this is not routine intubation for the surgical case).
▶ The patient is transferred to another acute care facility.
▶ The patient dies.

▶ The patient miraculously and unexpectedly improves. As in all these exceptions, physician documentation is critical.

CASE EXAMPLE OF TWO-MIDNIGHT INPATIENT STAY

The patient was a same-day surgical admit for a scheduled tracheostomy (CPT code 31600), *an outpatient Medicare procedure*. Medical history included tracheal stenosis, status posttracheal resection with reanastomosis and secondary dyspnea because of tracheomalacia. The planned hospital stay was documented in the EMR to be at least 4 days. Because of the medical history and the expected 4-day postoperative stay, an inpatient preoperative order was entered in the EMR by the provider. Postoperatively, the patient was admitted to the PACU in an inpatient status. The PACU case manager had a decision to make: Was the correct order inpatient or extended recovery based on outpatient procedure code for Medicare? The PACU case manager spoke with the provider who had signed the inpatient certification and confirmed the intended LOS indicated in the EMR. A joint decision was made to allow the inpatient order in the EMR to stand. The case manager in the PACU informed the case manager on the receiving floor of the intended LOS and asked that he or she continue to follow up for possible care plan changes that might warrant a condition 44. Subsequently, the patient was transferred to the intermediate/step-down unit for 1 day and then to a medical/surgical floor for an additional 5 days. The patient remained on 10 L of oxygen per minute through the tracheal collar for the duration of the hospital stay, and tube feeds were initiated. Per the CMS guidelines, the patient met inpatient criteria. The patient required continuing services and monitoring beyond two midnights, and the patient's condition was severe enough to require inpatient treatment that was documented in the EMR by the provider. Inpatient was the correct status for this Medicare patient, even though the patient had an outpatient procedure done per Medicare guidelines (Coulter and VanGelder, 2014).

▶ Recovery Audit Contractors

The Recovery Audit Program is contracted by the CMS to identify and correct Medicare overpayments made on claims of healthcare services provided to Medicare beneficiaries, and also to identify underpayments to providers. The program was started in 2005 as a 3-year demonstration project and included only three states: California, Florida, and New York. Even before the project concluded, the CMS extended the RACs to three other states: Arizona, Massachusetts, and South Carolina. This was due to the amount of dollars recouped by the program; RACs were successful in allowing the CMS to recoup Medicare overpayments during the demonstration run between 2005 and 2008. The RACs resulted in over $900 million in overpayments being returned to the Medicare Trust

Fund and nearly $38 million in underpayments returned to healthcare providers. As a result, Congress required the Secretary of the Department of Health and Human Services to institute (under Section 302 of the Tax Relief and Health Care Act of 2006) a permanent and national Recovery Audit Program to recoup overpayments associated with services for which payment is made under part A or B of title XVIII of the Social Security Act. Section 1893(h) mandated that the Recovery Audit Program expanded to all the states in January 2010.

Of interest is how Recovery Auditors (RAs) are paid. As required by Section 1893(h) of the act, RAs are paid on a contingency-fee basis. The amount of the contingency fee is a percentage of the payment recovered from, or reimbursed to, providers. The RAs negotiate their contingency fees at the time of the contract award. The base contingency fees ranged from 9% to 12.5% for all claim types, except durable medical equipment (DME). The contingency fees for DME claims ranged from 14% to 17.5%. The RA must return the contingency fee if an improper payment determination is overturned at any level of appeal. For the fiscal year, 2014, the Recovery Audit Program returned over $1.6 billion to the Medicare Trust Funds. Inpatient hospital patient status reviews previously accounted for a substantial portion of RA corrections (CMS, 2016b).

In fiscal year, 2014, the RAs identified and corrected $2.57 billion in improper payments. There were $2.39 billion collected in overpayments and $173.1 million in identified underpayments paid back to providers. In FY 2014, program corrections were $1.2 billion, or 31.5% below program corrections in FY 2013. The CMS attributes some of the decrease in corrections from previous years to the limited reviews that took place during the closeout process of the existing RA contracts (CMS, 2016b).

In fiscal year ending September 30, 2015, $359.7 million in overpayments were collected and $81.0 million in underpayments were returned to providers. According to the FY2015 Agency Financial Report, RACs have collected a net of $8.9449 billion since the start of fiscal year 2010 (American Society of Anesthesiologists, 2016).

Each RA is responsible for identifying overpayments and underpayments in approximately one-quarter of the country. The Recovery Audit Program awarded by the CMS as of October 2016 is (CMS, 2017d):

▶ Region 1—Performant Recovery, Inc.
▶ Region 2—Cotiviti, LLC
▶ Region 3—Cotiviti, LLC
▶ Region 4—HMS Federal Solutions
▶ Region 5—Performant Recovery, Inc.

The RACs in Regions 1 to 4 will perform postpayment review to identify and correct Medicare claims that contain improper payments (overpayments or underpayments) that were made under Part A and Part B, for all provider types other than Durable Medical Equipment, Prosthetics, Orthotics, and Supplies (DMEPOS) and Home Health/Hospice. The Region 5 RAC will be dedicated to the postpayment review of DMEPOS and Home Health/Hospice claims nationally.

RACs, now known as RAs, and the QIOs determine many "denials" (also called "overpayments") at all levels of care. There has been much contention over the years about the subjected overpayments, how they were done, and how RAs are paid. Employing case managers or UM nurses to primarily focus on patients' eligibility for inpatient admissions, medical necessity reviews, and evaluation of the appropriateness of observation status and outpatient care is the best weapon against denials. Case managers/UM nurses work to ensure compliance with Medicare payment procedures, and provision of services in the appropriate setting and at the right level of care.

▶ Changing Patient's Status

Changing patient's status of hospital patients must be done on the basis of the insurance the patient currently has, regulations, benefits, authorizations, and, of course the medical necessity; these are some of the multiple issues that the case manager must keep in mind.

Commercial payors and some MAPs do not follow the directions and regulations of the CMS. For example, during, or even after a hospital stay, a commercial payor may suggest that they will reimburse the entire hospital stay at an observation level, rather than an inpatient level. It is up to the case manager to confer with the UR committee, the attending physician, and the PA about the medical issues. If agreement is reached, the order can be written—back to time and date of the original inpatient order—for observation status. The same may hold true if the patient medically demonstrates that an inpatient status is more appropriate. If all concur, the admission orders/statuses will match the determination of the insurance, the attending physician, and the PA. These days, carve-outs of statuses have been made (for example the health insurance company will pay for observation for the first and last day and for inpatient status on days 2 to 4). These days, there are fewer patients who follow an expected path and less health insurance companies that follow the easy path.

For commercial surgeries, authorization is key to the patient status. However, if more surgery is done than planned or if the patient does not respond as expected, that authorization may be challenged. The work of the NCM in these instances is to accurately document all clinical details and use a set of evidence-based criteria before calling the health insurance company. If the insurance company does not agree (maybe because they use a different set of criteria), gather the physicians and ask for a peer-to-peer review.

Medicare is different and has precise rules about the timing of orders and the regulations that revolve around each status change action. For example, when a Medicare patient is converted to inpatient status after receiving observation services, it is important to note that all charges associated with the outpatient stay roll into the DRG assignment. The hours spent receiving observation services, however, do not roll into the inpatient admission, and LOS capture begins at the time the admission order is written (ACMA, 2016a). Backdated Medicare admission orders are not allowed. Some of the details are given in the following sections on CC44 and the *MOON* notice.

CONDITION CODE 44: MEDICARE INPATIENT CHANGED TO OBSERVATION STATUS

CC44 is a term that refers to changing an inpatient admission to an outpatient status after care has been rendered and upon internal review; the hospital determines that inpatient services did not meet medical necessity criteria and admission status should be changed to observation. This is a Medicare regulation and is not required by commercial payors or some MAP. CC44 has been in use since 2004 and is billed under Medicare Part B. Prior to CC44, the hospital's only option when it found a patient did not meet inpatient criteria was to self-deny the claim and bill for ancillary services. With CC44, the change from inpatient to observations is permissible provided that the following conditions are met:

1. The change in status was made prior to the patient's discharge or release from the hospital.
2. The hospital has not submitted a claim to Medicare for the inpatient admission.
3. The attending physician concurs with the UR committee determination.
4. The physician's concurrence with the determination is documented in the patient's chart.

The patient's medical record must contain orders and notes that indicate why the change in status was made, what care was furnished to the Medicare beneficiary, and the participants making this decision to change the status. In these situations, the entire episode of the hospital admission must be treated as an outpatient encounter. The claim should clearly reflect the change and should always adhere to the required paperwork; that is, using the exact forms as designated by Medicare. Case managers and UM nurses can play an effective role in reviewing such events and in ensuring that hospitals submit appropriate claims to Medicare. Such careful reviews allow a hospital to maintain compliance with the Medicare CoP and to reduce reimbursement errors and denial rates.

When the status is changed to observation and CC44 is initiated, the beneficiary must be notified via the *MOON* notice.

MEDICARE OUTPATIENT OBSERVATION NOTICE (MOON)

One of the most significant changes that affect case managers since the two-midnight rule is the current (and evolving) regulation known as the *MOON*. Prior to this regulation, when a hospital placed a Medicare beneficiary in observation status, or changed the beneficiary's status to observation, a notice was required to be given to the beneficiary. Nearly every US hospital had its own version of the observation notice. Two major changes have occurred with the MOON:

1. The patient/family must sign the MOON notice or can refuse to sign. If the patient or representative refuses to sign, the hospital staff member should sign the document and indicate the patient's refusal to sign. The details are spelled out in the MOON instructions.
2. Hospitals and critical access hospitals are required to furnish a CMS-developed, standardized notice and oral explanation of the MOON, to a Medicare beneficiary who has been receiving observation services as an outpatient for more than 24 hours and no later than 36 hours after observation services are initiated (CMS, 2016c).

This is not unlike the IM, which is standardized and requires a signature. The reasons these changes were initiated include:

1. Complaints from Medicare beneficiaries (sticker shock, if you will) when receiving hospital bills for observation services, especially if they thought they were inpatient at the time. The MOON will inform more than one million beneficiaries annually of the reason(s) they are in outpatient settings receiving observation services and the implications of such status with regard to Medicare cost sharing and coverage for posthospitalization SNF services.
2. There was no standardization of this regulation; now there is.

There are two time frames in a patient's hospital stay that case managers must be aware of the MOON notice: when a patient is bedded as an observation patient initially and when a Medicare patient's status is changed to observation from inpatient (and a CC44 is initiated).

The MOON notice may reduce the number of surprises about the qualifying 3-day inpatient stays ("What? I am not inpatient and must pay for my SNF?"). Another change is that the notice (at this time) contains information about medication costs. For many years, hospitals have been put in a tough position about outpatient medications when a patient is under observation status. Essentially, the observation situation is that, if a patient is taking a medication at home and also is receiving it during an observation hospital stay, the beneficiary is charged an unexpected Medicare Part B copay for these medications; they were never actually admitted into the hospital and the drugs, therefore, are not covered under Part A. Here lies the problem for the beneficiary; the hospital charges much more (for example, for an aspirin) than the local drug store does. Here is the dilemma for the hospital; they are aware about this, but mostly will not allow patients to take their own medications from home—and for valid 'risk' reasons. This issue will likely become more publicized in the coming years and may also be a case management task—to speak to the patients about these potential costs.

DISCUSSION QUESTIONS

1. What is the difference between prior, concurrent, and retrospective review? Authorization or certification?

2. Under what circumstances is a case manager able to achieve certification/authorization for continued or extended LOS?

3. Compare and contrast InterQual criteria and MCG Health guidelines. For which populations is each commonly used?

4. How can a case manager best apply the criteria or guidelines in the UM activities? Discuss the application differentiating admission, from continued stay, from discharge.

5. What makes case management plans/clinical pathways effective? What makes them ineffective?

6. What conditions are considered inappropriate for a hospital to claim reimbursement from Medicare? Differentiate present on admission from hospital-acquired conditions.

7. What is outpatient observation status? Discuss the benefits and disadvantages of observation status.

8. What documentation is required when changing a patient's status from observation to inpatient?

9. Why does the CMS focus on reviewing payments/reimbursements?

▶ REFERENCES

American Case Management Association. (2016a). *Compass: Directional training for case managers.* Version 3.0. Little Rock, AR: Author.

American Case Management Association. (2016b). *Compare AD: Avoidable delay and utilization management (UM).* Little Rock, AR: Author.

American Case Management Association. (2016c). *ACMA scope of services & standards of practice for hospital/health system case management.* Little Rock, AR: Author.

American Society of Anesthesiologists. (2016). *Updates to the recovery audit program. Timely topics: Payment and practice management.* Retrieved September 30, 2016, from https://www.asahq.org/~/media/sites/asahq/files/public/quality-and-practice-mgt/2016-06-21-updates-to-the-rac-program.pdf?la=en

Anonymous. (1997). Extended care pathway development process can help manage disease across the continuum. *Post Acute Care Strategy Report,* 2(11), 9–12.

Case Management Society of America. (2016). *Standards of practice for case management.* Little Rock, AR: Author.

Case Management Society of America. (2017). *Core curriculum for case management* (3rd ed.). Philadelphia, PA: Author.

Chawla, A., Westrich, K., Matter, S., Kaltenboeck, A., & Dubois, R. (2016). Care pathways in US healthcare settings: Current successes and limitations, and future challenges. *The American Journal of Managed Care,* 22(1), 54–62.

Coulter, E., & VanGelder, M. E. (2014). Recent changes in the innovative postanesthesia care unit gatekeeper role. *Professional Case Management,* 19(5), 205–213.

Centers for Medicare & Medicaid Services. (2016a). *Recovery audit program.* Retrieved September 29, 2016, from, https://www.cms.gov/research-statistics-data-and-systems/monitoring-programs/medicare-ffs-compliance-programs/recovery-audit-program/

Centers for Medicare & Medicaid Services. (2016b). *Recovery auditing in medicare for fiscal year 2014 FY 2014 report to congress as required by Section 1893(h) of the Social Security Act.* Retrieved September 30, 2016, from, https://www.cms.gov/Research-Statistics-Data-and-Systems/Monitoring-Programs/Medicare-FFS-Compliance-Programs/Recovery-Audit-Program/Downloads/RAC-RTC-FY2014.pdf

Centers for Medicare & Medicaid Services. (2016c). Hospital Inpatient Prospective Payment System (IPPS) and Long Term Acute Care Hospital (LTCH) Proposed Rule Issues for Fiscal Year (FY) 2017. Retrieved October 1, 2016, from, https://www.cms.gov/Newsroom/MediaReleaseDatabase/Fact-sheets/2016-Fact-sheets-items/2016-08-02.html

Centers for Medicare & Medicaid Services. (2016d). *Medicare fee for service recovery audit program.* Retrieved February 28, 2016, from, https://www.cms.gov/Research-Statistics-Data-and-Systems/Monitoring-Programs/Medicare-FFS-Compliance-Programs/Recovery-Audit-Program/

InterQual Level of Care Criteria. (2016). *Adult care.* Newton, MA: Author.

McKesson. (2016a). *InterQual acute criteria: Increased quality care over decreased cost equals value.* McKesson: Newton

McKesson. (2016b). *Innovating to meet emerging demands in care management.* McKesson: Newton

McKesson. (2016c). *InterQual evidence-based criteria portfolio: Enabling shared, clinical decision support.* McKesson: Newton

MCG Health. (2016). *Milliman care guidelines.* Retrieved September 28, 2016, from, http://www.careguidelines.com

Miodonski, K. (2012). *Aligning case management processes with the revenue cycle.* Retrieved September 29, 2016, from, http://www.beckershospitalreview.com/finance/aligning-case-management-processes-with-the-revenue-cycle.html

Ollapally, V. (2016). CMS eases restrictions imposed under the two-midnight rule. *Bulletin of the American College of Surgeons.* Retrieved October 1, 2016, from, http://bulletin.facs.org/2016/03/cms-eases-restrictions-imposed-under-the-two-midnight-rule/

Panella, M (2003). Reducing clinical variations with clinical pathways: do pathways work? *International Journal for Quality in Health Care.* 15(6), 509–521. Retrieved September 28, 2016, from, http://intqhc.oxfordjournals.org/content/15/6/509.full

Powell, S. (2013). Is it time to retire (or at least semi-retire) observation? *Professional Case Management Journal.* 18(2), 56–63.

Quality Improvement Organization. (2016). History of the QIO program. Accessed on 9/29/16 from the world wide web at http://qioprogram.org/qionews/articles/history-qio-program

VanGelder, M. E., & Coulter, E. (2013). An innovative case management gatekeeper model for Medicare surgeries. *Professional Case Management,* 18(3), 112–119.

Vanhaecht, K., Panella, M., Van Zelm, R., & Sermeus, W. (2016). History of clinical pathways. *International Journal of Care Pathways.* Retrieved September 29, 2016, from, https://perswww.kuleuven.be/~u0035350/00000097390f70c01/000000097390f92209/00000097391054203/index.html

Zander, K. (1992). Physicians, Care Maps™, and collaboration. *Definition,* 7(1), 1–4.

CHAPTER 6

Transitional Planning: Understanding Levels and Transitions of Care

LEARNING OBJECTIVES

Upon completion of this chapter, the reader will be able to:

1. Define the terms discharge planning, transitional planning, transitions of care, and levels of care.
2. Discuss the relationship between transitions of care and levels of care.
3. Differentiate between the various care settings across the healthcare continuum.
4. Differentiate skilled from nonskilled care.
5. Explain the relationships among transitional planning, utilization management, and reimbursement.
6. Describe the role of the case manager in the various practice settings.
7. Report the impact of case management on care quality and patient safety during transitions of care.

ESSENTIAL TERMS

Accountable Care Organizations • Advanced Life Support (ALS) Ambulance • Air Ambulance • Basic Life Support (BLS) Ambulance • Custodial Care • Discharge Planning • Extended Care Facility • Grievance Process • Home Health Services • Hospice • Hospital-Issued Notice of Noncoverage (HINN) • Important Message from Medicare • Intermediate Care • Long-Term Care (LTC) • Medicare Outpatient Observation Notice (MOON) • Nonskilled Services • Notice of Discharge and Medicare Appeal Rights (NODMAR) • Notice of Noncoverage (NONC) • Patient-Centered Medical Home • Polypharmacy • Quality Improvement Organization (QIO) • Rehabilitation Services • Skilled Care • Skilled Nursing Facility (SNF) • Specialty Pharmacy Providers • Subacute Care • Three-Nights Rule • Transfer Diagnosis-Related Groups (DRGs) • Transitional Planning • Transitions of Care

Transitional planning, discharge planning, and safe transfers of patients to alternative levels of care or home are a major case management responsibility. These require a basic understanding of the levels of care, reimbursement methods and rules, and health insurance coverage. Case managers have earned the reputation of being transitional and discharge planning experts; therefore, their roles in patient advocacy, safe discharge, and transitional planning are significant.

Transitional planning is defined as a dynamic, interactive, collaborative, and interdisciplinary process of assessment and evaluation of the healthcare needs of patients and their families or caregivers during or after a phase of illness and an episode of care. It aims to transition patients from one level of care to another, usually to a lesser acuity setting, including the patient's home. It also includes the assessment of the patient's and family's needs and the planning and brokering of the necessary services identified on the basis of the patient's condition (Cesta & Tahan, 2017). In addition, the process ensures that services are provided at the appropriate level of care—at the right time, in the right amount, by the right provider, and in the right setting.

In contrast, discharge planning is integral to and subsumed in transitional planning. It basically focuses on discharging patients from an inpatient hospital setting to another facility or home (Cesta & Tahan, 2017). The use of the term *transitional planning* became more common with the advent of managed care and the need for utilization management/review, where criteria for care provision (i.e., medical necessity) in each of the various levels of care (e.g., acute care hospital, subacute, skilled nursing facility [SNF], home care, hospice, wellness and prevention, etc.) were reinforced through the health insurance authorization/certification process.

ACCREDITATION AND REGULATORY PERSPECTIVE

Despite the difference in the use of the terms *transitional planning* and *discharge planning*, regulatory and accreditation standards continue to focus mainly on discharge planning. For example, The Joint Commission (TJC) requires hospital policies and procedures on discharge planning. It also requires policies and procedures on patient flow that indirectly implies standards around transitional planning despite the lack of use of such terms. In January 1995, the Centers for Medicare & Medicaid Services (CMS), known then as the Health Care Financing Administration (HCFA), gave more powers to TJC (also known then as The Joint Commission on Accreditation of Healthcare Organizations [JCAHO]) requirements when the CMS *Conditions of Participation for Hospitals—Discharge Planning Regulations* stated that "the hospital must arrange for the initial implementation of the patient's discharge plan" (CMS, 2009a, b). Today, TJC's guidelines for the provision of care and services including discharge planning consist of the following standards (TJC, 2017):

◗ The hospital accepts for care, treatment, and services only those patients whose identified care, treatment, and services it can meet.

◗ The development of a plan for care, treatment, and services is individualized and appropriate to the patient's needs, strengths, limitations, and goals.

◗ Care provision and services must be according to the plan of care.

◗ Coordination of care, treatment, and services provided to a patient as part of the plan of care, treatment, and services must be consistent with the hospital's scope of care, treatment, and services.

◗ The patient/family/caregiver receives education and training specific to his or her needs and as appropriate to the care, treatment, and services provided. Education and training are specific to the patient's abilities. For patients who are children and youth, academic education must be provided as needed while they are hospitalized.

◗ The patient/family/caregiver receives information about the postdischarge services including durable medical equipment (DME) and follow-up care appointments.

◗ Patients may be discharged home from the hospital or transferred to another level of care, treatment, and services to different health professionals or to other settings for continued services. The process of transfer or discharge must be based on the patient's assessed needs.

◗ To facilitate a discharge or transfer, the hospital assesses the patient's needs, plans for discharge or transfer, facilitates the discharge or transfer process, and helps ensure that the continuity of care, treatment, and services is maintained.

◗ The discharge/transition planning process must start upon admission to allow healthcare professionals to anticipate the patient's ongoing care needs, especially those necessary post discharge. Early planning allows healthcare professionals more time to work with the patient/family/caregiver to identify resources available and find services to better meet the individualized needs of the patient.

◗ The discharge/transitional planning process must address the need for coordination of care and continuing care, treatment, and services after discharge or transfer from the hospital. An ideal process is one that employs case management concepts and addresses the following:

◗ The reasons for transfer or discharge.

◗ The conditions under which the transfer or discharge can occur.

◗ Shifting responsibility for the patient's care from one clinician/provider of care, organization, clinical program, or service, to another.

◗ A mechanism for appropriate and safe transfer: internally within an organization (e.g., from one patient care unit to another or from a generalist to a specialist provider) and externally from one organization to another (e.g., from a hospital to an SNF or from a hospital to a subacute care rehabilitation facility).

◗ The accountability and responsibility for the patient's safety during transfer of both the organization/provider initiating the transfer and the one receiving the patient.

◗ The patient's transfer or discharge occurs based on the patient's needs and where best these needs can be met, especially after the patient no longer meets medical necessity criteria for acute/hospital care.

◗ The discharge/transitional planning process must allow for noting reasons and conditions for the patient's discharge/transfer and the method for shifting responsibility for the patient's care from one clinician, hospital, program, or service to another. The hospital here must have a process in place to share and receive important information (handoff communication) when the patient is discharged or transferred to another care setting or provider.

For a hospital to ensure that an effective discharge planning process is in place, the following standards and expectations must be carefully considered. Case managers can play an essential role in ensuring that the provision of care adheres to the standards described in the previous paragraphs as well as the nine listed in the following paragraphs, cited on the basis of the Medicare's Conditions of Participation (CoP).

1. Hospitals must identify, at an early stage of hospitalization (preferably at the time of admission and no more than 24 hours), patients who are likely to suffer adverse health consequences if discharged without adequate discharge planning.

2. Hospitals must provide a discharge planning evaluation for patients identified under the requirement listed earlier and for other patients on the request of the patient or his or her representative.

3. Any discharge planning evaluation must be made on a timely basis to ensure that appropriate arrangements for posthospital care will be made before discharge and to avoid unnecessary delays in discharge.

4. This discharge planning evaluation must include the patient's likely need for and the availability of appropriate posthospital services. It must be included in the patient's medical record for use in establishing an appropriate discharge plan, and the results of the evaluation must be discussed with the interdisciplinary care team involved in the care, the patient, and/or his or her representative.

5. The discharge planning evaluation must include an assessment of the patient's capacity for self-care and self-management or of the possibility of the patient being cared for in the environment from which he or she entered the hospital.

6. Hospitals must reassess the discharge plan if there are factors that may affect continuing care needs or the appropriateness of the discharge plan.

7. Hospitals must provide the patient with a list of agencies and/or facilities that are appropriate to the identified care needs and are Medicare participating (e.g., a list of home care agencies or a list of skilled care facilities). In the case of Medicare Advantage plans, a list of those contracted with the plan must be provided.

8. If a transfer or referral is needed, hospitals must transfer or refer the patient along with the necessary medical information to the appropriate facility, agency, or outpatient services as needed for follow-up and ancillary care.

9. A registered professional nurse (RN), social worker (SW), nurse case manager, or other appropriately qualified staff member must develop or supervise the development of the discharge planning evaluation or discharge plan.

Point Number 9 is interesting in that most (although not all) case managers who perform this function at the acute level of care have one of the two licensures listed. The law supports what nurses, case managers, and SWs do. The responsibility for discharge planning, then, based on the Medicare's CoP, should be interdisciplinary; it should not be restricted to one specific health discipline or professional. A case manager may play a primary role in discharge planning, but he or she should work collaboratively with the rest of the interdisciplinary healthcare team.

As utilization management criteria continue to tighten, patients with increased physiologic needs are more than ever being moved to lower levels of care. The sooner the case manager can start the assessment process for a patient's actual and potential discharge needs, the more time can be spent matching appropriate services to these needs. When considering discharge planning, all levels of care options should be explored. Discharging a patient home with family support is preferable in most cases. If the family is unavailable, friends, neighbors, religious affiliation volunteers, or community referrals can sometimes provide the needed link between the patient's independence and his or her having to go to a supervisory or foster care setting. Social services can be an invaluable asset in care and discharge planning with this type of patient.

If more skilled care is required than can be provided by family or volunteers, perhaps the patient is safe to go home with the addition of home nursing services. Consider the use of home RN visits for care, teaching, or assessments; home physical therapy (PT); occupational therapy (OT) and speech/language therapy (ST); home aides (restrictions may apply on the basis of the health insurance plan benefits); home psychiatric nursing; or home social services. Many health insurance plans provide home health services only if the patient's condition and needs meet certain criteria such as being homebound; this is an important point to assess. Also, determine just what the patient's health insurance plan provides; many plans allow only a few intermittent visits, which do not always meet the patient's total needs.

If a patient is not homebound or can easily be transported by family members or volunteers, consider the use of outpatient services such as outpatient rehabilitation departments, which provide physical, speech, and occupational therapies. Freestanding clinics may provide a wide range of services from wound care to the administration of IV antibiotics or chemotherapy. When sending patients home, one needs to assess outpatient pharmaceutical benefits, especially prior to, or close to, the time of discharge. This is necessary because one of the primary causes for readmission to the acute care hospital setting is improper medication regimen and administration or lack of adherence to medications. Educational deficits may contribute to this problem; reviewing the medication reconciliation process and assessing knowledge deficits relating to medications are important case management responsibilities, especially in the case of polypharmacy. Another underlying contributor to the problem may be financial; not all insurance plans have adequate prescription coverage and some people cannot afford the prescriptions. For example, patients with traditional Medicare have few pharmaceutical benefits. Detective-like work by the case manager may be needed to see whether the patient's plan covers the necessary medications.

Until recently, traditional Medicare did not cover home IV antibiotics. Sending a Medicare patient home with IV antibiotics was nearly impossible unless the patient could personally finance the medications. This situation has changed now. If the Medicare plan is one of the "risk" contracts that pays for hospitalizations on a per diem or capitated basis (instead of the case rate applied in the diagnosis-related groups' [DRGs] prospective payment system [PPS]), it is financially beneficial to the plan to send the patient home with IV medications. Another option depending on the dosage and frequency is that a patient may be discharged home with follow-up in ambulatory infusion centers where the IV medications can be administered. Therefore, the health insurance company (i.e., the insurance-based case manager) often works with the provider-based case manager on the discharge plan to make sure it is cost-effective, safe, and meets the patient's discharge needs. Under the traditional Medicare DRG reimbursement, only the hospital is financially penalized for keeping a patient in-house for a long time for antibiotic administration, which is why traditional Medicare has little incentive to change this benefit.

If the health insurance company does not pay for home IV antibiotics and the patient is otherwise stable for discharge, assess whether the patient can receive the antibiotics at a freestanding clinic or at the doctor's office. It may be necessary to set up an observation admission or an outpatient admission on weekends for administering the dosage. Sometimes rare emergency departments can be used for this purpose; however, this should be discouraged, be a last resort, and done with the facility's approval. Traditional Medicare will pay for the nurse to administer the medication, so if the patient can afford the drug, this plan sometimes works (refer to Chapter 3, Reimbursement Concepts, for more information on drug benefits).

Medicaid plans generally pay for most prescriptive needs. It often has a "negative formulary" disallowing certain prescriptions. Some newer, expensive medications may need prior approval. No over-the-counter medications are covered (this also applies to most of the other insurance plans). Managed care pharmacy benefits may vary from the member paying 100% to the insurance company paying 100% (although rare); often members are required to pay about 20% of the cost of the medications and 100% when a cap amount of expenses has been met. This cap varies with every health insurance plan. Some members must purchase prescription riders on their policies to receive their benefits. Usually, the benefits require a copayment of $3 to $50 per prescription, an annual deductible, or a 20% coinsurance fee. The patient may also be reimbursed only at a generic rate if a generic equivalent is available (Kongstvedt, 2003). Another consideration is that many insurance plans with pharmaceutical benefits require the member to fill the prescription at designated contracted pharmacies. The case manager may need to find out where these pharmacies are if the patient does not know. A common option today is mail delivery of medications to the patient's home and for a 3-month at a time for medications to be taken for life. This option has shown to save money for the patient.

Discharging patients home is often the best plan of care for the patient and is also the least resource-intensive plan for the health insurance company. However, this is not always safe or possible. Discussions about the alternatives—nursing homes, rehabilitation, long-term care (LTC), and hospice—along with more details on home coverage follow. In all discharge plans, insurance verification of coverage is essential. Occasionally, nonbenefit options can be negotiated, but in all cases prior authorization should be obtained.

Early discharge or transitional planning, even in the preadmission phase, has been emphasized several times. Even with a good plan and prior authorization, the discharge or transitional plan may fall through or may require certain modifications. The patient's medical stability may change; family members may change their minds 30 minutes before transfer or discharge time; and various other surprises may pop up. Sometimes the case manager already had a nagging feeling that something was going to delay the discharge and therefore had an alternate plan in mind. A case manager's intuition is a useful skill and it prepares us for sudden stops and detours.

If a mentally competent patient decides to go home refusing all available services, documentation may be all that is needed. If there is a question of mental competency and the patient would be unsafe with his or her chosen discharge/transitional plan, a psychiatric consultation may be necessary to assess the patient's mental capacity.

▶ NOTICES OF NONCOVERAGE

Medicare beneficiaries are granted exceptional rights under the Medicare statutes. All Medicare beneficiaries enrolled in any of the Medicare health plans, including fee-for-service, health maintenance organizations (HMOs), Medicare Advantages plans, and other Medicare options, must receive the "Important Message from Medicare" at the time of admission to an acute care hospital. The message outlines beneficiaries' rights to discharge planning and their right to pursue a grievance process if they feel that they are being discharged too soon or without adequate posthospital care arrangements. The message must include details on how a patient or family member could request a review or an appeal by the relevant Quality Improvement Organization (QIO).

In reality, unfortunately, the day of admission is not the best time for patients or their families to read long legal notices, so they may not fully understand their rights. The hospital is responsible for informing patients of their rights and implementing these rights; as a patient advocate, the case manager should make sure that the patient understands these documents. Notices of Noncoverage (NONCs) deny coverage in hospitals, rehabilitation facilities, SNFs, or for various special services. Within acute care hospitals, there can be preadmission/admission notices, continued stay notices, or notices for days at the end of the stay. These are called Hospital-Issued Notices of Noncoverage (HINNs) for traditional Medicare beneficiaries. They used to be called Notice of Discharge and Medicare Appeal

Rights (NODMAR) for patients covered by Medicare Advantage Plans. Today the same notice is used for all Medicare beneficiaries regardless of the type of plan to which the beneficiary belongs.

In 1998, the CMS, known then as the HCFA, reinterpreted the regulations on NONCs. Beneficiary advocates were concerned that patients did not know their rights and were not sufficiently informed of these rights at the time of hospital discharge. In the past, notices were issued only if a dispute arose or when one was anticipated. Recently, the new interpretation of the regulations required that every Medicare HMO enrollee admitted to the hospital receive a NODMAR at least 24 hours prior to discharge. Today, however, the CMS has extended this rule to HINNs for all Medicare beneficiaries (not just those in HMOs).

Implementation of these rules has created problems for HMOs and their enrollees and for providers of care to Medicare beneficiaries. Because of short lengths of hospital stays, many enrollees do not receive the notice in a timely fashion or prior to discharge as was intended; some do not receive one at all. The documents are written by expert lawyers and are not easily understood by ill and recovering Medicare beneficiaries; all they read is that their Medicare benefits have been cut off or denied. Worried Medicare beneficiaries tend to sit on the QIOs' doorsteps on Monday mornings after having spent a weekend upset over these legal documents. Therefore, as a service to their patients, case managers can prepare patients by informing them of their rights to receive necessary hospital services, discharge plans, and the impending notice. It is important to engage in such preparation as early in a hospital stay as the day of admission. This way you avoid any surprises and the patient or family have had enough time to ponder the issues, prepare for the discharge, raise questions or concerns, and arrange for any necessary plans at home.

The most common conflict leading to a QIO review of an NONC occurs when the Medicare beneficiary requires custodial care, which Medicare does not cover. The family may not be able to take care of the patient's medical and activities of daily living (ADLs) needs, but it does not understand the difference between skilled and nonskilled care. As a case manager, you can avoid possible conflict by educating patients and families early in the hospital stay about Medicare coverage, benefits, and possible patient needs, including the difference between skilled and nonskilled care.

Medicare mandates that discharge planning begin at the time of admission. From the case manager's perspective, careful documentation of the patient's medical, financial, psychosocial status, and adequate discharge or transitional planning are needed; in fact, the HINN may be denied if the discharge plan is not clearly documented in the patient's medical record and in place. This documentation should show good faith and evidence that the patient is medically stable, is aware of the plan of care (including the discharge plan), and is aware that the discharge is based solely on medical status and is not related to a DRG payment. The discharge plan should be the result of collaboration with the patient, family, attending physician of record, and other healthcare providers, especially consultants. If the patient or family is uncooperative or unrealistic, the case manager should document in the record the attempts to make a reasonable discharge plan and health education activities performed to ensure the patient's or family's informed decision making. Medicare expects that every reasonable effort be made to ensure a safe, comprehensive plan for continuity of care. If this is not possible because of financial or social reasons, your only mantra should be "document, document, and document." Occasionally, the Medicare beneficiary will refuse to sign the NONC. Signature, although encouraged, is not required; however, informing the patient or family of the plan is required. The NONC is still valid even without a signature. Backup documentation is imperative to show that the notice was issued and that the patient refused to sign. The case manager may also want to call the QIO if the patient refuses to sign as additional good faith; the QIOs can then immediately start the review process so that all parties are given coverage and attention.

▶ Highlights of the Important Message from Medicare

The Important Message (IM) from Medicare has been around for many years; however, the CMS revised the IM and a new version went into effect as of July 2, 2007. The revisions grew out of a ruling on a lawsuit filed against Medicare (*Weichardt v. Leavitt*, C-03-5490 VRW). The revised IM streamlined the information to be communicated to patients and their families regarding their right for services and the process that can be followed if they disagree with the discharge plan or the date/time of discharge. The message is intended for all beneficiaries with Medicare, Medicare and Medicaid (dual eligible), Medicare and another insurance program, and Medicare as a secondary payor. When Medicare enacted this statue, it was thought it would improve the efficiency, effectiveness, economy, and quality of services delivered to Medicare beneficiaries.

The revised IM (Display 6-1) highlights the following (Powell, 2007):

▶ The Medicare beneficiary's right to services as a hospital inpatient and for posthospitalization (discharge). Hospital in this case refers to any inpatient facility.

▶ The Medicare beneficiary's right to request an expedited review and determination of the discharge decision. The IM also includes a detailed description of the QIO's review and appeal process to be followed, and the availability of other appeals processes if the beneficiary fails to meet the deadline for an expedited review/determination. This also

Department of Health & Human Services
Centers for Medicare & Medicaid Services
OMB Approval No. 0938-0692

Patient Name:

Patient ID Number:

Physician:

An Important Message From Medicare About Your Rights

As A Hospital Inpatient, You Have The Right To:

- Receive Medicare covered services. This includes medically necessary hospital services and services you may need after you are discharged, if ordered by your doctor. You have a right to know about these services, who will pay for them, and where you can get them.

- Be involved in any decisions about your hospital stay, and know who will pay for it.

- Report any concerns you have about the quality of care you receive to the Quality Improvement Organization (QIO) listed here:

_____

Name of QIO

_____

Telephone Number of QIO

_____

Your Medicare Discharge Rights

Planning For Your Discharge: During your hospital stay, the hospital staff will be working with you to prepare for your safe discharge and arrange for services you may need after you leave the hospital. When you no longer need inpatient hospital care, your doctor or the hospital staff will inform you of your planned discharge date.

If you think you are being discharged too soon:
- You can talk to the hospital staff, your doctor and your managed care plan (if you belong to one) about your concerns.

- You also have the right to an appeal, that is, a review of your case by a Quality Improvement Organization (QIO). The QIO is an outside reviewer hired by Medicare to look at your case to decide whether you are ready to leave the hospital.

  - **If you want to appeal, you must contact the QIO no later than your planned discharge date and before you leave the hospital.**

  - If you do this, you will not have to pay for the services you receive during the appeal (except for charges like copays and deductibles).

- If you do not appeal, but decide to stay in the hospital past your planned discharge date, you may have to pay for any services you receive after that date.

- Step by step instructions for calling the QIO and filing an appeal are on page 2.

To speak with someone at the hospital about this notice, call _____ .

Please sign and date here to show you received this notice and understand your rights.

Signature of Patient or Representative	Date/Time

Form CMS-R-193 (Exp. 03/31/2020)

(continued)

IMPORTANT MESSAGE FROM MEDICARE (*continued*)

Steps To Appeal Your Discharge

- **Step 1**: You must contact the QIO no later than your planned discharge date and before you leave the hospital. If you do this, you will not have to pay for the services you receive during the appeal (except for charges like copays and deductibles).

  - Here is the contact information for the QIO: _____

    Name of QIO (in bold)

    _____

    Telephone Number of QIO

    _____

  - You can file a request for an appeal any day of the week. **Once you speak to someone or leave a message, your appeal has begun.**

  - Ask the hospital if you need help contacting the QIO.

  - The name of this hospital is : _____

Hospital Name	Provider ID Number

- **Step 2**: You will receive a detailed notice from the hospital or your Medicare Advantage or other Medicare managed care plan (if you belong to one) that explains the reasons they think you are ready to be discharged.

- **Step 3**: The QIO will ask for your opinion. You or your representative need to be available to speak with the QIO, if requested. You or your representative may give the QIO a written statement, but you are not required to do so.

- **Step 4**: The QIO will review your medical records and other important information about your case.

- **Step 5**: The QIO will notify you of its decision within <u>1 day after</u> it receives all necessary information.

  - If the QIO finds that you are not ready to be discharged, Medicare will continue to cover your hospital services.

  - If the QIO finds you are ready to be discharged, Medicare will continue to cover your services until noon of the day <u>after</u> the QIO notifies you of its decision.

If You Miss The Deadline To Appeal, You Have Other Appeal Rights:

- You can still ask the QIO or your plan (if you belong to one) for a review of your case:

  - If you have Original Medicare: Call the QIO listed above.
  - If you belong to a Medicare Advantage Plan or other Medicare managed care plan: Call your plan.

- If you stay in the hospital, the hospital may charge you for any services you receive after your planned discharge date.

For more information, call 1-800-MEDICARE (1-800-633-4227), or TTY: 1-877-486-2048.

CMS does not discriminate in its programs and activities. To request this publication in an alternate format, please call: 1-800-MEDICARE or email: <u>AltFormatRequest@cms.hhs.gov</u> .

Additional Information:

display 6-1

Notice Instructions: The Important Message From Medicare

Completing The Notice

Page 1 of the Important Message from Medicare

A. Header

Hospitals must display "Department of Health & Human Services, Centers for Medicare & Medicaid Services" and the OMB number.

The following blanks must be completed by the hospital. Information inserted by hospitals in the blank spaces on the IM may be typed or legibly hand-written in 12-point font or the equivalent. Hospitals may also use a patient label that includes the following information:

Patient Name: Fill in the patient's full name.

Patient ID number: Fill in an ID number that identifies this patient. This number should not be, nor should it contain, the social security number.

Physician: Fill in the name of the patient's physician.

B. Body of the Notice

Bullet number 3 – Report any concerns you have about the quality of care you receive to the Quality Improvement Organization (QIO) listed here _____.

Hospitals may preprint or otherwise insert the name and telephone number (including TTY) of the QIO.

To speak with someone at the hospital about this notice call: Fill in a telephone number at the hospital for the patient or representative to call with questions about the notice. Preferably, a contact name should also be included.

Patient or Representative Signature: Have the patient or representative sign the notice to indicate that he or she has received it and understands its contents.

Date/Time: Have the patient or representative place the date and time that he or she signed the notice.

Page 2 of the Important Message from Medicare

First sub-bullet – Insert name and telephone number of QIO in bold: Insert name and telephone number (including TTY), in bold, of the Quality Improvement Organization that performs reviews for the hospital.

Second sub-bullet – The name of this hospital is: Insert/preprint the name of the hospital, including the Medicare provider ID number (not the telephone number).

Additional Information: Hospitals may use this section for additional documentation, including, for example, obtaining beneficiary initials, date, and time to document delivery of the follow-up copy of the IM, or documentation of refusals.

SOURCE: Centers for Medicare & Medicaid Services. (CMS). Hospital Discharge Appeal Notices, Important Message from Medicare. Accessed 8/7/2017. Available online at
https://www.cms.gov/Medicare/Medicare-General-Information/BNI/HospitalDischargeAppealNotices.html

includes contact information of the QIO to whom the patient must report the concerns.

▶ The circumstances under which a beneficiary will or will not be financially liable for charges for continued hospital stay.

▶ The Medicare beneficiary's right to receive additional detailed information and as needed.

▶ The Medicare beneficiary's signature requirement to indicate that he or she has received the notice and comprehends its contents.

The Medicare beneficiary's rights as a hospital patient include receipt of necessary hospital services covered by Medicare; information about any decisions made by the hospital, his or her doctor, the health plan, or anyone else involved about the hospital stay; and who will pay for it. The rights also include the hospital's obligation to arrange for services the patient will receive postdischarge such as home care or transfer to a subacute care facility or SNF. In addition, the patient also has the right to be informed in advance about the name of the agency to provide the services and who will be paying for these services. Although patients always had these rights in the past, the rights were not consistently placed in front of patients the way they are now.

Today, the CMS dictates that hospitals provide patients, in writing (i.e., the IM from Medicare Notice), with the information about their rights for services within two calendar days of the day of admission to the hospital, obtain the patient's signature, and keep a copy of the IM in the patient's record. Hospitals are also required to inform patients in writing of their discharge plan, again as soon as possible prior to the discharge from the hospital, but no more than two calendar days before discharge. In cases where the delivery of the initial IM occurs within less than 2 days of the date of discharge, the hospital is not required to issue a new IM. For Medicare beneficiaries who request an appeal, the hospital is obligated to deliver a detailed notice to the patient. To clarify the timeline of this process, let us consider a situation where a patient is admitted to the hospital on Monday, given the initial IM notice on Wednesday, and discharged on Friday; the second IM notice will not be required. However, if the patient was admitted to the hospital on the 10th of the month, received the initial IM notice on the 12th of the month, and was discharged on the 16th, the patient would require a second IM notice be given no earlier than the 14th of the same month.

Timing of the initial IM notice can be prior to the hospital admission date in elective admissions. In such cases, the notice can be given during the preadmission or preregistration visit but not more than seven calendar days prior to admission. However, one should avoid routine delivery of the second/follow-up IM notice to the patient on the day of discharge. The IM notice that a hospital should deliver to a patient should be the standardized notice available on the CMS's website. The form is known as CMS-R-193. Hospitals are not allowed to modify the notice; however, they are allowed to add their names, logos, addresses, and contact information. The CMS requires that the patient sign the notice; however, if he or she refuses, the date of refusal should be documented as the date of receipt of the notice. A copy is usually given to the patient and another is kept in his or her medical record.

The IM from Medicare does not apply in the case of swing beds, outpatient departments such as emergency services, outpatient observation status, and changes in a patient's status from inpatient to outpatient. Medicare beneficiaries where the IM rule applies include enrollees in the original Medicare and Medicare Advantage plans, dual eligible Medicare and Medicaid individuals, and other beneficiaries where Medicare is a secondary payor.

▶ The Review Process

The Medicare beneficiary is guaranteed the right to an independent review by the QIO in the event the beneficiary or his or her family believes he or she is being asked to leave the hospital too soon or that the postdischarge services are inadequate. The grievance process starts when the attending physician and the case management department (or utilization review department if separate from case management) believe the patient no longer meets medical criteria for the acute hospital level of care. If the patient or family disagrees with the discharge decision/notice, they can appeal such notice with a prompt telephone call to the QIO by noon of the next business day after receiving the IM from Medicare Notice. This call starts the grievance (review and appeal) process (Display 6-1). The QIO's decision of the appeal is communicated to the patient or family using another Medicare form called the "Detailed Notice of Discharge." The hospital uses this form as a patient letter to communicate the QIO's decision (Display 6-2). Without the telephone call to the QIO, the patient or family may be liable for hospital charges, starting on the third day after receiving the NONC. If the QIO agrees with the original NONC, the patient may be billed for all charges beginning on the day after he or she received the QIO's final decision. If the patient/family continues to disagree with the discharge provisions, a request for reconsideration can be made. Hospitals are obligated to communicate to the patient the QIO's decision about the review/appeal filed by the patient. Display 6-2 includes the letter given to patients describing the QIO's decision about the discharge appeal.

If the patient feels that the NONC is in error, the case manager must be able to articulate the review/grievance process. This is no easy task, as many specific details apply according to the person who gives the NONC, who receives it, and when it is received. It is recommended that the case management department find a contact person in the QIO in its state for such situations.

Patient Name: OMB Approval No. 0938-1019

Patient ID Number: Date Issued:

Physician:

{Insert Hospital or Plan Logo here}

Detailed Notice Of Discharge

You have asked for a review by the Quality Improvement Organization (QIO), an independent reviewer hired by Medicare to review your case. This notice gives you a detailed explanation about why your hospital and your managed care plan (if you belong to one), in agreement with your doctor, believe that your inpatient hospital services should end on _____ . This is based on Medicare coverage policies listed below and your medical condition.

This is not an official Medicare decision. The decision on your appeal will come from your Quality Improvement Organization (QIO).

- Medicare Coverage Policies:

    _____ Medicare does not cover inpatient hospital services that are not medically necessary or could be safely furnished in another setting. (Refer to 42 Code of Federal Regulations, 411.15 (g) and (k)).

    _____ Medicare Managed Care policies, if applicable: _____ _____ {insert specific managed care policies}

    _____ Other _____ {insert other applicable policies}

- Specific information about your current medical condition:

- If you would like a copy of the documents sent to the QIO, or copies of the specific policies or criteria used to make this decision, please call _____{insert hospital and/or plan telephone number}.

CMS does not discriminate in its programs and activities. To request this publication in an alternative format, please call: 1-800-MEDICARE or email: AltFormatRequest@cms.hhs.gov.

According to the Paperwork Reduction Act of 1995, no persons are required to respond to a collection of information unless it displays a valid OMB control number. The valid OMB control number for this information collection is 0938- 1019. The time required to complete this information collection is estimated to average 60 minutes per response, including the time to review instructions, search existing data resources, gather the data needed, and complete and review the information collection. If you have comments concerning the accuracy of the time estimate(s) or suggestions for improving this form, please write to: CMS, 7500 Security Boulevard, Attn: PRA Reports Clearance Officer, Mail Stop C4-26-05, Baltimore, Maryland 21244-1850.

CMS 10066 (Exp. 10/31/2019)

(continued)

display 6-2

Instructions for Completing the Detailed Notice of Discharge
CMS 10066

This is a standardized notice. Hospitals may not deviate from the content of the form except where indicated. Please note that the OMB control number must be displayed on the notice. Insertions must be typed or legibly hand-written in 12-point font or the equivalent.

Hospitals or plans may modify the following sections to incorporate use of a sticker or label that includes this information:

> **Patient Name:** Fill in the patient's full name.
>
> **Patient ID number:** Fill in the patient's ID number. This should not be, nor should it contain, the patient's social security or HICN number.
>
> **Physician:** Fill in the name of the patient's physician.
>
> **Date Issued:** Fill in the date the notice is delivered to the patient by the hospital/plan.

Insert logo here: Hospitals/plans may elect to place their logo in this space. However, the name, address, and telephone number of the hospital/plan must be immediately under the logo, if not incorporated into the logo. If no logo is used, the name and address and telephone number (including TTY) of the hospital/plan must appear above the title of the form.

BLANK 1: "**This notice gives you a detailed explanation of why your hospital and your managed care plan (if you belong to one), in agreement with your doctor, believe that your inpatient hospital services should end on** _____. In the space provided, fill in planned date of discharge.

First Bullet: "**Medicare Coverage Policies:**" Place a check next to the applicable Medicare and/or managed care policies. If necessary, hospitals may also use the selection "Other" to list other applicable policies, guidelines or instructions. Hospitals or plans may also preprint frequently used coverage policies or add more space below this line, if necessary. Policies should be written in full sentences and in plain language. In addition, the hospital or plan may attach additional pages or specific policies or discharge criteria to the notice. Any attachments must be included with the copy sent to the QIO as well.

Second Bullet: "**Specific information about your current medical condition**" Fill in detailed and specific information about the patient's current medical condition and the reasons why services are no longer reasonable or necessary for this patient or are no longer covered according to Medicare or Medicare managed care coverage guidelines. Use full sentences and plain language.

Third Bullet: "**If you would like a copy of the documents sent to the QIO, or copies of the specific policies or criteria used to make this decision, please call** _____." The hospital/plan should also supply a telephone number for patients to call to get a copy of the relevant documents sent to the QIO. If the hospital/plan has not attached the Medicare policies and/or the Medicare managed care plan policies used to decide the discharge date, the hospital should supply a telephone number for patients to call to obtain copies of this information.

Hospitals or plans may add space below this section to insert a signature line and date, if they so choose.

SOURCE: Centers for Medicare & Medicaid Services. (CMS). Hospital Discharge Appeal Notices, Detailed Notice of Discharge. Accessed 8/7/2017. Available online at
https://www.cms.gov/Medicare/Medicare-General-Information/BNI/HospitalDischargeAppealNotices.html

The QIO can be a resource for Medicare information for you and your patients. If Medicare beneficiaries do not accept information from you, then the QIO, the fiscal intermediary (Part A), or other Medicare organizations may be able to educate the beneficiary. Educate yourself about Medicare information sources and materials. The Medicare (www.medicare.gov) and the CMS (www.cms.hhs.gov) websites are a good source of information; and *The Medicare Handbook* is a valuable resource for patients and professionals. The *Handbook* can be obtained from Social Security, your state's QIO, your Area Agency on Aging, or other organizations; it is also available on the CMS website.

The IM from Medicare includes information about the process a Medicare beneficiary would use in case of a review or appeal. The information must use the specific language as mandated by the CMS. (Refer to Display 6-1 for more information.) The notice must also include directions that a beneficiary would follow if he or she desires to file an appeal with the QIO. The IM from Medicare notice contains additional information about the patient's other appeal rights; for example, missing an appeal deadline but still wishing to file an appeal. Patients can still appeal as long as the request for review and appeal is made within 30 calendar days of the discharge date.

The four HINN include the following:

1. The Preadmission/Admission HINN is used to notify the patient that Medicare is not likely to pay for the admission because it is not considered medically necessary or it could be furnished safely in another setting.
2. The HINN 11, Notice for Noncovered Services in a Covered Stay, is used to notify patients that their physician has ordered specific services that are potentially not covered during a hospital stay even if the hospital stay is covered. For example, this notice is issued in the event the physician ordered a diagnostic or therapeutic procedure or service that is not part of the care of the condition for which the patient is admitted to hospital. In this case the procedure cannot be bundled into payment or treatment for the diagnosis that justifies the inpatient stay. HINN 11 certifies the patient's consent to accept financial liability for the noncovered procedure.
3. The HINN 12, Notice for Noncovered Continued Stay, is used to notify patients that the hospital believes Medicare may not pay for the continued stay in the hospital beginning on a certain date. The notice would include the estimated cost of the continued stay.
4. The Notice of Hospital Requested Review (NHRR) is used when a hospital requests a QIO review for a discharge decision when the attending physician does not concur with the hospital's opinion that the

patient is ready for discharge. The NHRR notifies patients that the hospital has requested a medical opinion from the QIO because it had determined that the patient's condition no longer meets Medicare criteria for continued hospital stay; that is, the hospital stay is no longer medically necessary but the physician disagrees. This notice alerts patients that the QIO may contact them and that the QIO will be reviewing the facts and determine whether there is a need for continued stay.

▶ Notice of Noncoverage in Outpatient Observation Status

OUTPATIENT OBSERVATION STATUS

Observation care is often characterized as a component of emergency medicine that allows hospitals to triage patients who do not immediately require hospital inpatient admission but are too sick to be discharged. There are no clear standards or criteria as to when certain patients should be placed under outpatient observation status rather than admitted as an inpatient, so hospitals and emergency departments often rely on the admitting physician's judgment. Experientially speaking, however, one may describe outpatient observation care as a set of specific and clinically appropriate services, including ongoing short-term treatment, assessment, and reassessment, that patients receive while a decision is being made regarding whether they will require further treatment as hospital inpatients or whether they are well enough to be safely discharged from the hospital.

Observation care may be offered in dedicated observation units within the hospital, in medical or surgical units/beds, or in an extension of or within the emergency department area. Regardless of location, however, case managers are instrumental in monitoring the status of these patients and ensuring that the utilization review procedures and requirements for these types of patients are met. Such role reduces the hospital's financial risk which may result from submitting claims with wrong patient status (or level of care) to Medicare for reimbursement and getting denied.

Observation services are commonly ordered for patients who present to the emergency department, and based on an assessment by the healthcare provider, determines whether these patients require a significant period of treatment or monitoring to effectively evaluate the presenting symptoms and condition. Then, the provider can confidently decide whether to admit to the hospital, discharge home, or transfer to another facility or level of care.

Studies have shown that the number of Medicare beneficiaries receiving outpatient observation care have been increasing over the past few years. In response to concerns regarding long observation stays and short inpatient admissions, the CMS finalized a policy often referred to as the "Two-Midnight Rule" on August 19, 2013. This rule was intended to address concerns about and provide clarification on when hospital inpatient admissions and hospital outpatient observation services are generally appropriate. This change increased the importance of case management services and added to the role of case managers the need to review patients' status (level of care) for appropriateness before a claim is submitted to Medicare for reimbursement. The purpose of such review is to ensure that the claim reflects the correct patient's status and such is justified on the basis of the medical record's documentation. Additionally, to provide greater clarity to the Medicare beneficiary receiving outpatient observation care, the CMS also developed the Medicare Outpatient Observation Notice (MOON) which was signed into law on August 6, 2015. The act requires hospitals to notify a beneficiary if he or she has been under observation for more than 24 hours and to communicate the implications of such status, including the eligibility for SNF coverage.

MEDICARE OUTPATIENT OBSERVATION NOTICE

The MOON is a standardized notice to inform Medicare beneficiaries (including Medicare Advantage/health plan enrollees) that they are outpatients receiving observation services and are not inpatients of a hospital or critical access hospital (CAH) (Display 6-3). The MOON is mandated by the Federal Notice of Observation Treatment and Implication for Care Eligibility Act (NOTICE Act, P.L. 114-42), and went into effect from March 8, 2017. The NOTICE Act requires all hospitals and CAHs to provide patients with written and oral notification about their care being provided under observation status.

When delivering the MOON, hospitals and CAHs are required to explain the notice and its content, document that an oral explanation was provided, and answer all beneficiary questions to the best of their ability.

The NOTICE Act notes that the MOON must be given to beneficiaries in Original Medicare (fee-for-service) and Medicare Advantage enrollees who receive observation services as outpatients for more than 24 hours. The notice must also be provided to beneficiaries who do not have Medicare Part B coverage, those who are subsequently admitted as inpatients prior to the required delivery of the MOON, and those for whom Medicare is either the primary or secondary payor. The hospital or CAH must provide the MOON no later than 36 hours after observation services as an outpatient begin. However, hospitals and CAHs may deliver the MOON to an individual receiving observation services as an outpatient before such individual has received more than 24 hours of observation services. Allowing delivery of the MOON before an individual has received 24 hours of observation services affords hospitals and CAHs the flexibility to deliver the MOON consistent with any applicable state law that requires notice to outpatients receiving observation services within 24 hours after observation services begin.

The start time of observation services, for the purpose of determining when more than 24 hours of observation services have been received, is the actual time when observation services are initiated as documented in the patient's medical record, in accordance with a physician's or provider's order. In the event the Medicare beneficiary refuses to sign the MOON, and there is no representative to sign on behalf of the beneficiary, the staff member of the hospital or CAH who has presented the written notification must sign the notice. The staff member signing the notice must also indicate his or her name and title, a statement certifying that the notification was presented, and the date and time of such presentation. The staff member must annotate the "Additional Information" section of the MOON form with these requirements. The date and time of refusal is considered the date of notice receipt.

In the event the Medicare beneficiary's representative is not available in person, a staff member from the hospital or CAH may present the MOON notice telephonically. In this case the staff member also annotates the "Additional Information" section of such delivery and then mail a paper copy of the completed form to the representative on the same day the notice was delivered telephonically. The hospital or CAH must retain a copy of the MOON notice in the patient's medical record, regardless of how it was completed. The hospital or CAH must also provide the patient or representative with a copy of the completed MOON notice.

▶ LEVELS OF CARE

Interpretations vary about what constitutes skilled, subacute, intermediate, or custodial levels of care, causing confusion that at times extends to reimbursement issues. A definition of skilled care in one SNF may constitute the subacute level in another facility. Hospice benefits are interpreted differently among hospice companies. Home health may be provided by one agency, whereas another agency may feel the care is too technical. Appropriate assessment of a patient's needs is essential and may provide clues to the case manager as to whether insurance will pay for the planned level of care and services. These definitions and criteria may vary from facility to facility, so clarification may be needed. For explanation purposes, this chapter separates the levels of care into three phases: preacute, acute, and postacute care.

I. Preacute. This level includes:
   a. Health promotion, wellness, and prevention services
   b. Ambulatory care clinics, including primary and specialty care clinics
   c. Patient-centered medical home.
   d. Accountable care organizations—community based

MEDICARE OUTPATIENT OBSERVATION NOTICE

(Hospitals may include contact information or logo here)

Medicare Outpatient Observation Notice

Patient name: _____   Patient number: _____

You're a hospital outpatient receiving observation services. You are not an inpatient because:

_____

Being an outpatient may affect what you pay in a hospital:

▶ When you're a hospital outpatient, your observation stay is covered under Medicare Part B.
▶ For Part B services, you generally pay:
  ● A copayment for each outpatient hospital service you get. Part B copayments may vary by type of service.
  ● 20% of the Medicare-approved amount for most doctor services, after the Part B deductible.

Observation services may affect coverage and payment of your care after you leave the hospital:

▶ If you need skilled nursing facility (SNF) care after you leave the hospital, Medicare Part A will only cover SNF care if you've had a 3-day minimum, medically necessary, inpatient hospital stay for a related illness or injury. An inpatient hospital stay begins the day the hospital admits you as an inpatient based on a doctor's order and doesn't include the day you're discharged.
▶ If you have Medicaid, a Medicare Advantage plan or other health plan, Medicaid or the plan may have different rules for SNF coverage after you leave the hospital. Check with Medicaid or your plan.

NOTE: Medicare Part A generally doesn't cover outpatient hospital services, like an observation stay. However, Part A will generally cover medically necessary inpatient services if the hospital admits you as an inpatient based on a doctor's order. In most cases, you'll pay a one-time deductible for all of your inpatient hospital services for the first 60 days you're in a hospital.

_____

If you have any questions about your observation services, ask the hospital staff member giving you this notice or the doctor providing your hospital care. You can also ask to speak with someone from the hospital's utilization or discharge planning department.

You can also call 1-800-MEDICARE (1-800-633-4227). TTY users should call 1-877-486-2048.

Form CMS 10611-MOON   Expiration 12/31/2019 OMB approval 0938-1308

Your costs for medications:

Generally, prescription and over-the-counter drugs, including "self-administered drugs," you get in a hospital outpatient setting (like an emergency department) aren't covered by Part B. "Self-administered drugs" are drugs you'd normally take on your own. For safety reasons, many hospitals don't allow you to take medications brought from home. If you have a Medicare prescription drug plan (Part D), your plan may help you pay for these drugs. You'll likely need to pay out of pocket for these drugs and submit a claim to your drug plan for a refund. Contact your drug plan for more information.

_____

If you're enrolled in a Medicare Advantage plan (like an HMO or PPO) or other Medicare health plan (Part C), your costs and coverage may be different. Check with your plan to find out about coverage for outpatient observation services.

If you're a Qualified Medicare Beneficiary through your state Medicaid program, you can't be billed for Part A or Part B deductibles, coinsurance, and copayments.

_____

Additional Information (Optional):

_____

Please sign below to show you received and understand this notice.

_____

Signature of Patient or Representative   **Date / Time**

CMS does not discriminate in its programs and activities. To request this publication in alternative format, please call: 1-800-MEDICARE or email: AltFormatRequest@cms.hhs.gov.

Form CMS 10611-MOON Expiration 12/31/2019   OMB approval 0938-1308

Adapted from CMS. *Medicare Outpatient Observation Notice (MOON)*. Retrieved from, https://www.cms.gov/Medicare/Medicare-General-Information/BNI/

display 6-4

HEALTH INSURANCE BENEFITS AND RULES OF COVERAGE

All insurance plans have their own rules for coverage. At all times obtain verification of coverage and authorization for services because:

▶ The insurance coverage may not have the specific benefit that the case manager, interdisciplinary healthcare team, or patient requests.

▶ The insurance coverage may not be adequate to cover the medical needs and support services of the patient.

▶ A patient may have already exhausted, or partially exhausted, the needed benefit(s).

II. Acute care. This level includes:
   a. Acute care hospitals
   b. Inpatient acute rehabilitation hospitals
   c. All services within these hospitals (such as emergency department and intensive or critical care).

III. Postacute care. This includes the following services:
   a. SNFs (freestanding and hospital based)
   b. Hospice (freestanding and hospital based)
   c. Rehabilitation units (freestanding and hospital based) that are not considered acute
   d. Home health agencies
   e. Specialty pharmacy providers.

Within the three phases, various types of services can be provided; there are no definite lines separating the real care of patients. This is the reason why case management that focuses on the patient rather than the level of care provides the greatest benefits. A home health patient may require acute care; an acute care patient may require hospice care; or an LTC patient may require hospitalization, custodial care, or home health and assisted living. However, a basic understanding of what constitutes custodial care, intermediate care, skilled nursing care, and LTC are important when matching a patient to a potential next level of care; it is also imperative to understand these levels when dealing with reimbursement issues. It is essential to understand health insurance coverage of various medical levels of care; however, many health insurance plans have their own customized rendition of what is covered or excluded (i.e., carved out). Some coverage is disappointing, whereas other coverage may be surprisingly generous. Medicare insurance criteria have been used as an example in most cases in this chapter for the following three reasons:

1. Medicare is the largest supplier of medical coverage in the United States.
2. Medicare criteria are often used as a basis for private health insurance coverage.

3. Medicare reimbursement changes usually precede reimbursement changes in other health plans (See "The Incentives of Change" later in this chapter).

Medicare coverage rules are usually taken from the traditional form of Medicare. The managed Medicare plans provide wide variations in their coverage. At all times, obtain verification of coverage and authorization for services; all insurance plans have their own rules for coverage (Display 6-4).

▶ Custodial Care

Custodial care also is referred to as personal care, supervisory care, or assisted living. Group homes and foster homes may also be included at this level of care. The CMS definition of custodial care is care that is primarily for the purpose of helping patients with their personal care needs such as ADLs; this care could safely and reasonably be supplied by persons without professional skills or training. Examples include helping patients get out of bed, eating, and bathing.

Custodial care requires the least skilled personnel of all the levels of extended care. We have never had a health insurance company pay for a patient who needed only custodial care (LTC patients may be an exception). The rule of thumb for Medicare and most insurance companies is as follows:

▶ If custodial care is the only kind of care needed, Medicare will not pay.
▶ If skilled care is required, custodial care can be included in the services and Medicare pays.

The custodial level of care is generally characterized by patients who can:

▶ Ambulate independently with or without assistive devices such as walkers, wheelchairs, or canes.
▶ Transfer from the bed to a chair or toilet with standby assistance.
▶ Accomplish ADLs such as eating, dressing, grooming, or bathing with only minimal assistance. Food preparation may be needed.
▶ Be considered continent of bowel and bladder although may require minimal assistance in caring for indwelling urinary catheters or colostomy appliances.
▶ Take own medications with general staff monitoring; no sliding scale or adjusted dosages.
▶ Interact socially. These patients may have intermittent episodes of confusion, impaired judgment, or agitation but do not require restraints to control behavior.

Sometimes home health nursing and an assisted living arrangement can be provided if, for example, an otherwise custodial care patient needs help only with sliding scale insulin or PT. Call the home's main caretaker or owner.

Many of such patients are considered family in their group homes, and the staff will work with the case manager in discharge planning.

▶ Intermediate Care

The patient needing intermediate care requires moderate assistance with ADLs and restorative nursing supervision for some activities. Such persons are not as independent as those classified under custodial care, and in some facilities the distinction between the two levels of care is blurred. Health insurance companies usually do not pay for this level of care unless skilled care is also required. The intermediate level of care is generally characterized by a patient who:

- Needs no more than one person for transferring from a bed to a chair or toilet.
- Needs assistance with ambulation but can self-propel a wheelchair.
- Requires a moderate amount of assistance in bathing, grooming, eating, and dressing.
- May need restraints.
- Has routine medications and treatments that can be provided for with general monitoring by others.
- May be intermittently incontinent of bowel or bladder and may need help with an indwelling Foley catheter or colostomy.
- Can socially interact but may have periods of confusion, agitation, or emotional outbursts that can be controlled with moderate intervention.

▶ Skilled Nursing

In some SNFs, the delineation between skilled nursing care and subacute care is one of progressing complexity of the patient's medical and functional needs. This level of care is considered the most intensive in the SNF system. Patients may require maximum assistance with ADLs, may be totally incontinent of bowel and bladder, and may be disoriented, confused, combative, or even obtunded. Yet these characteristics alone will not qualify a patient for health insurance coverage. For an insurance company to pay for care at an SNF level, a care need from a skilled licensed professional provided daily and the assessment that this care must take place at the SNF level for reasons of patient safety and economy are also required. The skilled services in the following paragraphs represent some services covered under many health insurance plans. A patient with injections, more frequent or complex dressing changes, or more invasive tubes may be considered to need subacute rather than skilled care.

Even if a patient is medically stable, SNFs may not be able to provide the level of care needed (due to staffing restraints), especially if the care is too complex in nature. A transitional hospital should be considered in such complex cases.

Skilled nursing services may include (but are not limited to):

- Daily injections: IV fluids, IV medications, intramuscular injections, and subcutaneous injections (such as sliding scale insulin or heparin).
- Daily wound care requiring aseptic technique.
- Tube feedings or tube care: nasogastric tube, duodenostomy tube, gastrostomy tube, jejunostomy tube, tracheostomy care (initial teaching and care).
- Frequent observation and assessment by licensed personnel to prevent deterioration of the patient's condition or complications; this change would require prompt nursing response.
- Treatment of skin injuries including decubitus ulcers (severity of stage 3 or worse) and severe skin conditions or deep tissue injuries.
- Initial phases of a regimen that involves the administration of medical gases such as bronchodilator therapy.
- Early postoperative care and teaching for colostomies, ileostomies, Hickman catheters, and other tubes.
- Therapy: PT and possibly adjunctive ST or OT.
- Teaching a patient with newly diagnosed diabetes about diet, sliding scale insulin injections, foot care, and other preventive measures.

▶ LONG-TERM CARE

The expression *long-term care* (LTC) used to be synonymous with nursing home placement. This is no longer the case; chronically impaired people who are dependent on others to care for them can be found in homes, foster homes, day care centers, and a variety of other institutional and noninstitutional settings.

There is no single regulatory definition of LTC, but most emphasize the dependence and chronicity of the patient. In general, LTC is targeted at persons with functional disabilities that may present as a physical or mental problem. The goal of LTC is to promote or maintain as much independence and quality of life as possible. If the patient is terminally ill, the goal is to maintain comfort, dignity, and peaceful death. A broad spectrum of services is provided, depending on the unique needs of the individual and family. Private LTC coverage is available, and the number of individual LTC policies grew exponentially in the 1990s. It is rarely financed with company insurance policies, and the consumer must usually pay for the entire, somewhat expensive premium (Kongstvedt, 2003). State coffers provide LTC to persons who can pass the strict medical and financial requirements. Consider the changing demographics of the United States: chronically ill patients are living longer and the number of elderly people and younger people with multiple chronic diseases such as end-stage renal disease, diabetes, and heart failure is increasing. These factors are making a significant impact on the LTC budget. With the currently aging baby boomers, this trend is likely to continue. This is also why LTC policies are being sold in increasing numbers.

Candidates qualifying under the definition of LTC generally fall into one of two groups: (1) those requiring complex care and extensive convalescence, such as a major trauma victim, and (2) those with chronic and multiple medical, mental health, and social problems who are unable to care for themselves. Some patients with diagnoses such as severe mental retardation, cerebral palsy, or spastic quadriplegia fall into the chronic category. They live in group homes where all their needs are met. If these patients need hospitalization, health insurance authorization is not usually required to return them to that facility. In many cases, LTC patients have fairly stable transitions and discharge dispositions. There is no inherent limit to the number of medical or custodial resources that a LTC patient can consume.

Many patients have acute medical insurance and short-term extended care benefits. The case manager needs to see beyond these benefits and assess the need for LTC. Even if a patient meets the strict state requirements, the process to qualify for state LTC coverage can take up to 90 days; again, early assessment and planning can avoid future problems.

▶ PREACUTE LEVEL OF CARE

The preacute level of care consists of those settings that are available in the community which an individual may encounter. Specific settings will be considered based upon the health or diagnosis with a specific disease, and whether the patient's condition is stable and they are managing well in the community. People access health promotion, wellness, and prevention services on a proactive and routine basis. In this level of care, such people may receive the following services:

▶ Routine health checks and physical assessments,
▶ Health promotion awareness,
▶ Health instructions,
▶ Health risk behavior assessment or screening, and
▶ Counseling for healthy lifestyle behavior.

Healthy people may access health promotion and wellness services through their health insurance benefit plans either telephonically, or by completing health risk assessments online, or upon visiting their primary care providers for annual physicals or upon demand. These services are usually least expensive, and users of these services may incur a copay (often $15 or more per encounter) on the basis of the plan's benefits. The copay may be higher in the case of tests, other than those that are routinely performed during an annual check-up.

▶ Primary Care Clinics

Primary care clinics are community based and accessed by individuals on an ambulatory care basis, often for routine care. They are the day-to-day providers of healthcare services. These clinics are offered by providers such as physicians, nurse practitioners, and physician assistants in the form of individual private practices or group practices. Primary care clinics may also be associated with integrated healthcare systems or stand-alone hospitals. They tend to be staffed with experienced and board-certified providers (i.e., general or family practitioners) who today act as the point of entry into the healthcare system. Additionally, these clinics accept most health insurance plans and offer a variety of services such as the following.

▶ Annual physicals
▶ School physicals
▶ Well-woman services
▶ Well-baby services
▶ Vaccines and injections
▶ Internal, family, pediatric, and/or geriatric care
▶ Routine preventive and urgent medical care
▶ Health risk screenings and disease prevention
▶ Health maintenance
▶ Health counseling
▶ Patient education
▶ Diagnosis and treatment of acute and chronic illnesses

Primary care clinics may offer routine physical assessments, and simple blood and radiologic tests. When services such as radiology tests are not available on-site, they are arranged for with affiliated facilities and followed up by the primary care provider in the clinic. Primary care involves the widest scope of healthcare, including all ages of patients, patients of all socioeconomic and geographic origins, patients seeking to maintain optimal health, and patients with all manner of acute and chronic physical, mental, and social health issues, including multiple chronic diseases. Consequently, a primary care practitioner must possess a wide breadth of knowledge in many areas. During the past decade, the provision of chronic disease management services has become more common in these primary care clinics. Therefore, the presence of case managers in such chronic care management clinics has increased in popularity, especially because of the complex health conditions of patients and the diverse services provided in the primary care clinics, including the coordination of consults with specialty care providers.

▶ Patient-Centered Medical Home

The Agency for Healthcare Research and Quality recognizes that revitalizing the primary care system in the United States is foundational to achieving high-quality, accessible, and efficient health care for all Americans. The primary care medical home, also referred to as the patient-centered medical home (PCMH), medical home, advanced primary care, and the healthcare home, is a promising model for transforming delivery of primary care. The PCMH is a model of care delivery that puts patients and their families at the center or forefront of care by building effective, respectful, and trusting relationships between people and their clinical care providers. It is a philosophy or model of care that is designed to provide patient-centered, comprehensive (holistic), team-based, coordinated, and accessible, care that is focused on quality, safety, and cost-consciousness (Cesta & Tahan, 2017). Research has shown that such context of care delivery improves quality, patient experience, and staff satisfaction, while reducing healthcare costs.

The American Academy of Pediatrics introduced the medical home concept in 1967, and in 2007 leading primary care-oriented medical professional societies released the Joint Principles of the PCMH. In 2008, the National Commission of Quality Assurance (NCQA) commenced its PCMH Recognition (accreditation/certification) program, the first evaluation program in the country based on the PCMH model. These activities have contributed to increased popularity and recognition of the PCMH. As of March 2017, the NCQA has accredited more than 12,000 primary care practices (with more than 60,000 clinicians) as PCMHs, whereas 43 states have embraced the PCMH model (NCQA, 2017).

According to NCQA (2017), successful PCMHs have six characteristics as described herewith. These are also featured in the accreditation standards offered by the NCQA for PCMHs.

1. *Team-Based Care and Practice Organization* which helps structure a practice's leadership, care team responsibilities, and how the practice partners with patients, families, and caregivers.
2. *Knowing and Managing Patients* using best practices to set standards for data collection, medication reconciliation, evidence-based clinical decision support, and other activities.
3. *Patient-Centered Access and Continuity of Care* which guides practices to provide patients with convenient access to clinical advice and counseling, to ultimately ensure continuity of care.
4. *Care Management and* Support which emphasizes clinicians' use of care management protocols to identify patients who need and benefit from close management of their conditions and services.
5. *Care Coordination and Care Transitions* to ensure that primary and specialty care clinicians are effectively sharing information in a timely manner, and managing patient referrals to specialty services minimize cost, confusion, and inappropriate care and resource utilization.
6. *Performance Measurement and Quality Improvement* which include the development of innovative ways to measure performance, set goals, and develop activities that will improve performance of the practice and ultimately impact positively on the patient's health condition and experience of care.

Case managers have become integral members of interdisciplinary healthcare teams within the PCMH care setting. The primary focus of these case managers is care coordination and appropriate utilization of resources and therefore facilitating the patient's timely access to care and resources to ultimately prevent unnecessary progression of illness (disease process) and the need for costly acute care resources. It is a common practice in the PCMH to risk-stratify patients (i.e., low, moderate, high, or very high risk) into groups and deliver case management services on the basis of the degree of risk of the group. For example, case managers may provide routine risk screening, wellness, and health prevention services (perhaps telephonically) to those in the low-risk group compared with frequent in-person/face-to-face assessments and counseling with complex care coordination activities to those in the high or very high-risk groups.

Health homes, which are similar to the PCMH, have also become recently increasingly popular as a result of the Patient Protection and Affordable Care Act. However, health homes are state funded and available exclusively for the Medicaid beneficiaries. The purpose of these Medicaid health homes is the provision of comprehensive care coordination services for those Medicaid beneficiaries with one or more chronic conditions and often requiring behavioral health and social support services in addition to medical care. These settings have also witnessed a rise in the use of case managers and case management services.

▶ Accountable Care Organizations

Accountable Care Organizations (ACOs) are shared savings programs offered by Medicare to reduce the costs of care and improve quality and safety of the Medicare beneficiary. ACOs have been implemented as part of the Patient Protection and Affordable Care Act of 2010, under the CMS Center for Innovation. They are models of care where groups of doctors, hospitals, independent practice associations, integrated healthcare delivery networks, and other healthcare providers come together voluntarily to provide coordinated, high-quality, patient-centered care to the Medicare patients. The goal of coordinated care is to ensure that patients, especially those who suffer from one or more chronic health conditions, access the right care at the right time, while avoiding unnecessary duplication of services, and preventing medical errors. When an ACO succeeds both in delivering high-quality care and spending healthcare dollars more wisely, it will share in the savings it achieves for the Medicare program.

As value-based purchasing becomes more prominent, healthcare providers will increasingly need to focus on the whole patient or on populations of patients, encouraging and requiring teamwork among the various clinicians and across specialties. They will also need to focus on coordination of services and resources among healthcare organizations and providers of all types across the continuum of care (e.g., physician groups, hospitals, health systems, payors, and vendors). This will require all parties to relinquish their traditional siloed views and adopt a more expansive and collaborative model of care delivery—respecting the talent and experience brought to the table by all stakeholders. The need for this level of collaboration and coordination is characteristic of ACOs.

Participating in an ACO is purely voluntary for healthcare providers. Different organizations are at different stages in their ability to move toward an ACO model. Organizations across the country have already transformed the way they deliver care, in ways similar to those of the ACOs Medicare supports. There are different models of participation which include the following:

1. *Medicare Shared Savings Program*—a program that helps a Medicare fee-for-service program provider become an ACO.
2. *Advance Payment ACO Model*—a supplementary incentive program for selected participants in the Shared Savings Program.
3. *Pioneer ACO Model*—a program designed for early adopters of coordinated care. This type is no longer available today; it was limited to those ACOs that participated in the initial demonstration models and before such approaches became more widely available.

An ACO may use a range of payment methods which include: (a) fee-for-service with or without shared savings arrangements, (b) capitation for specific defined populations (e.g., diabetes), (c) global capitation based on a payment per person, rather than a payment per service provided, and (d) capitation on a per member per month fee structure. The traditional transaction-based payment method (i.e., fee-for-service) does not provide the incentives required to support ACOs and population health. As the reimbursement methods migrate completely toward payment for value (value-based purchasing), the ACO arrangement will also change. It is anticipated that ACOs will increasingly be reimbursed under a capitated method that incentivizes optimal quality, safety, efficiency, and health outcomes for populations of patients.

Fee-for-service Medicare patients who see providers that are participating in a Medicare ACO maintain all their Medicare rights, including the right to choose any doctors and providers that accept Medicare. Whether providers choose to participate in an ACO or not, their patients with Medicare may continue to see them. ACOs coordinate and integrate Medicare services, with success being evaluated using over 30 quality measures organized in four domains. These domains are: patient experience, care coordination and patient safety, preventive health, and at-risk populations. It is likely that a fifth domain be added; it is thought to address claims-based measures and focus on resource utilization. The higher the quality of care providers deliver, the more shared savings their

ACO may earn, provided they also lower growth in healthcare expenditures. Ultimately, ACOs are focusing on the goals of achieving the triple aim of improving care delivery, improving health, and reducing growth in costs through improvement of care delivery (https://www.cms.gov/Medicare/Medicare-Fee-for-Service-Payment/ACO/).

▶ ACUTE LEVEL OF CARE

Acute care services are self-explanatory, with the exception of various rehabilitation services and transitional hospitals, which are explained in more detail herewith.

▶ Rehabilitation Services

Rehabilitation services, PT, OT, and ST can be provided at various levels of care depending on the patient's functional ability and support system. Home PT/OT/ST can also be provided on an intermittent basis. For daily rehabilitation needs, an SNF level may be required. Inpatient acute rehabilitation facilities generally require that the patient can tolerate 3 hours of combined rehabilitative services daily and follow at least one- to two-step commands. Transitional hospitals can take patients at any level of rehabilitation needed and can generally move them within the hospital structure to the appropriate level and therapies.

A trauma or stroke patient in an acute hospital often requires an inpatient rehabilitation consultant. If the patient is said to be at "too high a level" for inpatient rehabilitation, it means that he or she does not require the intense focus of this level of care. An SNF level or even home care with home therapy services may be more appropriate. If the patient is said to be at "too low a level" for inpatient rehabilitation, it may mean that he or she cannot follow commands or cannot yet tolerate 3 hours of intense rehabilitation. Again, an SNF level may be more appropriate, with the hope and intention of the patient improving enough to graduate to an inpatient facility.

Again, health insurance coverage is the key in most cases. Some companies cover their members at varying degrees of dysfunction in the different rehabilitative levels.

There is a Medicare exception to the 3 hours of rehabilitation daily. If the patient has a complicating condition that prevents him or her from participating for 3 hours, but inpatient rehabilitation is the only reasonable means by which even a low-intensity rehabilitation program can be safely carried out, it may be authorized. Documentation and appropriate consultation with a physiatrist must support the claim.

▶ Inpatient Rehabilitation Centers

Inpatient rehabilitation care is covered under many major insurance plans, but strict criteria must be met because this is a cost-intensive setting. The criteria listed in the following paragraphs follow reimbursement guidelines under Medicare. As in any discharge plan, consult the patient's insurance coverage or request that the rehabilitation hospital/unit of the patient's choice examine the coverage. Most admission departments (or intake coordinators) can let the case manager know about coverage within 24 hours of a request. It is also beneficial to contact the insurance-based case manager or other representatives and discuss the patient's situation and plan of care. Some health insurance plans use stricter guidelines than the Medicare criteria. If the provider-based case manager and the rehabilitation physician feel strongly that the patient is an excellent rehabilitation candidate but the health insurance company is reluctant to cover services, try negotiation. Sometimes a short stay can be agreed on, with frequent monitoring of the patient's progress toward self-care.

INSURANCE CRITERIA

Four main categories of criteria reflect Medicare requirements for authorization in an inpatient rehabilitation facility. Other insurance companies may use the same general criteria.

1. Admitting diagnosis must include at least one of the following conditions:
   ▶ Amputation
   ▶ Arthritis
   ▶ Cardiac conditions
   ▶ Chronic pain
   ▶ Congenital disorder
   ▶ Cerebral vascular accident (CVA)
   ▶ Diabetes mellitus
   ▶ Fracture
   ▶ Head trauma/brain injury
   ▶ Multiple trauma
   ▶ Musculoskeletal disorder
   ▶ Neurologic disorder
   ▶ Orthopedic condition
   ▶ Pulmonary condition
   ▶ Spinal cord injury.
2. The primary problem must include a recent functional loss, whereas before the illness or accident, the patient must have been independent in that function. There must also be dependence on the assistance of another person to carry out that function. Some functional categories include the following:
   ▶ Bladder dysfunction—incontinence, use of external catheter;
   ▶ Bowel dysfunction—incontinence, maintenance of an excretory pattern;
   ▶ Communication—major receptive or expressive aphasia;
   ▶ Cognitive dysfunction—change in the patient's attention span, memory, or intelligence;
   ▶ Medical monitoring—the patient's medical status requiring intensive medical monitoring

or nursing attention at least once daily because of a cardiovascular, gastrointestinal, urologic, endocrine, or neurologic disorder. This is in addition to the primary diagnosis as stated in the first point;
   ▶ Medical safety—the patient either exhibits or is at risk for secondary complications such as decubitus ulcers, contractures, urinary tract infections, or major spasticity;
   ▶ Mobility dysfunction—the patient must learn safe transfers to chair/bed/toilet/shower, walking (usually with appliances), negotiating stairs, wheelchairs, and so on;
   ▶ Pain control—pain severely prohibits active motion or functional use;
   ▶ Personal safety—the patient is physically unsafe alone;
   ▶ Self-care activities—ADLs must be renegotiated, such as feeding, drinking, dressing, grooming, brace and prosthesis care, bathing, toileting, and perineal care.
3. The physician must document the expectation of significant improvement in functional ability within a reasonable time frame.
4. If a patient was previously in a rehabilitation program with an unsuccessful outcome, this patient must have some change in condition or circumstances that would indicate that progress is now possible; otherwise, he or she will not be eligible.

Other important criteria for admission to an inpatient rehabilitation unit include medical stability, mental ability to follow one- to two-step commands, and ability to withstand at least 3 hours of therapies daily and five times per week. The 3 hours can consist of any combination of PT, OT, and ST.

A patient may be discharged from a rehabilitation unit for several reasons, including:

   ▶ The stated goals of rehabilitation have all been met.
   ▶ There has been no progress toward the stated goals after an adequate trial (usually 1 week without any appreciable headway).
   ▶ A severe complication develops, necessitating a transfer to acute care.
   ▶ A complication develops, inhibiting the multidisciplinary approach for more than 1 week. In this case, it is sometimes necessary and reasonable to transfer the patient to an SNF level of care until the rehabilitation treatment modalities can be reinstated.

▶ Transitional Hospitals

Although uncommon today, it is still important for the case manager to be aware of transitional hospitals and to understand their characteristics. Transitional hospitals are acute care hospitals for medically stable patients with long rehabilitative needs and care that are too complex for SNFs to handle/meet.

These hospitals usually have a lower price structure than traditional acute care hospitals, mainly because fewer specialists are on staff and the facilities contain only basic diagnostic or surgical equipment. They usually do not have expensive and sophisticated equipment such as CT scanners or MRI, but do have the basics such as x-ray capabilities. Major surgeries are not done on-site, but simple surgical procedures such as surgical feeding tube placement or tracheostomies can be performed. These hospitals are lower in price, patient acuity, and intensity or complexity of services because of the nonacute nature of the patient's needs. RN staffing is reported to be determined the same way as at other acute care hospitals; that is, it is dependent on the patient's acuity levels and care needs.

These hospitals can handle patients just below the (ICU) level with multiple complex medication regimens and treatments, which may include:

▶ Ventilator-dependent patients, including weaning patients;
▶ Use of total parenteral nutrition (TPN) or hyperalimentation;
▶ Extensive wound care;
▶ Infectious disease management;
▶ IV medication therapies;
▶ Burn care;
▶ All rehabilitation modalities (OT/PT/ST);
▶ Hemodialysis patients;
▶ Prehospice patients—pain control therapies;
▶ Coma recovery, cognitive rehabilitation, neurobehavioral rehabilitation;
▶ Most other treatments that can be done at other acute hospitals or levels of care.

In the early 1990s, one patient with AIDS also developed Guillain-Barré syndrome and became ventilator dependent for many months. It took almost 1 month to obtain placement in an SNF that handled ventilators because of the long waiting periods. A Gallup poll in 1991 revealed that there was an average waiting period of 35 days between the time that a chronic ventilator–dependent patient could be discharged from an acute care hospital and the availability of an appropriate bed (Anonymous, 1991). Such circumstances facilitated the proliferation of transitional hospitals at the time. It now takes less time to place a patient with a complex medical condition in an SNF. Additionally, some SNFs today are able to handle complex supportive care and services such as dialysis, TPN, and mechanical ventilation dependency.

If a patient's condition is very complex but "too low a level" for inpatient rehabilitation, transitional hospitals should be considered. For example, a patient came in for a coronary catheterization, suffered a stroke and a cardiac arrest during the procedure, and required a tracheostomy. Eventually, this patient was weaned from the mechanical ventilator. She was alert and oriented but too weak to tolerate intensive rehabilitation modalities. She also required more frequent tracheal suctioning than SNFs can usually handle. The transitional hospital further stabilized the respiratory function and strengthened her. Later this woman was placed in an inpatient rehabilitation unit, where she did very well.

▶ POSTACUTE LEVEL OF CARE

▶ Definitions of Subacute Care

Subacute care fills in the gap between acute hospitalization and LTC. Patients who are eligible for subacute care may also require intense care and services. However, they do not require the complex diagnostic workups or treatments, usually characteristic of acute care hospitals, and are considered medically stable with a fairly constant treatment plan. Sometimes the term *postacute care* is used; this includes all levels of care below acute hospitalization, including home healthcare. Subacute care has received an enormous amount of attention as a cost-saving level of care, yet few will agree on what it is or even where it is. The delivery of care may be in either inpatient settings (as in the definitions given in the following paragraphs) or outpatient settings. Some feel subacute care is a transitional phase between the acute stage and the rehabilitation stage, or a service that fills the gap between acute care and skilled home care (Display 6-5). TJC and the Commission on Accreditation of Rehabilitation Facilities have developed subacute accreditation standards for inpatient facilities.

Subacute care is comprehensive inpatient care designed for the person who has had an acute illness, injury, or exacerbation of an existing health condition or disease process. It requires the coordination of services by an interdisciplinary healthcare team of physicians, nurses, and other professionals including respiratory therapist, PT, OT, and/or ST. TJC (2017) has defined subacute care as:

Care that is rendered immediately after, or instead of, acute hospitalization to treat one or more specific, active, complex medical/health conditions or to administer one or more technically complex treatments in the context of an individual's underlying long-term condition and overall situation.

The National Association of Subacute/Postacute Care (NASPAC) emphasizes the following definition:

Subacute care is a comprehensive, cost-effective inpatient level of care for patients who:

▶ have had an acute event from injury, illness, or exacerbation of a disease process.
▶ have a determined course of treatment.
▶ though stable, require diagnostics or invasive procedures, but not intensive procedures requiring an acute level of care (NASPAC, 2009).

SUBACUTE LEVELS OF CARE

display 6-5

Levels of Care	Subacute and Rehabilitation	Skilled Nursing	Intermediate Care	Assisted Living/ Custodial Care
Medical stability	Can be complex and unstable; requires ongoing monitoring by RNs; complex care for multimedical problems may be provided	Can be complex and generally stable; requires skilled nursing observation and modification of care plan to prevent further deterioration	Client medically stable; intermittent nursing and medical services needed to maintain medical stability	Client medically stable
Injections	Complex IV therapy regimen; multiple IV medications requiring infusion pumps	IV push therapy; simple IV therapy; central line care	IM and SC injections	No IV, IM, SC injections; may retain home health nurses to provide these services
Medication regimen	Complex medication regimen because of unstable conditions; at least 5 medication changes per week by the attending physician may be required to meet this level of care	Medication regimen requiring some adjustments in dosages or frequency of medication; done through observation and assessment of vital signs or laboratory data	Administration of routine medication; RN or LPN monitoring may be necessary with occasional dose or frequency changes when ordered by attending physician	Stable regimen of oral medications; home health nurses may be hired to monitor more complex medications such as sliding scale insulin
Respiratory treatments	Some facilities care for patients on respirators, including frequent suction and SVN PRN treatments	May have oxygen, SVN treatments, inhaler therapies	Routine oxygen administration and a stable respiratory therapy regimen	May have home oxygen, simple oxygen, simple inhalers
Suctioning	Frequent (more than every 4 hours) tracheal suctioning allowed; new tracheostomy care	Nonsterile suctioning or intermittent sterile suctioning	Simple, routine nonsterile suctioning	No suctioning
Invasive tube care	Can handle complex tube care including tracheostomy tube, gastrostomy tubes, jejunostomy tubes, ileostomies, colostomies, indwelling tubes, T tubes, catheters; may include irrigation, monitoring, replacement PRN, site care, and self-care instructions	Same as subacute, but patient and care must be fairly stable; patients at this level with several types of tubes not accepted at some facilities	Routine maintenance and care of uncomplicated catheters, tubes, ostomies; may do intermittent irrigations	Empty drainage tubes and do simple, routine care (more complex care may require intermittent home health nursing visits)
Wound care/ dressings	Complex treatments and wound care; Criteria: treatment over 20 minutes, performed by RN level nurse, 2 or more times per 8-hour shift	Will perform complex, sterile, and frequent dressing changes or wound cases needing close monitoring (wounds can be infected and acute)	Will perform routine care for noninfected, chronic wounds and skin conditions	May perform simple care such as salves and simple dry dressing; may call in a home health RN for further care
Rehabilitation	Usually requires a minimum of 2 therapies (physical, occupational, or speech) and the patient's ability to tolerate at least 3 hours of therapy daily	Rehabilitation therapy needed on a daily basis and performed by a licensed therapist	May be supervised by a licensed therapist (restorative nursing); may include assistance with ambulation. range of motion, positioning, and so on	Not a safe level of care if the patient requires rehabilitation, unless home health is involved in a noncomplex case

(continued)

SUBACUTE LEVELS OF CARE (continued)

Mobility	Requires complex assistance from licensed personnel	Usually requires assistance of more than 1 person in mobility, transfers to chair, bed, toilet, or bath; unable to help very much in these activities; assistive devices may be used	Patient possibly able to participate in mobility and transfers to chair, bed, toilet. or bath; assistive devices may or may not be needed	Often allows wheelchair-bound clients, but must be independent in getting to and from bathroom and eating areas and independent in getting in and out of bed
Patient education/ health teaching	Teaching needs identified and taught by licensed professional staff; administration of medications, self-care of tubes, wounds, use of equipment is taught on ongoing basis in preparation for discharge to a lesser level of care	Teaching needs identified and taught by licensed professional staff; administration of medications, self-care of tubes, wounds, use of equipment, and other needs taught on an ongoing basis in preparation for discharge to a lesser level of care	Simple teaching done by nonlicensed professionals but under the supervision of licensed staff; may teach basic ADL support, feeding techniques, use of assistive devices, and so on	No teaching skills at this level of care; home health nurses may be retained if needed
Nutrition	Can accommodate TPN, IV fluids, use of infusion pumps, tube feedings with residual checks	TPN and IV fluids accommodated at some facilities; tube feeding with or without infusion pump and maximum assistance with oral feeding accommodated	Requires some assistance with self-feeding	Most require the client to be able to get to the dining room and feed self
Personal hygiene and toileting	Can accommodate total care of personal hygiene and toileting, including disimpaction when needed and perineal care	Can accommodate total care of personal hygiene and toileting, including disimpaction when needed and perineal care	Assists with toileting, perineal care, bathing, and grooming	Most require the client to be continent; some accept indwelling catheters and assist with dressing and grooming efforts
Behavioral/ mental		May be confused, disoriented, combative; may need physical or chemical restraints for safety of patient or others; patients with active, serious psychological disorders are not legally allowed at this level of care in many states	May be intermittently confused or disoriented, requiring staff intervention and possibly restraints for protective purposes; patients with active, serious psychological disorders not legally allowed at this level of care in many states	May be slightly forgetful; not a safe level of care for confused, disoriented clients

ADL, activities of daily living; IM, intramuscular; PRN, as needed; SC, subcutaneous; SVN, small volume nebulizer; TPN, total parenteral nutrition.

The severity of the patient's condition requires:

▶ active physician direction with frequent on-site visits.
▶ professional nursing care.
▶ significant ancillary services.
▶ an outcomes-focused interdisciplinary approach utilizing a professional team.

▶ complex medical and/or rehabilitation care (NASPAC, 2009).

The American Health Care Association, a national organization representing nursing and residential care facilities, defines subacute care as:

A comprehensive inpatient program designed for the individual who has had an acute event as a result of illness, injury, or exacerbation of a disease process; has a determined course of treatment; and does not require intensive diagnostic and/or invasive procedures.

The severity of an individual's condition requires an outcome-focused interdisciplinary approach utilizing a professional team to deliver complex clinical intervention (medical and/or rehabilitation). These highly specialized programs promote quality care by utilizing healthcare resources efficiently and effectively.

Subacute care requires the coordinated services of an interdisciplinary team of care providers such as a physician, case manager, nurse, physical therapist, occupational therapist, SW, and others. It is generally more intensive than traditional care provided in an SNF and less intensive than care provided in an acute care/hospital setting. Moreover, it requires frequent patient assessments that could vary from daily to weekly depending on the condition being treated. In addition, it involves a review of the clinical course of treatment and plan for care for the time period until the condition being treated is stabilized or the predetermined treatment course is completed (TJC, 2017). Integral to the provision of care in a subacute care facility TJC identified seven characteristics that are described in Display 6-6.

There are four general categories of subacute patients classified on the basis of their projected length of stay (LOS) and intensity of service.

1. *Transitional subacute.* The estimated (LOS) is 3 to 30 days. The intensity of rehabilitation and/or nursing care is 5 to 8 hours per day. The conditions of the patients of this category are rather intense, such as those requiring chemotherapy, postsurgical interventions, and IV antibiotics. The care can be rendered in a hospital-based or a freestanding SNF.

2. *General subacute.* The estimated LOS is 10 to 40 days. The intensity of rehabilitation and/or nursing care is 3 to 5 hours per day. A stroke patient may require this level of care depending on the residual deficit. Care can be rendered in a freestanding SNF.

3. *Chronic subacute.* The estimated LOS is 60 to 90 days. The intensity of rehabilitation and/or nursing care is 3 to 5 hours per day. Patients of this category may have intensive but chronic conditions, for example, a stable mechanical ventilator–dependent patient or one with a medical and a cognitive deficit such as Alzheimer's disease or a total hip replacement. Care facilities will require careful choice; not all skilled care environments are staffed for this level of care.

4. *Long-term transitional subacute.* The estimated LOS is 25 days or more. The intensity of rehabilitation and/or nursing care is 6 to 9 hours per day. It is most likely that this type of subacute care will end in placing the patient in an LTC facility. Here the care is more intensive than LTC as patients may be developmentally impaired with head trauma or birth defects.

Subacute rehabilitation services can be divided into three general categories according to Carr (2000) which are still relevant to and applicable in today's healthcare environment. These are:

1. Short-term rehabilitation for patients with significant medical and nursing needs but too ill to tolerate rigorous rehabilitation therapy in an acute care setting. These patients also require high use of PT, OT, and ST services. Common medical problems include orthopedics such as total hip or

---

display 6-6

CHARACTERISTICS OF THE PROVISION OF SUBACUTE CARE ACCORDING TO THE JOINT COMMISSION

1. Time: Care is rendered immediately after, or instead of, an acute care hospital stay.
2. Reason: Treatment of one or more specific, active, complex, or unusual medical conditions or administration of one or more technically complex treatments in the context of the patient's underlying long-term conditions and overall situation.
3. Care Providers: Requirement of the services of an interdisciplinary team of healthcare professionals who are trained and knowledgeable in the assessment and management of the specific conditions and performance of the necessary procedures.
4. Care Setting: Care is provided in an inpatient setting.
5. Frequency: Care requires frequent patient assessment and review of the clinical course and treatment plan, perhaps weekly or more often.
6. Intensity of Services: Care is provided at a level that is generally more intensive than a traditional SNF/nursing home and less intensive than that provided in an acute inpatient care unit/hospital.
7. Duration of Services: Care may last for a limited time or until a condition is stabilized or a predetermined treatment course is completed (e.g., IV antibiotics course). The time period may vary from several days to several months depending on the course of treatment and the patient's progress.

Adapted from The Joint Commission. (2017). *Comprehensive accreditation manual for hospitals.* Oakbrook Terrace, IL: Author.

knee replacements, and neurology such as stroke, brain, or spinal cord injury.

2. Short-term rehabilitation for patients with complex medical conditions. These patients require intense medical and nursing management. These patients also require a high use of respiratory, laboratory, and pharmacy services as well as medical supplies. Common medical problems include cardiology, oncology, pulmonary, dialysis, complex wounds, IV fluid therapy, and parenteral nutrition.

3. Long-term or chronic rehabilitation for patients who have experienced extended acute care stays, are medically stable but have relatively high nursing needs and ancillary services. Common medical conditions include head injuries, coma, multiple trauma, and mechanical ventilation dependency.

▶ Skilled Nursing Facilities

SNFs offer a level of care that is below acute hospitalization, in which the patient still requires ongoing skilled care from licensed personnel (e.g., nurses, SWs, OT, PT, ST) on a daily basis. Other terms include nursing home, nursing home placement, intermediate care facility, or extended care facility.

The use of acronyms is fine for medical personnel, but it is best to use the entire term when talking to patients or their families. We sometimes use the term "extended care facility" and explain that this is an extension of the hospital care the patient is now receiving but at a less intense pace. We do not like using the term "nursing home" or "convalescent center." These terms often bring up unfavorable images or frightening memories of neglect or of loved ones dying.

Most communities have reference books and brochures listing their SNFs, along with contact names, addresses, and telephone numbers. Other information such as ratings, level of care offered, quality and safety measures/performance, and Medicare certification is usually provided. Not all facilities provide the same levels of care or even quality of care. It is worth a visit to these sites for a thorough understanding of the level of skilled care each one can provide. These visits can be real eye-openers. We learned about an SNF in which a licensed professional nurse was on duty only from 6 am until 10 pm; the case manager, therefore, could not send to this facility anyone with even a "to keep open" IV line in case it needed attention at 2 am. However, this SNF had a good PT department; if that was the patient's sole need, this facility would be a good match.

Remember to offer the patient and family options. It is important for them to be aware of what is available, at least in their geographical area of interest. Engage with them in a discussion about the various options and ensure that the final decision is theirs to make. This maintains their

right to choice and self-determination. Make them aware that, although they have selected the top three options, the payor may require you to accept the first facility that approves the patient's transfer. Keep the following factors (questions) in mind when choosing an SNF:

▶ Does the facility's skill level meet the assessed needs of the patient?
▶ Will the patient/family agree to this facility? Is it an acceptable location for visiting purpose?
▶ Does the patient's primary physician go to this facility? If not, would the physician prefer another SNF that is also acceptable to the patient/family? Perhaps the physician, family, and patient would agree to have another physician follow-up on the patient while at the SNF of choice.
▶ Is the chosen SNF a contracted facility with the payor?
▶ Will the services that the patient needs be covered at the SNF level of care by the payor?

INSURANCE CRITERIA

Traditional Medicare patients (those reimbursed under the DRG system) may enter an SNF level of care when certain criteria have been met:

▶ The patient must be in the hospital for three consecutive days, also referred to as the 3-Midnight Rule (This criterion is not required for the Medicare Advantage Plans.); refer to the section on the 3-Midnight Rule for more information.
▶ The 3-day stay must have been medically necessary.
▶ The SNF reason for admission must also be congruent with the reason the patient was in the hospital; or
▶ Posthospital SNF placement may take place within 30 days of hospital discharge. The 3-day rule applies.

The SNF benefit has been included in Medicare Part A to provide extended skilled nursing care for patients who were recently hospitalized but no longer needed the intensive treatments of an acute care/hospital setting. Under Part A, Medicare provides payment for 100 days of skilled nursing care, including medical and therapy services, for each episode of illness. These skilled nursing services typically are provided in a LTC facility. For SNF stays that are not covered by Medicare Part A, Part B may provide coverage, however, for a limited amount of services such as therapy care.

The 3-day hospital stay requirement is for an inpatient status only; patients admitted under outpatient observation status do not qualify. If it appears that the patient will need SNF placement and meets acute inpatient medical necessity criteria, ask the physician for an order to change the patient to inpatient status. In addition, Medicare and other health insurance plans also mandate the following criteria before a patient can be admitted to an SNF:

- The medical condition requires daily, skilled services of a licensed healthcare professional.
- Those services cannot be provided at a lesser level of care or it would be impractical, uneconomical, or inefficient to do so.
- The care provided must be based on physician orders.

COVERAGE OPTIONS

The following SNF coverage options are specifically for Medicare-reimbursed patients, but many health insurance companies have the same or similar provisions. Major SNF services covered under Medicare Parts A and B include:

- Nursing care provided by or under the supervision of a RN;
- Bed and board (semiprivate room and meals, which may include special diets);
- Therapy services (PT, OT, ST) furnished by the SNF or by others under special arrangements made by the facility;
- Blood transfusions (additional fees may be required);
- Medical social services;
- Drugs, biologicals, supplies, appliances, and equipment, furnished for use in the SNF, as are ordinarily furnished by such facility for the care and treatment of residents/inpatients;
- Medical services provided by a physician (which may include an intern or resident-in-training of a hospital with which the facility has in effect a transfer agreement under an approved teaching program of the hospital), and other diagnostic or therapeutic services provided by a hospital with which the SNF has such an agreement in effect;
- Use of DME such as walkers or wheelchairs;
- Other services necessary to the health of the residents (patients) as are generally provided by an SNF, or by others under arrangements.

Some SNF services not covered by Medicare include:

- Personal convenience items such as televisions and telephones (not all SNFs provide them unless the patient requests them and rents them);
- Private duty nurses;
- The extra charge necessary for a private room, unless the private room is deemed to be medically necessary.

▶ Hospice

Hospice programs began in Great Britain many decades ago. The concept reached the United States in the 1970s and has recently gained much respect and popularity. The philosophy of hospice is that terminally ill patients should be allowed to maintain their final days of life comfortably, with respect and dignity. Ideally, these last days take place at home in the presence of family members, friends, and loved ones, if desired. Hospice may be the plan of care of choice when nothing further can be done medically for the patient, the patient and family agree that death is imminent, and the patient and family want only palliative and comfort measures taken, not aggressive curative measures. Hospice does not hasten or postpone death but allows nature to take its course. The hospice philosophy reminds case managers that this dying person is a living person and deserves a peaceful and dignified death.

Often families and medical staff are confused about the difference in services between home health services and hospice. Although hospice is similar to home health services in many ways, it differs in some important aspects. The following are some differences between Medicare home health coverage and Medicare hospice coverage services as the standard guideline. Be aware that health insurance companies other than Medicare may or may not include hospice benefits; if they have the hospice benefit, they may include different covered services.

In 1995, a new revision was added to the Medicare hospice regulations. It states: "A discharge planning evaluation must include an evaluation of a patient's likely need for appropriate post-hospital services, including hospice services and the availability of those services" (Hamilton & Thomsen, 1998).

Payment for hospice services under Medicare is based on four levels of care. Depending on the intensity of services, the per diem rate is adjusted. The four levels are as follows (Hamilton & Thomsen, 1998):

1. Routine home care;
2. Continuous home care (24 hours in a crisis situation);
3. Inpatient respite care (not to exceed five consecutive days at a time); or
4. General inpatient care (for pain control or other symptom management that would be difficult to control in lesser levels of care/settings).

COMPARISON BETWEEN HOSPICE COVERAGE AND HOME HEALTH COVERAGE

- *Skilled nursing services are provided on an intermittent basis.* Both home health and hospice provide skilled nursing services, but hospice covers these services on a 24-hour, 7-day-a-week, on-call basis.
- *Nonskilled services.* Most home health agencies do not provide nonskilled nursing services because they are rarely covered under health insurance plans or agreements. Nurse aides may be covered under Medicare for two to three 1-hour visits per week for personal care, but only under strict criteria. Hospice can provide 12 to 16 hours of personal aides per week if needed, including some homemaker services.

▶ *Physician services.* Both home health and hospice care must be under the guidance of an ordering physician.

▶ *Bereavement services and counseling (including spiritual counseling).* This is perhaps the most important distinction between home health services and hospice services. Bereavement and counseling services are often offered to the family for several months after the death of the patient. More importantly, if hospice is called in early enough, these trained persons help prepare the family for the impending death, often averting shock and crisis situations.

▶ *Social services and volunteers.* With hospice, social service personnel and volunteers are part of the multidisciplinary staff. Home health agencies are allowed very limited social service attention at home.

▶ *Homebound requirement.* Under home health criteria, the patient must be homebound or must undergo an unusual hardship to get care through outpatient facilities. Although terminal hospice patients are often homebound, this is not a mandatory requirement for hospice care.

▶ *Prescription drugs for symptom management and pain control.* Traditional Medicare rarely pays for prescription medications at home (exceptions are noted in "Medicare" in Chapter 3). Under the hospice benefit, prescription medications to manage symptoms and control pain are covered. There is a 5% or $5 or more charge (copay) toward each prescription, whichever is less.

▶ *DME and home oxygen.* Medicare has strict criteria for many types of DME, including oxygen (see home oxygen criteria in "Home Care Services"). Hospice guidelines for various types of DME are more lax and can be provided for the comfort of the patient.

▶ *Respite care.* This is not a covered service under home health. With hospice, limited respite care in an SNF allows the family to take care of needed business or take a break so that it does not get overwhelmed with the extensive care that most terminal patients require. The respite is limited to five consecutive days per benefit quarter.

▶ *Physical, occupational, and speech-language therapy.* These therapies are carried out for the purpose of symptom control or to allow the patient to maintain basic ADL function. Both home health and hospice benefits cover this service.

▶ *Continuous care during periods of medical crisis.* Only hospice carries this benefit. For some families, continuous care during this period is the key benefit that allows the patient to die at home with dignity.

▶ *Deductibles.* There are no deductibles under the hospice benefit.

MEDICARE HOSPICE CRITERIA

The hospice benefit may be used by a Medicare beneficiary if all the three following criteria are met:

1. A physician certifies that the patient is terminally ill.
2. The patient (or family) chooses to use the hospice benefit.
3. The hospice agency is Medicare certified.

If these three criteria are met and the patient is in the hospital, a physician order for hospice will be needed. After a call is made to refer this patient to hospice, a representative will come to the hospital, meet the patient and family, and answer questions. A hospice referral can also be made while a patient is at home, but also with the above-mentioned criteria.

Although a patient chooses to forego standard Medicare benefits in lieu of hospice benefits, standard benefits begin if treatment for a problem unrelated to the hospice condition is needed. For example, if a patient with terminal AIDS falls and breaks a leg, then the necessary care for this accident will be paid for by standard Medicare.

HOSPICE BENEFIT PERIODS

Special benefit periods apply to the hospice portion of Medicare. When a patient opts for the hospice benefit, the benefit periods define the extent of his or her coverage (see "Medicare" in Chapter 3 for standard Medicare benefit periods). Part A will pay for two 90-day benefit periods and unlimited 60-day benefit periods. Extension periods of indefinite duration protect the patient in the event of long terminal stages of illness.

Patients can choose to cancel hospice and return to Medicare benefits or vice versa as long as there are remaining benefit periods; when someone cancels the hospice benefit, the remaining days in the benefit period are lost. If any benefit periods remain, they may still return to hospice and use these periods.

MYTHS AND REALITIES

Perhaps because hospice is so similar to home health or because it is simply misunderstood, myths about hospice abound. The following are some myths that are commonly heard from patients and families.

Myth: Hospice is only for terminal cancer patients.

Reality: Hospice is for any terminal condition: chronic obstructive pulmonary disease (COPD), AIDS, cystic fibrosis, and any end-stage disease (cardiac, liver, renal, Alzheimer's disease, to name a few terminal conditions).

Myth: The patient must have only 6 months to live.

Reality: Although in general the prognosis for life expectancy should be in months rather than years, it is often difficult to say for certain how long a patient will live. Unfortunately, this misunderstanding has caused healthcare teams to wait until the last minute before calling in hospice, thereby losing valuable time in which patients and families could be receiving care and counseling that could improve the quality of the remaining time. Also, remember that Medicare allows 210 days (two benefit periods of 90 days and one benefit period of 30 days), which equals 7 months; add to that the indefinite extension. This is fact enough that demise is not "required" in 6 months.

Myth: A 24-hour caregiver is required.

Reality: This one requires careful assessment. We know some patients who had been admitted to hospice who were still independent, although this is rare. Others do well with the 12 to 16 hours of assistance provided. If a patient is terminal, is dependent on others, and does not have a strong support system, then an SNF for terminal care (under Medicare Part A) may be a better choice.

Myth: Nursing home patients cannot receive hospice care.

Reality: Medicare does not pay for the room and board of an SNF under the hospice benefit. However, if the family can fund the room and board or the patient's private insurance policy covers this, as some do, then hospice can be used at the SNF level of care. The bereavement and counseling portion of hospice can then be used; it is an important part of terminal care.

Myth: To be accepted into hospice, all further medical treatment must be forfeited.

Reality: The important distinction here is whether the care is for aggressive, curative purposes or for palliative, comfort means. Radiation therapy has been used for palliation treatment. If someone may have several months to live and cannot tolerate food or tube feedings, TPN has been authorized. The main question to ask is why the care is being given. Hospice patients in distress are readmitted into the hospital; often they are stabilized and sent back home with hospice again. Conditions not related to the hospice condition are treated under Medicare Part A. However, if a patient wants to try chemotherapy with the hope of a cure, he or she will have to leave the hospice benefit period and opt for standard Medicare benefits.

PALLIATIVE CARE

One cannot discuss hospice care without addressing palliative care; it is more frequent today to have a patient consider palliative care long before hospice care. Palliative care can be delivered concurrently with life-prolonging measures and may begin at the time a life-threatening and debilitating illness is diagnosed. Similar to hospice, palliative care is an interdisciplinary approach to care delivery with the main focus of relief of suffering and improvement in the patients' quality of life. Both hospice and palliative care address the physical, intellectual, emotional, social, and spiritual needs of patients and their families.

The five goals of palliative care are:

1. Pain control and management;
2. Sharing of appropriate information with the patient and family, especially that which is essential for informed decision making regarding treatment options;
3. Coordination and facilitation of care activities, especially during transitions from one care setting to another or from one provider of care to another;
4. Preparation of the patients and their families for dignified death;
5. Provision of bereavement support to patients and families.

Palliative care is provided in all care settings, including acute care hospitals, rehabilitation facilities, SNFs, outpatient clinics, home, assisted living facilities, and others. Care is provided at two levels: primary and specialized. The primary level refers to the provision of palliative care and services by the same multidisciplinary team responsible for the management of the patient's medical condition. The specialized level refers to palliative care and services provided by a multidisciplinary care team trained, specialized, and credentialed in palliative care.

▶ Home Care Services

Most patients who have been living independently before the present episode of illness prefer to return to their own homes. Perhaps they are not completely independent or back to their baseline condition, but have family support for their basic needs. Sometimes home care services provide the vital link to a patient's independence. A thorough social and medical assessment can evaluate the safety of a home health plan of care. For example, if the patient is a debilitated 94-year-old mother who lives with her daughter, the daughter also needs to be assessed to see if she can still safely care for her mother (the daughter will likely be in her seventies).

Home health agencies are public or private organizations that specialize in providing both skilled and nonskilled services in a patient's home. This line of service is not new, and several agencies have already celebrated their centennial. Display 6-7 describes a variety of services that may be offered in the home setting; however, reimbursement for these services is based on the health insurance plan and benefits that the patient may possess. Changes in the way that America is delivering healthcare are having a significant effect on the home healthcare industry. There is an increase in patients being sent home, necessitating more care from RNs or other licensed professionals such as PT. Patients have more medical needs than ever before, requiring clinically and technically astute nurses with developed critical thinking skills and advanced practice degrees.

SKILLED AND NONSKILLED SERVICES

Skilled Services: Healthcare services that require delivery by a licensed professional such as a registered nurse, physical therapist, occupational therapist, respiratory therapist, social worker, and speech therapist. Examples are wound care, vital signs assessment, health education, psychosocial counseling, catheter care, physical rehabilitation, and IV medication administration.

Nonskilled Services: Healthcare services that can be provided by a paraprofessional or an unlicensed person such as a home aide. Examples are close observation, bathing, feeding, and transferring from bed to chair.

Custodial Care: Care provided to patients to assist them in meeting the activities of daily living such as bathing and feeding. It also includes the services of a homemaker or housekeeper who can assist a patient in cleaning his or her home, food/meal preparation, or complete grocery shopping. This is a term sometimes used interchangeably with nonskilled care.

Respite Care: Care provided in an inpatient setting such as a hospital or an SNF for the purpose of offering the patient's usual caregiver (family member, friend, or another relative) the opportunity to get some rest. This type of care is common in the case of hospice patients and it is usually of the nonskilled type of services.

More patients are being sent home on weekends and late in the day, necessitating staff that is available and flexible.

Perhaps the most far-reaching change is occurring because of the Medicare risk contracts or Medicare Advantage Plans. Although this chapter discusses the criteria requirements of the traditional Medicare model, these risk contracts are touching all areas of healthcare, including home health agencies. As more members choose the Medicare HMOs, more hospitals, physician groups, and home health agencies are agreeing to capitation as a means of reimbursement (see Chapter 3: Reimbursement Concepts for further discussion on capitation). Although this puts home health agencies at some risk, it has some advantages over the traditional Medicare model. One must also remember that Medicare Advantage plans are obliged to provide at a minimum what traditional Medicare would have provided. Therefore, applying necessity criteria for home health services before such services are confirmed assures reimbursement and reduces financial risk on the provider and/or patient.

HEALTH INSURANCE CRITERIA

In the traditional Medicare model, both Part A and Part B cover home health services. Home health visits are authorized only if all of the following five criteria are met:

1. The patient is homebound, which means that he or she is confined to the home or that it would be a great hardship to come to an outpatient facility for treatment.

2. The care required includes intermittent (not necessarily daily, as in the SNF criteria) skilled nursing services and possibly physical, occupational, and speech therapies. These services should be offered on a part-time basis.

3. The care and services must be reasonable and necessary; that is, must be needed on the basis of the patient's health condition and appropriate for provision in the home environment.

4. The patient is under the care of a licensed physician who has set up a home health plan of care and oversees it. The plan is reasonable and necessary and is reviewed at least every 60 days.

5. The home health agency is Medicare certified, which means that the strictest federal standards are met.

HEALTH INSURANCE COVERAGE

It is doubtful whether this basic criteria set will change. However, the following covered and noncovered services should also be considered. Under the traditional Medicare model, covered home services (if the above-mentioned criteria are met) include those in the following discussion:

1. *Part-Time or Intermittent Skilled Nursing Care.* This may include up to 8 hours of reasonable and necessary care per day for up to 21 consecutive days (more, under some circumstances). Few cases are allotted 8 hours per day, and the key phrase is "reasonable and necessary." Most patients who need 8 hours of skilled nursing care are not in the home environment. Occasionally, this does happen. For the most part, stress this point to your patients that an average home visit from an RN lasts 45 minutes to 1 hour, not 8 hours, and that the services must be skilled.

2. *Physical or Speech Therapy.* PT and ST may be added if skilled nursing services have been assessed and they are deemed reasonable and necessary. This also opens the gate for OT and home health aide services.

3. *Home Health Aide Services.* If skilled nursing services have been assessed as necessary and physical or speech therapies have also been deemed necessary, the patient may qualify for intermittent home health aide services. Aide visits occur 2 to 3 times per week to help with personal care such as bathing, grooming, and changing linen. Home health aide services are rarely covered under private health insurance plans; check your patient's coverage for the exception.

4. *Home Social Services.* If skilled nursing services have been assessed, the patient may qualify for home social services. This is at times more effective than a SW seeing the patient in an acute or subacute facility. The patient is seen and assessed in his or her own environment, and this often elicits a more realistic appraisal of the social situation.

5. *Medical Supplies.* Supplies, such as dressings, will be made available if needed by the RN for the patient's care.

6. *DME.* DME must be approved, because not all equipment is covered under Medicare (Display 6-8). Medicare Part B covers medically necessary DMEs that a patient's physician prescribes for use in the home. To be covered, the DME must meet the following criteria:

   ❭ Durable (can withstand repeated use),
   ❭ Used for a medical reason,
   ❭ Not usually useful to someone who is not sick or injured,
   ❭ Used in the patient's home setting, and
   ❭ Has an expected lifetime of at least 3 years.

The amount a beneficiary pays for equipment varies on the basis of the type of equipment needed. A beneficiary is expected to pay an annual deductible for Medicare Part B services and supplies before Medicare begins to pay its share. After exhausting the deductible, a beneficiary may still be responsible for 20% coinsurance. For Medicare to cover DME, any needed equipment must be purchased from a Medicare participating supplier. *DME* or *home medical equipment* (HME) are terms that are used for a wide variety of products, services, and equipment. They are often classified into four general groups:

1. Basic mobility aids such as walkers, canes, and crutches;
2. Assistive devices to increase independence for ADLs, such as bathroom equipment (shower chairs, hand rails), kitchen equipment, ostomy supplies, or wound care supplies;
3. Mobility aids such as wheelchairs or electric beds;
4. High-technology equipment such as ventilators, IV pumps, parenteral and enteral nutrition, continuous chemotherapy infusion machines, apnea/sleep monitors, and technology that is custom-designed for quadriplegia/paraplegia/rehabilitation patients.

If a patient is in the hospital or another facility and DME is ordered, the CMS will allow 2 days before discharge for delivery of the equipment if the purpose of the delivery is to teach the patient how to use the equipment properly; the DME must also be for subsequent use in the patient's home. In the past, early delivery sent up red flags to the CMS. Case managers should document why the DME was delivered early and include the related patient/family teaching sessions. On the billing side, no bills must be rendered for the DME before the date of the patient's discharge from the facility to the home; the date of discharge is deemed to be the date of delivery. It is advisable that case managers coordinate the delivery of a DME to the hospital setting or patient's home in a timely manner that avoids the need for additional hospital days.

7. *Oxygen Therapy.* Some DME, such as oxygen, have strict criteria that must be met. The home oxygen criteria are added here because very many patients, such as those with COPD, diffuse interstitial lung

---

display 6-8

LIST OF DURABLE MEDICAL EQUIPMENT/SUPPLIES COVERED BY MEDICARE

a. Air-fluidized beds and other support services
b. Blood glucose monitoring devices and related supplies such as test strips
c. Canes (except for the blind)
d. Commode chairs
e. Continuous passive motion machines
f. Crutches
g. Dialysis machines
h. Home oxygen equipment and supplies
i. Hospital beds
j. Infusion pumps and related supplies (and some medicines used in infusion pumps if considered reasonable and necessary)
k. Nebulizers (and some medicines used in nebulizers if considered reasonable and necessary)
l. Ostomy supplies
m. Patient lifts (to lift patients from bed to wheelchair by hydraulic operation)
n. Sleep apnea and continuous positive airway pressure devices and accessories
o. Suction pumps
p. Therapeutic shoes
q. Traction equipment
r. Walkers
s. Wheelchairs (manual and power mobility devices)
t. Wound care supplies

disease, cystic fibrosis, bronchiectasis, or widespread lung cancer, need it for comfort and survival. (If the patient is admitted into hospice, the oxygen guidelines are not as strict as those for home care.)

Medicare may cover oxygen for home use provided it is (a) a part of the eligibility benefits under the Medicare insurance category; (b) reasonable and necessary for the diagnosis or treatment of illness or injury, or to improve the functioning of a malformed body organ; (c) ordered by a physic/provider; (d) furnished by a supplier who is enrolled in the Medicare program; and (e) in compliance with all applicable Medicare statutory and regulatory requirements.

Oxygen therapy coverage may include the following systems for furnishing oxygen, tubing, and related supplies for the delivery of oxygen, vessels for storing oxygen, and oxygen contents. Reasonable and necessary oxygen items and equipment for home use must also meet all of the following criteria:

1. The treating physician or other qualified provider (e.g., a nurse practitioner, physician assistant) has examined the patient and determined that the patient's condition is potentially expected to improve with oxygen therapy. Example of eligible conditions are: severe lung disease (e.g., COPD, diffuse interstitial lung disease, cystic fibrosis, bronchiectasis, and widespread pulmonary neoplasm) or hypoxia-related symptoms or findings (e.g., pulmonary hypertension, recurring congestive heart failure because of cor pulmonale, erythrocytosis, impairment of cognitive process, nocturnal restlessness, and morning headache).
2. The treating physician, a qualified provider, Medicare-certified supplier of laboratory services, or a hospital has conducted qualifying blood gas studies confirming the need for oxygen treatment.
3. The qualifying blood gas study values were obtained under specific conditions such as (a) during an inpatient hospital stay, however closest to but no earlier than 2 days prior to the hospital discharge date, with home oxygen therapy beginning immediately following discharge; or (b) during an outpatient encounter, but within 30 days of the date of initial certification while the patient is in a chronic stable state, at a time when the patient is not in a period of acute illness or of an exacerbation of his or her underlying disease.
4. The treating physician tried or considered alternative treatments and they were deemed clinically ineffective.

For initial certification for home oxygen therapy, the patient's blood gas study (either an arterial blood gas or an oximetry test) values must meet one of the three criteria groups described in Display 6-9.

Medicare also requires a face-to-face encounter with a healthcare provider as a condition for payment. On the basis of the Patient Protection and Affordable Care Act of 2010, one of the treating practitioners (providers) who perform a face-to-face assessment of the patient and an examination of the need for oxygen therapy must include either a physician (medical doctor, doctor of osteopathy, or doctor of podiatric medicine), nurse practitioner (NP), clinical nurse specialist, or physician assistant (PA). The following face-to-face encounter requirements must be met:

1. The treating provider must perform an in-person examination with the patient on or before the date of the Written Order (Prescription) Prior to Delivery (WOPD) and within the 6 months prior to date of the WOPD. It must also be on or before the date of delivery for the item(s) prescribed.
2. The treating provider must document that the patient was evaluated and/or treated for a condition that supports the need for the order for DME item(s) that pertain to home oxygen therapy.
3. A new face-to-face examination must be performed each time the provider orders a new prescription for one of the specified items of oxygen therapy.

Medicare requires a new prescription for all claims for payment of purchases or initial rentals for items not originally covered (or reimbursed) by Medicare Part B. Claims for items obtained outside of Medicare Part B (e.g., from another payor prior to Medicare participation, including Medicare Advantage plans) are considered new initial claims for Medicare payment purposes. A new prescription is also required when there is a change in the oxygen therapy order or needed supplies, if coverage determination requires periodic prescription renewal, and upon replacing an item or a supplier.

The patient's medical record must contain sufficient documentation of the patient's medical condition to substantiate the need for oxygen therapy in the home, including the type and quantity ordered and frequency of use. Such documentation must meet the coverage determination requirements and be included on the Certificate for Medical Necessity for Oxygen Therapy. The information in the patient's medical record may include the following:

- Patient's diagnosis;
- Duration of the medical condition;
- Patient's clinical course, whether worsening or improving, and prognosis;
- Results of the blood gas study;

CRITERIA GROUPS FOR ELIGIBILITY FOR INITIAL OXYGEN THERAPY UNDER MEDICARE BENEFITS PROGRAM

display 6-9

Group I Criteria:

Initial coverage of home oxygen therapy is limited to 12 months or the treating physician-specified length of need for oxygen, whichever is shorter. Criteria here include:

1. Patient is on room air while at rest (awake) when tested and the Arterial Oxygen Saturation is at or below 88%, or the arterial partial pressure of oxygen (PO_2) is at or below 55 mm Hg.
2. Patient tested during exercise and, if during the day while at rest, Arterial PO_2 is at or above 56 mm Hg or an Arterial Oxygen Saturation is at or above 89%, Arterial PO_2 is at or below 55 mm Hg or an Arterial Oxygen Saturation is at or below 88%, and documented improvement of hypoxemia during exercise with oxygen therapy.
3. Patient tested during sleep and if Arterial PO_2 is at or above 56 mm Hg or an Arterial Oxygen Saturation is at or above 89% while awake. Additional testing must show that Arterial PO_2 is at or below 55 mm Hg or an Arterial Oxygen Saturation is at or below 88% for at least 5 minutes taken during sleep. Or, a decrease in Arterial PO_2 of more than 10 mm Hg or a decrease in Arterial Oxygen Saturation more than 5% for at least 5 minutes associated with symptoms or signs more than 5% from baseline saturation for at least 5 minutes taken during sleep associated with symptoms or signs reasonably attributable to hypoxemia.

Group II Criteria:

Initial coverage of Group II home oxygen therapy is limited to 3 months or the length of time the treating physician specifies oxygen is needed, whichever is shorter. Such therapy may include portable oxygen systems if the patient is mobile within the home and the qualifying blood gas study is performed at rest while awake or during exercise. Medicare will deny portable oxygen as not reasonable and necessary if the only qualifying blood gas study is performed during sleep. Criteria here include:

1. Patient on room air at rest while awake when tested and an Arterial Oxygen Saturation of 89% at rest (awake) or an Arterial PO_2 of 56–59 mm Hg and (a) dependent edema suggesting congestive heart failure; (b) pulmonary hypertension or cor pulmonale, determined by the measurement of pulmonary artery pressure, gated blood pool scan, echocardiogram, or pulmonale on EKG (P wave greater than 3 mm in standard leads II, III, or AVF); or (c) erythrocythemia with a hematocrit greater than 56%.
2. Patient tested during exercise showing an Arterial Oxygen Saturation of 89% or an Arterial PO_2 of 56–59 mm Hg and (a) dependent edema suggesting congestive heart failure; (b) pulmonary hypertension or cor pulmonale, determined by the measurement of pulmonary artery pressure, gated blood pool scan, echocardiogram, or pulmonale on EKG (P wave greater than 3 mm in standard leads II, III, or AVF); or (c) erythrocythemia with a hematocrit greater than 56%.
3. Patient tested during sleep for at least 5 minutes showing an Arterial Oxygen Saturation of 89% or an Arterial PO_2 of 56–59 mm Hg and (a) dependent edema suggesting congestive heart failure; (b) pulmonary hypertension or cor pulmonale, determined by the measurement of pulmonary artery pressure, gated blood pool scan, echocardiogram, or pulmonale on EKG (P wave greater than 3 mm in standard leads II, III, or AVF); or (c) erythrocythemia with a hematocrit greater than 56%.

Group III Criteria:

Arterial Oxygen Saturation at or above 90% or Arterial PO_2 at or above 60 mm Hg.

Home oxygen therapy items and equipment may be covered for patients who are enrolled subjects in the following clinical trials as approved by the Centers for Medicare & Medicaid Services (CMS):

1. Long-term oxygen therapy: Patients in this clinical trial sponsored by the National Heart, Lung, and Blood Institute must have an arterial PO_2 from 56 to 65 mm Hg or an oxygen saturation at or above 89%.
2. Cluster headaches: Patients in this clinical trial are treated for cluster headaches when they have had at least 5 very severe unilateral headache attacks lasting 15–180 minutes when untreated.

- If portable oxygen therapy is needed, an indication that the patient is mobile within the home. This should include a detailed order for the oxygen therapy.
- Nature and extent of the patient's functional limitations;
- Other therapeutic interventions and results;
- Patient's past experiences with oxygen therapy and related items.

8. *Home Medications.* Some IV antibiotics, and other select medications, are now offered by Medicare in the home setting (see "Medicare" in Chapter 3 for further discussion).
9. *Psychological Nurse Assistance Under Specific Criteria.* This service may be needed by mental and behavioral health patients or for social support and counseling for patients immediately after discharge from a hospital stay.

10. *Services Not Covered.* Services that are not covered under traditional Medicare in the home setting include the following:

▶ General homemaker services such as shopping, cleaning, laundry, and meal preparation;

▶ Standby services such as 24-hour nurse or nurse aide care at home so the patient will not be left alone;

▶ Blood transfusions;

▶ Medications—except when specifically authorized; for example, medications used in a nebulizer and known to be medically necessary.

These strict criteria have been somewhat lifted with the Medicare Advantage Plans. They provide more freedom to choose and use whatever services best meet the patient's healthcare needs and the plan's financial needs. These Medicare plans act more like independent HMOs or even some Medicaid plans; criteria such as a 3-day hospitalization being required before a patient can be placed in an SNF or IV antibiotics not being provided for in the home setting no longer make any fiscal sense.

The previous regulations and limitations on Medicare patients are being lifted with Medicare Advantage Plans. The contracts allow "in lieu of" services. This means, for example, that if a patient could be discharged sooner from the hospital if he or she had, in addition to skilled nursing services, some personal care and provisions for meals, the home health agency has the flexibility to use in lieu of services. The hospital (which may also be capitated on these plans) may choose to reimburse the home health agency for these services in lieu of an extended hospitalization. This allowance of services is carefully monitored. Many studies have been developed to see if Medicare Advantage Plans are providing enough services. These studies have not been conclusive, and although some beneficiaries love the managed plans, others have found them to be inadequate.

Occasionally, the distinction between skilled services and nonskilled services becomes blurred. Essentially, a skilled service is one that is performed by a licensed professional such as an RN, physical therapist, respiratory therapist, occupational therapist, or speech therapist. The care given must be for the purpose of patient safety or medical stability. Display 6-10 shows some examples of skilled care and nonskilled care; these may be appropriately applied in any level of care.

Home health agencies are becoming more sophisticated, and many furnish almost any service that can be provided at the acute care level as long as the patient is medically stable. Even if the patient needs blood products (red blood cells [RBCs], fresh frozen plasma [FFP]), many home health agencies can accommodate such treatment/service; often this requires a 24-hour advance notice. However, emergency transfusions must be handled at a higher level of care. It is helpful to know which agencies can provide specified services. Like SNFs, home health agencies differ in their level of acuity. It is important to secure insurance authorization before calling an agency. Many insurance companies use only specific contracted agencies; calling the correct one at the onset can save a hospital day and a dose of aggravation.

When a case manager evaluates a patient for home health, a balance must be considered between what amount of self-care (with or without family help) can be safely attained and what other options are available from the payors. For example, sending a patient home with infusion services requires careful consideration. The patient or family must have cognitive and motor skills to perform the infusion safely, and motivation must be high to minimize poor compliance (especially in long protocols or ones in which there are uncomfortable side effects). Working with the infusion nurses and the patient is a value-added benefit to the case manager. An infusion nurse may also supply much of the patient education and instruction. Psychosocial issues that may only show up "in person" may be revealed. Ongoing on-site supervision is required with many central IV lines and also to keep the patient on track; it is also imperative when any type of drug abuse is suspected.

When making a referral to home health, the case manager must be aware of the patient's insurance benefits, limitations, and the amount of benefits already used. Knowing the insurance coverage used and how much remains will assist the coordination of care by preserving enough benefit for the full term (when possible); some very debilitated patients can take their benefits down to the wire by the end of the fiscal year. Although the home health agency must check these benefits (as they are dependent on payment), the case manager must provide the home health agency with some basic information including the patient's name, age, diagnosis, brief medical history, address, telephone number, insurance identification number, Social Security number (which may be different than the insurance identification number), date of birth, and the service(s) requested.

Some rules about referring patients to home health or other agencies and facilities affect case management. One rule, "Nondiscrimination in Post-Hospital Referral to Home Health Agencies and Other Entities," went into effect in 1997. On the basis of this rule, some issues that apply include:

▶ If any Medicare-certified agency requests to be put on a hospital's referral list, the hospital must comply. However, case managers must know what clinical expertise the patient may require and which facilities have those capabilities.

▶ The hospital cannot specify or recommend any particular home health agency to a patient. However, it is within the case management/patient advocate responsibilities to point out which facilities or agencies are in a patient's preferred network and

COMPARISON OF SKILLED AND NONSKILLED SERVICES

Service Provided	Skilled Care	Unskilled Care
Vital signs	Takes vital signs; may record and report worrisome vital signs to physician; observes cardiopulmonary stability; teaches caregiver how to take and record vital signs and when to call physician	Takes vital signs; may record and report to appropriate person
Medications	Administers medications, injections, sliding scale insulin, suppositories, eye drops; teaches families about medication, side effects, what to do for side effects, observation of the client's ability to comply with medication prescriptions, perhaps teach to give injections; assesses for negative side effects such as toxic levels	May assist in giving medications by reminding the client of the times to take them or helping open the lid
Skin care	Teaches diabetic skin and foot care; assesses skin for breakdown; performs aseptic wound care that may include packing, wet to dry dressings, dry dressing with sterile technique, irrigations; teaches family wound care; takes wound cultures, reports negative assessment to the physician or any negative change in skin condition; provides care for grade 3 or worse decubitus ulcers	Gives baths; applies lotions, ointments, creams, powders; applies nonsterile dressings; may reinforce dressings; provides treatment for chronic, noninfected surgical wounds and minor skin problems
Diet and nutrition	Instructs in special diets such as a low sodium, diabetic, renal, administer TPN, or tube feedings; instructs in the administration of TPN or tube feedings; assesses nutritional status, monitors and teaches fluid restriction or fluid status; teaches and assesses fluid intake and output; replaces some indwelling tubes	Helps prepare meals; assists with feeding
Elimination	Inserts straight catheter or Foley; teaches straight catheterizing procedure; observes and teaches signs of urinary tract infection; provides bowel or ladder training; provides care, observation, and teaching of new ostomy; assesses and reports skin breakdown	Cleans perineal area; empties drainage bags such as colostomies, indwelling Foley; measures urine; tests urine for sugar and acetone; assists client on and off commode; treats incontinence with diapers or rubber sheets; provides general care of colostomies or ileostomies including assisting in appliance changes in stable ostomy
Respiratory	Teaches and administers medical gases in the initial stages; in tracheostomy clients, suctioning and tracheostomy care; instructs client/family in tracheostomy self-care; observes and reports signs of respiratory distress or infection; administers oxygen; respiratory therapists may make ventilator changes per doctor's orders; provides small volume nebulizer and chest physiotherapy treatments and instruction	Administers medical gases after initial stages; provides small volume nebulizer and chest physiotherapy treatments after initial phase; assists in the tracheostomy care of a stable tracheostomy patient
Rehabilitation	Assesses and instructs in the use of assistive devices, range-of-motion exercises, gait training, transfers; administers hot packs, ultrasound treatments, TENS units, whirlpools in compliance with the doctor's prescriptions; the speech therapist assesses and helps with communication problems and swallowing difficulties	Supervises exercises taught to client; performs passive and active range of motion in conjunction with the physical therapist; assists in applying and removing prosthesis; assists with the use of canes, walkers, wheelchairs, and Hoyer lifts
Miscellaneous	Assesses any complex set of unskilled needs that requires putting together an overall picture of the patient for that patient's medical safety	

geographic region of residence; the patients should also be aware that they can choose outside their network, although the costs to them will likely be higher.

▶ If there are any financial interests, the hospital must make this clear on the referral lists.

Compliance with the above-mentioned rules is necessary for all Medicare-certified facilities and agencies. Therefore, documentation of these conversations is important. Some hospitals have entered their referral lists—including home health agencies, DME companies, hospice providers, SNFs, transportation companies, emergency response centers (Lifeline), hemodialysis centers, and nutrition programs—into laptop computers or hand-held devices; some even include maps, Medicare-specific qualifications, addresses, telephone numbers, and the clinical abilities of each company. Having such tools in place makes it easier for case managers to share such information with the patient and family; the tools allow easy access to such information at the point of care/patient's bedside and enhance consistency in the approach to discharge and transitional planning. Documentation should demonstrate which options were discussed, the physician or ordering provider recommendations, which agencies/facilities are financially related to the parent hospital, and the patient/family response to the choices.

▶ SPECIALTY PHARMACY PROVIDERS

Case managers are constantly looking for new ways to assist patients in maintaining the quality of their lives. One way to do this is to expedite as much personal independence as possible. In recent years, specialty pharmacy providers have been a case manager's ally in meeting this goal. Pharmacy management is often complex and requires round-the-clock expertise when anxious patients and families perceive something is wrong or unsure about how/when to administer a medication. A quality specialty pharmacy provider will enhance the case managers' clinical and financial expertise; trained professional pharmacists, nurses, and reimbursement experts add to the case manager's pool of resources when seeking the best alternative to high-cost, specialty biotherapy treatment.

Specialty staff provides teaching about medications as well as ongoing monitoring and evaluating of the patient's pharmacy needs. The additional clinical support enhances other case/disease/chronic care management goals in patients receiving injectable medications, especially those with complex regimens. It also:

▶ Increases patient compliance with recommended therapy.
▶ Increases patient education and knowledge of condition and treatment.
▶ Reduces the potential for patient errors in dosing and medication administration.
▶ Decreases patient's family caregiver and patient anxiety.
▶ Reduces the overall cost of delivery.
▶ May assist the case management organization/department in the collection of medication-related data.

Case managers will find working with these professionals to be of major assistance, but they should first make sure that the use of this level of provider is part of the patient's health benefits/insurance plan or can be negotiated. When a case manager makes a referral to a specialty pharmacy provider, the following sequence commences. The physician's office calls, electronically transmits, or faxes the patient's prescription to the company. The company's intake nurse calls the patient to explain the program and provide education on the medication, self-injection, side effects, and potential drug interactions. Because this is often provided "long distance," a visit or two from a home health agency may be needed for hands-on teaching about the medication and the self-injection. All deliveries in prefilled syringes or single dose vials are made to the patient's home. Following the initial prescription delivery, the patient is routinely contacted by a patient care coordinator who:

▶ Assesses patient compliance and progress.
▶ Inquires regarding the side effects from the medication.
▶ Arranges the next scheduled delivery.
▶ Verifies the shipping address.
▶ Refers the patient to the clinical staff for any clinical questions necessitating the need for follow-up.

The company's pharmacists and nurses are available for ongoing consultation with the patient, patient's family or caregiver, physician, and case manager 24 hours a day. This service has been very successful with long protocols of 12 to 18 months of medications with annoying side effects, and it has appeared to increase compliance. These providers have stringent quality programs. The pharmacies used should be those accredited through TJC.

▶ POLYPHARMACY

Although specialty pharmacy and home-based administration of complex IV medications have been in existence for a couple of decades, over the past several years, the use of acute care pharmacists for the patient's safe transitions of care has become increasingly popular. This service is known to have great benefits when a patient is placed on a complex regimen and multiple medications, often referred to as *polypharmacy*. An example is the prescribing of a statin, an ACE inhibitor, a beta-blocker, aspirin, and an antidepressant in the first year after a myocardial infarction. This does not even include any other medications for the treatment of conditions that are common with the incidence of cardiac disease such as poor renal function, increased cholesterol blood levels, and/or hypertension.

Polypharmacy is defined as the use of multiple medications (usually four or more) by a patient for two or more chronic health conditions. Generally, adults aged over 65 years of age experience polypharmacy; therefore, this situation is more common in the elderly. Over 40% of older adults living in their own homes or SNFs experience polypharmacy; some also suffer an intellectual disability that increases the risk for unsafe medication management practices. Unfortunately, there are many negative consequences associated with polypharmacy. Specifically, the burden of taking multiple medications has been associated with greater healthcare costs and an increased risk of adverse drug events (ADEs), drug interactions, medication nonadherence, reduced functional or cognitive capacity, and multiple geriatric syndromes (e.g., falls, urinary and bowel incontinence, diminished ability to perform ADLs and IADLs). Therefore, healthcare professionals, including case managers, must consider polypharmacy a special situation that requires careful assessment and monitoring to prevent significant ADEs, drug and drug interactions, unnecessary prescribing, or unsafe medications administration practices resulting in avoidable readmissions to the acute care/hospital setting.

The role of pharmacists has recently witnessed increased popularity as the issue of polypharmacy continues to grow in importance because of the aging population, as a result of the baby boomer generation getting older and an increased life expectancy associated with the ongoing improvements in healthcare services and technological advances. This is also complicated by the fact that the elderly tends to suffer from multiple chronic illness requiring an increased number of medications. Pharmacists, especially in the acute, ambulatory, and home health care settings, have become integral members of interdisciplinary healthcare teams managing the diverse and complex needs of the elderly patients and others who suffer complex and chronic health conditions. They are recognized for their knowledge of the pharmacologic profiles of complex drugs and the effects these drugs have on the individual patients. The roles pharmacists play may include the following:

▶ Deciding whether and how to reduce a list of medications a patient may have been prescribed;
▶ Thoughtful review of the list of prescribed medications and the development of a plan for safe administration and handling;
▶ Collaboration with other healthcare providers within and across case settings in the management of safe transition of care activities;
▶ Patient and family education and counseling to enhance self-management skills and knowledge. This has been demonstrated to prevent suboptimal (or unsafe) transitions of care practices and the need for unnecessary readmissions to the hospital setting or visits to the emergency department.

▶ MEDICARE EXTENDED CARE BENEFIT: THE 3-MIDNIGHT/3-DAY RULE

Within the Medicare list of benefits for beneficiaries is the "extended care benefit," commonly referred to as the 3-Midnight Rule or 3-Day Rule. This benefit means that

fee-for-service Medicare beneficiaries are entitled to the extended care benefit only if they have been in an acute inpatient care setting (i.e., hospital) for three consecutive calendar days. The days are counted on the basis of the number of times a patient appears on the hospital's midnight census. The 3-Midnight Rule applies only to patients who need posthospital skilled services in an SNF. Such patients tend to require extended care from an acute care stay. The 3-Midnight Rule does not apply to patients whose postacute care stay requires services from a home healthcare agency, or can be transferred to a LTC facility for posthospital rehabilitation (Birmingham, 2008).

The decision of the 3-Midnight Rule was made in the late 1960s on the basis of a national review of care patterns of Medicare patients. This review revealed that patients usually are in an acute care setting for 3 days on average before a discharge plan, including the identification of posthospital services needed, is developed. Although this review is very old, it is currently statutorily mandated and the requirement stands. Case managers must be careful about this rule and ensure compliance when they develop the discharge plans for their patients (Birmingham, 2008). The 3-Midnight/3-Day Rule is described in 42 CFR, §409.30 of the Social Security Act:

> A claim for extended care benefits generally qualifies for Medicare reimbursement only if the admission to SNF level of care is preceded by an inpatient hospital stay of at least three consecutive calendar days, not counting the date of discharge, and is within 30 calendar days after the date of discharge from a hospital.

In addition to the 3-Midnight Rule to qualify for an SNF admission, a patient must require "daily therapy." This means that the patient must receive skilled nursing services, skilled rehabilitation services, or a combination of both on a 7 days-a-week basis. In the event a patient whose care in an SNF is based solely on the need for skilled rehabilitation rather than skilled nursing services or both, he or she would meet the "daily basis" criteria when he or she receives the skilled rehabilitation services for at least 5 days a week. If the rehabilitation therapy services are provided less than 5 days a week, the "daily" requirement would not be met and the patient would not qualify for the extended care benefit (Birmingham, 2008).

It is important for case managers to track the number of days a patient is in the acute care setting before they finalize a patient's discharge plan to an SNF. For example, if a patient was transferred from another acute care facility where he or she has spent 1 day, this day counts in the new facility toward the 3-Day Rule extended care benefit. In contrast, however, if a patient spends time in the emergency department or at an observation level of care (i.e., "observation status") prior to an admission to a hospital, the time spent in these levels does not count toward the 3-Day Rule even though the patient is in an acute care setting. Another area that is of importance for case managers when deciding whether a patient meets the 3-Day Rule is examining the patient's previous acute care stays; perhaps the most recent discharge from a hospital setting occurred less than 30 days prior to the current admission.

Case managers must be aware that although Medicare beneficiaries are generally entitled to coverage for care they receive in an SNF, they can still be liable for substantial cost sharing related to the care they receive in an SNF if that care is not preceded by a hospital inpatient stay of at least 3 days. This is of great importance because Medicare beneficiaries are at increased financial risk for failing to meet this 3-day inpatient stay requirement, especially after the introduction of the outpatient observation status which may result in confusion when it is appropriate to begin to count the 3-day rule. Such events are likely to happen because patients today are receiving shorter inpatient hospital stays and overnight observation care as hospital outpatients, often for days at a time, which does not qualify for Medicare Part A-covered SNF care.

▶ HOSPITAL READMISSION REDUCTION PROGRAM

In October 2012, the CMS began to reduce its reimbursement (Medicare payments for inpatient PPS) for hospitals with excessive readmissions as compared to readmissions of other similar hospitals and nationally. This reduction in payment is viewed as a penalty under the value-based purchasing program, part of the Patient Protection and Affordable Care Act of 2010. The program is referred to as the Medicare Hospital Readmission Reduction Program (HRRP). Although it is communicated as an incentive program for those hospitals with commendable performance (competitive readmission rate), it is set up as a reimbursement reduction in a penalty structure for those with poor readmission rates.

The reimbursement reduction is not arbitrary; it applies a complex methodology that considers expected readmission rates and compares these with actual or observed rates for each of the diagnoses included in the program. It calculates the penalty on the basis of the amount of Medicare reimbursement received by the hospital for the excess readmissions. Medicare collects the excess payments from the hospital by applying a percentage reduction in the base Medicare inpatient claims payments related to the five diagnoses and not to exceed a certain cap amount. The percentage penalty in 2017 may reach up to 3% of the affected payments. In fiscal year 2013, the percentage penalty was 1%. Medicare applies a time period of three full years of hospital data in calculating the incentive or penalty. For example, the 2017 incentives or penalties are based on hospital readmissions that occurred from July 2012 through June 2015. There is always a time lag in these retrospective determinations which makes it more

of a challenge for case managers and other providers to improve performance of its readmission reduction efforts.

At the inception of the Medicare's HRRP, the focus was on readmissions occurring after *initial* hospitalizations for patients with three select diagnoses which included: acute myocardial infarction (AMI), heart failure (HF), and pneumonia. The current focus has expanded to include COPD, total hip and total knee replacement procedures, and coronary artery bypass graft surgery. To calculate a hospital's readmission rate for a diagnosis, the hospital must have discharged 25 Medicare beneficiaries or greater with that diagnosis. The CMS collects hospitals' overall readmission rates (regardless of initial diagnoses), but these overall rates are not currently used in the HRRP to calculate readmission penalties.

Hospitalization can be a disappointing event for anyone; they are even more concerning when they result in subsequent readmission(s). A hospital readmission occurs when a patient returns to the hospital setting for care as an inpatient within a specified time period after being discharged from the earlier (initial) hospitalization. For the Medicare benefits program, this period is defined as 30 days, and includes readmissions to any hospital, not just the hospital at which the Medicare beneficiary was originally hospitalized. Medicare today uses an "all-cause" definition of readmission, meaning that hospital stays within 30 days of a discharge from an initial hospitalization are considered readmissions, regardless of the reason for the readmission. This all-cause definition is used in calculating Medicare's national average readmission rate and each hospital's specific readmission rate. Starting in 2014, the CMS began making an exception for *planned* hospitalizations (such as a scheduled coronary angioplasty) within the 30-day window; these are no longer counted as readmissions.

Readmissions, especially those that happen for the same reason as prior admissions and within a short period of time such as 30 days, are stressful for everyone: the patient, healthcare provider, the case manager, and the payor. While many readmissions are unavoidable, wide variations in hospitals' readmission rates suggest that patients admitted to certain hospitals are more likely to experience readmissions compared with other hospitals. Higher readmission rates may also indicate quality and safety concerns, the likelihood of inadequate discharge/ transitional planning activities, and improper postdischarge services.

The Kaiser Family Foundation conducted a review of the impact of the HRRP. It studied the years since the program went into effect. The review showed the following observations (Boccuti & Cassillas, 2017):

▶ Total Medicare penalties assessed on hospitals for readmissions will increase to $528 million in 2017, $108 million more than in 2016. The increase is thought to be related mostly to more medical conditions being measured (increase from 3 to 5 conditions).

▶ Hospital penalties will average less than 1% of their Medicare inpatient payments compared with the maximum expected penalty of 3% in 2017. This is likely because of the strategies these hospitals have implemented to counter the financial risk imposed on the basis of the HRRP.

▶ In 2017, 78% of Medicare patient admissions are projected to be cared for in hospitals receiving either no readmission penalty or penalties of less than 1%. Fewer than 2% of Medicare patient admissions will be in hospitals receiving the maximum financial penalty of 3%.

▶ Nationally, beneficiary readmission rates started to fall in 2012, and have continued the same trend ever since. For example, readmission rates for AMI dropped from 19.7% in the period July 2008 to June 2011 to 17% in the period July 2011 to June 2014; while HF dropped from 24.7% to 22% and pneumonia dropped from 18.5% to 16.9% for the same time periods.

▶ Across all 5 years of the HRRP, certain types of hospitals are more likely than others to incur penalties. These include hospitals with relatively higher shares of low-income Medicare beneficiaries and major teaching hospitals. Neglecting to factor the social determinants of health into the risk adjustment methodology and the calculation of readmission rates and ratios of actual to expected has been a major area of contention among hospitals caring for the Medicare beneficiaries. On the bright side, however, Congress recently enacted legislation to incorporate a socioeconomic adjustment in how hospital performance is measured, on the basis of each hospital's share of inpatients who are dually qualified for Medicare and Medicaid. The benefit of such change remains to be evaluated.

Because of the HRRP, the CMS has been able to pressure hospitals to improve their transitional/discharge planning programs for the Medicare beneficiaries and reduce their readmission rates. Some of the strategies hospitals have implemented and found to be beneficial include, but are not limited to, the following:

▶ Integrating discharge and transitional planning into case management programs and roles;

▶ Approaching discharge/transitional planning as an interdisciplinary process that is characterized by collaboration among the various members of the healthcare team;

▶ Rounding on patients as an interdisciplinary care team daily, focusing on discussing the "plan for day, plan for the stay, and plan for post discharge/transition" with the patient and family and ensuring they are informed participants;

▶ Addressing the patients' nonmedical needs such as available transportation for postdischarge follow-up appointments with primary care providers, ability to obtain the medications prescribed including affordability, and the presence of the social support system to assist in self-care management. These needs if left unaddressed have been known to cause avoidable hospital readmissions or returns to emergency departments.

▶ Providing health education and counseling, especially regarding "red flags" or symptoms requiring immediate attention by healthcare providers (i.e., primary care provider) and healthy lifestyle behavior change (e.g., special diet, exercise program, and giving up smoking or alcohol consumption);

▶ Using personal health record where the patient's important health and personal information is stored and remains accessible at all times; for example, online via the World Wide Web.

▶ Communicating post discharge with the patient/family/caregiver to ensure continuity of care and that the patient is able to safely manage self-care. Successful communications are happening within 48 to 72 hours of discharge from the hospital. Other benefits of such communication are following up on medications and other prescribed treatments, confirming that appointments with primary care providers are finalized, assuring that home health services and DME are in place, and answering questions.

▶ Establishing partnership and collaborations across care settings and providers especially between the hospital and the postacute services. These efforts focus on improving handoff communications and assuring continuity of care.

▶ Establishing "transitions of care bridge" clinics to follow up on patients who do not have primary care providers. These patients are seen in these bridge clinics for up to 30 days while follow-up appointments with newly arranged primary care providers are confirmed. These clinics fill the gap that has been known to increase the need for readmissions because of delayed follow-up care.

▶ Assessing the patient's risk for readmission using valid and reliable tools. Such tools allow case managers to score patients on the basis of several elements/parameters (e.g., age over 65 years, gender, the number of prescribed and over-the-counter medications, the number of comorbidities, and health insurance status) that have demonstrated the ability to predict the likelihood for readmission. On the basis of the score, case managers then stratify patients into risk categories and employ specific case management activities appropriate for the risk category. These tools have recently become available in electronic documentation systems for ease of access and use. Some hospitals are applying these tools at multiple points throughout the patient's hospital stay; for example, upon admission, mid-stay, and day before discharge/transition.

▶ Assigning a coach or advisor to the patient to support the patient coping with the postdischarge course of care and enhancing adherence to complex medical regimens.

▶ Initiating the patient's discharge/transitional plan upon admission and reassessing the appropriateness of the plan regularly throughout the hospital stay to ensure it continues to meet the patient's needs and the required care after discharge from the hospital.

▶ Contacting the patients' primary care providers and notifying them of patients' admissions to the hospital and discharge from the hospital and informing them of any changes made to medications and treatments, and the need for timely follow-up care.

▶ Sharing data with all involved, including those attached internally and externally to the hospital. For example, holding a monthly meeting with postacute care providers to review performance relevant to discharge/transitional planning such as the number of patients transferred, turnaround time to accept a patient's transfer, the number of patients declined transfer, reasons for delays or declinations, and so on. In such meetings, opportunities for improvement and the development of improvement plans are discussed.

It is evident in all these strategies that case management is a key success factor. It is also important to recognize the value of well-organized discharge/transitional planning process in preventing avoidable hospital readmissions or visits to the emergency department, enhancing patients' experience of care, and increasing patients' self-management abilities. Additionally, such processes improve the quality of care, reduces healthcare costs/spending, and increases the hospital's likelihood to receive an incentive from the CMS as part of the Medicare HRRP.

Discharge/transitional planning has become a "continuous" process for all patients regardless of need rather than an occasional activity more relevant for only those with complex conditions. Because of the financial penalties associated with the HRRP, the view of healthcare providers and administrators of this process has also shifted to one of revenue-producing event rather than an expense. The process starts earlier in a patient's admission (sometimes even before admission to the hospital) and continues throughout the hospital course of care and across care settings and providers especially those the patient would require after discharge from the hospital. This reflects the true continuum of healthcare and provides the focus that case management practices have come to demonstrate and recognize as best practice.

Optimal discharge/transitional planning processes are those that involve various interdisciplinary members (e.g., physicians, NPs, PAs, case managers, SWs, nurses, dietitians, pharmacists, therapists, postacute care representatives, and DME agents, and others as indicated on the basis of patient/family needs). Most importantly, however, is the active participation of patients, families, and their caregivers. Clear roles and responsibilities are important for communicating the accountability of each team member. For example:

▶ Physicians, NPs, PAs, and nurses provide the patient/family information about medications, treatments, and follow-up care.

▶ Case managers set up home health services or coordinate the patient's transition to an SNF.

▶ SWs help a patient/family/caregiver navigate the emotional, social, and financial needs and concerns, especially as they relate to the health condition and hospitalization.

▶ Pharmacists educate the patient about the complex medications regimen (polypharmacy), strategize with the patient/family/caregiver how best to manage the complex medication schedule, and complete medication reconciliation.

▶ Therapists review the activity and exercise regimen with the patient/family/caregiver and strategize how best to manage ADLs.

▶ Dietitians counsel patients/families/caregivers about the special diet and how to adhere to it.

Additionally, effective discharge/transitional planning processes are those that consider the social determinants of health and their effects on the patient's care, health condition, quality of life, and well-being. In this regard, the team, including case managers and SWs, take the time to get to know patients personally and as human beings, understand their concerns, sensitive issues, and the barriers that have (or may in the future) affected their abilities to successfully self-manage their own health. Here, case managers are able to move from "doing to" or "doing for" to "doing with" the patient/family to improve patient activation, empowerment, and self-management knowledge, skills, and abilities. Case managers may also evaluate the patient's home environment for safety and appropriateness (e.g., availability of electricity, heat, and air-conditioning), affordability to secure the prescribed medications, concern for food insecurity, and the challenge of transportation to follow-up care appointments.

▶ THE INCENTIVES OF CHANGE

▶ Prospective Payment Systems

The Balanced Budget Act (BBA) of 1997 has created new reimbursement rules for postacute services. All postacute services that are reimbursed through Medicare have changed, from the cost-based system to the PPS. These include home healthcare, SNFs, rehabilitation facilities, subacute care facilities, and outpatient services/ambulatory care. At this time, there are no plans to limit beneficiaries of the traditional Medicare health plan to panels of contracted providers; however, the Medicare Advantage Plans still use managed care strategies.

Methods of Medicare reimbursement have often been the forerunner of reimbursement changes in other insurance arenas; therefore, it is important for the case manager to see what is changing and formulate strategies to assist patients to secure needed resources. In addition to the changes that occurred in the home health, rehabilitation, ambulatory care, and SNF sectors, case managers must also be well aware of the definition of a hospital discharge for top 10 diagnoses (see "The Discharge/Transfer Rule—The Top 10 DRGs" in this chapter). In domino fashion, this change will affect case management plans through the continuum of care/health and human services.

Reimbursement rates, in the form of PPS, DRGs, and per diem methods (Display 6-11), motivate healthcare agencies and facilities to practice patient care under various incentives. It is the incentive behind the game plan that must be understood for the case manager to truly advocate for the patient and family.

Per diem rates tailor the reimbursement to the number of days a patient stays in a healthcare facility for care; a set price is paid for each day without regard to actual costs incurred. Traditionally, per diem rates encouraged longer stays, up to the use of all possible days, and there was less incentive to discharge a patient home or transfer to another facility for continued care. However, under the recent federal payment structures, this type of thinking is no longer considered a successful strategy. When a facility is paid on a fixed per diem rate, it must make careful choices of admitting patients who clearly require less expensive and lower levels of medical care. Ventilator-dependent patients in SNFs, for example, may be reimbursed as low as $185 per day in some geographic locations. With this level of reimbursement, keeping a patient in a facility longer will not equate to more dollars. Per diem reimbursement also supports the incentive to use the least amount of resources per day. Cost-efficient care is critical to survival; however, quality of care must also be maintained.

REIMBURSEMENT METHODS

display 6-11

▶ *Cost-based reimbursement* is based on the actual costs of a patient's care.
▶ *PPS/DRG* is a method of payment to providers at a preestablished rate, regardless of the providers' actual costs.
▶ *Per diem reimbursement* is a fixed daily rate based on the acuity of the patients.

The PPS in a subacute level now tailors the payment to the level of the patient's functional status. This is different from the PPS reimbursement method (i.e., DRGs) applied in the acute care setting, which tailors the payment to the diagnosis. When the PPS was instituted in the hospital setting in the 1980s, the hospital incentive was discharge of the patient as early as possible, sometimes bordering on premature discharge. The hospital was essentially paid a set amount (i.e., the DRG case rate) for the episode of care; keeping the patient in the hospital cost the facility more money, but no more funds would be reimbursed. This incentive to move the patient to another level of care as quickly as possible caused the proliferation of subacute centers where care could be rendered to still fairly sick patients.

The result was that the subacute sector of healthcare grew at an alarming rate. In 1996 subacute care in the United States cost about $28 billion; today, the number exceeds $55 billion. At this rate of growth, the Medicare funds simply cannot sustain the costs. Something has to be done. The reimbursement changes we have seen or are now seeing are attempts to stay the tide.

Subacute care has basically been paid on the old fee-for-service model. External case managers who must negotiate costs when moving patients down the continuum of care have, on occasion, come up against a situation in which the subacute costs quoted exceeded the ICU or floor costs in the hospital. These are not isolated cases and explain why the PPS has moved into the postacute arena. From a subacute perspective, this meant a huge change in reimbursement from more than $1,000 per day to perhaps $300 less per day; this is certainly an incentive to be more efficient in providing care.

The CMS and Congress felt that these changes would affect two situations:

1. At least for a set of hospital discharge DRGs, described in the following paragraphs, incentives for early discharges would be affected. The incentive would change, as the hospital would not have the incentive to discharge/transfer the patients as quickly. In the future, it will be interesting to note if, for these DRGs, more patients go home rather than to SNFs after the hospital because of the few extra days in acute care.
2. It would control costs at the subacute level.

Changes in the reimbursement structure of the home health industry were also destined to happen; the cost of that care has risen dramatically. For example, in 1990, $3 billion was billed for home health services; in 1997 this escalated to $20 billion. In 1998, at least 3.8 million Medicare beneficiaries received some form of home care. The home health fee-for-service reimbursement structure encouraged providers to use as many services and visits as possible. By changing the reimbursement structure to the PPS (and including some cap limits), there is no longer an incentive to prolong services; rather, the intelligent choice would be to structure the care for efficient healing and independence of the beneficiary. Today, risk is even more complicated with the advent of bundled payment structures and value-based purchasing approaches to reimbursement.

Some of this growth was because patients are using home healthcare as a reasonable and correct level of care; some of the cost has become the target of Medicare's fraud, waste, and abuse examinations. It is estimated in some areas of the country that 40% of payments made by Medicare for home health services were improper. Consider that the original intent of Medicare home health benefits was short-term assistance. As many case managers are aware, traditional Medicare patients have received home health services for much longer than originally intended. This is not always inappropriate, and those patients may otherwise suffer.

Were the reimbursement changes necessary or unfair? Critics of the new reimbursement structure feel that there are many inequities in the home health reimbursement fee schedule. One major complaint is that the reimbursement is based on very old data, a time when patients were not sent home as medically intensive as they are today. Some home health agencies and SNFs (whose per diem rates are based on old data as well) are feeling the impact to such a degree that they may not survive. However, the changes had to happen; the healthcare funds could no longer sustain the growth. Through governmental agencies, healthcare providers will be observed for fraud and abuse. Underneath it all, the CMS is looking for the right incentives: to promote access to care and to provide quality care—the same incentives as case managers. One thing is clear: case management is being mentioned time and again as a critical piece to balance the incentives, control costs, and ensure quality and safe patient care.

▶ The Postacute Discharge/Transfer Rule—The Transfer DRGs

The CMS became concerned with the lessening of lengths of stay over the years. The DRG-based payment system was originally formulated on reimbursement for a Medicare LOS that was approximately 40% higher than was experienced in 1998. The tremendous numbers of transfers to the subacute arena did not go unnoticed. As an outgrowth of the BBA of 1997, and beginning in October 1998, there were 10 DRGs (initial number of transfer DRGs) that would no longer be considered a discharge from an acute care setting and an admission to a postacute setting; rather, they were labeled Transfer DRGs. The CMS would reimburse hospitals for patients that fell into one of these DRGs under a "post-acute care transfer payment policy." The postacute care settings included in the transfer policy are:

- ▶ LTC hospitals
- ▶ Rehabilitation facilities
- ▶ Psychiatric facilities
- ▶ SNFs
- ▶ Home healthcare when the patient receives clinically related care that begins within 3 days after the hospital stay
- ▶ Rehabilitation distinct part units located in an acute care hospital or CAH
- ▶ Psychiatric distinct part units located in an acute care hospital or CAH
- ▶ Cancer hospitals
- ▶ Children's hospitals.

The original Transfer DRGs were chosen because of their high volume of use in postacute transfers and included strokes, amputations for circulation disorders, skin grafts, hip procedures, and tracheostomies. This ruling also included "swing beds," which was not a popular rule with the American Hospital Association. The Transfer DRGs at the time accounted for about 30% of the Medicare patients, each representing between 2% and 6% of the total Medicare volume. The number of Transfer DRGs has increased over time; there were 29 Transfer DRGs in Fiscal Year (FY) 2004; 182 by October 1, 2005 (or FY 2006); 190 by FY 2007; 273 by FY 2008; and today a total of 275 DRGs are impacted by this rule. It is reported that today over 6 million Medicare hospital discharges per year fall into the Transfer DRGs, accounting for about 42% of the total Medicare annual discharges.

Patients who fall in one of the Transfer DRGs are considered transfers if:

- ▶ The patients subsequently receive care in an SNF or a home health agency after discharge from the hospital.
- ▶ The services are related to the hospitalization.
- ▶ The services are provided within 3 days of the hospitalization.

From a hospital's fiscal viewpoint, this translates into a situation in which the transfer of any Medicare patient who falls into one of the Transfer DRGs before the "geometric mean day" of the DRG would result in the hospital being penalized. The reduction in reimbursement follows a complicated formula that depends on the patient's actual LOS and the geometric mean LOS for that DRG. It is not possible for a hospital to increase its Medicare revenues; the best it can do is minimize its reduction in payments. Case managers in the acute care settings play an essential role in the review and prevention of potential discharges that are thought to fall within the transfer DRGs. Their role is considered integral to reducing or preventing a hospital's financial risk and standing with the CMS—in the form of adherence to the standards and CoP.

An early transfer patient is one who is discharged more than 1 day sooner than the geometric mean LOS of patients in that DRG. The hospitals are paid 50% when the patient is admitted; the remaining 50% is divided by the geometric mean LOS and paid as a per diem. Fiscally sophisticated hospitals analyze the expenditures of the last few days before the geometric mean day to determine if the per diem losses are more—or less—than the actual cost of care. In some cases, it may even be fiscally smarter to transfer sooner (assuming the patient is stable) to a lesser level of care; however, incentives that result in clinically compromising situations would be a poor choice and likely to be noticed. Under the PPS, hospitals are given financial incentives to minimize Medicare patients' LOS; however, these early transfers actually increase Medicare costs because Medicare pays for care in both the acute and postacute settings.

The acute strategies must complement the needs on the subacute care side; with the reimbursement changes at the subacute level, this could pose problems. If lower acuity patients are admitted to SNFs because the hospital kept the patient in acute care until the geometric mean day, their reimbursement level may be less. Networks of acute and subacute providers will be best equipped to work out solutions that are good for everyone. However, it is the case manager, as a patient advocate, who must be aware of any subtle strategies that may not be in the patient's best interests.

Hospital case management can play a huge role in keeping this rule a relatively minor inconvenience. With fraud, waste, and abuse monitoring going on at all levels of care, hospitals are being watched for inappropriate transfers to postacute care settings. When a patient is discharged, the hospital may bill under the total DRG rate. When a patient is transferred, the hospital must bill under the per diem rate; if home health or SNF care is ordered, the hospital must bill as a transfer rather than a discharge. This can be a problem because physicians may arrange for SNF placement or home healthcare after a patient is discharged from the hospital. If this happens with these Transfer DRGs, and the hospital bills for the total DRG, it could be considered fraud in the eyes of Medicare. Therefore, hospitals must be aware of orders for postacute services for these patients, even if they are ordered 1 to 3 days after discharge. Case managers are the link between the ordering physician and the proposed care; postacute follow-up care becomes even more essential.

The transfer DRGs could be a useful tool for case managers. A hospital with very few early transfers might need to reexamine its LOS controls and its transfer policies. A hospital that is keeping a large fraction of its Medicare patients longer than the Medicare geometric mean LOS may be losing money under the inpatient PPS. Some of the strategies case managers may implement to prevent financial risk and suspicion of fraud and abuse include the following:

▶ Implementation of tighter utilization review and management controls;

▶ Considering some form of partnerships with other SNFs, home health agencies, or rehabilitation facilities;

▶ Taking a new look at any clinical pathways for these Transfer DRGs;

▶ In addition to optimal care, considering the geometric mean day for the most appropriate timing of the transfer to a subacute level of care, such as home health or SNF;

▶ Avoiding an early discharge, unless if it is necessary and appropriate, because it could lessen the hospital reimbursement;

▶ An otherwise transferable patient should not be kept in the hospital for fiscal reasons; these are the types of fiscal strategies that the CMS is monitoring. If all this sounds like a "between a rock and a hard place" scenario, it may be.

A patient's early transfer may be a safe alternative that may fiscally benefit the SNF level of care; it may also penalize the hospital financially. Holding the patient until the geometric mean day will admit a patient to an SNF with less acuity and less SNF reimbursement; it may even leave the SNF out of the loop if the patient is well enough to go home directly. In such instances, home health agencies may surface as the winners. These are the situations that are destined to twist the already convoluted healthcare system into another curve.

From the inception of the Postacute Transfer Rule, the CMS acknowledged that errors can occur with discharge status assignment by hospital personnel. Audits by the Office of Inspector General which started in 2004 have confirmed that hospitals were significantly overpaid and edits were finally implemented. Today, the CMS allows hospitals to edit the discharge status assignment even after claims submission. The Medicare contractors are responsible for identifying "overpayment" situations after the receipt of claims from the hospital and postacute providers. The CMS has made it clear from the start that the development of edits would apply only to overpayments; hospitals would have to perform their own validation of proper discharge status code assignment to detect incidents of underpayments. Although such situations are likely to occur, recovering the underpayment amounts from the CMS remains a challenge.

In the past several years, the CMS has developed the Recovery Audit Contractor (RAC) program to identify overpayments for claims, including those impacted by the Postacute Transfer Rule. This remains a controversial issue today, as ironically the RACs identify underpayments through a computer algorithm and do not validate the level of care with postacute providers. The RACs are "recovering" Transfer DRG overpayments, whereas the hospitals/providers are left to uncover underpayments themselves. There are a number of reasons for Postacute Transfer DRG underpayments. For example:

▶ When assigning the discharge status code to the patient's claim, the hospital does not always have enough information available to make the proper assignment. The discharge plan may lack the level of care specificity that is needed in order for the proper assignment to occur. In this situation, assumptions may be made on the basis of the name of the postdischarge care provider.

▶ Many postacute care providers furnish multiple disciplines of care. Without accurate documentation, the wrong discharge status code may be selected, leading to an underpayment.

▶ Sometimes, home health services are planned for the patient's postdischarge course of care, but the patient or family makes other arrangements or delays these services. For example, instead of home health care by a licensed home health agency, the patient's family may cancel the services and decide to take care of the patient at home themselves. The hospital remains unaware that the patient's plan of care has changed, and as a result, the hospital is reimbursed at a lower level, and an underpayment has occurred.

▶ Some discharge status codes are used infrequently, and occasionally a hospital billing system is missing a particular code. In this case, the "next best" code will likely be assigned, and this code may inappropriately trigger the Postacute Transfer Rule when the CMS determines the hospital's reimbursement for that claim.

▶ HOME HEALTHCARE SERVICES

Over the past two decades, many changes have taken place in Medicare benefits, especially in the areas of home health and SNF benefits. The cost-based (or fee-for-service) system has been replaced with the PPS, which controls reimbursement to home care agencies; it does not cap the number of visits that a patient can receive or limit the amount of money that can be spent on any one patient. As a result, home health agencies need to look more closely than ever before at what the cost of each patient may be. Admitting practices and policies are likely to change because of the PPS, and case managers may find that some patients are harder to place in home care than in the past. Case managers need to know how much home health benefits have been used for each patient. For many Medicare beneficiaries, this may entail looking at usage in various states, as many retired people live in different places in the winter and summer (such people are called "snowbirds" in Arizona and Florida). A critical eye on the quality of care is more important than ever, as is the choice of agency. Just as there are various levels of clinical efficiency within the SNF level of care, home health agencies may start to become more expert in some areas and with certain types of patients than before.

▶ Specific Benefit Changes

VENIPUNCTURE

In the past, any Medicare beneficiary who qualified for home blood draws (venipunctures) was automatically considered eligible for an extensive selection of home services. A new venipuncture plan closes what the CMS felt was an expensive loophole. Home blood draws are still a covered item. However, two issues have been addressed: (1) the blood draws are provided by a laboratory technician rather than a home health nurse (unless there are no laboratories in rural areas) and (2) laboratory draws are no longer an automatic trigger that allows all other home care services to be initiated. Any homebound Medicare patient who requires home blood draws will receive them; any homebound Medicare patient who requires blood draws and other home healthcare services will not be denied those benefits. For example, an 82-year-old man was confined to bed after hip surgery. He also suffered from severe rheumatoid arthritis and was status-post stroke. He was eligible for home venipuncture, home PT, and probably some home aide services.

DIABETIC SUPPLIES

Effective July 1998, Medicare coverage for glucose monitors and testing strips expanded. All diabetics now qualify for glucose monitoring devices (under the DME benefit), strips, lancet devices, lancets, glucose control solutions for checking the accuracy of the test strips, and monitors. This applies, regardless of insulin intake, if a Medicare patient's diabetes would be better controlled through testing blood sugar. However, a 20% coinsurance applies on all diabetes supplies. The patient should ask his or her physician to write a prescription, which should state how often the blood sugar is to be tested; this will indicate how many test strips will be dispensed. Medicare covers the quantity of test strips ordered.

▶ What to Do If You Are an External Case Manager

▶ Remember that the physician is the key decision maker. It is ultimately the physician who will assess the patient and determine whether the patient's care is still medically necessary and therefore may still qualify for home healthcare.

▶ Be realistic: Some benefits have been generously provided for in the past; with new reimbursement methods, companies will have to be managing more comprehensively if they are to survive. Personal care services may be one area that will be monitored closely by home health agencies.

▶ Keep current about Medicare reimbursement and benefit changes: This knowledge is needed if you are to strategize about how best to meet the needs of your patients.

▶ If the patient/family or another case manager calls with home health concerns, reassess the medical condition to evaluate the appropriate level of services. If you feel that the home healthcare that has been ordered remains medically necessary, detail the orders again and document them carefully in the medical record.

▶ What to Do If You Are Employed in a Home Health Agency

▶ Educate employees about the new changes in benefits and reimbursement. They must understand reimbursement challenges to help plan for care and services in a way that is beneficial for all parties. Assist employees with ways to handle beneficiary questions about changes in services. SWs, trained in role-playing, can be valuable for this function. Emphasize that the patients and families may be traumatized by the impending changes. This may be especially true for fee-for-service beneficiaries who have been receiving ample services; they have a point of comparison and may not like the cutbacks.

▶ Use proven strategies to provide quality services in a cost-efficient manner. These may include the use of:
a. Case management (strongly recognized in the literature as an important strategy).
b. Clinical pathways/case management plans, especially those that cross levels of care.
c. Disease or chronic care management strategies.
d. Protocols, guidelines, and care plans.
e. Coordination of care across multiple providers and settings (those involved in the care of a patient or settings being considered for continued care).

▶ Monitor provider behavior: It may appear to be an intelligent strategy to admit only low-cost beneficiaries (i.e., "cherry picking") and discharge patients quickly. These strategies present their own challenges, legally and ethically. Overextending services to non-Medicare patients may also lead to negative consequences.

▶ Determine new strategies to cope with consolidated billing rules. This may include partnering/contracting with other service providers or using staff strategies such as outsourcing (see "Consolidated Billing" later in this chapter).

▶ Use proven case management strategies for quality, cost-efficient patient care. This includes providing the appropriate number of visits, the duration

of visits, the skill level of the caregiver, and the appropriate use of DME and supplies.

▶ Focus on the patient.

▶ SKILLED NURSING FACILITY CHANGES

▶ Reimbursement Changes

Since the 1980s, Medicare has reimbursed the SNF level of care on a cost-based/fee-for-service system. Essentially, this meant that SNFs would bill for the costs of care plus a markup; this left little incentive to control costs. The old fee-for-service has now been changed, and traditional Medicare is looking more like managed care. Reimbursement today is based on a PPS method. This level of care (SNFs) and the related PPS reimbursement method has revealed a growth in case management use. There are three reasons for this:

1. SNFs are reimbursed by the PPS. The CMS has been monitoring for any changes in quality of care that potentially accompany the reimbursement changes. Like hospitals that have experienced the PPS, SNFs require the skills of case managers to ensure quality of care for the residents, while containing costs.
2. The demographics are changing; baby boomers are aging (more demand for SNFs).
3. Life expectancy is increasing (more demand for SNFs), especially because of technological and treatment advances. The elderly population today also suffers from increasingly complex and chronic health conditions that require higher intensity of healthcare resources.

SNF survival requires some significant changes in the way it does business. Unlike the diagnosis-based DRGs that are used to reimburse acute care (hospitals), resource utilization groups (RUGs) base their SNF payments on the use of resources. The RUGs adjust the federal rate calculated for SNF reimbursement. The payment is based on a per diem and reflects routine care, rehabilitation, and other ancillary costs (e.g., laboratory tests, radiographs, medications, etc.) of covered SNF services furnished to beneficiaries under Medicare Part A. The reimbursement is adjusted for case mix and geographic variation in wages using the hospital wage index. Case mix adjustment is completed using the resident classification system (RUGs IV) on the basis of data from resident assessments (the Minimum Data Set [MDS] 3.0) and relative weights developed from staff time data.

The RUG IV model consists of eight major categories (Display 6-12) and 66 specific groups. For example, the highest major category, Rehabilitation Plus Extensive Services, includes 23 groups, representing 10 different levels of rehabilitation services. In the 66-group model, the residents in the Rehabilitation Plus Extensive Services

display 6-12

CHARACTERISTICS OF THE RESOURCE UTILIZATION GROUPS IV

Major RUG IV Categories	Characteristics
Rehabilitation plus extensive services	Residents in this category have a minimum activity of daily living (ADL) dependency score of 2 or more; are receiving physical therapy, occupational therapy, and/or speech-language pathology services while being a resident; and receiving complex clinical care for needs involving tracheostomy care, ventilator/respirator, and/or infection isolation.
Rehabilitation	Residents in this category are receiving physical therapy, occupational therapy, and/or speech-language pathology services while being residents.
Extensive services	Residents in this category have a minimum ADL dependency score of 2 or more and are receiving complex clinical care and have needs involving: tracheostomy care, ventilator/respirator, and/or infection isolation while being residents.
Special care—high	Residents in this category have a minimum ADL dependency score of 2 or more, and are receiving complex clinical care or have serious medical conditions involving any one of the following: comatose, septicemia, diabetes with insulin injections and insulin order changes, quadriplegia with a higher minimum ADL dependence criterion (ADL score of 5 or more), chronic obstructive pulmonary disease with shortness of breath when lying flat, fever with pneumonia, vomiting, weight loss, or tube feeding meeting intake requirement, parenteral/IV feeding, or respiratory therapy.
Special care—low	Residents in this category have a minimum ADL dependency score of 2 or more, and are receiving complex clinical care or have serious medical conditions involving any of the following: cerebral palsy with an ADL dependency score of 5 or more, multiple sclerosis with an ADL dependency score of 5 or more, Parkinson's disease with an ADL dependency score of 5 or more, respiratory failure and oxygen therapy, tube feeding meeting intake requirement, ulcer treatment with 2 or more ulcers like venous ulcers, arterial ulcers, or Stage II pressure ulcers, ulcer treatment with any Stage III or IV pressure ulcer, foot infections or wounds with the application of dressing, radiation therapy, or dialysis while being residents.
Special care—clinically complex	Residents in this category are receiving complex clinical care or have conditions requiring skilled nursing management, interventions, or treatments involving any of the following: pneumonia, hemiplegia with an ADL dependency score of 5 or more, surgical wounds or open lesions requiring treatment, burns, chemotherapy, oxygen therapy, IV medications, or transfusions while being residents.
Behavioral health symptoms and cognitive performance	Residents in this category have a maximum ADL dependency score of 5 or less and behavioral or cognitive performance symptoms, involving any of the following: difficulty in repeating words, temporal orientation, or recall, difficulty in making oneself understood, short-term memory, or decision making, hallucinations, delusions, physical behavioral symptoms toward others, verbal behavioral symptoms toward others, rejection of care, or wandering.
Reduced physical function	Residents in this category primarily have a need for support with activities of ADLs and general supervision.

Compiled from North Dakota, Department of Human Services, Medical Services Division. (2013, October). *A step by step guide to assigning a classification for RUG IV*. North Dakota: Author.

groups have the highest level of combined nursing and rehabilitation need, whereas residents in the Rehabilitation groups have the next highest level of need. Therefore, on the basis of the intensity of the level of need, the 66-group model has the Rehabilitation Plus Extensive Services groups first followed by the Rehabilitation groups, the Extensive Services groups, the Special Care High groups, the Special Care Low groups, the clinically complex groups, the Behavioral Symptoms and Cognitive Performance groups, and the Reduced Physical Function groups.

The SNF resident assessment instrument (RAI) helps nursing home staff in gathering definitive information on a resident's strengths and needs, which must be addressed in an individualized plan of care. It also assists staff with evaluating goal achievement and revising the plans accordingly by enabling the nursing home to track changes in the resident's status. Involving health and professional disciplines such as nursing, dietary, social work, PT, OT, speech-language pathology, and pharmacy in the RAI process fosters a more holistic approach to resident care and strengthens team communication. The RAI consists of three parts: the MDS version 3.0, the Care Area Assessment (CAA) process, and the RAI Utilization Guidelines. Utilization of the three parts of the RAI yields information about a resident's functional status, strengths, weaknesses, and preferences. It also offers guidance on further necessary assessment once problems have been identified.

The *MDS* is a core set of screening, clinical, and functional status elements, including common definitions and coding categories. These form the foundation of a comprehensive assessment for all residents of SNFs that are certified to participate in Medicare or Medicaid benefit programs. The items in the MDS standardize communication about resident problems and conditions within SNFs and with outside agencies. The MDS assessments are of various types, including the comprehensive admission, quarterly, discharge, entry tracking, and PPS item sets.

The *Care Area Assessment Process* is designed to assist the clinician to systematically interpret the information recorded on the MDS. Once a care area has been triggered, SNF providers use current, evidence-based clinical resources to assess this potential problem and determine whether to develop a plan of care for it. The CAA process helps the clinician to focus on key issues identified during the assessment process, so that decisions as to whether and how to intervene can be explored with the resident. Specific components of the CAA process include:

- Care Area Triggers (CATs) which are specific resident responses for one or a combination of MDS elements. The triggers identify residents who have or are at risk for developing specific functional problems and require further assessment.
- CAA is the further investigation of triggered areas, to determine if the CATs require interventions and care planning.
- CAA Summary Section which provides a location for documentation of the care area(s) that have triggered from the MDS and the decisions made during the CAA process regarding whether to proceed to care planning.

The *Utilization Guidelines* provide instructions for when and how to use the RAI. These include instructions for completion of the RAI as well as structured frameworks for synthesizing the MDS and other clinical information.

The MDS consists of 21 sections and over 100 items; originally the MDS was more of a care plan and clinical assessment than a billing mechanism (CMS, 2009a, b; 2016). The assessment established by the MDS 3.0 determines under which of the 66 RUGs a patient will be classified. The RUGs group then sets the prospective per diem rate that each SNF will be paid by Medicare for treating a particular patient. The RUGs IV are based on:

- A hierarchy of eight major resident (i.e., the patient) types;
- The resident's functionality; and

- The intensity of services or additional problems or services.

Resident functionality is measured through ADLs that are calculated on the basis of the assessment in the MDS 3.0; assessment includes functional levels such as bed mobility, transfers, toilet use, and eating (parenteral vs. IV vs. tube feeds). All RUG IV categories are classified using an ADL score; this score can range from 0 to 16, depending on the response to the MDS 3.0 questions. The RUGs IV score is not only important on admission to the SNF; the prior activity of the patient may also affect the RUGs rate. The patient may fall under the extensive care category if:

- He or she received IV or parenteral feeding in the past 7 days, or
- He or she received IV medication, suctioning, tracheostomy care, or ventilator treatment in the past 14 days.

In effect, the SNF would receive "credit" for prior services rendered to this patient. This is why an on-site preadmission screening by the case manager is so important before admission to the SNF. Although the SNF will have an assessment period, it will still be advantageous to know as much about the patient as possible before admission. This task will certainly require a case manager with the skills of Sherlock Holmes and one who has a reputation with the SNFs of being a trusted professional. Any information used to place a patient in a particular RUGs IV category must have adequate backup documentation both in the SNF and before the SNF admission (7- to 14-day activity). This preadmission screening will be a valuable tool to assess if the patient is deemed skilled by Medicare's standards. Accepting a patient into an SNF with misinformation could cost the facility financially and have painful consequences for the patient and family. The case manager must carefully review all pertinent information and make decisions involving the multidisciplinary care required.

The MDS assessments must be done accurately and on time. Penalties in the form of the lowest default rates are imposed for late assessments; there are no exceptions. When a Medicare beneficiary enters the nursing home for the first time:

- A comprehensive, multidisciplinary assessment must be completed by the 5th or 14th day (this day can be chosen by the SNF).
- A 5-day assessment must have an assessment reference date of any day between day 1 and 8 (and must be completed by day 14).
- A 14-day assessment is required with an assessment reference date that may be as early as day 11 or as late as day 19, because there is a 5-day grace period.
- Other assessments are due on days 30, 60, and 90.

▶ PT, OT, ST, AND RESPIRATORY THERAPY CHANGES

In FY 1995, CMS data showed that in SNFs, almost 50% of the charges are for room and board; 30% are for rehabilitation services. In light of these data, many changes have been made under the PPS in the rehabilitation services area. The PPS reimbursements mandate that the whole rehabilitation service area looks at the way it delivers care. The RUGs IV categories include reimbursement for the minutes of therapy delivered directly to the patient. The time required to perform an initial evaluation, develop treatment goals, and create the plan of care for the patient cannot be counted as minutes of therapy received by the patient. Because actual minutes of therapy delivered directly to the patient are so important for the RUGs IV level, many therapists have been told to carry stopwatches. Inaccuracy of minutes could result in a lower RUGs IV level, which could equate to $30 per day in lost reimbursement for a 1-minute difference. Rounding off the minutes or poor documentation will be a red flag for reviewers. The two highest therapy levels are:

- ▶ Ultra high level: a minimum of 720 minutes of therapy per week.
- ▶ Very high level: a minimum of 500 minutes of therapy per week.

The RUGs IV classification pays for minutes of therapy and is not tied to who delivers the therapy. Therefore, as a strategy to optimize reimbursement and reduce labor costs, many SNFs will use "therapy extenders" such as PT assistants or rehabilitation aides. These staff members must be supervised by a licensed or certified individual. Another strategy will be the use of group therapy sessions. This will enhance the ability to deliver many minutes of therapy to patients, while using only one staff person/therapist. However, Medicare mandates that only four residents per therapist session, and no more than 25% of the patient's total therapy minutes, can be spent in group therapy.

▶ Reimbursement Changes

Beginning in January 1999, Medicare imposed an annual financial cap on outpatient PT, OT, and ST covered under Medicare Part B. One potential problem that could arise is if a patient receives therapies from unknown sources and the present agency submits a bill in excess of the cap. This is another important reason for case management continuity; a case manager who knows the total expenditures of his or her patient is invaluable. This knowledge is expected for many external case management positions; these case managers must keep track of the amount of benefits the patients have and the amount of benefits that have been exhausted. Can the claims payors help determine how much the patient has used in therapies? Sometimes. However, if the claim has not yet been submitted (and billing may be months behind), then the total expenditures will be incomplete. Sometimes an accurate guesstimate must be made on the total; this may involve going to the individual billing departments of the agencies the patient used for therapies (or other services or DME).

Medicare helps pay for medically necessary outpatient OT, PT, and ST services when the physician or therapist sets up the plan of treatment and the physician periodically reviews the plan to see how a patient is progressing and for how long the therapy will be needed. These services may be obtained from a Medicare participating outpatient provider such as a hospital-based clinic, home health agency, or comprehensive outpatient rehabilitation facility. In private practice settings, Medicare pays for OT and PT services but not for services given by a speech-language pathologist. In these settings and services, the beneficiary remains responsible for 20% coinsurance.

Respiratory therapy is another area that is scrutinized under the PPS. Before January 1999, respiratory therapy was a reimbursable service provided to clinically appropriate patients. Medicare would pay a licensed respiratory therapist for the assessment, evaluation, care plan, and respiratory treatments of the patient. In the newer structure, respiratory therapy is included in the per diem rate. The RUGs IV grouping takes respiratory therapy into consideration in the three nonrehabilitation groups: extensive services, special care, and clinically complex patients. The MDS 3.0 qualifies respiratory therapy as coughing and deep breathing, "heat nebulizers," aerosol treatments, and mechanical ventilation. These treatments must be provided by a qualified professional; however, it no longer has to be a licensed respiratory therapist. As a result, nurses are being required to perform the respiratory treatments; licensed respiratory therapists will be used more frequently in a part-time, consulting role to set up the respiratory plan of care. Again, documentation to support the RUGs IV level is necessary for correct reimbursement.

▶ Suggestions for Managing Therapies

- ▶ Patient and family health education must begin as soon as feasible to assist in the therapy process. Patient self-care management has always been a basic case management premise; now it is essential.
- ▶ In the SNF level of care, 14 of the 18 highest reimbursement categories under the RUGs require rehabilitation services. Patients utilizing these services may become very important to the fiscal health of SNFs. However, this is one area that is being closely monitored.
- ▶ It must be decided whether hiring therapists or using contracted therapists is in your best fiscal interest. This is a complex and individualized situation that must take many variables into consideration.
- ▶ PT, OT, and ST have always been covered. However, because of perceived or actual abuses of

these services, they will be examined in greater detail. Whether the patient resides in an SNF (thus referenced on the RAI and MDS assessments) or is at home, documentation in the medical record should support the following:

a. That the services were ordered by a physician;

b. That a qualified therapist performed an evaluation and plan of care;

c. That the services were provided by or directly supervised by an appropriately licensed individual;

d. That the services were medically necessary;

e. That the services were provided with appropriate frequency and duration;

f. That the plan includes realistic and measurable goals for the patient.

▮ Focus on the patient.

▮ What to Do If You Are Employed in a SNF

▮ Become part of an integrated network. This can open up financial options that may be necessary for survival. Strategies to deal with the acute care Transfer DRGs and the transfer to postacute care payment policy (see "The Discharge/Transfer Rule" earlier in this chapter) will benefit from an integrated network. Optimal transfer strategies will require quick and easy access to other levels of care. Several SNFs could unite to share ancillary staff or pharmacy needs, order supplies through group purchasing, or combine staff training efforts.

▮ Educate employees about the new changes in benefits and reimbursement. They must understand reimbursement challenges to help plan care that is both cost-effective and provides safe, quality care for the residents.

▮ Monitor admission requests.

a. Whereas previously the intake coordinator may have spoken to the hospital nurse or case manager and read parts of the medical record, it may be that the admissions nurse should go to the site and actually see the patient; there is often a difference between the "paper patient" and the "actual patient."

b. With the new discharge/transfer rules, the acuity of patients for those particular DRGs may be less on admission to the SNF (because the hospital may keep the patient an extra day or two); the admission of a less acute patient may mean a lower RUG classification and a lower reimbursement level.

c. Under a RUGs-based PPS reimbursement system, one survival strategy may be to control the clinical mix of patients being admitted to the facility. The screening criteria that each SNF sets up, will be important for their fiscal survival. However, a little thought here will bring to light many potential legal, ethical, and business dilemmas; only time will tell what the consequences of using any strategy will be.

d. Another RUG strategy may be to place the patient in the highest RUG category, while providing the lowest use of resources possible. This "survival" strategy has been cited in the literature as a method to "level the playing field" because the patient's medical condition often changes and can cause higher resource use; however, RUG reimbursement does not change with the patient's condition unless the patient's functional level also changes. Again, this strategy should be used with caution.

▮ Use proven strategies to provide quality services in a cost-efficient manner. These include the use of:

a. Case management (strongly recognized in the literature as an important strategy).

b. Clinical pathways/case management plans, especially those that cross levels of care.

c. Disease management strategies.

d. Protocols, guidelines, and care plans.

e. Coordination of care across multiple providers and settings (those involved in the care of a patient or settings being considered for continued care).

▮ Prove your worth. Learn about outcomes and document cost and quality savings.

▮ Use physician assessment before transfers back to acute care. If a patient is transferred back to the hospital and it is determined that the SNF could have handled the problem, the SNF may be responsible for footing the bill.

▮ Summarize the MDS accurately and thoroughly. This is the critical tool that will determine revenue entitled to the facility.

a. Train pertinent staff members to use these documents accurately and thoroughly. A team effort (the nurse case manager, SW, OT/PT/ST rehabilitation professionals, etc.) may be required to demonstrate fully the range of care provided.

b. Do not overestimate patient needs; this will be picked up during the fraud and abuse examinations. However, completely document all the care ordered by the physician to maximize reimbursement.

c. Demonstrate that the care must be provided on a daily basis.

d. Complete the MDS within the stated time frame. If not done in a timely manner, default per diems will be reimbursed.

▶ Continue appropriate care and services to non-Medicare residents. Overutilization of services to non-Medicare patients will continue to be monitored.

▶ Know your facility's patient mix. Each facility has a unique blend of clinical and cultural situations. Examine where costs are heaviest and look for potential waste. Start a quality improvement program to set up the most efficient and effective means to achieve quality and financial goals.

▶ Revisit the details of your system. Reevaluate all policies, procedures, clinical pathways, documentation, invoicing, billing, forms, transitions of care and handoff practices, and software systems to ensure they comply with consolidated billing requirements and good PPS survival strategies.

▶ Update software systems if necessary; it is mandated for MDS. It will also be essential to adequately document and calculate RUG groupings and electronically transmit the data. With consolidated billing, the software systems will also assist in the tracking of ancillary services and DME/supplies. Lastly, software can assist in outcomes studies, which are more important for survival than ever.

▶ Determine new strategies to cope with consolidated billing rules. This may include partnering/contracting with other service providers or using staff strategies such as outsourcing.

▶ Use proven case management strategies for quality, cost-efficient patient care. As in acute care, perform concurrent review, observe for quality issues, effect and document utilization management strategies, and start post-SNF discharge planning early.

▶ Focus on the patient.

▶ What to Do If You Are a Hospital or External Case Manager

▶ Develop good relationships with the referring facilities. SNFs depend on honest assessments of patients for quality of care and financial survival. Report the patient assessment in an objective and thorough manner. The trust between the hospital and SNF case managers is important. Not every patient will "get in," but on some frantic Friday afternoon, when there is a last-minute SNF bed desperately required, the SNF case manager will know you are not giving an unrealistic report of a patient just to get that person admitted.

▶ Understand the clinical and reimbursement issues of RUGs, RAIs, and MDS assessments. There is a good chance that it may be more difficult to find placements for high-cost patients. The higher-based per diems translate into less medical costs and more ADL needs. Rehabilitation services may also be in demand. This "cherry picking" could

cause ill feelings and frustration all around; work together and understand the constraints that the SNFs are under.

▶ Remember that the physician is the key decision maker. It is ultimately the physician who will assess the patient and determine whether the patient's care in an SNF is still medically necessary. However, reimbursement can become a barrier, and advance planning is more important than ever before.

▶ Be realistic. Some benefits have been generously provided for in the past; with new reimbursement, companies will have to be managing more comprehensively if they are to survive. Also, be realistic about the patient's potential for improvement.

▶ Watch for inappropriate denial of SNF admissions. Current literature states that any SNF can produce reasons for refusing patients (e.g., they have no beds, they cannot take that level of acuity, they currently do not have the staff, etc.). The truth is that many SNFs may turn to privately insured patients to offset the CMS PPS reimbursement system as a survival strategy, or facilities may determine the policy about which patients are/are not to be accepted. The reasons will likely be financial; the underlying fear may be related to survival.

▶ Keep current about Medicare reimbursement and benefit changes (Display 6-13). This knowledge is needed if you are to strategize about how best to meet the needs of your patients.

▶ If the patient/family or another case manager calls with SNF care concerns, reassess the medical

display 6-13

HELPFUL INTERNET SITES: NAVIGATING MEDICARE REIMBURSEMENT CHANGES

Some internet sites that may be helpful in navigating the Medicare reimbursement changes include the following:

https://www.congress.gov/
This site includes current and pending legislative activities.

http://www.loc.gov
This site will take you to Library of Congress where the Balanced Budget Act of 1997 can be located. This site has legislative information of all types.

https://www.cms.gov/Medicare/Quality-Initiatives-Patient-Assessment-Instruments/NursingHomeQualityInits/index.html?redirect=/NursingHomeQualityInits/25_NHQIMDS30.asp

http://www.dhs.state.tx.us/proj/mds.html (this site requires registration)
These sites have information on the MDS—the patient acuity measurement tool that SNFs use (with the PPS reimbursement, accurate assessment using this tool is essential for survival).

condition to evaluate appropriate level of services. If you feel that the SNF care remains medically necessary, detail the reasons for this level of care and document them carefully in the medical record.

▶ Remember that the transfer/discharge orders must be very specific. This is good patient care. It is also necessary for full reimbursement for the SNF. An order for a "PT evaluation" is no longer enough.

▶ Try to move patients to SNFs early in the day. The SNFs must heed strict MDS assessment and treatment time limits, and the day of admission is now day 1.

▶ Focus on the patient.

▶ OTHER DURABLE MEDICAL EQUIPMENT

Some DME changes have already been discussed, such as glucose monitoring devices and testing strips for patients with diabetes. However, the BBA of 1997 and the Deficit Reduction Act of 2005 have created other new changes that the case manager should be aware of to perform cost-efficient, quality care, and be a support to other members of the healthcare team. DME has been deemed "abused," and will be scrutinized carefully. Some changes include:

▶ Physicians must provide ICD-10 codes (which are diagnostic) for DME, orthotics, prosthetics, and supplies billed to the DME arm of the CMS.

▶ Reimbursement has changed from reasonable charges to a fixed payment for such items as parenteral and enteral nutrition as well as home dialysis equipment.

▶ Although glucose monitors and testing strips are covered for patients with diabetes regardless of insulin requirements, a deductible and coinsurance still apply.

▶ Reimbursement for oxygen supplies is also reduced.

▶ Orthotics and prosthetics reimbursement will increase 1% annually.

▶ Mandatory beneficiary ownership of capped rental items of DME after the 13th month of rental.

▶ Mandatory beneficiary ownership of oxygen equipment rental after the 36th month of rental.

▶ Beneficiary paying for service maintenance of DME when such is actually provided.

▶ Beneficiary having a "first month purchase option" for power wheelchairs.

The PPS per diem rate is all-inclusive, and case managers must be aware that most orthotics, prosthetics, and mobility appliances will not be provided in the SNF. The reason for this is simply one of survival: if a prosthetic device costs $10,000, even the highest RUGs IV reimbursement rate will not be profitable. Because the SNF would not make a profit, it may not even survive.

It is imperative that the case manager use all available resources for the benefit of the patient.

Case managers must be more aware than ever of what is going on behind the scenes. DME and HME companies are also realizing deep cuts; in response, they may have to cut some of the value-added services that case managers have taken for granted. For example, oxygen suppliers typically have provided an extra follow-up visit to the patient to ensure that he or she understood the proper use of the equipment and to check for compliance issues. More teaching will have to go on in the inpatient setting. As nurses and respiratory therapists are delivering small volume nebulizer (SVN) or other treatments, they will also need to be teaching the patients at the same time. Case managers will be required to stay on top of these sessions and document them carefully. The same will hold true for all ancillary services; nurses, respiratory therapists, physical therapists, occupational therapists, and speech therapists will need to start home teaching earlier and with more intensity. Although this was always supposed to be done, safe care now depends on it.

Technological advances in home equipment are other changes that are sweeping the world. Case managers must be knowledgeable about the best equipment, the pros and cons of each type of equipment, and the patient's benefits (what will be a covered service). The quality of life and independence of our patients depend on it. This is a challenging part of case management; it can be made easier through working with experts in their fields. Unfortunately, not all contracted companies hire the most knowledgeable employees who will be of assistance in case management decisions; therefore, it is important to find companies that can answer DME—and state-of-the-art—questions when needed.

The CMS always monitors the payment/reimbursement systems in all settings, including the SNFs. Some of the issues being watched (and some also apply to home care) include:

▶ Incentives will be dramatically changed from the past. Do any incentives practiced have the potential to negatively affect quality of care and/or patient's access to services?

▶ Are there changes in the types of patients who are being admitted to SNFs?

▶ Are there changes in the average LOS?

▶ Are appropriate services being provided to patients in SNFs? Are there distinctions between patients who receive rehabilitation therapies versus those who do not? PT/OT/ST reimbursement in SNFs has also been undergoing changes.

▶ Why are some patients with similar medical conditions and nursing needs discharged from acute care settings to an SNF, whereas others go home with or without home health care services? Are there differences in patient criteria or conditions?

Is there evidence that reflects that the more clinically complex patients go to the more intensive level of care?

▶ Are there incentives to discharge patients before addressing and treating underlying chronic problems?

▶ What are the reasons for readmission to acute care? Are they preventable? Is there care needed after hospitalization that is not being addressed?

▶ Do SNFs have the clinical staffing skill to meet the needs of the complexity of patients they admit, especially those requiring rehabilitation services or care resources for those with unusual and complicated health conditions such as ventricular assist devices?

All these changes may catapult healthcare to where it always needed to be: focusing on the patient. As it becomes more difficult to "win" the reimbursement game, there may be only one thing left to do. Going back to an old nursing medication rule: provide the right care, in the right setting, at the right amount, and for the right reasons.

▶ TRANSFERRING PATIENTS

▶ Transitions of Care

Today, most healthcare needs of patients with chronic and complex medical conditions are being handled in multiple care settings and require the involvement of many healthcare providers, often during a single episode of illness/care. Those involved in the care are not limited to the professionals from one single organization where the patient is admitted for care. Others external to the organization are also involved based on the patient's care needs, especially those that are necessary for continued care and postdischarge services such as from an acute care facility. For example, a patient may be admitted to an ICU for a couple of days until his or her condition is stable enough for transfer to a telemetry floor or a regular patient care unit. A few days later, the patient may need a transfer to an SNF or subacute rehabilitation care setting for continued services. While in the hospital setting, this patient may also require the care of a specialist depending on the medical condition being addressed (e.g., cardiologist, endocrinologist, diabetologist, neurosurgeon, etc.). As this patient moves across settings and levels of care, or is seen by multiple physicians and other healthcare professionals (e.g., case manager, SW, physical therapist, etc.), he or she experiences transitions of care.

The term *transitions of care* is defined as a process of moving patients from one level of care to another, usually from most to least complex; however, depending on the patient's health condition and needed treatments/services, the transition may occur in the other direction as well—from least to most. Transitions may also include a handover from one healthcare provider to another such as from a generalist to a cardiologist or neurosurgeon.

Some healthcare professionals believe that a change in a patient's plan of care, even if it is as simple as changing the dosage of or discontinuing a medication means a transition of care situation; that is because it changes or interrupts one or more care patterns for the patient.

Tahan (2007) explains that transitions of care cannot take place without an act of "handoff." A handoff, according to Tahan, is an action that facilitates the transfer of responsibility for the care of a patient from one provider to another, from one care setting to another, or from one level of care to another. Although the term *handoff* has been widely used, some healthcare professionals currently are advocating for the use of the term *handover* instead. Some critics claim that handoff may inadvertently imply the termination of care and accountability, whereas handover may mean continuity. Regardless of which term one uses, it is essential to relinquish active participation in the care of a patient only after ensuring that the transfer of responsibility and accountability for care has occurred effectively, accurately, safely, at the right time, and to the right person or setting.

A single care transition may constitute multiple handoff/over acts. For example, when a patient is transferred from the hospital setting to an SNF, it requires transitioning the responsibility of care from the hospital team to the SNF team; sharing information about the plan of care, medications, treatment regimens, allergies, and so on; and communicating about the patient's medical history, interests, health insurance status, and numerous other aspects of the care to be provided at the SNF. The following are the five main contexts during which care transitions take place:

1. Transfer of responsibility for care from one healthcare provider to another, such as from a primary care to a specialist physician, from one nurse to another, or from one case manager to another.
2. Change in the environment of care within a healthcare facility, such as moving a patient from the emergency department to the ICU setting.
3. Change in the environment of care from one facility to another, including hospitals, SNFs, outpatient clinic, and others.
4. Change in the plan of care, such as adding a new, or discontinuing an existing, medication.
5. Change in the payor or health plan, such as changing from a fee-for-service Medicare Plan to Medicare Advantage Plan.

Transitions of care occur during a time when a patient journeys through the healthcare system. This journey may result in vulnerable situations and require an increased need for coordination and continuity of care. During care transitions, patients face significant challenges; they are usually at a higher risk for medical errors, poor quality care, and unsafe experiences. Some of the reasons for these events include system inefficiencies, lack of appropriate follow-up, and poor communication. Transitions of care should be well planned and adequately timed; they must enhance the continuity of care and involve a two-way interaction. Case managers can play an important role in planning and executing transitions of care activities. They are integral to preventing poor outcomes and negative experiences. Safe transitions of care depend on a system approach to care as well as a culture of healthcare professionals working together regardless of place, time, and space boundaries. Case managers are known to be integrators of care and to function in ways that transcend organizational boundaries.

Care coordination, a component of case management, is an effective strategy case managers proactively use in the event of care transition encounters to ensure that care is uninterrupted and patients experience positive outcomes. Additionally, case management is essential for effective care transitions; the case management process (refer to Chapter 4) has been known to facilitate the integration and coordination of healthcare services across consumers of healthcare, providers of care, payors for services, and care settings; that is, across people, space, and time. Contextually speaking, case management facilitates effective collaboration and communication among healthcare team members and across settings, before, during, and after an act of handoff/over or a care transition. These critical interactions ensure patient safety and optimal care outcomes.

Patients at increased risk during transitions of care or handoffs/overs include children with special care needs, the frail elderly, persons with cognitive impairments, persons with complex medical conditions and treatment regimens, persons with disabilities, persons at the end of life, the uninsured, those with low income or poor social networks, and those with mental/behavioral health issues. When such patients are transferred to another provider, another level of care, or to another acute hospital, specific information must accompany them. The general transfer packet should include the following:

- Physician transfer orders
- Chest radiograph (preferably within 30 days)
- Medical history and physical examination results
- Laboratory results
- ECG results
- Urinalysis results
- Preadmission screening (PAS), preadmission screening and annual resident review (PASAAR) forms
- Assessments from nursing, PT, OT, and ST (as needed)
- Social service assessments
- Advance directives, do not resuscitate forms (if appropriate), living wills, medical power of attorney
- Copies of important information such as results of CT scans, echocardiograms, Dopplers, MRIs, miscellaneous cardiodiagnostic tests, and so on

- A transfer note or summary that provides comprehensive information of the patient's status, the course of treatment received, and the plan for continued care (Display 6-14).

A complete and thorough transfer packet is necessary for continuity of patient care and avoids much trouble and many unnecessary problems. Patients have been returned to emergency departments for not having a chest radiograph accompany them to the facility. SNFs must ensure that their residents are free from tuberculosis, and the necessity of a chest radiograph is usually nonnegotiable. Patients with a positive Mantoux skin test may also need a signed and dated letter from the physician stating that the resident is free from pulmonary tuberculosis or that three consecutive sputum cultures have shown negative results for 3 days in a row.

Another required form in many states is the PAS document. It is also known as a PASAAR form. This program, started by Medicaid in the mid-1980s, was originally designed as a technique to manage LTC costs and utilization of services in nursing homes. It includes an on-site (or hospital) assessment of the patient's needs. In some states, this assessment is extensive and includes an evaluation of physical and mental health, functional status, and formal and informal social supports. Although the PAS program was not deemed successful as a utilization control measure, it was praised for its ability to help assess the level of care and type of facility that is best for the patient. Some PAS programs contain a level I and level II. Level I is essentially used to assess medical necessity for an SNF. Level II indicates whether a psychological referral is needed. This may hold up a transfer to an SNF for a week or more. State laws prohibit SNFs or supervisory homes from accepting patients with active mental illnesses that may cause them to be a danger to themselves or other residents in the SNF. If a patient might need to pass a level II PAS, the paperwork should be started early in the admission.

One last detail: a patient must have an accepting physician at the SNF. If the patient's primary physician cannot follow up at the SNF, the facility often helps to find a physician who can.

▶ Transportation

Safe patient transportation between levels of care is an important consideration for the case manager. Several levels of transportation are available for transferring patients to an outside destination, and the patient's needs must be matched to the appropriate mode of transportation. In many instances, the patient or family is responsible for the cost of transportation. Some rare insurance policies pay for expensive forms of transportation, so if the patient claims to have such a policy rider, this needs to be checked out. Some family members may request a more

KEY INFORMATION THAT MUST BE COVERED IN THE TRANSFER NOTE

I. Background Information

   a. Patient's name and date of birth
   b. Next of kin and contact information
   c. Address and telephone number
   d. Primary language spoken and need for interpretation, health literacy
   e. Health beliefs
   f. Name of primary care provider and contact information
   g. Name of specialist care provider(s) and contact information
   h. Presence of advance directive, healthcare proxy, living will, do not resuscitate order
   i. Living situation and social support system
   j. Employment status.

II. Medical History

   a. Allergies
   b. Chief complaint and summary of current healthcare encounter
   c. Medical problems complicating management of the current condition
   d. Past medical history including any comorbidities (chronic illnesses)
   e. Comprehensive list of medications: prescription and over-the-counter drugs including the use of herbal products and vitamins. Medication reconciliation including a medication list which should contain name of drug, frequency of intake, dosage, and special precautions or instructions
   f. Current or past surgical procedures
   g. Use of durable medical equipment, supplies, and assistive devices
   h. Other important health information.

III. Health Insurance Benefits

   a. Insurance benefits/health plan–related information such as name, policy number, and expiration date
   b. Provider network
   c. Coverage
   d. Any other necessary information.

IV. Plan of Care

   a. Care goals
   b. Long-term and short-term treatment plans
   c. Areas that require special attention; for example, health education, the use of devices such as a "glucometer"
   d. Medication regimen
   e. Precautions and isolation status; for example, the presence of MRSA or c-diff
   f. Psychosocial issues/concerns
   g. Barriers to achieving goals
   h. Wishes regarding end-of-life care; for example, life-sustaining measures
   i. Caregiver and ability and willingness to provide ongoing care for the patient
   j. Community-level support
   k. Transitional plan of care.

V. Health Education and Engagement Plan

   a. Areas that the patient and/or caregiver knows well
   b. Areas that need further attention or specific follow-up
   c. Plan regarding medication intake
   d. Plan regarding skilled services or treatment regimen
   e. State of self-management including activation level
   f. Counseling regarding healthy lifestyle behaviors and areas needing continued focus.

VI. Functional Status

   a. Self-care ability
   b. Ability to make own decisions
   c. Level of dependence or independence
   d. Cognition: impaired, alert/oriented, disoriented

KEY INFORMATION THAT MUST BE COVERED IN THE TRANSFER NOTE (continued)

    e. Ability to dress, especially lower extremities
    f. Bathing
    g. Toileting
    h. Ambulation: use of aids such as walker, crutches, prosthesis
    i. Transferring from bed to chair and vice versa
    j. Need for transportation services
    k. Housekeeping assistance.

VII. Home Health Services

    a. Name of agency and contact information, if any
    b. Use of home health aide, visiting nurse service, allied health professionals (e.g., physical therapy, social worker)
    c. Frequency and type of visits
    d. Skilled care: wound care, dressing changes, IV therapy.

VIII. Durable Medical Equipment

    a. Current needs
    b. Previous use
    c. Name of vendor and phone number
    d. Patient's/caregiver's knowledge and ability of use.

intensive level of transportation than the case manager has assessed, and may be willing to pay for it. In one instance, a case manager had assessed that a patient could safely be transported to another hospital using a stretcher van. The family wanted an advanced cardiac life support (ACLS) ambulance plus an RN. Therefore, even when planning the mode of transportation, the patient and family must be included in the decision.

PRIVATE VEHICLES

Private vehicles are the most common mode of transportation. The patient is usually accompanied by family or friends, but occasionally drives him- or herself to the hospital. In such a case, arrangements must be made for the vehicle if the physician feels it is unsafe for the patient to drive. The simplest solution here is for a family member or neighbor to be dropped off at the facility to drive the vehicle and patient home. The facility's personnel can help get the patient into the vehicle. The case manager should assess whether there is enough help at the destination to get the patient inside safely. Assessment is also needed for any equipment needs for the trip. For example, many patients have their portable oxygen tanks at home and must make prior arrangements to retrieve them before they leave the facility. Also, assess the length of the trip and the possible need for more than one oxygen tank. Assess whether the patient can remain sitting for the trip: very ill patients and some orthopedic procedures make this mode of transportation unrealistic. Assess whether the patient has stairs to climb at the other end. If the patient cannot negotiate stairs, a car, taxi, or wheelchair van will not work and a stretcher van should be considered; the stretcher van personnel will take the patient up the stairs and help him or her to get settled.

TAXICAB

Ask some of the same questions as aforementioned for taxis, realizing that cab drivers are often less helpful at the other end than family members because of their legal constraints. Also, find out whether the patient can afford a taxi. Many hospitals have funds or cab vouchers to help needy people. From a fiscal perspective, a cab ride is less expensive than a day in the hospital if a patient cannot get someone to take him home until the following day.

WHEELCHAIR VAN

Wheelchair vans are a good choice for several types of patients. If patients who are quadriplegic or who have cerebral palsy use a wheelchair at home, they often have their own wheelchair at the hospital. Notify the van company whether it needs to provide a wheelchair or whether the patient has one. If a patient can sit up for a designated length of time but may be slightly confused, he or she may need to be restrained. Careful assessment is imperative when sending a patient needing restraints in a wheelchair van. For example, it would be safer to use a higher level of transportation if the patient is combative or requires maximum restraining. (Consider what the risk management issues would be if the patient is maximally restrained and the van catches fire or goes over the side of a road!) Orthopedic patients can often use wheelchair vans with adaptive equipment such as leg lifts. Specify what equipment is required when ordering the van. Again, assess the whole medical picture before deciding on this level of transportation.

STRETCHER VANS

Stretcher vans allow a patient to lie down for the entire ride. The patient is transferred from the facility bed to the stretcher and taken to the destination, even transported up or down stairs, in the same position. Very ill, debilitated patients who cannot sit for any length of time are candidates for stretcher vans, as are some orthopedic patients or those who must stay on their abdomen or back because of medical considerations such as skin flaps or graft procedures. No form of cardiac monitoring is included in this mode of transportation.

AMBULANCES

There are two types of ambulances: basic life support (BLS) and advanced life support (ALS). BLS ambulances include a BLS paramedic and limited cardiac monitoring. Psychiatric patients or suicidal patients who are being transferred to a mental health unit minimally require this level of care; if the transfer is involuntary and the patient is likely to become combative, extra help should be requested and restraints may be necessary. In general, assess the patient's medical stability and decide whether it would be beneficial to have a BLS paramedic on board.

ALS ambulances include paramedics trained in ACLS procedures. Cardiac monitoring and a drug box are available for use. Any patient who has a running IV line or who requires medications (including potassium) will minimally require this level of care.

AIR AMBULANCE

Air transport is the most cost-intensive type of transportation available, often costing thousands of dollars for even short flights. When an unstable patient is being transferred to another acute care facility and speed is of the essence, it may be the only safe mode of transfer. As in an ALS ambulance, the air ambulance has cardiac monitoring, a medication box, and ACLS-trained personnel, including an RN.

Almost any patient can be transferred safely, when necessary, with enough support. Some cases require careful consideration and advanced planning. Insurance companies often require their medically stable patients to be transferred to contracted hospitals. One patient had a chest tube and needed an ALS ambulance with an RN on board. Because most ambulance companies retain only a few nurses, it took an extra day to provide the required services. Other patients require detailed coordination of oxygen, stretcher vans, air transport, and accepting facilities. Patients with certain conditions cannot be transferred safely in air transports because of the pressure changes at high altitudes. Transportation needs can be tricky and require early team coordination and planning.

CONSIDERATIONS IN PLANNING TRANSPORTATION

Further important considerations to assess when planning a mode of transportation are as follows.

TUBES AND LINES Most tubes can be capped off for shorter rides and require only a physician's order to do so. This may include IV lines (peripheral or central), feeding tubes, suction tubes such as nasogastric tubes or percutaneous endoscopic gastrostomy tubes, gastrostomy tubes, or jejunostomy tubes. Most modes of transportation—even taxis—allow capped-off tubes, although that is not to say that a taxi is the safest vehicle assessed. If a tube cannot be capped off, an ambulance may be the lowest level of transportation allowed. If, for example, IV fluid containing potassium is running, then an ALS ambulance must be used. The transportation company can clear up any questions, because they carry on their business under legal guidelines.

OXYGEN Some state laws mandate that oxygen cannot be supplied by the transportation company for wheelchair or stretcher vans. The company can provide oxygen only in a BLS or ALS ambulance. However, if the patient has his or her own portable oxygen tank, a wheelchair van or stretcher van may be provided in conjunction with the patient's personal equipment. The van personnel are not allowed to adjust the oxygen, so that the patient's ability to care for his or her own portable tank must be considered.

PRICES OF TRANSPORTATION Because the patient is responsible for the cost of transportation in many instances, the case manager may want to compare the prices of various companies for the best rate. Ambulance prices are essentially set by the government, but taxi, wheelchair van, and stretcher van prices may vary.

TRANSPORTATION REIMBURSEMENT Insurance companies often reimburse for transportation between two medically necessary levels of care; they usually do not reimburse for transportation to the patient's home. Medicare reimbursement for transportation is very strict and includes only ground ambulance or air ambulance transport.

▶ Ground ambulance may be reimbursed under Medicare Part B for a medically necessary transfer if:
   1. The ambulance, equipment, and personnel meet Medicare requirements and approval.
   2. Any other mode of transportation could endanger the patient.
   3. The destination is to or from a hospital or SNF. This does not include such destinations as hemodialysis facilities, doctor's offices, or ambulatory surgery centers.
   4. The transportation is to a local facility (usually). If the facility is outside the local area, Medicare will help pay for the transportation to the nearest appropriate facility.
▶ Air ambulance may be reimbursed by Medicare if:
   1. The medical condition seriously endangers the member's life.
   2. Immediate medical attention is necessary for the person's survival or necessary to avoid severe health damage.
   3. Land ambulance is unavailable or would be so time-consuming that health or life would be further endangered.

DISCUSSION QUESTIONS

1. Discuss the importance of discharge planning regulations and accreditation standards for the role of the case manager.

2. Discuss how discharge planning is affected on the basis of the differences between traditional Medicare and the newer risk Medicare contracts. Do you see these changes positively or negatively?

3. Discuss the IM from Medicare and its related appeals review process. How would you handle a family/patient who disagrees with the hospital discharge date or postdischarge services? What steps would you take? What are the financial implications when a patient or hospital does not adhere to the IM from Medicare process?

4. Explain the Medicare Outpatient Observation Notice (MOON) and how it applies to patient care. Discuss under what circumstances the MOON notice applies and what to do in the event the patient declines to sign the notice.

5. Give examples of patients who are appropriate for the custodial level of care, the intermediate level of care, and the skilled and subacute levels of care. Discuss possible pay sources for each level of care.

6. What might constitute a patient being at too high or too low a level for inpatient rehabilitation?

7. Cite an example of a good candidate for a transitional hospital.

8. Cite an example of a good home healthcare patient. Give reasons that may be contrary to home health services.

9. Compare and contrast home health services with hospice care.

10. Cite examples matching patients' needs to safe transportation.

11. Discuss the role of the case manager in safe transitions of care. What can a case manager do to enhance patient safety when a patient is transferred from one provider to another? From one service to another? From one setting/organization to another?

▶ REFERENCES

Anonymous. (1991). CMs find innovative options for patients between the ICU and the acute care bed. *Case Management Advisor, 2*(8), 113–117.

Birmingham, J. (2008). Understanding the Medicare "extended care benefit" a.k.a. the 3-midnight rule. *Professional Case Management, 13*(1), 7–16.

Boccuti, C., & Cassillas, G. (2017, March 10). *Aiming for fewer hospital U-turns: The Medicare Hospital Readmission Reduction Program*. [Online]. Retrieved June 25, 2017, from http://www.kff.org/medicare/issue-brief/aiming-for-fewer-hospital-u-turns-the-medicare-hospital-readmission-reduction-program/. Kaiser Family Foundation (KFF)

Carr, D. D. (2000). Case management for the subacute patient in a skilled nursing facility. *Lippincott's Case Management, 5*(2), 83–92.

Centers for Medicare & Medicaid Services. (2007). *CMS manual, Medicare claims processing*. Transmittal Number 1257 (May 25, 2007). [Online]. Retrieved March 3, 2008, from http://www.cms.hhs.gov/Transmittals/downloads/R1257CP.pdf.

Centers for Medicare & Medicaid Services. (2009a). *Conditions of participation for hospitals, chapter IV: Discharge planning*. [Online]. Retrieved April 13, 2009, from www.cms.hhs.gov/CFCsAndCoPs/06_Hospitals.asp#TopofPage

Centers for Medicare & Medicaid Services. (2009b). *Minimum data sets 2.0*. [Online]. Retrieved April 13, 2009, from www.cms.hhs.gov/MinimumDataSets20

Centers for Medicare & Medicaid Services. (2016, October). *Long term care facility resident assessment instrument 3.0 user's manual, version 1.14* [Online]. Retrieved June 25, 2017, from https://downloads.cms.gov/files/MDS-30-RAI-Manual-V114-October-2016.pdf

Cesta, T., & Tahan, H. (2017). *The case manager's survival guide: winning strategies in the new healthcare environment* (3rd ed.). Lancaster, PA: DEStech Publications.

Hamilton, M., & Thomsen, T. (1998). Removing the label. *Continuing Care, 17*(9), 26–29, 40.

Kongstvedt, P. R. (2003). *Essentials of managed health care* (4th ed.). Gaithersburg, MD: Aspen Publishers.

National Association of Subacute/Postacute Care. (2009). *Frequently asked questions*. [Online]. Retrieved April 13, 2009, from http://www.naspac.net/faq.asp.

National Committee of Quality Assurance. (2017). *Patient Centered Medical Home (PCMH)*. [Online]. Retrieved June 25, 2017, from http://www.ncqa.org/programs/recognition/practices/patient-centered-medical-home-pcmh/why-pcmh

Powell, S. (2007). An important message from Medicare, new rules on July 1, 2007. *Professional Case Management, 12*(2), 1–3.

Tahan, H. A. (2007). One patient, numerous healthcare providers, and multiple care settings. *Professional Case Management, 12*(1), 37–46.

The Joint Commission. (2017). *Comprehensive accreditation manual for hospitals*. Oakbrook Terrace, IL: Author.

PART 3

Key Concepts in Case Management Practice

"Quality is never an accident; it is always the result of high intention, sincere effort, intelligent direction and skillful execution; it represents the wise choice of many alternatives."

WILLA A. FOSTER

CHAPTER 7

Quality Management and Outcomes Evaluation

"Quality is never an accident; it is always the result of high intention, sincere effort, intelligent direction and skillful execution; it represents the wise choice of many alternatives."

WILLA A. FOSTER

LEARNING OBJECTIVES

Upon completion of this chapter, the reader will be able to:

1. Define performance management, outcomes management, risk management, and core measures.
2. Describe the relationship between case management and quality management.
3. Discuss the relationship between the National Quality Strategy, the National Quality Initiative, Hospital Value-Based Purchasing Program, and quality core measures.
4. Describe the process of quality reviews.
5. Explain the role of the case manager in quality and outcomes management.
6. List five strategies in case management practice that enhance patient safety.
7. Describe the role of the case manager in the reporting of outcomes (core measures).
8. Explain the value of clinical documentation improvement programs.

ESSENTIAL TERMS

Adverse Patient Outcome (APO) • Clinical Documentation Improvement • Core Measures • Important Aspects of Care • Incident • Incident Report • Indicators • National Quality Initiative • National Quality Strategy • Occurrence Report • Outcomes • Outcomes Management • Patient Safety • Pay-for-Performance • Performance Improvement (PI) • Performance Management (PM) • Potentially Compensable Event • Quality Assurance (QA) • Quality Improvement (QI) • Quality Management (QM) • Quality of Care • Risk Management (RM) • The Quadruple Aim • The Triple Aim • Total Quality Management (TQM) • Value-Based Purchasing (VBP) • Variances

The present healthcare climate contains several factors that leave it open to accusations of compromised patient safety and quality of care and wasted resources. Among these factors are utilization review and management criteria that are becoming stricter every year and that demand prompt transitioning of patients to lower levels of care. Additional factors are the increased scrutiny of the use and allocation of healthcare resources; health insurance capitation and risk contracts that place hospitals and other types of healthcare organizations at increased fiscal risk; and cost-cutting activities resorted to by organizations in an effort to be cost-effective, activities that ultimately change the professional staff-to-patient ratios. Most importantly, however, today's consumers of healthcare services are demanding to receive full value from the systems of care that are evident not only in clinical outcomes, quality of life, and well-being, but in optimal experience of care as well.

Quality improvement (QI)—also referred to as quality management (QM) and traditionally referred to as quality assurance—has long been a function mandated by regulatory (e.g., Department of Health and Human Services) or accreditation agencies such as The Joint Commission (TJC), previously known as The Joint Commission on Accreditation of Healthcare Organizations (JCAHO). Some TJC requirements that improve various aspects of quality care include the creation of hospital policies and procedures; job descriptions; personnel performance evaluations; credentialing of professional staff; professional licensure verification, background checks, the provision of educational programs to ensure that knowledge, competencies, and clinical skills are up-to-date; and continual monitoring activities. TJC mandates the demonstration of interdisciplinary performance improvement (PI) efforts using specific indicators and processes. Rather than merely emphasizing quality assurance, which is often episodic in its assessments, today the emphasis is on the concepts of QI and performance management (PM) (TJC, 2017a). Gleaned from the industrial sector that is typical of the Japanese automotive management philosophies since World War II, QI attempts to meet or exceed the customer's needs. The customer is no longer the patient only but everyone associated with the healthcare industry, those who work for your organization and for other organizations (Fanucci, Hammil, Johannson, Leggett, & Smith, 1993) across the continuum of care.

The continuous QI (CQI) concept, sometimes referred to as total quality management (TQM), has gained strength in the healthcare industry and is closely related to QI processes and risk management (RM) activities. The intent of all improvement processes, whether labeled QI, QM, PI, or another acronym, is to provide excellent care in the first place, evident through patient safety and quality of care, thus lessening chances of adverse events that will need RM attention. QI and PM emphasize a proactive rather than a reactive approach; they provide the compass that leads the way to quality services. The result—excellent quality, safe, and affordable care—is the measuring rod.

Another frequently used term for similar activities is *performance improvement*, which uses the processes of assessment, design, improvement, measurement, and control.

- ▶ The *assessment* step focuses on measuring the extent of the issue of interest or the process in need for improvement. This step assists professionals in understanding the magnitude of the various factors contributing to the concerns and prioritizing which one(s) must be addressed first.
- ▶ The *design* step is responsible for designing new (or modifying existing) functions, processes, and services on the basis of the mission and vision of the organization, the concerns identified, the expectations and needs of the customers, and the most up-to-date information regarding the focus of improvement.
- ▶ The *improvement* step emphasizes the need to implement the strategic and well-thought-out changes prompted by the identified concerns or problems and the desired outcomes.
- ▶ The *measurement* step evaluates the effectiveness of the redesigned process(es); thus, identifying opportunities for further improvement/modification as necessary. The focus of measurement includes areas of care that are high volume, high risk, high cost, and problem prone. Integral to the measurement step is a reassessment that provides a systematic approach to determine whether the goals and priorities for the redesigned process have been met and how further improvements can be made.

- ▶ The *control* step includes the implementation of specific activities or strategies to maintain and sustain the improvement and the redesigned process. This is important for ensuring that the improvements achieved become part of the regular process.

The following quote from Kongstvedt still holds true today. It emphasizes the movement from a punitive quality assurance model (find the bad apple) to the QI model of quality performance.

> Effective quality management is both a continuous and a systematic endeavor. Instead of centering on crisis, wrongdoing by individuals, and conformity to correct processes established by experts, quality management should engage everyone in the organization in continuous efforts to raise the organization's level of performance. (Kongstvedt, 1993, p. 167)

This ideal of a high level of performance is the goal of QI and RM programs. Unfortunately, because mistakes do take place, we must also continue to focus on crises when they occur and to monitor potential or actual problems. This troubleshooting is done through safety checks, infection control surveillance, incident reports, RM activities, care evaluations, outcomes management, case management assessments, and use of tools such as evidence-based practice guidelines or clinical pathways. Quality assurance cannot "assure" that risks and maloccurrences will not happen, but through the previously mentioned activities and prompt identification of problems, the risk (and quality) manager can initiate the appropriate intervention to minimize crescendoing consequences.

RM and QI are closely related programs with similar goals. This chapter clarifies the similarities and differences of traditional QI-RM programs, discusses the National Quality Strategy and value-based purchasing (VBP), illustrates the importance of the case manager's role to QI-RM activities, and describes circumstances, claims categories, and indicators that warrant close attention. Through the course of a case manager's responsibilities, chart reviews and discussions with others on the healthcare team often expose potential problems in care or services.

▶ QI AND RM RESPONSIBILITIES

Traditional QI is a process that determines whether the care provided meets medical and nationally recognized and accepted standards (Sederer, 1987). QI activities are designed to monitor, prevent, and correct quality deficiencies. In that sense, QI is a proactive model. It is a continuous effort to raise the healthcare organization's quality level and performance. This is accomplished through quality assessment, which is the process by which quality of care is examined and evaluated. It is also achieved through the implementation of tools, methods, or strategies so that quality of care and patient safety are assured at all times. In this regard, quality assurance activities are performed on an ongoing basis, with the goal of QI. However, this traditional effort of quality assurance has changed, routinely incorporating more QI, QM, PI, and RM techniques, which is having the effect of making quality assurance even more proactive. The first step is no longer monitoring, but rather doing it right the first time and all the time.

Traditional RM is the "art and science of how not to be successfully sued" (Sederer, 1987, p. 214). Ideally, the major emphasis is on the identification of potential risk areas and on interventions that will enhance patient safety and prevent losses, including untoward events, before they occur. In reality, however, many organizations call in the RM department after the undesirable event has occurred. Its function then is to control and minimize losses through legal methods and public relations efforts. Because of this, RM sometimes has been characterized as the "damage control" entity: "an attempt to remedy the effects of internal failures before they can become external [and costly] embarrassments" (Kongstvedt, 1993, p. 166).

In this sense, RM is a reactive model, but risk cannot always be prevented. Some adverse events do not become apparent until after the fact. Consider a case in which a patient received standard treatment for a disease and in which patient care was of high quality during the treatment phase: good QM. Unfortunately, the disease was misdiagnosed: poor RM potential. This case is not likely to be reported through routine QI channels at the time of misdiagnosis.

To avoid the reactive nature of RM activities, healthcare organizations have implemented risk mitigation programs that allow them to identify proactively potential risks or failures and to implement specific interventions (checks and balances) to prevent these potential problems from occurring. The following are examples of risk mitigation activities:

▶ Skin or tissue injury (previously referred to as pressure ulcer) prevention programs.
▶ Falls risk assessment and injury reduction programs.
▶ Infection control surveillance: screening for Methicillin-Resistant Staphylococcus Aureus (MRSA), central line–associated blood stream infections, catheter-associated urinary tract infection, incision/surgical site infection, hand hygiene, and testing for water safety.
▶ Prevention of complications: anticoagulation therapy, deep vein thrombosis prophylaxis, ventilator-associated pneumonia prophylaxis, early recognition of sepsis protocol.
▶ Failure mode analysis: examining processes of care to identify potential risk for failure and instituting an intervention to prevent such risk; for example,

requiring two-person check for chemotherapeutic agent use/administration or requiring two-person check for blood and blood product administration; use of an MRI safety checklist.
▶ Daily review of throughput and patient flow activities: among other indicators, this involves bed capacity evaluation, bed management, an examination of emergency department patient volume, hours of diversion, and percentage of "waiting to be admitted" patients; an examination of postanesthesia care unit patient volume and length of stay; and turnaround time for admitting patients to an inpatient bed.
▶ Utilization management activities: these consist of reviewing whether patients have met the medical necessity criteria for the level of care in which they are being cared for; examining whether the utilization review procedures of the health insurance company are adhered to; and obtaining authorizations/certifications for services before they are provided to patients as appropriate. These activities tend to primarily focus on preventing financial risk.

▶ HOW QI AND RM CONTRAST AND COMPARE

Like case management, the direction in QI emphasizes looking at the big picture and efficiently coordinating the whole system of care delivery. Classic QI, with its inherent limitations and flaws, is still necessary and required by regulatory agencies such as TJC. Therefore, an understanding of how QI and RM differ, and how they work together, is important.

RM and QI differ in the following ways:

▶ Their focuses are different. RM is concerned with acceptable care from a legal and financial perspective and attempts to minimize the costs of liability insurance and the liability of claims. QI emphasizes patient care issues and related outcomes rather than financial concerns.
▶ RM looks at all hospital exposures: environmental, patient safety, visitor safety, and so on. QI emphasizes patient-care–focused issues, which include all services involved in patient care: optimal quality of care, adherence to professional standards, and reasonable and prudent delivery of care.
▶ RM focuses on loss prevention activities. QI facilitates the improvement of the processes of care and ultimately their associated outcomes.
▶ Overall, RM aims to reduce the probability of adverse patient outcomes (APOs). QI, on the other hand, aims to increase the probability of quality patient outcomes.

The following are areas of common concern in RM and QI:

▶ Both are concerned with anything that may cause risk of injury to the patient. Both attempt to identify and avoid APOs.

▶ Both involve the monitoring of trends to identify risk patterns or problems in patient care.

▶ Both require and emphasize the need for complete and clear documentation.

▶ Although it is more important in the case of RM, transparency with the patient/family when an error occurs applies to both RM and QI.

▶ Both require cooperation and information from the interdisciplinary team to assess trends and resolve problematic issues. This is of particular importance to case managers, who play an integral role in RM, especially identifying potential risk while engaged in medical record review as well as communication with members of the interdisciplinary team. Being on the front lines, case managers often are privy to discovering impending or completed adverse occurrences.

▶ Many of the tools used are effective for both QI and RM purposes.

▶ Both attempt to correct identified problems by educational methods, changes in policies and procedures, or disciplinary action.

▶ QI AND RM TERMINOLOGY

Some terms frequently used during QI and RM activities are self-explanatory: *mishap*, *patient safety problem*, *error*, *maloccurrence*. Others require further definition.

▶ Outcomes

Outcomes describe the results and consequences from the care received; outcomes also result from care that was not received. Outcome studies look for trends and patterns, and potentially adverse events. Poor outcomes revealed through outcome studies often lead to policy and procedural changes and additional training and education of personnel to minimize a problem. Sometimes they may result in a change of job descriptions.

Outcomes are the end result of a process or an activity. They are used as indicators of quality and are often measurable in nature. Additionally, they can be manipulated or changed as a result of a focused intervention. Experts have classified outcomes into categories as follows:

▶ Clinical
▶ Financial (utilization, cost, and revenue)
▶ Physical and cognitive functioning
▶ Experience of care
▶ Quality of life
▶ Well-being

▶ Outcomes Management

Outcomes management is a process that applies outcomes research to practice, allowing the delivery of evidence-based care and treatments. It involves assessment and measurement of performance (based on specific indicators) at one point in time; monitoring and evaluation of performance using the same outcomes over time and at specific intervals (longitudinal approach); analysis and interpretation of the results to identify issues or concerns; and taking specific or strategic actions to improve quality and performance.

Combining outcomes and case management enables us to improve our patient care practices and performance by highlighting opportunities for:

▶ Improving patient care quality and safety.
▶ Implementing evidence-based standards, protocols, guidelines, and treatment options.
▶ Conducting systematic evaluation of performance, including the effectiveness of programs such as case management.
▶ Understanding performance associated with VBP core measures and implementing focused improvement plans.

Case managers are frequently involved in the evaluation of the effectiveness of the case management programs of which they are a part. Such activities cannot be done without focusing on identifying key and strategic case management–related outcome indicators and on doing the following: assessing, measuring, and monitoring these indicators; analyzing and interpreting the data; and finally improving the effectiveness of case management where the opportunity for improvement exists. These activities are nothing but outcomes management in itself. Only with these activities, case managers are able to improve the quality of the care patients receive and ensure that it is also safe.

Examples of outcome indicators/measures case managers evaluate include those listed in Display 7-1. Healthcare organizations report their performance on these outcomes on a regular basis (e.g., monthly or quarterly) using a report card, dashboard, or scorecard format. They usually trend their performance over time (longitudinal approach) and compare it against predetermined targets, using either internal or external benchmarks, or both. Executives of case management programs also use these reports to communicate the contribution of case management to patient care quality, safety, and outcomes, including return on investment. Such reports are perceived as powerful tools to demonstrate the effectiveness of case management and its impact on patient care and healthcare services.

▶ Adverse Patient Outcome (APO)

An *APO* is defined as any adverse patient occurrence that, under optimal conditions, is not a natural consequence of

EXAMPLES OF OUTCOME MEASURES RELEVANT TO CASE MANAGEMENT PROGRAMS

Category	Examples of Outcome Measures	Category	Examples of Outcome Measures
Cost	▶ Length of stay ▶ Cost per case ▶ Cost per day ▶ Cost per diagnosis-related group ▶ Cost per service or product line ▶ Cost per encounter or visit	Clinical	▶ Achievement of intermediate outcomes (e.g., switching from IV to oral medications) as expected on the basis of the clinical pathway or guideline ▶ Achievement of discharge outcomes (e.g., no fever for 24 hours prior to discharge) as expected in the clinical pathway ▶ Morbidity/complication rates (e.g., nosocomial infections) ▶ Mortality rates ▶ Relief of signs and symptoms of a disease condition ▶ Compliance rates with core measures (refer to table 7.2 for additional information) ▶ Medical errors or significant events ▶ Pain management ▶ Value-based purchasing core measures
Utilization	▶ Average number of laboratory tests (e.g., complete blood count, chemistry, pathology) per case ▶ Average number of radiologic tests (e.g., chest x-ray, CT scan, MRI) per case ▶ Denials of services rate ▶ Appeals conversion rate (by case manager) ▶ Appeals conversion rate (by physician advisor) ▶ Number of avoided days ▶ Conversion of observation status to inpatient status ▶ Volume of one-day admissions ▶ Turnaround time on tests ▶ Turnaround time on procedures ▶ Surgical delays ▶ Surgical cancelations ▶ Number of hospital admissions per 100 persons (population) ▶ Number of emergence department visits per 1,000 persons (population)	Care experience and satisfaction	▶ Patient and family experience scores ▶ Satisfaction scores ▶ Patient and family health knowledge ▶ Pain and comfort ▶ Self-management abilities ▶ Physical ability and level of independence ▶ State of well-being ▶ Health perception ▶ Health literacy level ▶ Quality of life
Transitional planning and throughput	▶ Delays in discharge ▶ Readmissions within 72 hours of discharge ▶ Readmissions within 1 week of discharge ▶ Readmissions within 30 days of discharge ▶ Volume of discharge to home without services ▶ Volume of discharge to home with home care ▶ Volume of discharge to another facility (e.g., skilled nursing facility, acute or subacute rehabilitation facility) ▶ Returns to operating room ▶ Returns to ICU ▶ Turnaround time on admissions from emergency department ▶ Turnaround time on admissions from postanesthesia care unit ▶ Appropriateness of the level of care ▶ Effective handoffs/handovers: completion of transfer of key information (verbal and written) from one provider or setting to another	Variance/delay in care	▶ Patient- and family-related variances (e.g., refusal of discharge or care) ▶ System-related variances (e.g., radiology test is unavailable because of equipment malfunction) ▶ Community-related variances (e.g., bed in skilled nursing facility is unavailable) ▶ Practitioner-related variances (e.g., medication error) ▶ Left without being seen (emergency department) ▶ Timely access to care (e.g., delay in completion of a specialty provider consult) ▶ Routine screening (e.g., percentage of mammogram completion)

the patient's disease process or the end result of a procedure or a care activity. Such events happen during the normal course of healthcare services. APOs may include an injury that was caused by medical management rather than the underlying disease; perhaps the injury also prolonged the patient's hospitalization because of the need for further care that otherwise would have been unnecessary, or produced a short-term or permanent disability at the time of discharge. Experts, such as the Institute for Healthcare Improvement (IHI), have defined APOs as unintended physical injury including death because of medical care (including the absence of indicated medical treatment), which requires additional monitoring, treatment, or hospitalization.

Many organizations detail a severity coding system for APOs. In general, severity ratings separate acceptable and unacceptable ranges of outcomes. For example:

▶ *Level I.* There is a confirmed quality problem with minimal potential for significant adverse effect(s) on the patient. The problem may be a discharge with mild bacteriuria and pyuria and without follow-up plans for further evaluation. Events that are predictable within an expected standard of care may also be included in level I; these are events such as urinary retention after a total abdominal hysterectomy.

▶ *Level II.* There is a confirmed quality problem with the potential for significant adverse effect(s) on the patient. Perhaps the wrong intravenous fluid or medication was administered but was quickly discovered and corrected before any harm occurred.

▶ *Level III.* There is a confirmed quality problem with significant deviation from expected levels of care, resulting in an unexpected injury to patients. These events represent gross departures from expected standards and may result in serious impairment such as loss of a limb or function of a body part, psychological injury, or death. An example would be operating on the wrong side, such as the left instead of the right hip, or removing the wrong kidney.

Adverse patient occurrences are of many types (Display 7-2); they may be preventable or nonpreventable. Preventable APOs are avoidable by any available means at the time of occurrence unless that means was not considered a standard of care. Preventable APOs, on the other hand, are care activities or interventions that fell below the standard expected of healthcare professionals under similar circumstances. These events are usually relevant to both healthcare providers and patients/families alike. For healthcare providers, adverse events and outcomes may reduce the quality of their care and increase costs because of the need for additional services. For patients and their families, adverse events bring about a suboptimal experience of care and may increase the burden of disease and recovery.

It is important for case managers to remain alert to the incidence of APOs and take immediate action to prevent further serious damage to patients because of these events. It is also necessary for them to carefully assess the situation and determine the implications of the events. Additionally, case managers must understand that the adverse outcomes may not always be noted during the patients' hospitalization; rather, outcomes may not be visible until 30 days after discharge or transfer to another care setting or provider. The intended result of treatment, the likelihood of the adverse outcome occurring, and the presence or absence of a medical error causing it are all irrelevant in identifying an adverse outcome. APOs that are of special significance for case managers are those included in the VBP Program under the safety domain; for example, incidence of healthcare-associated conditions/infections.

Healthcare organizations have a process in place for identifying, reporting, investigating, and correcting such adverse events. An example is a root cause analysis (RCA) process which may also be known as an event review, which involves an interdisciplinary team that includes representation from RM and quality and patient safety departments in addition to the clinicians involved in the event and other experts. Today, however, the presence of representatives from human factor engineering departments has been gaining momentum. These professionals contribute greatly to the review process because of their

---

display 7-2

TYPES OF ADVERSE PATIENT OCCURRENCES

▶ *Preventable adverse events:* those that have occurred due to error or failure to apply an accepted strategy for prevention.

▶ *Ameliorable adverse events:* events that, while not preventable, could have been less harmful if care had been different.

▶ *Adverse events because of negligence:* those that have occurred due to care that falls below the recognized or established standards expected of clinicians under similar conditions.

▶ *Near miss:* an unsafe situation that is indistinguishable from a preventable adverse event except for the outcome.

A patient is exposed to a potentially harmful situation, but does not experience the harm at all either because of luck or because of early detection. Often near misses are discovered before they reach the patient.

▶ *Error:* a broader term referring to any act of commission (i.e., doing something wrong) or omission (i.e., failing to do the right thing or not doing something at all) that exposes patients to a potentially harmful situation. The outcome may vary from being of high significance or serious in nature to being insignificant or with no untoward consequences at all.

specialized knowledge and skills in carefully examining the systems of care and the interface of the professionals with the environment, equipment, and health information systems and technology. Some of these events may require reporting to your state's Department of Health and Human Services and/or to accreditation agencies such as TJC. Usually your organization will have an administrative procedure in place describing these events, the RCA process, and the reporting process.

The RCA process may include the following:

▶ Study of the involved environment, systems, and processes to identify the critical steps and decision points;
▶ Identification of the personnel, actions, and equipment necessary for the proper functioning of the system or process, and critical to its outcomes;
▶ The finding of links between variables involved in performance;
▶ The ranking of the frequency of causes;
▶ Peer review by other healthcare professionals, commonly recognized as experts in the field.

Investigating APOs by applying the RCA review process almost always results in recommendations for improving a patient care flow process, enforcing a process, adding a new process, or eliminating an existing one. In addition, it may result in additional training and education of certain personnel, especially those intimately involved in the process. After a change has been implemented, monitoring of outcomes is usually necessary.

▶ Potentially Compensable Event

A potentially compensable event is one in which the end result could be litigation. For more information, refer to Chapter 8. These events are usually reviewed and managed by RM specialists and legal counsel.

▶ Incident

An incident is an accident, error, or the discovery of a hazardous condition that is inconsistent with the standards of care or standards of practice either established by the healthcare organization or advocated for by healthcare-related professional associations.

▶ Incident Report (Also Known as Occurrence Report)

An incident report is a communication tool to record adverse events or unusual occurrences. Incident reports assess potential liabilities, are used for discovering existing problems, and help identify the need for revising current standards, processes of care, policies, or procedures. State law determines whether they are confidential or discoverable in court. It is not advisable to document in the medical record that an incident report has been filled

out, although the events of the incident may be recorded in the patient's chart if they are important to future care and treatment. The case manager should be objective, factual, clear, and complete. He or she must refrain from speculation, subjectivity, or drawing judgment. This is important because incident reports may be discoverable in court.

Today's incident reporting systems are available in an electronic manner with specialized software applications that allow for sophisticated data analyses and reporting. Special features of these applications may include the ability to:

▶ Analyze large data sets applying quantitative methods.
▶ Analyze "free text" content applying qualitative methods.
▶ Identify the trends and patterns of events.
▶ Assist in determining priorities for special PI efforts.
▶ Report events in an anonymous manner where necessary.

▶ Variances

Variances are deviations from expected care or standards. Four types of variances exist: practitioner, system/institutional, community, and patient/family (see "Lag Days and Variances" in Chapter 5 for a more complete discussion).

▶ Important Aspects of Care

These aspects of care occur frequently, affect large numbers of patients, or place patients at risk for serious consequences if not provided for optimally. These aspects of care are often the target of PI activities and therefore must be measurable.

▶ Core Measures and Other CMS-Related Measures

Core measures are a national, standardized performance measurement system that was implemented to improve the quality of healthcare services and delivery systems. First begun by TJC in 1997 as a voluntary effort for the management of the quality and performance of healthcare organizations, they were known as the ORYX measures and later renamed "core measures." Over a decade ago, the Centers for Medicare & Medicaid Services (CMS) implemented a core measures system that is in alignment with TJC. The CMS system is also known as National Quality Measures and endeavors to help hospitals improve the quality of patient care by focusing on the actual results (outcomes, consequences) of care. The measures are medical information retrieved from patients' records and converted into a rate or percentage that shows how well hospitals care for their patients. Recently, the CMS turned the National Quality Measures into pay-for-performance and in 2010 to the VBP Program.

HOSPITAL VALUE-BASED PURCHASING PROGRAM

The Patient Protection and Affordable Care Act of 2010 established the Hospital VBP Program, which applied to Medicare reimbursement payments beginning in fiscal year (FY) 2013 and affected payment for inpatient hospital stays in more than 3,000 hospitals across the United States. Under this program, Medicare makes incentive payments to hospitals on the basis of either how well they perform on each of the measures included in the program or how much they improve their performance on each measure compared with their performance during a baseline period.

The Hospital VBP Program has shifted the focus of quality from volume to value and allowed Medicare beneficiaries to have a choice about where to receive care. Choice has become easier for patients since the performance of participating hospitals on the VBP Program measures is available online for anyone to access at the Hospital Compare website: https://www.medicare.gov/hospitalcompare/search.html. The program's core measures focus on the following:

▶ Mortality and complications,
▶ Healthcare-associated infections,
▶ Patient safety,
▶ Patient experience,
▶ Processes of care including care coordination,
▶ Clinical outcomes of care, and
▶ Efficiency and cost reduction (CMS, 2015).

The CMS bases hospital performance on an approved set of measures and dimensions grouped into specific quality domains. The measures pertain to specific diagnosis-related groups (DRGs). Both the measures and domains vary depending on the program's FY. Display 7-3 provides the applicable domains for FY 2016 through FY 2018 and the specified weights allocated for each domain. The weights are used for hospitals' performance-scoring purposes. Displays 7-4 and 7-5 list the measures for FY 2017 and 2018 (CMS, 2015).

The Hospital VBP Program rewards acute care hospitals with incentive payments for the quality of care they provide to Medicare beneficiaries. Conversely, if the quality of care is found not to meet the target benchmarks, or hospitals do not demonstrate improvements in the measures, the program penalizes the hospitals financially in the form of a percentage reduction of Medicare reimbursement payments under the inpatient prospective payment system. Therefore, the Hospital VBP Program is designed to encourage hospitals to improve the quality of care and experience of patients. Hospitals can achieve better quality of care and experience by implementing the following strategies:

▶ Eliminating or reducing healthcare errors and adverse events that result in patient harm.
▶ Adopting evidence-based care standards and protocols that ensure the best outcomes for patients.

display 7-3 · HOSPITAL VALUE-BASED PURCHASING PROGRAM'S DOMAINS AND ASSOCIATED WEIGHTS, 2016 TO 2018

Fiscal Year	Applicable Domains and Weights (%)
2016	▶ Clinical Process of Care (10%) ▶ Patient Experience of Care (25%) ▶ Outcome (40%) Efficiency (25%)
2017	▶ Patient and Caregiver-Centered Experience of Care/Care Coordination (25%) ▶ Safety (20%) ▶ Clinical Care (30%) ▶ Clinical Care—Outcomes (25%) ▶ Clinical Care—Process (5%) ▶ Efficiency and Cost Reduction (25%)
2018	▶ Patient and Caregiver-Centered Experience of Care/Care Coordination (25%) ▶ Safety (25%) ▶ Clinical Care (25%) ▶ Efficiency and Cost Reduction (25%)

SOURCE: Department of Health and Human Services, & Centers for Medicare & Medicaid Services, & Medicare Learning Network. (2015, September). *Hospital value-based purchasing*. Retrieved July 1, 2017, from https://www.cms.gov/Outreach-and-Education/Medicare-Learning-Network-MLN/MLNProducts/downloads/Hospital_VBPurchasing_Fact_Sheet_ICN907664.pdf

NOTE: Beginning with FY 2017, the CMS reclassified the quality domains to align more closely with its National Quality Strategy (NQS). The NQS serves as a blueprint for healthcare stakeholders across the country and helps prioritize QI efforts, share lessons learned, and measure collective success.

▶ Changing hospital-based systems and processes of care delivery to ensure optimal care experiences for patients.
▶ Increasing care transparency for consumers.
▶ Recognizing hospitals that provide high quality and safe care at a lower cost to Medicare beneficiaries (CMS, 2015).

The incentive (or penalty) payment methodology included in the Medicare's Hospital VBP Program is complex. Hospitals in the VBP Program may earn 2 scores on each measure: one for their achievements of quality of care (performance or achievement) and another for the degree of progress (PI) demonstrated in the quality of care as compared to performance in baseline measurement period. The final score awarded to a hospital for each measure is the higher of these 2 scores. Generally, for each measure included in the Program, the CMS considers a threshold of 50th percentile performance (achievement score) and a benchmark determined as the mean of the top decile performing hospitals for the same measure (improvement score). Hospitals may earn an

display 7-4

CORE MEASURES/NATIONAL QUALITY MEASURES (HOSPITAL VALUE-BASED PURCHASING MEASURES—FY 2017)

Measure Code	Core Measures	Measure Type
CAUTI	Catheter-associated urinary tract infection	Safety
CLABSI	Central line–associated blood Stream infection	Safety
CDI	*Clostridium difficile* Infection (*C. difficile*)	Safety
MRSA	Methicillin-resistant *Staphylococcus aureus* Bacteremia	Safety
AHRQ PSI-90 Composite	Complication/ patient safety for selected Indicators (composite)	Safety
SSI	Surgical site infection (SSI): ▶ Colon ▶ Abdominal hysterectomy	Safety
MORT-30-PN	Pneumonia (PN) 30-day mortality rate	Clinical care: outcomes
MORT-30-AMI	Acute myocardial infarction (AMI) 30-day mortality rate	Clinical care: outcomes

Measure Code	Core Measures	Measure Type
AMI-7a	Fibrinolytic therapy received within 30 minutes of hospital arrival clinical care—processes	Clinical care: outcomes
MORT-30-HF	Heart failure (HF) 30-day mortality rate	Clinical care: outcomes
IMM-2	Influenza immunization	Clinical care: processes
PC-01	Elective delivery prior to 39 completed weeks gestation	Clinical care: processes
MSPB-1	Medicare spending per beneficiary (MSPB)	Efficiency and cost reduction
HCAHPS survey	▶ Communication with nurses ▶ Communication with doctors ▶ Responsiveness of hospital staff ▶ Pain management ▶ Communication about medicines ▶ Cleanliness and quietness of hospital environment ▶ Discharge information ▶ Overall rating of hospital	Patient and Caregiver-centered experience of care/care coordination

SOURCE: Department of Health and Human Services, & Centers for Medicare & Medicaid Services, & Medicare Learning Network (2015, September). *Hospital value-based purchasing.* Retrieved July 1, 2017, from https://www.cms.gov/Outreach-and-Education/Medicare-Learning-Network-MLN/ MLNProducts/downloads/Hospital_VBPurchasing_Fact_Sheet_ICN907664.pdf

achievement score of 1 to 10 points and an improvement score of 1 to 9 points. A hospital will earn no points on each of the achievement or improvement scores if it does not demonstrate better performance compared with the baseline period (CMS, 2015).

The CMS adjusts a part of the hospitals' Medicare payments on the basis of a total performance score that reflects on a measure-by-measure basis how well the hospital has performed (achievement score) compared with all the other participating hospitals, or how much the hospital has improved its performance (improvement score) compared with the performance demonstrated during a prior measurement period. This approach reflects the importance that the CMS places on the value of care rather than the quantity. Essentially, on the basis of the Hospital VBP Program, the CMS withholds participating hospitals' Medicare payments by a percentage specified by law. It then uses the estimated total amount of those payment reductions to fund the value-based incentive payments to the participating hospitals as required on the basis of their performance. In this regard, the CMS applies the

net result of the payment reduction and the incentive as a claim-by-claim adjustment factor to the base operating Medicare severity DRG (MS-DRG) payment amount for Medicare fee-for-service claims in the FY associated with the performance period. The CMS usually withholds a percentage of its Medicare payments to hospitals and then uses the withheld amount to disperse as incentive payments to eligible hospitals. The applicable withheld percentage has been increasing over time starting with 1% in 2013, 1.25% in 2014, 1.50% in 2015, 1.75% in 2016, and 2.00% in 2017 and beyond. This process increases a hospital's financial risk and therefore enhances the essential role of case management (CMS, 2015).

Case managers have played an important role in reducing a hospital's financial risk on the basis of the Hospital VBP Program. They engage in daily activities with the interdisciplinary healthcare teams that aim to ensure the care the Medicare beneficiaries (and other patients) receive is safe and of utmost quality and meets the VBP requirements (core measures), and demonstrate optimal patient experience of care and ongoing improvements.

CORE MEASURES/NATIONAL QUALITY MEASURES (HOSPITAL VALUE-BASED PURCHASING MEASURES—FY 2018)

display 7-5

Measure Code	Core Measures	Measure Type
CAUTI	Catheter-associated urinary tract infection	Safety
CLABSI	Central line–associated blood Stream infection	Safety
CDI	*Clostridium difficile* infection (*C. difficile*)	Safety
MRSA	Methicillin-resistant *Staphylococcus aureus* Bacteremia	Safety
AHRQ PSI-90 composite	Complication/patient safety for selected Indicators (composite)	Safety
SSI	Surgical site infection (SSI): ▶ Colon ▶ Abdominal hysterectomy	Safety
PC-01	Elective delivery prior to 39 completed weeks gestation	Safety
MORT-30-PN	Pneumonia (PN) 30-day mortality rate	Clinical care: outcomes

Measure Code	Core Measures	Measure Type
MORT-30-AMI	Acute myocardial infarction (AMI) 30-day mortality rate	Clinical care: outcomes
MORT-30-HF	Heart failure (HF) 30-day mortality rate	Clinical care: outcomes
MSPB-1	Medicare spending per beneficiary (MSPB)	Efficiency and cost reduction
HCAHPS Survey	▶ Communication with nurses ▶ Communication with doctors ▶ Responsiveness of hospital staff ▶ Pain management ▶ Communication about medicines ▶ Cleanliness and quietness of hospital environment ▶ Discharge information ▶ Care transitions ▶ Overall rating of hospital	Patient and caregiver-centered experience of care/care coordination

SOURCE: Department of Health and Human Services, & Centers for Medicare & Medicaid Services, & Medicare Learning Network (2015, September). *Hospital value-based purchasing.* Retrieved July 1, 2017, from https://www.cms.gov/Outreach-and-Education/Medicare-Learning-Network-MLN/MLNProducts/downloads/Hospital_VBPurchasing_Fact_Sheet_ICN907664.pdf

The measures and domains of the Hospital VBP Program have evolved over time. It is expected that these continue to change on the basis of future performance of hospitals and the CMS quality strategy. Some measures have been discontinued since the program first started in FY 2013. Others have been added. It is important to note that as hospital performance on a measure demonstrates optimal improvements and such improvements are sustained over time, the CMS often drops that measure from the VBP Program. Although such a measure is dropped from the quality reporting and incentive payment calculation, hospitals continue to focus on sustaining the improvement achieved in such a measure. These efforts maintain the focus on the value rather than the volume of care.

Reflecting on the measures included in FY 2018 compared with those of FY 2017 (refer to Displays 7-4 and 7-5), one may notice that PC-01, Elective Delivery Prior to 39 Completed Weeks Gestation was moved to the safety dDomain from the Domain of Clinical Care; measure IMM2, Influenza Immunization was removed from the Clinical Care Domain; and HCAHPS Survey, Care Transitions was added to the Patient and Caregiver-Centered Experience of Care/Care Coordination Domain. These changes may not be as dramatic as those that occurred in the prior FY. For example, when comparing FY 2016 with FY 2017, one notices that in FY 2017, the CMS added the following three measures to the Hospital VBP Program:

1. PC-01, Elective delivery prior to 39 completed weeks gestation (Clinical care—Process subdomain).
2. CDI, *Clostridium difficile* infection (safety domain).
3. MRSA, Methicillin-resistant *Staphylococcus aureus* (safety domain).

It is also evident that the CMS eliminated the following six measures from the Program in FY 2017 compared with those of FY 2016 (CMS, 2015):

1. PN-6, Initial antibiotic selection for community acquired pneumonia (CAP) in immunocompetent patient.
2. SCIP-Card-2, Surgery patients on a beta-blocker prior to arrival that received a beta-blocker during the perioperative period.
3. SCIP-Inf-2, Prophylactic antibiotic selection for surgical patients
4. SCIP-Inf-3, Prophylactic antibiotics discontinued within 24 hours after surgery end time.

5. SCIP-Inf-9, Postoperative urinary catheter removal on postoperative day 1 or 2.
6. SCIP-VTE-2, Surgery patients who received appropriate venous thromboembolism prophylaxis within 24 hours prior to surgery to 24 hours after surgery.

PUBLIC REPORTING OF PERFORMANCE DATA

Today, participation in the public reporting of data on these core measures is an expectation laid down by the CMS. Although public reporting of data on core measures is not mandatory, if a hospital (for example) does not publicly report its data, its reimbursement by the CMS will be affected. Therefore, hospitals tend to report their data to maintain acceptable reimbursement rates. The core measures are derived largely from a set of quality indicators defined by the CMS. These have been shown to reduce the risk of complications, prevent recurrences, and improve the quality of care for patients who come to a hospital for treatment of a condition or illness. Under each category, key actions are listed that represent the most widely accepted, research-based care process for appropriate care in that category.

Other CMS-related measures are the Hospital Outcome of Care Measures, which include 30-day risk-adjusted death (mortality) rates and are produced from Medicare claims and enrollment data using a complex statistical model. The model predicts patient deaths for any cause within 30 days of hospital admission for heart attack, or heart failure, or pneumonia, whether the patients die while still in the hospital or after discharge. Thirty-day mortality is used because this is the time when deaths are most likely to be related to the care patients received in the hospital. Deaths that occur outside the hospital within 30 days are included along with deaths that occur in the hospital, because some hospitals discharge patients sooner than others. By *risk-adjusted* we mean that the model calculates a death (mortality) rate that adjusts for the kinds of patients who go to that hospital, so that hospitals that take care of sicker patients won't have a worse rate just because their patients were sicker before they arrived at the hospital.

As part of the ongoing effort to improve the quality of care, the CMS also developed the first readmission outcome measure for hospitals in 2008: a 30-day risk-standardized readmission measure for heart failure (HF) patients. This measure responds to the call by the Medicare Payment Advisory Commission to develop readmission measures, with HF as a priority condition. The measure includes fee-for-service Medicare beneficiaries of at least 65 years of age with a principal discharge diagnosis of HF. In September 2008, the CMS conducted a national "dry run" of the implementation of the 30-day HF readmission measure. The dry run was designed to educate hospitals about the HF readmission measure and to test the public reporting of outcomes on this measure. Like the 30-day-risk-adjusted-death rates, the readmission measure will also affect hospital reimbursement. Today

similar measures apply for patients with acute myocardial infarction (AMI) and pneumonia as evident in the Hospital VBP Program.

The 30-day-risk-adjusted-death rates and the HF readmission measure, in addition to the rest of the core measures, are important for case managers. The role case managers play in transitional and discharge planning relates directly to these outcomes. For example, if a patient were discharged prematurely from the hospital, or if a patient's care needs after discharge were not appropriately coordinated, resulting in an unsafe discharge, the patient would have a much higher chance of experiencing serious deterioration in health condition and therefore an increased risk for death after discharge.

In addition, the CMS requires hospitals to evaluate patient and family experience of care received, using the Hospital Consumer Assessment of Healthcare Providers and Systems (HCAHPS) measure. This is a national, standardized survey of hospital patients. The HCAHPS was created to publicly report the patient's perspective on hospital care. The survey asks a random sample of recently discharged patients about important aspects of their hospital experience. Included in this assessment of patients' experiences are questions about how prepared they were for discharge and how informed they were about new medications—two important case management responsibilities. Similar to data on the core measures, the HCAHPS results are also publicly reported and posted on the Hospital Compare website to allow consumers of healthcare to make fair and objective comparisons of hospitals and of individual hospitals with state and national benchmarks. For more on HCAHPS information, visit the official HCAHPS website (www.hcahpsonline. org). Today, patient and family experience measures have been expanded to other care settings including ambulatory care and long-term care.

▶ THE NATIONAL QUALITY STRATEGY

Healthcare spending in the United States has exceeded $2.5 trillion a year, the highest per capita in the world. Despite the increased spending, the country experiences shorter life expectancy and higher infant mortality rates than other developed countries do. These performance outcomes suggest that increased spending has not translated into better care. The Patient Protection and Affordable Care Act of 2010 has required the United States Department of Health and Human Services to establish a National Strategy for Quality Improvement in Health Care, known today as the National Quality Strategy (NQS). Congress approved the strategy on March 21, 2011.

The Agency for Healthcare Research and Quality (AHRQ) has led this strategy on behalf of the U.S. Department of Health and Human Services. The NQS is the first policy to set national goals to improve the quality of healthcare in the United States. It also sets standards and regulations to measure the quality of healthcare and its impact on public health. The strategy has established three objectives:

1. To make healthcare more accessible, safe, and patient-/family-centered;
2. To address environmental, social, and behavioral influences on health and healthcare; and
3. To make care more affordable for all.

The National Quality Strategy development applied a transparent and collaborative process where input from a diverse group of stakeholders was obtained, including healthcare professionals and patient advocacy groups. The NQS was then presented online for public review and feedback where more than 300 groups, organizations,

and individuals, representing all sectors of healthcare services and the public, provided comments. On the basis of this input, the NQS finally established a set of three overarching strategies which built on the IHI's Triple Aim: better care (individual related), better health (population related), and lower cost. Recently a fourth dimension was added, and this focuses on the experience of healthcare provider (satisfaction with the care environment); thus, the transition to the Quadruple Aim has taken place. The NQS strategies were also supported by six principles or priorities to address the most common health concerns that Americans face. The NQS also identified nine levers for stakeholders to use in align their core functions to drive improvement on the aims and aligning principles/priorities (Display 7-6) (AHRQ, 2017).

display 7-6

THE NATIONAL QUALITY STRATEGY

Aspect	Highlights
Aims	1. Better Care ▶ Improve the overall quality, by making healthcare more patient centered, reliable, accessible, and safe. 2. Healthy People/Healthy Communities ▶ Improve the health of the US population by supporting proven interventions to address behavioral, social, and environmental determinants of health in addition to delivering higher-quality care. 3. Affordable Care ▶ Reduce the cost of quality healthcare for individuals, families, employers, and government.
Principles/priorities	1. Making care safer by reducing harm caused in the delivery of care and services. 2. Ensuring that each person and family is engaged as partners in their care. 3. Promoting effective communication and coordination of care across healthcare providers and care settings. 4. Promoting the most effective prevention and treatment practices for the leading causes of mortality, starting with cardiovascular disease. 5. Working with communities to promote the wide use of best practices to enable healthy living. 6. Making quality care more affordable for individuals, families, employers, and governments by developing and spreading new healthcare delivery models.

Aspect	Highlights
Levers	1. Measurement and Feedback ▶ Provide performance feedback to health insurance plans and healthcare providers to improve care. 2. Public Reporting ▶ Compare treatment results, costs, and patient experience of care for consumers of healthcare services. 3. Learning and Technical Assistance ▶ Foster learning environments that offer training, resources, tools, and guidance to help healthcare organizations achieve quality and safety improvement goals. 4. Certification, Accreditation, and Regulation ▶ Adopt or adhere to approaches to meet safety and quality standards of healthcare provision. 5. Consumer Incentives and Benefit Designs ▶ Help consumers adopt healthy behavioral lifestyle and make informed decisions about their health and healthcare. 6. Payment ▶ Reward and incentivize providers to deliver high-quality, patient-centered care to patients and their families. 7. Health Information Technology ▶ Improve communication, transparency, and efficiency for better coordinated health and healthcare. 8. Innovation and Diffusion ▶ Foster innovation in healthcare quality improvement, and facilitate rapid adoption within and across organizations and communities. 9. Workforce Development ▶ Invest in people to prepare the next generation of healthcare professionals and support lifelong learning for healthcare providers.

SOURCE: Agency for Healthcare Research and Quality. (2017, March). About the National Quality Strategy. Rockville, MD: Author. Retrieved July 1, 2017, from http://www.ahrq.gov/workingforquality/about/index.html

▶ The aims (better care, affordable care for the individual, and healthy people/healthy communities) are used to guide and assess local, state, and national efforts to improve health and the quality of healthcare.

▶ The principles/priorities are intended to advance the three aims and improve health and healthcare quality.

▶ Each of the levers represents a core healthcare organizational business function, resource, and/or action that stakeholders can use to align to the NQS and implement to improve the quality of care (AHRQ, 2017).

Improving health and healthcare quality is everyone's top priority. Desirable and rewarding improvements can successfully be achieved when all involved stakeholders (e.g., individuals, family members, family caregivers, payors, healthcare providers, employers, regulatory and accreditation agencies, and communities) make it their mission and priority. No doubt, these stakeholders have already been engaged in healthcare quality improvement activities; although they may not be necessarily applying the NQS aims and principles and using the levers, these already existing efforts make it easier for stakeholders to realign their activities to the NQS rather than starting anew.

▶ The Centers for Medicare & Medicaid Services' Quality Strategy

The CMS quality strategy is built on the foundation of the United States Department of Health and Human Services' NQS that was developed and is being overseen by the AHRQ. The CMS quality strategy guides the collaborative activities of all agencies within CMS toward healthcare transformation. Like the NQS, the CMS quality strategy was developed through a participatory, transparent, and collaborative process that included the input of a wide range of stakeholders. For more than a year, a group of leaders from across the CMS met and developed the strategy. This group also sought advice and input from other agencies of the United States Department of Health and Human Services, the healthcare community, and CMS beneficiaries to inform the development of the final strategy as we know it today (CMS, 2017).

The Quality Strategy prioritizes six goals for success and illustrates the continued collaboration and transparency among key stakeholders. The CMS vision for this strategy is: optimize health outcomes by improving quality and transforming the health system. The strategy's six goals are summarized herewith on the basis of the CMS Medicare Quality Initiatives Program (CMS, 2017).

1. *Make care safer by reducing harm caused in the delivery of care.* This goal aims to improve and support a culture of safety in the environment of healthcare delivery; reduce inappropriate and unnecessary care that can lead to harm; and prevent or minimize harm in all healthcare settings. This goal can be achieved through (a) improving communication among patients, families, and healthcare providers; (b) empowering patients to become more engaged in their health and healthcare; (c) promoting better coordination of care within and across healthcare settings; (d) implementing evidence-based safety best practices wherever care is provided; and (e) supporting payment systems that incentivize healthcare organizations and providers that minimize patient harm from inappropriate care.

2. *Strengthen person and family engagement as partners in their health and healthcare.* This goal ensures that healthcare delivery and services incorporate the person and family preferences. It also aims to improve the patient and family experience of care and promote patient's self-management knowledge skills and abilities. This goal can be achieved by (a) actively encouraging patients and their family engagement across the healthcare continuum; (b) promoting the use of tools and strategies that promote self-determination and achieve individuals' goals, values, and preferences; (c) creating an environment of care where the individual, as the center of the interdisciplinary healthcare team, can create health and wellness goals that are accessible, appropriate, effective, and sufficient; and (d) identifying patient and family engagement best practices and techniques and integrate these practices into care delivery systems with the opportunity to improve the experience of care for patients and their families on a large scale.

3. *Promote effective communication and coordination of care.* This goal emphasizes the need to reduce admissions and readmissions to the acute care setting (e.g., Hospital Readmissions Reduction program [HRRP]) and apply best practices in care coordination and readmission reduction to enable successful transitions of care across settings and providers. These activities should enable effective healthcare system navigation by patients and their families. It is thought that this goal is best achieved by (a) encouraging the implementation of care coordination across the healthcare continuum; (b) promoting a patient- and family-centered approach to coordination of care; and (c) recognizing the importance of sharing critical information about the patient/family across care settings and providers and the impact on such information on continuity of care, safety and quality.

4. *Promote effective prevention and treatment of chronic disease.* This goal aims to increase the appropriate use of screening and prevention services and the need to strengthen interventions to prevent heart attacks and strokes. It also addresses the importance of improving

the access and quality of care (and outcomes) for people with multiple chronic conditions, behavioral health concerns, and perinatal care. These aims are best achieved through (a) collaboration across various stakeholders (e.g., healthcare providers, state and federal health-related agencies, nongovernmental agencies, payors, and patient advocacy groups) to increase awareness of current and new preventive healthcare services available to Medicare, Medicaid, and Children's Health Insurance Program (CHIP) beneficiaries; (b) raising the importance of preventive services in improving beneficiary health; and (c) reducing disparities in access to and utilization of primary and specialty healthcare services, and preventive care for all populations.

5. *Work with communities to promote best practices of healthy living.* This goal promotes the need to partner with and support federal, state, and local public health improvement efforts and improve access within communities to best practices of healthy living. It also encourages the use of evidence-based community interventions and community-based social services to prevent and treat chronic disease. This goal can be realized through two main strategies: (a) building and strengthening relationships with various stakeholders to better link Medicare, Medicaid, and CHIP beneficiaries, and the healthcare providers that serve them, with community-based resources and organizations that support good health; and (b) encouraging healthcare providers to also partner with local and state public health improvement efforts, so that these beneficiaries can benefit from the high-quality, community-based programs and services that support healthy living.

6. *Make healthcare affordable.* This goal encourages the development and implementation of payment systems that reward value over volume such as the Hospital VBP Program. It also supports the use of cost analysis data to inform payment policies and methods (e.g., Accountable Care Organizations, shared risk programs, and bundled payment). This goal can be realized by (a) establishing common measures that will help assess the cost impact of new programs and payment systems; (b) improving data systems by encouraging and supporting health information exchanges for administrative simplification, and making data available to healthcare providers across organizations and settings; (c) making healthcare costs and quality more transparent to consumers and providers, enabling them to make better choices and decisions; and (d) implementing national quality improvement programs and initiatives to systematically spread known best practices to reduce costs and improve healthcare services and outcomes.

The six goals and their associated objectives, interventions, and implementation strategies highlight the contribution of case management programs and case managers especially in the areas of discharge and transitional planning, use of electronic medical record–based tools for communication with providers and across settings, and outcomes management and improvement. The goals and interventions are inherently interrelated and demonstrate characteristics of case management programs. This has recently increased the value of case management and its contribution to healthcare organizations' bottom lines. This has also allowed case managers to assume an essential role as primary drivers of change for better healthcare services, including quality and safety outcomes, and reduction in costs through effective allocation and utilization of resources.

▶ Alignment of Measures of Care Quality

Since the inception of core measures and pay-for-performance, and today with the increased use of the VBP Program, the number of core measures continues to rise. This increase is also attributed to the adoption of measures by various health-related entities, including the following:

▶ *Professional organizations and societies* such as the Society for Hospital Medicine, the American Medical Association, the American College of Cardiology, the American Nurses Association, the American Academy of Nursing, and others.

▶ *Government affiliated organizations* such as the National Quality Forum and the AHRQ.

▶ *Nongovernment affiliated organizations* such as the National Committee for Quality Assurance, TJC, and the URAC, previously known as the Utilization Review Accreditation Commission.

The above-mentioned organizations and societies have also been known to develop quality and outcomes measures, some of which have been formally adopted in the Hospitals VBP Program and CMS National Quality Strategy and Quality Improvement Initiative. Such popularity has contributed to the development of a large set of quality or core measures, some of which is duplicative across organizations, whereas others are conflicting or confusing. Additionally, the effective management of these core measures has been a great challenge for all parties alike: healthcare providers, payors, accreditation agencies, and regulators.

The NQS has been addressing the rising number of clinical quality measures and the resulting duplication used in national programs. One of the NQS's main goal is to have measures that matter and minimize healthcare provider burden, while ensuring better quality of care to patients and their families, and at an affordable cost. For this purpose, the United States Department of Health and Human Services (USDHHS) convened the Measurement Policy Council in early 2012 to start aligning measures across the department. Composed of senior-level representatives from agencies and operating divisions across USDHHS, the group also addresses new measure development and implementation, and measurement policy. The Council has so far reviewed nine topics to date: hypertension control, hospital-acquired conditions/patient safety, HCAHPs, smoking cessation, depression screening, care coordination, HIV/AIDS, perinatal, and obesity/body mass index (BMI). The core measure sets that the Measurement Policy Council developed for each topic can be viewed here: https://www.ahrq.gov/sites/default/files/wysiwyg/workingforquality/mpcmeasures.pdf.

While these measures are used for federal programs, the Measurement Policy Council supports state and private sector efforts to adopt core measure sets for further harmonization and alignment across the healthcare industry.

▶ HOW CASE MANAGEMENT, QM, AND RM WORK TOGETHER

Case managers constantly oversee all aspects of patient care: assessing, reassessing, evaluating, monitoring, and reevaluating. For this reason, case managers are critical team members in the QI-RM process. Consider the following six high-risk areas for healthcare professionals, including nurses; after reviews of occurrences and actual claims against nurses, these deficits have been deemed areas of practice that can become major sources of liability. Many of these "failures" can be spotted through astute chart reviews; hopefully, this can prevent an APO from occurring and therefore avoiding patient harm.

1. Failure to take, or properly assess, a patient's history—*Example:* a missed medication allergy.
2. Failure to perform a nursing procedure according to nursing standards—*Example:* failure to properly administer medications.
3. Failure to follow a provider's/doctor's order promptly or correctly—*Example:* failure to follow the organization's chain of command if the nurse, case manager, social worker, or therapist thinks something is wrong or lacking in the orders. It may also be that the correct procedure was followed; however, it may not have been fully documented.
4. Failure to report deviations from accepted practice—*Example:* delay in the switch from intravenous to oral antibiotics, resulting in unnecessary prolonged hospital stay, or early signs of sepsis going unnoticed, resulting in a serious change in the patient's condition (otherwise preventable) and implementation of intensive care/services; again, these may also indicate a lack of complete documentation of what really transpired.
5. Failure to properly supervise the patient—*Example:* patient falls, IV line failures or infiltrates, patient

self-extubation. These may result from inadequate assessment and monitoring; these may also be due to staff handling more patients than is humanly possible.

6. Failure to summon the medical attending physician appropriately—*Example:* a related but frequent allegation is the failure to communicate appropriate and complete information to the physician and in a timely manner, resulting in a delay in progressing care.
7. Failure to share important information about a patient's condition and plan of care between healthcare providers and settings—*Example:* a patient transfer from a skilled nursing facility to an acute care or hospital, and transfer records are missing and the hospital is unable to reach providers at the prior setting. These factors resulted in a plan of care that did not address all of the patient's chronic illness and neglected to continue required medications.

Keeping these high-risk areas of concern in mind, consider how important a case manager's skills and responsibilities are from a QI-RM perspective. As patient advocates who are involved in all areas of patient care delivery and health services, case managers are always alert for any hindrances to optimal outcomes. Case management is a highly prized RM tool in many ways.

▶ Case Managers Identify and Anticipate Potential Problems

- ▶ Case managers are adept at identifying circumstances that make the patient vulnerable to high-risk incidents, optimally before they happen but certainly before they have done maximum (and sometimes irreparable) damage. Related to this is the identification of potential safety issues in confused and/or frail patients. For example, quality medical record reviews reveal that a patient had a high potassium level, yet no one on the interdisciplinary healthcare team attempted to discontinue the potassium supplement from the IV solutions. The review also shows that a medication that was listed under allergies was ordered for a patient.
- ▶ Case managers identify traits in patients and/or their families that could make them vulnerable to high-risk incidents and adjust the care plan for maximum safety.
- ▶ Case managers act as patient advocates; they function in a capacity in which they hear many patient and family complaints. Sometimes the case manager can appropriately intervene; sometimes it is important to call the RM department. The wise choice is always to practice good communication and documentation skills.

▶ Case managers act as liaisons among the patient, the organizations where they work, other providers of care, and the health insurance company. In this capacity, case managers assist in developing treatment and discharge/transition plans. The case manager ascertains the best plan to meet the individual needs of the patient—all within the constraints of the payor (health insurance company). This often takes thought, creativity, and negotiation skills in today's resource-conscious atmosphere. At times, it is necessary to do some bargaining to meet the basic needs of the patient. Perhaps without the case manager's assessment of the need for these services—and negotiation skills—this patient would be a future risk liability; many insurance companies realize this concept and are willing to cooperate by authorizing plans that have been negotiated by the case manager to enhance the patient's safety. The authorization may include more discharge supports than are normally covered, such as a noncovered service or piece of equipment.

▶ Quality Reviews

Quality reviews refer to screening the clinical content of the patient's medical record and treatment to determine if professionally and nationally recognized standards of care were met. Many times, a careful review of the patient's medical record will reveal issues or situations that warrant a closer inspection of the care provided. Any condition that may indicate poor or incomplete patient care, occurring either inside a facility or as an outpatient service, requires QI or RM notification. In general, the sequence for handling quality reviews goes as follows:

1. Identification of a quality and/or safety concern: This concern may be revealed in a patient's medical record review or in a discussion with a member of the interdisciplinary team or patient/family member.
2. Determination if a quality/safety problem indeed exists: If a significant breach of the standards of care is suspected, it must then be validated by appropriate professionals. The case manager must decide how to proceed, and this may depend on the type of organization and situation. For a hospital case manager, the first line of action is usually a call to the RM department; in a health maintenance organization or another organization, a medical director or administrator may need to be notified. The case manager should make details of the concern and appropriate documentation available to the medical director or another specialist to determine if there is, in fact, a problem. Organizations usually have policies and procedures that mandate the sequence of events that must take place when a quality of care or safety issue is suspect. Depending on the issue

or concern at hand, an RCA or a comprehensive event review may be completed.
3. Confirmation of the existence of a quality or safety problem: The organizational policy and procedure usually details how, in what time frame, and to whom the information is communicated.

When reviewing patients' medical records, paying careful attention to the quality of care and safety reflected in the documentation of the interdisciplinary healthcare team may reveal poor, suboptimal, incomplete patient care, or clues to possible delayed diagnoses, and admission concerns.

DELAYED DIAGNOSES

Be aware that reasons other than missed early signs and symptoms or clues—such as patient noncompliance, poor historian, or reluctance to share sensitive or perceived embarrassing information—can cause some of the following delayed diagnoses:

▶ First admission for advanced disease processes including, for example, advanced metastatic cancer, perforated ulcer, advanced tuberculosis.
▶ Diagnosis such as a perforated appendix when a chart review reveals an emergency department visit for abdominal pain 3 days before the current admission to the hospital for the management of the perforated appendix.
▶ Severe diabetic ketoacidosis (watch for noncompliance or "brittle" diabetes).
▶ Shock (various types), septicemia, or bacteremia: Perhaps a patient has visited the emergency department for early signs of sepsis that were not recognized a few days prior to current admission to the hospital's critical care unit for the management of shock, indicating avoidable deterioration in the patient's health condition.
▶ Possible poor monitoring of a patient's condition: Examples include pregnancy-induced hypertension (preeclampsia, eclampsia, and toxemia), exacerbation of HF, or chronic obstructive pulmonary disease.

ADMISSION CONCERNS

▶ Admissions for diseases for which immunizations are available: Did the pediatrician, family practitioner, or primary care physician offer the immunizations? Did the parent (or patient, if an adult) refuse them or not take the child to the primary care physician for availing them?
▶ Admissions from complications following an outpatient or emergency department procedure: Examples include poorly reset fractures, neurologic defects, and wound infections.
▶ Admissions for side effects of outpatient drug therapy: Did the patient take more, or less, than was

ordered? Did the physician or nurse improperly or incompletely educate the patient about the medication? Were the patient's blood levels adequately monitored for the medication? Examples include gastrointestinal bleeding resulting from the patient taking aspirin while also consuming Coumadin, or hypokalemia while the patient was taking a potassium-depleting diuretic.

▶ Readmission for the same condition within 2 weeks or 30 days of discharge from the hospital or long-term care facility for the same problem/chief complaint: This can happen with any condition or diagnosis. The causes may range from patient noncompliance (a woman with HF who goes home and eats pretzels) to poor outpatient monitoring or premature discharge.

▶ Issues of social determinants of health being poorly managed and dismissed for their impact on the patient's health condition when developing a plan of care for a patient: For example, a patient has a health insurance plan with limited coverage and is discharged with a list of medications some of which are not covered under the insurance plan and the patient cannot afford filling the prescription; a patient returns to the hospital with a deteriorating health condition that requires more costly services that otherwise would have been avoided. Another patient discharged with limited physical functioning ability and needs transportation to the outpatient dialysis treatment center; a patient ends up missing a dialysis treatment and lands in the emergency department after a deterioration in condition because the patient missed the dialysis on account of lack of transportation.

OTHER EXAMPLES OF QUALITY REVIEWS

Sometimes critical thinking and investigative work must precede the discovery of poor management of the care of a patient or the occurrence of adverse events that perhaps have not been reported to the appropriate parties/departments within the hospital, and no disclosure to the patient and/or family has taken place either. For example:

▶ During a gastrectomy, the spleen is removed. Because this is not standard protocol for a gastrectomy, the curious case manager would investigate the case. No explanation is found in the progress notes or in the operative procedure report. The pathology report states that the splenic artery had been injured, necessitating the removal of the spleen. The spleen tissue seemed to have been normal.

▶ Perhaps a hysterectomy patient returns postoperatively with bloody urine. A further review shows the ureter was inadvertently transected and repaired.

▶ A 6-week-old infant is admitted for seizures. A review of his birth chart reveals that labor was prolonged and difficult; it necessitated midforceps delivery. Documentation of the physical examination of the infant upon birth is found to be incomplete in the medical record.

▶ An infant with congenital heart disease develops severe bradycardia and arrhythmia and dies. An autopsy report shows his digoxin level was 10 times above the normal range. Medical record review reveals an order for a higher dose of digoxin than normal and there has been no documentation of digoxin level test to ensure therapeutic digoxin blood level.

▶ An infant with an Apgar score of 3 requires resuscitation. A review of the maternal predelivery record shows that the mother had been given excessive doses of narcotics.

▶ RM Recommendations and Prevention Skills

CONSULT A RISK MANAGER

When in doubt about anything that may preclude an RM event, call a risk manager in your organization for clarification and evaluation. Seek continuing educational sessions about risk management at your organization of employment; such sessions expand your knowledge in this area and enhance your skills. Your diligence and timely referrals of questionable situations to RM may prevent otherwise expensive lawsuits.

ALERT THE RM DEPARTMENT

A goal of RM is never to be served with a lawsuit of which the facility agency was previously unaware. Through proper alerts by the case manager, the RM department would have the time to flag the medical records, review the records carefully, attempt to intervene as appropriate, and possibly review court records.

DO NOT AVOID ANGRY CLIENTS

When a patient or family has complaints, listen and be responsive. Many families and patients are angry because they feel no one is listening to them or because they remain uninformed of the diagnosis or the plan of care. Listening may not avert all lawsuits, but it is true that people get angrier if they feel ignored; such anger may expedite consulting a lawyer and the filing of a lawsuit.

NOTIFY A RISK MANAGER OF POTENTIAL SUITS

If a patient or family member mentions a lawsuit or attorney, a call to the risk manager may be appropriate. Although unreasonable expectations may be the cause of the threat, it is still better to notify the RM department for its assessment. Sometimes involving the "patient advocate team" for early intervention may also avert escalation of a situation and unpleasant outcomes.

BE INCLUSIVE

Include the patient/family unit in the decision-making process about various aspects of care. Those inside the boat are less likely to rock it.

CAREFULLY CONSIDER READMISSIONS

Readmissions soon after a discharge from the hospital need careful consideration. This is especially true if the previous admission had the possibility of suboptimal treatment or an inappropriate discharge or transitional plan (either a premature discharge/transfer or the result of poor discharge planning). Understanding the reasons for readmissions allows case managers to identify, on the basis of the practice trends and patterns, opportunities for improvement and hopefully to prevent future avoidable readmissions because of suboptimal care.

PAY SPECIAL ATTENTION TO HIGH-RISK NEONATES

Adverse outcomes in neonates need attention. All parents reasonably expect a positive outcome—a healthy newborn; events that deviate from this expectation could benefit from an RM evaluation.

PRACTICE QUALITY DOCUMENTATION

Documentation is a vital aspect of RM. This theme surfaces often throughout this book. Its importance cannot be overstated and is especially critical in the courtroom when proving whether negligence or malpractice has occurred. The old adage, "If it's not documented, it did not occur," is important; what is documented versus what is not documented can determine the outcome of a case. Documentation in a medical record may be the only evidence available to indicate whether a standard of care has been met. Because there would usually have been a big time gap between the rendering of the actual care, the filing of a lawsuit, and ultimately the confirmation of the date of hearing by the court; without thorough documentation important details may be lost.

The RM department also depends on quality documentation for determining how to handle a case. What the old adage does not do is give specific guidelines that may be helpful if a case does go to litigation. The following are some further recommendations regarding documentation that case managers may find helpful:

▶ Ask yourself whether you would mind if your documentation was read aloud in court. If the answer is "yes" on any case, assess why you feel discomfort. For example, did subjectivity, judgment, or frustration show up in your notes? Were your notes incomplete? Use this assessment for personal growth and improvement.

▶ Document all communication between yourself, the patient/family, other healthcare professionals, and physicians. Include dates and times of calls you have initiated, response time, doctor's response to the reason for the call, your interventions, and any modifications you made to the plan of care. Number 6 in the previous list of high-risk areas for nurses was a failure to summon medical attention. Perhaps in some cases the physician was summoned but, without supporting documentation, the nurse had to assume the responsibility for a poor outcome. If a physician is paged and does not answer within a reasonable amount of time and after a reasonable number of attempts, go through the chain of command until a physician who will address the problem can be reached. Seek the support of administrators on duty or nursing supervisors as you deem appropriate. Document all efforts and their outcomes.

▶ Falls are a major cause of litigation, especially when there is failure to properly supervise a patient. Document close observation, falls risk assessment, implementation of fall prevention activities, supervised toileting, and visits to a patient's room for treatment and monitoring purposes. This is especially important for case managers who are also direct care nurses.

▶ Follow some basic record-keeping rules. To begin with, remember to include the date and time on all entries. This is especially true in emergency situations. Furthermore, state all information clearly, factually, objectively, and completely. This should ensure that standards of care are met. Note any measures used to prevent complications, because they may show good faith in the future. Avoid ambiguity and remain objective. "Feels warm," "high blood pressure," and "lower temperature" are too nonspecific. Chart the facts—the actual values. Use words that are not susceptible to multiple meanings and misinterpretation.

▶ In a court of law, the appearance of the medical record is often as important as the content. Use TJC-approved abbreviations and recommendations. If at your environment of practice paper medical records are still in use, remember that using a whiting-out agent to delete errors is not permissible in court and leaves room for suspicion of falsifying information. The record for one case involving whiting-out agent had to be x-rayed to determine what was underneath. Use a single line to cross out an error. Write "error" over the single line and initial it. Sign all completed entries. Also, make sure all blanks and boxes are filled in or checked. Always write legibly and with permanent black ink. Fortunately, today with the wide use of electronic documentation systems, these concerns may not be as common as they used to be over a decade ago.

▶ If electronic documentation is used, be aware that the time of documentation may not necessarily be the actual time of observation, treatment, or evaluation. Remember to include the time of such activities in your documentation to avoid the problem of wrong time entry and the need to explain this in a court of law; those who review the medical record may assume that the electronic and automated time stamp is the actual time if the time has not been amended in your notes.

▶ Good follow-through should be evident from the documentation in the record. If a critical laboratory value or change in patient condition is noted, as stated earlier, keep track of the person to whom you reported it and what the response was. Note all patient responses to any treatments or medications given (again, this is especially important for case managers with direct patient care responsibilities). If a physician's order is not carried out, explain the reason(s).

▶ When documenting complications or mishaps, be factual, thorough, and objective. Do not assign blame or fault. Do not document in the patient's record that an event occurrence report was completed.

▶ Threats and complaints can be documented, but it is best to quote if possible. Document follow-up actions to the threat or complaint; also document whether you had consulted anyone to help manage the situation and the outcomes observed.

▶ Patient or family concerns or worries can also be documented. Identify who expressed concern, what was said (quote if possible), your verbal responses, and any interventions that were done in response to the concern.

▶ Patient nonadherence or poor self-management needs to be documented, including what the patient is or is not doing. A patient with diabetes eating candy or a patient allowed nothing by mouth found munching on crackers is not an uncommon occurrence. Nevertheless, such situations can delay surgical procedures and extend length of stay. In many cases, nonadherence can harm a patient and interfere with optimal patient care and outcomes.

▶ Document informed consent about medical procedures (more on this subject is discussed in "Informed Consent" in Chapter 8).

▶ Document information about transferring patients to other facilities. Document in the patient's medical record who was spoken to and what was agreed upon. This may include conversations or telephone calls to the patient's family, the skilled nursing facility, and the attending physician. Note who made the decision to transfer, when the transfer took place, and who approved the transfer. If there is a suboptimal outcome during or after a transfer, and there is no documentation that the family and/or the payor supported the transfer decision, repercussions can occur.

▶ QUALITY INDICATORS

Quality indicators are measurable, specific, and clear guides for monitoring and evaluating important aspects of patient care. Indicators may be written for any area that enhances patient care, from ambulatory services and social services to nuclear medicine and case management. Each service has its own specific indicators to monitor potential problems or opportunities to improve patient care delivery and services. Ongoing monitoring should reveal trends and opportunities for improvement. Several years ago, one study revealed a high rate of pneumothorax after central line insertions. Astute detective work disclosed a problem with a discrepancy between the insertion site and the use of an appropriate length of catheter. As a result, standards/protocols to address the prevention of such problems are followed.

Appendix 7-1 includes several sample indicators from various clinical specialties and/or service lines. A visit to the facility's QI and patient safety (QIPS) department is likely to reveal several books on quality screens, review tools, and monitors. A review is recommended, especially in your specific service line or case management practice setting. Such reviews often raise red flags about certain situations, and the case manager can then alert the QIPS or RM departments. Appendix 7-2 displays sample clinical indicators of generic quality screens advocated for by accreditation agencies and the CMS. A review of the CMS generic screens demonstrates some circumstances that may signal inadequate quality of care. Appendix 7-3 includes a compilation of 10 types of claims categories gleaned from the National Practitioner's Data Bank. These categories are used by RM departments as a possible indication of suboptimal quality of care. A review of the indicators, the CMS generic screens, and the claims categories should arm the case manager with enough cues, so that an "off" case will signal further investigation and monitoring and possibly a call to the RM or QM departments.

Quality indicators also include those described earlier in this chapter: case management outcome indicators/measures (Displays 7-1, 7-4, and 7-5) and sample core measures (Display 7-7) based on the Medicare Shared Savings Program implemented as part of Accountable Care Organizations (ACOs). ACOs are required to completely and accurately report on the quality measures that are used to calculate and assess quality performance. To be eligible to share in any savings generated, an ACO must meet the established quality performance standard that corresponds to its performance year. The program is set up where in the first performance year of the first agreement period, an ACO must satisfy the quality performance standard by reporting complete and accurate data on all quality measures. This is referred to as pay for reporting and if complete and accurate the ACO is deemed to have qualified for the maximum shared savings rate. In subsequent performance years, quality performance benchmarks are

CORE MEASURES USED FOR ACOs AS PART OF THE MEDICARE SHARED SAVINGS PROGRAM

Domain	Measure	Measure Description
Patient/caregiver experience	ACO-1	CAHPS: Getting timely care, appointments, and information
	ACO-2	CAHPS: How well your providers communicate
	ACO-3	CAHPS: Patients' rating of provider
	ACO-4	CAHPS: Access to specialists
	ACO-5	CAHPS: Health promotion and education
	ACO-6	CAHPS: Shared decision making
	ACO-7	CAHPS: Health status/functional status
	ACO-34	CAHPS: Stewardship of patient resources
Care coordination and patient safety	ACO-8	Risk-standardized, all condition readmission
	ACO-35	Skilled nursing facility 30-day all-cause readmission measure (SNFRM)
	ACO-36	All-cause unplanned admissions for patients with diabetes
	ACO-37	All-cause unplanned admissions for patients with HF
	ACO-38	All-cause unplanned admissions for patients with multiple
	ACO-43	Chronic conditions
	ACO-9	Ambulatory sensitive condition acute composite (AHRQ prevention quality indicator
	ACO-10	[PQI] #91)
	ACO-11	Ambulatory sensitive conditions admissions: chronic Obstructive pulmonary disease
	ACO-39	or asthma in older adults (AHRQ PQI #5)
	ACO-12	Ambulatory sensitive conditions admissions: HF (AHRQ PQI #8)
	ACO-13	Percent of primary care providers who successfully meet meaningful use requirements
	ACO-44	Documentation of current medications in the medical record
		Medication reconciliation post discharge
		Falls: Screening for future fall risk
		Use of imaging studies for low back pain
Preventive health	ACO-14	Preventive care and screening: Influenza immunization
	ACO-15	Pneumonia vaccination status for older adults
	ACO-16	Preventive care and screening: Body mass index (BMI) Screening and follow-up
	ACO-17	Preventive care and screening: Tobacco use—screening and cessation intervention
	ACO-18	Preventive care and screening: Screening for clinical depression and follow-up plan
	ACO-19	Colorectal cancer screening
	ACO-20	Breast cancer screening
	ACO-21	Preventive care and screening: Screening for high blood pressure and follow-up documented
	ACO-42	Statin therapy for the prevention and treatment of cardiovascular disease
At-risk population	ACO-40	Depression: Remission at 12 months
	Composite	Diabetes mellitus: Hemoglobin A1c poor control; eye exam
	ACO-27	Hypertension (HTN): Controlling high blood pressure
	and 41	Ischemic vascular disease: Use of aspirin or another antithrombotic
	ACO-28	Heart failure (HF): Beta-blocker therapy for left ventricular systolic dysfunction
	ACO-30	Coronary artery disease (CAD): Angiotensin-converting enzyme (ACE) inhibitor or
	ACO-31	angiotensin receptor blocker (ARB) therapy—for patients with CAD and diabetes or
	ACO-33	left ventricular systolic dysfunction (LVEF < 40%)

ACO, accountable care organization; CAHPS, consumer assessment of healthcare providers and systems.

SOURCE: Centers for Medicare & Medicaid Services. (2016, December). *Medicare shared savings program quality measure benchmarks for the 2016 and 2017 reporting years*. Retrieved from https://www.cms.gov/Medicare/Medicare-Fee-for-Service-Payment/sharedsavingsprogram/Downloads/MSSP-QM-Benchmarks-2016.pdf

phased-in for the performance measures, and the quality performance standard requires ACOs to continue to report complete and accurate quality data on all the core measures. However, Medicare determines the ACO's final shared savings rate on the basis of the ACO performance compared with national benchmarks (CMS, 2016). Other examples are from the National Quality Forum (NQF) (Display 7-8). The CMS has adopted measures already endorsed by the NQF in its Hospitals VBP Program, HRRP, and ACOs.

When examining quality in your healthcare organization, look for all the indicators your organization reports on, whether they are directly or indirectly related to the case management program of which you are a part. Often you will find that going beyond the case management program leads you to a better understanding of the total

display 7-8

SAMPLE CORE MEASURES FROM THE NATIONAL QUALITY MEASURES

Disease Category	Core Measures
Pneumonia	▶ Pneumococcal vaccination ▶ Blood cultures performed within 24 hours prior to or 24 hours after hospital arrival for patients who were transferred or admitted to the ICU within 24 hours of hospital arrival ▶ Blood cultures performed in the emergency department prior to antibiotic administration in the hospital ▶ Adult smoking cessation advice/counseling ▶ Initial antibiotic received within 4 hours of hospital arrival ▶ Initial antibiotic selection for community-acquired pneumonia in immunocompetent patients ▶ Care transitions ▶ Avoidance of antibiotic treatment in adults with acute bronchitis (AAB) ▶ Flu vaccinations for adults ages 18 and older ▶ HIV/AIDS: Pneumocystis pneumonia (PCP) prophylaxis ▶ Hospital-wide all-cause unplanned readmission measure (HWR) ▶ Hybrid hospital-wide readmission measure with claims and electronic health record data ▶ Severe sepsis and septic shock: Management bundle (composite measure) ▶ Mortality 30-day post hospital discharge ▶ Readmission 30-day post hospital discharge
Surgical care improvement/ surgical infection prevention	▶ Prophylactic antibiotic received within 1 hour prior to surgical incision (or 2 hours if receiving vancomycin or fluoroquinolone) ▶ Prophylactic antibiotic selection for surgical patients ▶ Prophylactic antibiotic discontinued within 24 hours after surgery end time ▶ Cardiac surgery patients with controlled 6 AM postoperative blood glucose ▶ Colorectal surgery patients with immediate postoperative normothermia ▶ Surgery patients on beta-blockers therapy prior to admission who received a beta-blocker during the perioperative period ▶ Surgery patients who received appropriate venous thromboembolism prophylaxis ordered
Heart failure	▶ Discharge instructions (including diet, activity, follow-up, medications, symptoms worsening, and weight monitoring) ▶ Evaluation of left ventricular systolic function ▶ Angiotensin-converting enzyme (ACE) inhibitor or angiotensin receptor blocker (ARB) for left ventricular systolic dysfunction ▶ Adult smoking cessation advice/counseling ▶ Care transitions ▶ Excess days in acute care after hospitalization for heart failure (HF) ▶ Hospital 30-day, all-cause, risk-standardized mortality rate (RSMR) following HF hospitalization for patients aged 18 and older ▶ Hospital 30-day, all-cause, risk-standardized readmission rate (RSRR) following HF hospitalization ▶ Hospital-wide all-cause unplanned readmission measure (HWR) ▶ Hybrid hospital-wide readmission measure with claims and electronic health record data ▶ Long-term care hospital functional outcome measure: Change in mobility among patients requiring ventilator support ▶ Risk-standardized acute admission rates for patients with HF
Acute myocardial infarction/heart attack	▶ Aspirin at arrival ▶ Aspirin prescribed at discharge ▶ Angiotensin-converting enzyme (ACE) Inhibitor or angiotensin receptor blocker (ARB) for left ventricular systolic dysfunction ▶ Adult smoking cessation advice/counseling ▶ Beta-blocker prescribed at discharge ▶ Beta-blocker at arrival ▶ Median time to fibrinolysis ▶ Fibrinolytic therapy received within 30 minutes of hospital arrival ▶ Median time to primary percutaneous coronary intervention ▶ Primary percutaneous coronary intervention received within 90 minutes of hospital arrival ▶ LDL cholesterol assessment ▶ Lipid-lowering therapy for discharge ▶ 30-day all-cause risk-standardized mortality rate following percutaneous coronary intervention (PCI) for patients with ST segment elevation myocardial infarction (STEMI) or cardiogenic shock

SAMPLE CORE MEASURES FROM THE NATIONAL QUALITY MEASURES *(continued)*

Disease Category	Core Measures
	▶ Hospital 30-day all-cause RSRR following acute myocardial infarction (AMI) hospitalization. ▶ 30-day all-cause risk-standardized mortality rate following PCI for patients without STEMI and without cardiogenic shock ▶ AMI Mortality Rate ▶ Excess days in acute care (EDAC) after hospitalization for AMI ▶ Hospital 30-Day RSRRs following PCI ▶ Hospital 30-day, all-cause, risk-standardized mortality rate (RSMR) following AMI hospitalization for patients 18 and older ▶ Hybrid hospital 30-day, all-cause, RSMR following AMI ▶ In-hospital risk-adjusted rate of bleeding events for patients undergoing PCI ▶ In-Hospital Risk-Adjusted Rate of Mortality for Patients undergoing PCI
Pediatric asthma	▶ Pharmacological therapy for persistent asthma ▶ Relievers for inpatient asthma (age 2–17 years) overall ▶ Relievers for inpatient asthma (age 2–4 years) ▶ Relievers for inpatient asthma (age 5–12 years) ▶ Relievers for inpatient asthma (age 13–17 years) ▶ Systemic corticosteroids for inpatient asthma (age 2–17 years) overall ▶ Systemic corticosteroids for inpatient asthma (age 2–4 years) ▶ Systemic corticosteroids for inpatient asthma (age 5–12 years) ▶ Systemic corticosteroids for inpatient asthma (age 13–17 years) ▶ Home management plan of care/document given to patient/caregiver ▶ Pediatric all-conditions readmission measure ▶ Asthma admissions rate ▶ Appropriate treatment for children with upper respiratory infection
Diabetes care	▶ Blood pressure control (<140/90 mm Hg) ▶ Eye Exam (retinal) performed ▶ Hemoglobin A1c (HbA1c) control (<8.0%) ▶ Hemoglobin A1c (HbA1c) poor control (>9.0%) ▶ Hemoglobin A1c (HbA1c) testing ▶ Medical attention for nephropathy ▶ Cholesterol: LDL-C control <100 mg/dL

SOURCE: Compiled from the National Quality Forum. (2017). *Where can I find a comprehensive list of NQF endorsed® measures? Quality positioning system.* Retrieved July 1, 2017, from http://www.qualityforum.org/Field_Guide/List_of_Measures.aspx

picture of quality and patient safety in your organization. Such understanding will also provide you with more appreciation for your role in, and contribution to, quality and the reputation of your organization. As you identify opportunities for improvement, you are better able to package a PI project beyond the immediate boundaries of your case management program, and therefore, you sell your improvement project idea to the executives in your organization, so that they can invest in making it happen. Communicating the value and benefits of your proposed improvement from the patient's perspective and experience and its potential impact on organizational performance are usually effective strategy for obtaining buy-in.

▶ PATIENT SAFETY AND CASE MANAGEMENT

Across the healthcare continuum and settings, patients are routinely transferred from one healthcare provider, service,

or setting to another. During these transitions, the risk of providing suboptimal care may exist. If case managers are careful during these transitions, exercise their patient/family advocacy role, and assume responsibility and accountability for ensuring patient safety, quality of care, and satisfaction with the care experience, then safe, optimal, and effective care is guaranteed. This "guarantee" is strengthened when case managers ensure the transfer of key and necessary information (both in verbal and written forms) between healthcare providers and settings. As a result, medical errors are prevented, safety is enhanced, continuity of care is maintained, and ultimately, quality is ensured.

Case managers integrate patient safety activities into every phase of the case management process: for example, advocacy, medication reconciliation, timeliness of care activities or treatments, timely completion of necessary tests, communication among providers of care, and communication with payors for authorization/certification of services. From assessment and planning, to monitoring and evaluation of outcomes, the case management process

display 7-9

KEY ORGANIZATIONS THAT FOCUS ON PATIENT SAFETY

- ▶ The Joint Commission: http://www.jointcommission.org
- ▶ National Patient Safety Foundation: http://www.npsf.org
- ▶ World Health Organization/World Alliance for Patient Safety: http://www.who.int/patientsafety/en/
- ▶ Agency for Healthcare Research and Quality/Patient Safety Network: http://www.psnet.ahrq.gov/
- ▶ Institute for Healthcare Improvement: http://www.ihi.org/IHI/Topics/PatientSafety/
- ▶ United States Department of Veterans Affairs/National Center for Patient Safety: http://www.va.gov/ncps/
- ▶ Consumers Advancing Patient Safety: http://www.patientsafety.org/
- ▶ United States Food and Drug Administration/Patient Safety News: http://www.accessdata.fda.gov/psn/index.cfm
- ▶ The National Quality Forum: https://www.qualityforum.org/
- ▶ The Centers for Medicare & Medicaid Services: https://www.cms.gov
- ▶ The National Quality Strategy: https://www.ahrq.gov/workingforquality/index.html

provides an excellent opportunity for implementing a proactive approach to patient safety by ensuring access to quality, safe, effective, timely, patient-centric/family-centric, and efficacious care and outcomes. Examples of organizations that focus on patient safety are listed in Display 7-9.

One of the original and most popular organizations to promote patient safety is TJC. It approved its first set of national patient safety goals (NPSGs) in July 2002. These goals included specific requirements for improving quality and patient care safety in healthcare organizations. Today, over 50% of TJC's standards are directly related to safety. Assessment of safety during an accreditation survey is "front and center" to the survey. The standards address specific issues that affect patient safety during an episode of care and illness. Case managers can play an important and integral role in assisting an organization to adhere to the standards and the NPSGs. For example, case managers can prevent accidental harm by ensuring that the medication reconciliation process is completed for every individual patient and that the handoff/handover communication, which includes the transfer of key information (e.g., medical regimen, medications, allergies, plan of care, etc.) from one provider or setting to another, is timely and complete.

The 2017 NPSGs for select care settings are listed in Display 7-10. The information shared reflects the applicability of each of the goals to three types of healthcare organizations: hospitals, ambulatory clinics, and home health agencies). TJC, however, also applies NPSGs to other settings, including behavioral health, critical access hospitals, nursing care centers, laboratory services, and physician's office-based surgery. Case management programs and the role of the case manager can affect these organizations' ability to adhere to the NPSGs. The goals where case management is most valuable may include those in the following areas:

- ▶ Communication among members of the interdisciplinary healthcare team, especially in reporting of test results (i.e., critical values) and handoffs or handovers.

- ▶ Use of evidence-based practice standards/protocols/guidelines such as anticoagulation therapy and deep vein thrombosis prophylaxis.
- ▶ Prevention of healthcare-associated infections, especially through the use of evidence-based practice standards/protocols (e.g., prevention of surgical site infection through use of antibiotic prophylaxis; prevention of central line–associated bloodstream infections).
- ▶ Medications reconciliation.
- ▶ Patient involvement in own safety through patient and family education of healthcare safety activities (e.g., hand hygiene, speak up campaign). Safety risks at home, especially if the patient is on oxygen therapy (e.g., oxygen therapy safety and prevention of fires) or of dependent physical functioning (e.g., barrier-free environment, risk for falling, and use of mobility-assist devices). This is best accomplished through the case manager's role in transitional/discharge planning and patient/family education.
- ▶ Recognition of changes in the patient's condition, which is achieved by engaging the right healthcare provider at the right time to address deterioration in patient health status, preventing delays in treatment, and enhancing patient's access to care.

▶ CLINICAL DOCUMENTATION IMPROVEMENT

Clinical documentation is at the center of every patient encounter regardless of care setting or the healthcare provider involved. It consists of the recording of findings from patients' assessments and diagnostic tests, plans of care, implementation of plans of care (i.e., treatments and interventions), monitoring and evaluation of care activities or services, including patients' responses to treatments. Clinical documentation also provides a rationale (justification) for the care and services provided. To be meaningful and beneficial, documentation must be accurate, timely, and reflect the scope of services that patients have received.

2017 NATIONAL PATIENT SAFETY GOALS IN SELECT CARE SETTINGS—THE JOINT COMMISSION

Goals	Description	Ambulatory	Hospital	Home Care
Identify patients correctly				
NPSG.01.01.01	Use at least two ways to identify patients. For example, use the patient's name and date of birth.	X	X	X
NPSG.01.03.01	Make sure that the correct patient gets the correct blood when he or she gets a blood transfusion.	X	X	
Improve staff communication				
NPSG.02.03.01	Get important test results to the right staff person on time.		X	
Use medicines safely				
NPSG.03.04.01	Before a procedure, label medicines that are not labeled. For example, medicines in syringes, cups, and basins. Do this in the area where medicines and supplies are set up.	X	X	
NPSG.03.05.01	Take extra care with patients who take medicines to thin their blood.	X	X	
NPSG.03.06.01	Record and pass along correct information about a patient's medicines. Find out what medicines the patient is taking. Compare those medicines to new medicines given to the patient. Make sure the patient knows which medicines to take when he or she is at home. Tell the patient it is important to bring an up-to-date list of medicines every time he or she visits a doctor.	X	X	X
Use alarms safely				
NPSG.06.01.01	Make improvements to ensure that alarms on medical equipment are heard and responded to on time.		X	
Prevent infection				
NPSG.07.01.01	Use the hand-cleaning guidelines from the Centers for Disease Control and Prevention or the World Health Organization. Set goals for improving hand cleaning. Use the goals to improve hand cleaning. Use proven guidelines to prevent infections that are difficult to treat. Use proven guidelines to prevent infection of the blood from central lines.	X	X	X
NPSG.07.03.01	Use proven guidelines to prevent infection after surgery.		X	
NPSG.07.04.01	Use proven guidelines to prevent infections of the urinary tract that are caused by catheters.		X	
NPSG.07.05.01		X	X	
NPSG.07.06.01			X	
Prevent patients from falling				
NPSG.09.02.01	Find out which patients are most likely to fall. For example, is the patient taking any medicines that might make them weak, dizzy, or sleepy? Take action to prevent falls for these patients.			X
Identify patient safety risks				
NPSG.15.01.01	Find out which patients are most likely to try to commit suicide.		X	
NPSG.15.02.01	Find out if there are any risks for patients who are getting oxygen. For example, fires in the patient's home.			X

(continued)

display 7-10

2017 NATIONAL PATIENT SAFETY GOALS IN SELECT CARE SETTINGS—THE JOINT COMMISSION (*continued*)

Goals	Description	Ambulatory	Hospital	Home Care
Prevent mistakes in surgery				
UP.01.01.01	Make sure that the correct surgery is done on the correct patient and at the correct place on the patient's body. Mark the correct place on the patient's body where the surgery is to be done.	X	X	
UP.01.02.01	Pause before the surgery to make sure that a mistake is not being made.	X	X	
UP.01.03.01		X	X	

SOURCE: Compiled from The Joint Commission. (2017b). *2017 National Patient Safety Goals®*. Retrieved July 1, 2017, from https://www.jointcommission.org/standards_information/npsgs.aspx

Clinical documentation helps justify the types of claims submitted to health insurance plans for reimbursement (payment) on the basis of the care provided. Insurance plans may deny processing some of the claims stating that the clinical documentation does not support these claims. Additionally, perhaps because of lack of knowledge and expertise, healthcare providers may be submitting claims for reimbursement, yet unaware of their inaccuracies. Although these claims are thought to reflect the patient acuity, severity of illness, and intensity of resources, they communicate a lower level of service and cost compared with the actual presenting patient condition and the services provided. These claims usually end up with erroneous codes (i.e., *ICD-9*, *ICD-10*, or *CPT* codes) because of the incomplete or inaccurate documentation. Clinical documentation improvement (CDI) helps correct these situations and has demonstrated that it can enhance revenue and adherence to regulatory and accreditation standards.

Successful CDI programs facilitate the accurate representation of a patient's clinical status and justify the needed services that translate into optimally coded data. This results in appropriate reimbursement amounts and ultimately expected revenues. Effectively coded data also contribute to quality reporting, healthcare provider/physician performance and report cards, reimbursement, public health data, and disease tracking (registries) and trending. A CDI program promotes clear, concise, complete, accurate, and compliant documentation which enhances reimbursement and revenue. These programs have been available for over a decade and are considered a common practice in healthcare organizations, especially hospitals.

The process of CDI consists of the analysis and interpretation of health/medical record documentation and coding procedures. It helps identify and rectify situations where opportunities for improvement exist. Examples of areas of focus in the CDI process are, but not limited to, the following:

▶ Insufficient or inaccurate documentation that does not support the patient's severity of illness and care;

▶ Principal diagnosis and procedure are not specific enough;

▶ Associated comorbidities or complications are missing;

▶ Treatments or procedures are incompletely recorded; and

▶ Coding for claim submissions is inaccurate, mostly reflective of lower reimbursement levels.

The process of CDI enhances the revenue of a healthcare organization or provider. It is considered a revenue cycle activity and entails the convergence of clinical care, documentation, coding, and billing processes. A CDI program promotes the documentation of medical necessity and appropriateness of the level of services to support the following:

▶ Admissions: inpatient vs. observation or outpatient treatment

▶ Readmission or continued stay

▶ Therapies, treatments, procedures, and specialty consults

▶ Appropriate coding through comprehensive and relevant documentation including complications and comorbidities

▶ Accurate case mix index (CMI)

▶ Correct payment and reduction of compliance risk

▶ Correct identification of the principal diagnosis and procedure, and secondary diagnoses and procedures

▶ Compliance with TJC accreditation standards, and regulatory requirements such as the Conditions of Participation

▶ Provision of evidence-based care and services

▶ Addressing the concerns of reimbursement denials, as appropriate

▶ Reporting of quality indicators and core measures: internally, externally, and publicly

▶ Benchmarking: regionally, nationally, or against the performance of other similar organizations.

CDI programs are often implemented as a function within case management departments or utilization review and management teams. Case managers in these programs collaborate with CDI specialists and together they assist in achieving the target improvements in documentation and reimbursement. Some organizations have embedded the CDI role as part of the case manager's responsibilities. This is more common among small and community hospitals. Others implemented CDI programs within the quality or health information management (HIM) (previously referred to as medical records) departments. Regardless, the CDI teams focus on target DRGs where the opportunity exists most; DRGs are identified on the basis of a review of the organization's performance compared with relevant benchmarks, including an examination of case volume by DRG; CMI; length of stay; use of complications and comorbidities, major CC, and present on admission codes; claims/reimbursement denials management; and excess days. Some of the improvement interventions are: development of documentation and coding training programs for clinicians and administrators, physician education, orientation for credentialing of new staff, *ICD-10* basics, coding standards and guidelines, shadowing clinicians while on the job for assessment and PI purposes, engagement of physician champions, and trending and reporting of data and performance.

A CDI program consists of a diverse team of people, processes, and technology that must work together to ensure success. Successful programs focus on assessing documentation requirements, codes assignment, coding guidelines, and quality reporting. They also have expert CDI specialists who analyze data, formulate physician queries, track CDI program performance, and successfully communicate with physicians, administration, HIM staff, and others as necessary. These professionals demonstrate a variety of professional backgrounds; the two who most often assume the CDI specialist role are health HIM professionals and registered nurses. They are credentialed as clinical documentation improvement practitioners through the American Health Information Management Academy or certified clinical documentation specialists through the Association of Clinical Documentation Improvement Specialists. Often CDI programs consist of the following key professionals, among others:

▶ *HIM professionals*, through their education, are familiar with documentation rules and regulations as well as accreditation standards that affect timely documentation. In addition, HIM professionals are familiar with important areas such as privacy, security, and confidentiality that also impact sharing of clinical information.
▶ *Registered nurses* demonstrate a strong clinical background which helps them identify gaps in the clinical evidence and documentation. They work with the healthcare providers on addressing these gaps and improve documentation, which in turn enhances reimbursement and quality reporting.
▶ *Physician champion* who has a strong rapport with physicians, is motivated to drive change in physician behavior, and possess the knowledge and skills necessary for the effective training of other providers.
▶ *Representative(s) from finance* dedicated for revenue cycle activities, who provide important financial reports to allow the identification of potential improvement opportunities.
▶ *Coding specialists* who are experts in coding, proficient in navigating the electronic health records, and demonstrate sufficient knowledge of coding-related policies, procedures, accreditation standards, and regulations, and who are excellent stewards of the coding process.

A CDI specialist reviews the medical record for any incomplete, ambiguous, or conflicting information. This specialist helps ensure that the medical record accurately captures the patient's condition, and that it supports the severity of illness and risk of mortality for the patient. When any documentation is incomplete, ambiguous, or conflicting, the CDI specialist seeks clarification from the medical team and ensures that corrections have been carried out as appropriate. The CDI specialists are the liaisons between the medical staff and the coding department, as they strive to have the most accurate and complete medical record available for coding and billing. They abide by the coding and reporting regulations set forth by the CMS and the National Center for Health Statistics using the International Classification of Diseases, tenth revision. Case managers are true partners in this regard.

DISCUSSION QUESTIONS

1. Describe a significant event or APO you identified in your practice that resulted in a RCA. How did you go about identifying the event? What was your role in the review process? What was the value of having case management represented on the RCA team?

2. What outcomes does your organization monitor and report on that relate to the case management program? How does your role as a case manager enhance your organization's performance in these outcomes?

3. How does your organization incorporate the NPSGs into the role of the case manager? If it does not, how do you suggest it should? Why?

4. How does the quality and safety core measures or indicators that your organization use relate to the NQS? The NQF? The Hospital Readmissions Reduction Program? The ACOs reporting and Shared Savings Program?

5. Discuss your role in enhancing the performance of your organization in the VBP Program or Pay-for-Performance.

6. Describe how the role of the case manager in transitional and discharge planning impacts quality, safety, outcomes, and core measures.

7. Describe how the role of the case manager in utilization review and management impacts quality, safety, outcomes, and core measures.

8. Explain the purpose of clinical documentation improvement programs and their relationships with utilization management. How do these programs contribute to QI opportunities and organizational bottom line? Who is best to assume the role of the clinical documentation specialist and why?

▶ REFERENCES

Agency for Healthcare Research and Quality. (2017, March). *About the National Quality Strategy.* Rockville, MD: Author. Retrieved July 1, 2017, from http://www.ahrq.gov/workingforquality/about/index.html

Centers for Medicare & Medicaid Services. (2015, September). *Hospital value-based purchasing.* Medicare Learning Network. Retrieved July 1, 2017, from https://www.cms.gov/Outreach-and-Education/Medicare-Learning-Network-MLN/MLNProducts/downloads/Hospital_VBPurchasing_Fact_Sheet_ICN907664.pdf

Centers for Medicare & Medicaid Services. (2016, December). *Medicare shared savings program quality measure benchmarks for the 2016 and 2017 reporting years.* Retrieved July 1, 2017, from https://www.cms.gov/Medicare/Medicare-Fee-for-Service-Payment/sharedsavingsprogram/Downloads/MSSP-QM-Benchmarks-2016.pdf

Centers for Medicare & Medicaid Services. (2017, March 11). *CMS quality strategy.* Retrieved July 1, 2017, from https://www.cms.gov/Medicare/Quality-Initiatives-Patient-Assessment-Instruments/QualityInitiativesGenInfo/CMS-Quality-Strategy.html

Fanucci, D., Hammil, M., Johannson, P., Leggett, J., & Smith, M.J. (1993). Quantum leap into continuous quality improvement. *Nursing Management,* 24(6), 28–30.

Kongstvedt, P. R. (1993). *The managed health care handbook.* Gaithersburg, MD: Aspen Publishers.

National Quality Forum. (2017). *Where can I find a comprehensive list of NQF endorsed® measures? Quality positioning system.* Retrieved July 1, 2017, from http://www.qualityforum.org/Field_Guide/List_of_Measures.aspx

Sederer, L. I. (1987). Utilization review and quality assurance: Staying in the black and working with the blues. *General Hospital Psychiatry, 9,* 210–219.

The Joint Commission. (2017a). *Comprehensive accreditation manual for hospitals.* Oakbrook Terrace, IL: Joint Commission Resources.

The Joint Commission. (2017b). *2017 National patient safety goals®.* [Online]. Retrieved July 1, 2017, from https://www.jointcommission.org/standards_information/npsgs.aspxw

Examples of Clinical Indicators (Not an Exhaustive List)

- Some of these indicators are "undeveloped" and lacking in specific criteria; your healthcare institution's indicators will likely contain objective criteria to match the needs of the organization.
- Many of these indicators are for inpatient and outpatient settings; indicators can be written for any organization.
- These indicators do not represent a complete list of potential complications; the case manager can use these as guideposts.

CARDIOLOGY AND CARDIOVASCULAR INDICATORS

- Readmission within 30 days of discharge
- Heart failure—not present on admission
- Pericarditis—not present on admission
- Pulmonary embolus—not present on admission
- Cardiac/respiratory arrest following cardiovascular (or other) procedure
- Postoperative neurologic deficits
- Complication of thrombolytic therapy
- Gingival bleeding
- Hematemesis
- Hematomas at puncture sites
- Unplanned transfer to special care unit
- Injury to organ/structure during cardiovascular procedure

- Return to operating room for postoperative thoracic bleeding
- Return for percutaneous transluminal coronary angioplasty (PTCA) of some lesion within 72 hours post procedure
- Post-PTCA complications such as hematoma at insertion site requiring evacuation or vascular intervention
- Patients undergoing nonemergent PTCA with subsequent occurrence of either an AMI or coronary artery bypass graft surgery needed within the same hospitalization
- Patients undergoing attempted or completed PTCA during which any lesion attempted is not dilated
- Mortality rate within 30 days of discharge or healthcare encounter

PEDIATRIC CARDIOVASCULAR INDICATORS

- Return to surgery for exploration of bleeding or another complication
- Infection of device or graft
- Sepsis with positive blood cultures and infection source/site
- Postoperative neurologic deficits
- Wound infection or dehiscence
- Pulmonary emboli not present on admission

- Cardiac or respiratory arrest
- Complication of device or graft such as occlusion or malfunction
- New-onset renal failure requiring dialysis
- Readmission for complication of surgical procedure within 30 days of discharge
- All deaths related to surgical procedures
- Mortality rate within 30 days of discharge or procedure

PEDIATRIC INDICATORS

- Apgar scores less than 6 at 1 minute and less than 8 at 5 minutes
- Newborn injuries
- Transfer to neonatal ICU after 24 hours of age
- Readmission to hospital within 72 hours of discharge
- Physical or sexual abuse

- Fever of unknown origin
- Errors in diagnosis and management
- Inpatient mortality including perioperative mortality
- Unscheduled admissions following ambulatory procedure
- Unscheduled return to ICU within 48 hours of transfer
- Uncontrolled asthma

NEUROLOGY AND NEUROSURGICAL INDICATORS

- Unplanned readmission within 15 days (and within 30 days) of hospital discharge
- Unplanned transfer to a special care unit
- Injury to an organ or structure during a procedure or treatment
- Pulmonary emboli or deep vein thrombosis (DVT) not present on admission
- More than five consultations
- Complication of neurodiagnostic procedures
- Neurologic deficits not present on admission
- Organ failure not present on admission
- Cardiac or respiratory arrest

- Discharge against medical advice (AMA) or patient/family dissatisfaction
- Deaths
- Unplanned return to operating room
- Unplanned removal, injury, or repair to an organ or structure during an operative procedure
- Acute MI during or within 48 hours of an operative procedure
- Wound infection or dehiscence
- Pulmonary edema not present on admission
- Unplanned transfusion of greater than 2 units of blood
- Acute hemorrhage or wound hematoma postoperatively
- Mortality rate within 30 days of hospital discharge
- Patients referred (and transferred) to postacute rehabilitation facility

INTERNAL MEDICINE INDICATORS

- Complications from invasive, diagnostic, or monitoring procedures
- Management errors including errors of omission or commission
- Death (see death indicators below)
- Delays or inadequacies in diagnosis increasing length of stay
- Adverse reactions to medications
- Unplanned admission to special care unit
- Pneumothorax following central line insertion
- Unrecognized early signs of sepsis

- Unplanned readmission for same reason within 30 days of discharge
- Unplanned transfer to special care unit
- Cardiac-respiratory arrest
- Patient/family dissatisfaction or AMA discharge
- Pulmonary emboli or DVT not present on admission
- Complications of anticoagulation therapy
- Organ failure not present on admission
- Urinary tract infection (nosocomial); catheter-associated urinary tract infection (CAUTI)
- Central line–associated blood stream infection (CLABSI)
- Mortality rate post 30 days of hospital discharge

UTILIZATION INDICATORS

- Hospital admission not meeting acute care medical necessity criteria
- Readmission within 30 days for incomplete management of problems of previous hospitalization
- Peer review organization/quality improvement organization issue needs attention (e.g., discharge appeals and notice of noncoverage)
- Hospital admissions converted to lower level of care before claims completion and processing
- Percentage completion of Medicare Notice of Outpatient Observation Status of Care

- Readmission within 15 days of hospital discharge for same diagnosis
- Readmission within 30 days of hospital discharge for same diagnosis
- All-cause readmissions within 30 days of hospital discharge
- Receipt of Medicare denial
- Number and percentage of denied hospital days
- Inappropriate outpatient observation status
- Delays in diagnosis increasing length of stay
- Percentage completion of Medicare Important Message (first notice and second notice)

ANESTHESIA INDICATORS

- Malintubation or reintubation
- Morbidity or mortality for complications such as hose disconnection, incorrect gas flow, or too much or too little medication
- Patient's developing postural headache within 4 post procedure days following use of spinal or epidural anesthesia administration

- Dental injury following procedure involving anesthesia care
- Ocular injury during procedures involving anesthesia care
- Unplanned admission within 2 post procedure days following outpatient procedures involving anesthesia
- Vocal cord paralysis after intubation that was not present before intubation

SOCIAL WORK INDICATORS

- Recognition of psychosocial needs such as crisis intervention
- Timeliness of interventions
- Quality of counseling/interventions

- Interdisciplinary collaboration
- Abuse (child and elder)
- Appropriateness of discharge or referrals
- Lack of health insurance

AMBULATORY INDICATORS

- Unscheduled returns to the emergency department within 72 hours
- Cancelation of ambulatory procedure on day of procedure
- Unplanned admission to acute care related to surgery or complication
- Patient not accompanied home by a designated person post ambulatory procedure

- Morbidity: Vascular, neurologic, pulmonary, cardiac, drug reactions, or infections
- Local anesthesia supplemented with general anesthesia
- Adequate patient education for safe self-care
- Lack of patient/family education
- Percentage completion of Medicare Notice of Outpatient Observation Status of Care
- Conversion rate from Outpatient Observation Status to inpatient admission

EMERGENCY SERVICES INDICATORS

- Registered patients in emergency department more than 6 hours or delayed evaluations or treatment
- Registered patients who leave emergency department before completion of treatment
- Percentage patients who leave emergency department with AMA discharges
- Transfers to another acute care facility

- Return visit for similar or same complaint
- Misadministration or adverse drug reaction
- Death after arrival and within 48 hours of admission
- Consultant responds within reasonable time
- Complications related to caseload
- Adherence to Emergency Medical Treatment and Labor Act
- Percentage completion of Medicare Notice of Outpatient Observation Status of Care
- Conversion from Outpatient Observation Status to inpatient care

DIETARY SERVICES INDICATORS

- Appropriateness of diet order versus diagnosis
- Adequacy of dietary counseling and teaching
- Adequacy of parenteral nutrition

- Duration of nothing by mouth status without nutritional support
- Adequacy of nutritional values of diets
- Diet orders/errors or ambiguous or improper dietary order

PATHOLOGY INDICATORS

- Monitoring unnecessary tests
- Evaluating appropriate sequencing and frequency of tests

- Evaluating inadequate or improper specimens
- Lost or inappropriately labeled specimen

NUCLEAR MEDICINE INDICATORS

- Turnaround time for studies
- Comparison between nuclear medicine and pathologic diagnosis for inconsistencies

- Appropriateness of study requested for the diagnosis
- Misadministration of, or adverse reaction to, radionuclide agents

RADIOLOGY INDICATORS

- Turnaround time for studies
- Number of "repeat" films
- Compare radiologic and pathologic diagnosis for any inconsistency
- Consistent reading by radiologist and nonradiologist (attending physician or others)
- Percentage of patients with reaction to IV administration of dye and contrast media

- Appropriateness of radiologic study to symptom/disease
- CT scan when headache is an isolated symptom
- Upper gastrointestinal (GI) series in asymptomatic duodenal ulcer patient
- Routine chest radiographs
- Studies meet utilization review criteria or guidelines

OBSTETRIC CLINICAL INDICATORS

- Any maternal death
- Fetal mortality in pregnancy over 20 weeks (stillborn)
- Delivery-related hemorrhage requiring transfusion
- Any Apgar score of less than 6 at 1 minute and less than 8 at 5 minutes
- Third- or fourth-degree birth canal laceration
- Malposition accidents and/or extractions
- Anesthesia-related problems
- Percentage of induced deliveries

- Intrahospital neonatal deaths of infants with birth weights 750 to 1,000 g who were born in a hospital with a neonatal intensive care unit (NICU) stay
- Readmissions of the mother within 2 weeks of delivery
- Infants weighing less than 1,800 gram delivered in a hospital without an NICU
- Unattended delivery
- Unplanned return to obstetric or surgery unit
- Newborn injuries
- Rate of scheduled/elective cesarean section

ICU INDICATORS

- Mortality
- Medication errors
- Appropriate admission and discharge criteria
- Patient returned to ICU/premature transfer
- Incidence of DVT
- Ventilator-associated pneumonia
- Delayed recognition of sepsis resulting in shock

- ICU psychosis
- Physician response time to calls
- Response time to "code blue" alerts (cardiopulmonary arrests)
- Complications of immobility
- Incidence of urinary tract infection (CAUTI)
- Incidence of MRSA
- Incidence of CLABSI
- Incidence of delirium

RESPIRATORY CARE INDICATORS

- Hypoxemia is documented for oxygen therapy (exception: myocardial infarction)
- Arterial blood gases (ABGs) criteria: Patient's clinical condition changes (exception: continuous ventilation therapy) For home oxygen authorization (room air ABGs)

- No oxygen as necessary (PRN)
- Mechanical ventilation is based on established criteria
- Premature extubation
- Self-extubation
- Reintubation
- Incidence of ventilator-associated pneumonia

REHABILITATION INDICATORS

- Timeliness of referral into rehabilitation unit
- Appropriateness and adequacy of treatment plan and goals
- Quality of treatment techniques
- Number and types of readmissions
- Delays in patient discharges because of lack of therapy on weekends

- Adequacy of interdisciplinary collaboration
- Patient's understanding of instructions
- Availability of inpatient and outpatient services
- Therapy sessions missed versus reasons
- Turnaround time for physical therapy assessment prior to referral for skilled nursing or rehabilitation (acute and subacute) facility transfer

PHARMACEUTICAL INDICATORS

- Time response to medications orders
- Accuracy of medication, dosage; dispensing errors
- Appropriateness of medication ordered
- Identification of interaction, compatibilities, adverse drug reactions, allergies

- Preparation of all mixtures
- Food or drug interactions or compatibilities
- PRN medications administered without documentation of effects
- Medication errors
- Percentage of patient with polypharmacy seen by a clinical pharmacist

DEATH INDICATORS—CRITERIA GUIDELINES

Note: If a patient meets 3 of the 4 expected death criteria (below), the death may not be a quality issue.

Note: for expected death, patient must meet 3 of the 4 criteria below [any combination])

Unexpected Death Criteria

1. Death within 24 hours of hospitalization
2. Death within 24 hours of a do not resuscitate (DNR) order
3. Death that occurs after a steady downhill course with multiple interventions
4. Death within 24 hours of surgery or other procedures

Expected Death Criteria

1. Clearly documented prognosis that death is expected
2. Patient/family/next of kin are aware of, and in agreement with, medical plan
3. Interventions are for comfort care only (hospice care)
4. DNR status is documented in orders and progress notes

ADEQUACY OF DISCHARGE/TRANSITIONAL PLANNING

- No documented plan for appropriate follow-up care or discharge planning as necessary, with consideration of physical, emotional, and mental status needs at the time of discharge or transfer to another level of care

- Handoff communication to healthcare providers at the next level of care lacks comprehensiveness in the information shared, resulting in suboptimal patient experience and safety concerns including inability to maintain continuity of care

MEDICAL STABILITY OF THE PATIENT AT DISCHARGE

- Blood pressure on day before or day of discharge: systolic, <85 mm Hg or >180 mm Hg; diastolic, <50 mm Hg or >110 mm Hg
- Oral temperature on day before or day of discharge >101°F or rectal, >102°F (38.3°C oral/38.9°C rectal)
- Pulse <50 beats/min (or <45 beats/min if patient is taking a beta-blocker) or >120 beats/min within 24 hours of discharge

- Abnormal results of diagnostic tests not addressed or explained in the medical record (e.g., pneumonia on chest X-ray, abnormal results of blood tests)
- IV fluids or medications on the day of discharge (excludes the ones that keep veins open, antibiotics, chemotherapy, or total parenteral nutrition)
- Purulent or bloody drainage of postoperative wound within 24 hours before discharge

DEATHS

- During or immediately after surgery
- After return to ICU, coronary care, or special care unit within 24 hours of being transferred

- Other unexpected deaths

NOSOCOMIAL INFECTIONS

- Temperature increase of more than 2°F more than 72 hours from admission
- Unrecognized early signs of sepsis resulting in development of septic shock

- Indication of infection after an invasive procedure (e.g., suctioning, central line insertion, Foley catheter insertion, tube feedings, surgery)

PATIENT FLOW

- Delay in admission to the hospital
- Admission to wrong level of care or patient care unit
- Lack of inpatient bed availability
- Diversion status in the emergency department (ED)
- ED overcrowding
- Premature transfer out of an ICU

- Premature discharge or transfer to another facility such as skilled nursing facility or subacute rehab
- Care is not provided at the right level such as staying in ED when requiring an ICU level of care

UNSCHEDULED RETURN TO SURGERY WITHIN SAME ADMISSION FOR SAME CONDITION AS PREVIOUS SURGERY OR TO CORRECT OPERATIVE PROBLEM (EXCLUDES STAGED PROCEDURES)

- Trauma suffered in the hospital
- Unplanned removal or repair of a normal organ (i.e., removal or repair not addressed in operative consent)
- Fall with injury or untoward effect (including but not limited to fracture, dislocation, concussion, laceration)
- Life-threatening complications of anesthesia
- Life-threatening transfusion error or reaction
- Hospital-acquired decubitus/pressure ulcer
- Care resulting in serious or life-threatening complications not related to admitting signs and symptoms, including but not limited to neurologic, endocrine, cardiovascular, renal, or respiratory body systems (e.g., resulting in dialysis, unplanned transfer to special care unit, lengthened hospital stay)
- Hospital-acquired urinary tract infection
- Hospital-acquired DVT (especially post surgery or procedure)
- Hospital-acquired ventilator-associated pneumonia
- Hospital-acquired MRSA or other types of infections

- Major adverse drug reactions or medication errors with serious potential for harm or resulting in special measures to correct (e.g., intubation, cardiopulmonary resuscitation, gastric lavage), including but not limited to the following:
  1. Incorrect antibiotic ordered by physician (e.g., inconsistent with diagnostic studies or patient's history of drug allergy)
  2. No diagnostic studies to confirm which drug is correct to administer (e.g., culture and sensitivity)
  3. Serum drug levels not measured as needed
  4. Diagnostic studies or other measures for side effects not performed as needed (e.g., blood urea nitrogen, creatinine, intake and output)

DIAGNOSIS RELATED

- Failure to diagnose (i.e., concluding that the patient has no disease or condition worthy of further follow-up or observation)
- Wrong diagnosis (misdiagnosis, i.e., original diagnosis is incorrect)
- Improper performance of tests

- Unnecessary diagnostic test
- Delay in diagnosis
- Failure to obtain consent or lack of informed consent
- Failure to recognize or account for conditions present on admission

ANESTHESIA RELATED

- Failure to complete patient assessment
- Failure to monitor patient
- Failure to test equipment
- Improper choice of anesthesia agent or equipment
- Improper technique or induction
- Improper monitoring of conscious sedation

- Improper use of equipment
- Improper intubation
- Improper positioning
- Failure to obtain consent or lack of informed consent
- Premature discharge post ambulatory procedure

SURGERY RELATED

- Failure to perform surgery
- Improper positioning
- Retained foreign body
- Wrong body part/surgery on the wrong site or side
- Improper performance of surgery
- Unnecessary surgery

- Delay in surgery
- Improper management of surgical patient
- Delay in postoperative care such as delay in extubation resulting in extended stay in the critical care unit
- Failure to obtain informed consent for surgery or lack of informed consent

MEDICATION RELATED

- Failure to order appropriate medication
- Wrong medication ordered
- Wrong dosage ordered of correct medication
- Failure to instruct on medication
- Improper management of medication regimen
- Failure to obtain consent for medication or lack of informed consent

- Failure to medicate
- Strong dosage administered
- Wrong patient
- Wrong route
- Improper technique
- Medication administration related (NOC)
- Failure to complete medications reconciliation
- Failure to continue necessary medications upon discharge

INTRAVENOUS AND BLOOD PRODUCTS RELATED

- Failure to monitor patient
- Wrong solution
- Wrong blood type
- Improper performance
- IV related (NOC)
- Failure to ensure contamination-free products

- Improper administration
- Failure to obtain consent or lack of informed consent
- Failure to monitor patient and identify early signs of an adverse reaction

OBSTETRICS RELATED

- Failure to manage pregnancy
- Improper choice of delivery method
- Improperly performed vaginal delivery
- Improperly performed cesarean section
- Delay in delivery (induction or surgery)
- Failure to obtain consent or lack of informed consent
- Improperly managed labor
- Failure to identify or meet fetal distress

- Delay in treatment of fetal distress (i.e., identified but treated in untimely manner)
- Retained foreign body—vaginal or uterine
- Abandonment
- Wrongful life or birth trauma suffered in the hospital
- Stillbirth

TREATMENT RELATED

- Failure to treat
- Wrong treatment or procedure performed (also improper choice)
- Failure to instruct patient on self-care
- Improper performance of a treatment or procedure
- Improper management of course of treatment
- Unnecessary treatment

- Delay in treatment
- Premature end of treatment (also abandonment)
- Failure to supervise treatment or procedure
- Failure to obtain consent for treatment or lack of informed consent
- Failure to refer or seek consultation

MONITORING RELATED

- Failure to monitor
- Failure to respond to the patient

- Failure to report on patient condition
- Failure to identify serious change in condition

BIOMEDICAL EQUIPMENT/PRODUCT RELATED

- Failure to inspect/monitor equipment
- Improper preventive maintenance
- Improper use of equipment
- Failure to respond to warning
- Lack of equipment

- Failure to instruct the patient on the use of equipment/product
- Malfunction or failure
- Wrong equipment used

MISCELLANEOUS

- Inappropriate behavior of clinician (i.e., sexual misconduct allegation, assault)
- Failure to protect third parties (i.e., failure to warn or protect from violent patient behavior)
- Breach of confidentiality or privacy including data breach

- Failure to maintain appropriate infection control practices
- Failure to follow institutional policy or procedure
- Others (provide detailed written description)
- Failure to review provider performance

NOC, not otherwise classified.

CHAPTER 8

Legal Considerations in Case Management Practice

Lynn S. Muller JD, BA-HCM, CCM, RN

"Law is a framework of authority directed by ethics"

LSM© 2011

LEARNING OBJECTIVES

Upon completion of this chapter, the reader will be able to:
1. Distinguish negligence from malpractice.
2. Recognize the importance of documentation in avoiding risk for litigation.
3. List four strategies to ensure appropriate patient discharge, transition, or case closure.
4. Describe the informed consent process.
5. Explain the role of legal documents in the planning and case management of patient's care.
6. Define the modern family.
7. Identify five strategies case managers may use to reduce legal risk.

ESSENTIAL TERMS

Administrative Law • Advance Directives for Healthcare • Affidavit of Merit • Breach Notification Rule • Competency • Confidentiality • Continuity of Care • Contract • Deposition • Discoverable/Discovery • Do Not Resuscitate (DNR) • Documentation • Elder Abuse • Employee Retirement Income Security Act of 1974 (ERISA) • Expedited Appeal • Expert Witness • Health Insurance Portability and Accountability Act of 1996 (HIPAA) • Implied Consent • Incompetence • Informed Consent • Interrogatory • Interstate Case Management • Living Will • Malpractice • Mandatory Reporting • Marijuana • Marriage Law • Modern Family • Negligence • Negligent Referral • Negligent Utilization Review • Patient Abandonment • Patient Self-Determination Act of 1990 • Patients' Bill of Rights • Power of Attorney (POA) • Pretrial • Professional Negligence • Reportable Events • Standard Appeal • Standard of Care • Standard of Practice • Statute of Limitations • Surrogate

The complex relationship between medicine and law requires healthcare providers to be careful about the way they deliver healthcare services to those who need them. Case managers are uniquely suited to work in a collaborative manner throughout the care continuum, having knowledge of both medical information and an educated appreciation for the law and its rules and regulations. Healthcare and case management have moved out of the shelter of hospitals into the community and virtually every setting of care. However, the concept of community is more global than ever before. The advent of advanced technology in both medicine and communication has opened opportunities for case management around the globe. With increased opportunity comes greater responsibility, and greater legal risks, to all players in the healthcare arena; as professionals, case managers are exposed to legal risks more than ever before. Each of the legal issues discussed in this chapter

repeatedly surfaces throughout the course of the case manager's responsibilities and the patient encounter with healthcare services.

This chapter starts with a description of general legal concepts that apply to case management and ends with a set of techniques case managers may employ to minimize liability exposure. Depending on the practice setting, not all types of legal exposure may apply to case management. For example, a hospital-based case manager who may or may not perform direct patient care duties has different potential risks than a telephonic case manager with a strong utilization management role.

Laws change and may vary from state to state. Even federal law can have different applications in the various states. The legalization of medical marijuana and recreational marijuana in a limited number of states brings an added onus for the case manager. Therefore, it is critical that case managers maintain their knowledge of statutes, rules and regulations for the state or states where they practice, especially because they are charged with the responsibility of knowing the law and acting in accordance with it, whether they know it or not. With the advent of the Internet, it is easier to find state and federal laws, particularly those legal issues that relate to nursing, social work, case management practice, rehabilitation counseling, vocational rehabilitation, disability management, pharmaceuticals, research, and other areas. However, it is important to remember that the law is not stagnant; it is an ever-changing and developing body of knowledge.

It is necessary to remain current. It is also important to participate where possible in the creation and maintenance of your institution's policies and procedures, particularly as they relate to case management practice and updates and changes in the law. If you have any doubt about a proper course of action, call your risk management department or legal counsel for assistance or guidance. You might also consider contacting an attorney familiar with medical-legal issues to obtain information on protecting your license while providing high-quality case management services. Additionally, you may consult with your professional organization, licensing agency, and certification body for an opinion on a situation you may be facing. Seeking expert advice is helpful when unsure of the best course of action.

▶ NEGLIGENCE

The very word *negligence* sends a chill down a healthcare professional's spine. Most people enter the healthcare field with a genuine sense of caring for others and a sincere commitment to doing the best job they can. Mistakes or oversights are far too common and occur even with the best of intentions or under the best circumstances. In your day-to-day life, such as in the case of driving your car, you are held to a simple or regular negligence standard. Negligence (Display 8-1) is the failure to act as a reasonable person

would in a given situation. The plaintiff, the individual who believes he or she was harmed by another (the defendant) and initiates a lawsuit by filing a complaint, must meet four very specific requirements to show that negligence has occurred. If one of these four elements is missing, the plaintiff will likely lose the case (Ovando & Thies, 1997); the court may consider the complaint unfounded.

Negligence is a tort, a civil wrong. It is distinguished from a crime in that it is one individual harming another, where money (known as dollar damages) can provide a remedy. Crime deals with victims who have been harmed by someone who has violated a state or federal statute. Victims leave the criminal courtroom empty-handed (Keaton, Dobbs, Keaton, & Owen, 1984). Many states provide for Victims' Funds, but these funds rarely give a victim more than a meager amount of money. Regular or simple negligence is a minimum standard and is based on a "reasonable person" standard. For example, when you are driving down the street you are expected to act in a reasonable and prudent manner, similar to the way other reasonable drivers would. A failure to do so, resulting in the injury of another, can subject you to liability; that is why we have automobile insurance.

▶ PROFESSIONAL NEGLIGENCE

Professional negligence, commonly referred to as *malpractice*, is a higher standard of obligation, a greater duty than simple or regular negligence. It is based on the idea that someone with specialized knowledge and skill, by virtue of education and experience, should know how to act in his or her specialized field. That special or superior knowledge is referred to as the Standard of Practice or Standard of Care (Display 8-2) (Keaton et al., 1984, § 32). The first level of scrutiny for a case manager's liability is the underlying profession of that individual case manager (e.g., nursing, physical therapy, medicine, vocational rehabilitation, and social work). If the case manager is a nurse, the Nurse Practice Act in the state of licensure is the controlling authority; a doctor would be viewed consistent with state law in his or her state of licensure. In addition, the so-called "geography rule" applies a standard to similarly situated professionals in the relevant geography/locale. For example, a practitioner in a remote and isolated village or Native American reservation with limited services would not be held to the same standard as a practitioner in a large metropolitan medical center with state-of-the-art equipment would be held. However, in the 21st century, with the advent of high-tech wireless and satellite communications, this distinction between these two types of practitioners is not as great as it once was. Within minutes, an ill or injured person can be transported from one location to another, even from the most remote area; therefore, the need for the geography rule appears to be diminishing. For links to all state boards of nursing and their Nurse Practice Acts, go to

---

display 8-1

THE FOUR ELEMENTS OF NEGLIGENCE

1. *Duty.* A legal obligation based on relationship or statute, such as parents' obligation to rescue their child; an obligation that a stranger does not share.
2. *Breach.* A failure to act in accordance with a recognized duty.
3. *Causation.* The required nexus or direct link between the breach of duty and the resulting harm; proof that the breach of duty actually caused the injury.
4. *Harm.* Injury experienced as a result of the breach. Some authorities add a fifth element, which is the requirement of proximate cause; a direct link between the breach of duty and the resulting harm (Cornell University Law School, 2017).

https://www.ncsbn.org/index.htm. For social work, refer to the National Association of Social Workers (NASW) (http://www.socialworkers.org). For certified case managers, refer to the Commission for Case Manager Certification (CCMC) (http://www.ccmcertification.org). Generally speaking, you may refer to the licensing services of your state education department for further information on your practice act as a licensed professional in your area of specialization.

▶ Affidavit of Merit

In most states, before a professional malpractice case can be filed in court (or shortly after filing), an Affidavit of Merit must also be filed; otherwise, the lawsuit will be dismissed. There is a growing body of case law discussing cases being rejected because of the failure to comply with the Affidavit of Merit requirement. In the Affidavit of Merit, a like-kind professional (nurse for a nurse, case manager for a case manager, etc.) must state under oath that there is reasonable probability that the case will succeed.

The following is an example of a law requiring an Affidavit of Merit.

> The plaintiff in a professional negligence case must prove the four elements of negligence: duty, breach, causation, and harm. The plaintiff also must prove that the healthcare professional deviated from a recognized and accepted standard of practice. In any action for damages for personal injuries, wrongful death, or property damage resulting from an alleged act of malpractice or negligence by a licensed person in his profession or occupation, the plaintiff shall, within 60 days following the date of filing of the answer to the complaint by the defendant, provide each defendant with an affidavit of an appropriate licensed person that there exists a reasonable probability that the care, skill, or knowledge exercised or exhibited in the treatment, practice, or work that is the subject of the complaint, fell outside acceptable or recognized professional or occupational standards or treatment practices. The court may grant no more than one additional period, not to exceed 60

days, to file the affidavit pursuant to this section, upon a finding of good cause. (N.J. ST. § 2A:53A-27 Affidavit of Merit, Rev., 2013)

There is no requirement that the professional who submits the Affidavit of Merit be the same individual who testifies at trial as an expert witness.

▶ Expert Witness

No medical or other professional negligence case can be litigated without an expert witness. The only way for the plaintiff to prove the case is to rely on the testimony of one or more expert witnesses. The Federal Rules of Evidence (adopted in whole or in part by most states) set forth the requirement that a like-kind expert testifies to the deviation from expected standards of practice and/or that no reasonable and similarly situated professional would have acted in the way that the defendant did, given similar circumstances (Fed. R. Evid. Article VII, Rule 703, 2011).

Some states have developed special panels or tribunals that examine the facts in an alleged malpractice case along with the Affidavit of Merit to determine whether the lawsuit can be filed at all (Gen. Laws Massachusetts, Part III, Title II, Ch. 231, § 60B). In those states, a preliminary hearing is conducted on the basis of the plaintiff's allegations contained in the complaint and documented by an expert witness. If the plaintiff fails at the panel stage, the lawsuit is dismissed before it starts. The composition of the panel typically includes lawyers, medical professionals, and lay people, representing the public.

▶ Case Manager Liability

The law is an ever-changing and growing body of knowledge. Nowhere is this truer than in case management practice. Case management is required by law in certain circumstances and states, such as Georgia, and some state-based workers' compensation laws and under federal law for certain beneficiaries of Tricare, the medical benefits system for the US military and its dependents. Failure to provide statutory case management services can be a violation of law in itself. For information about Tricare benefits, refer to http://www.tricare.mil/.

In most situations, case management services are provided through a contractual relationship. A client may have case management services through employment as either a direct benefit or through the state's workers' compensation system. Some businesses are using the services of absentee management companies that offer case management services as a component of a variety of health and wellness services for their employees. In recent years, case management as a component of acute care, within the traditional hospital setting, has grown tremendously. Transition across the care continuum to the most appropriate treatment level, as well as discharge

---

display 8-2

STANDARDS OF PRACTICE AND STANDARDS OF CARE

1. *Standards of Practice.* "Statements of acceptable level of performance or expectation for professional intervention or behavior associated with one's professional practice. They are generally formulated by practitioner organizations based on clinical expertise and the most current research findings."
2. *Standards of Care.* "Statements that delineate care that is expected to be provided to all clients [/patients]. They include predefined outcomes of care that clients can expect from providers and that are accepted within the community of professionals, based on the best scientific knowledge, current outcomes data, and clinical expertise" (Stanton and Tahan, 2017, p. 421).

planning and continuity of care services, provides new opportunities for case managers. Judges and juries decide cases on the basis of statute, case law, or both. With ever-changing practice settings, including telehealth, the law lags behind. Until a case comes through the courts identifying a new and different aspect of liability, the old rules still apply. Many cases are brought and settled out of court and the facts of those cases, even if known, do not change the body of case law.

Some examples of potential case management negligence are as follows:

▶ Failure to advocate on behalf of the patient/client/family/caregiver;
▶ Premature/Unsafe discharge from a hospital, home care, or skilled nursing facility (SNF);
▶ Negligent referral to alternate care centers;
▶ Negligent hiring and retention of employees;
▶ Inadequate communication with physicians or other healthcare professionals involved in patient care;
▶ Inadequate communication (e.g., withholding information) with a patient, family, and/or caregiver;
▶ Failure to comply with physician orders;
▶ Patient abandonment;
▶ Improper telephone triage;
▶ Failure to maintain medical record confidentiality;
▶ HIPAA Breach Notification;
▶ Adverse payment decisions, particularly those based on price alone, without an assessment of quality.

In addition to these concerns, case managers may also be placed in a precarious position due to competing pressures of the gamut of stakeholders. Healthcare has become an aggressively competitive market. There continue to be frequent mergers and acquisitions as well as bold and aggressive marketing ploys by companies; some even go so far as to market directly to consumers on television, in print media, and on the Internet. This may place case managers in a position where unrealistic expectations cannot be met or may be limited by contract. Marketing strategies can actually create a situation in which there is breach of contract, fraud, or misrepresentation.

The standards of professional practice are one of the gold standards that lawyers use to prove that the case manager did or did not breach the standard of care. However, keep in mind that case management remains a dependent credential—a supplement to one's primary profession.

▶ If You Are Named in a Lawsuit

If you are served with a summons and complaint, which are documents that initiate a lawsuit, you should follow the following do's and don'ts:

1. Don't refuse or avoid receiving these documents.
2. Don't argue with the process server.
3. Stop breathe and read the date of the alleged event.
4. Report receipt of the summons and complaint immediately to your attorney, your liability insurance company and your employer, as well as your insurance carrier and employer at the time in question, date of the alleged event, *if different*.
5. Obtain and review the record. Review it completely to refresh your recollection of the case. Lawsuits are typically filed up to 2 years after the incident, although this varies from state to state.
6. Follow your attorney's advice. If that individual is not fully familiar with your area of practice, explain your practice fully to that person, so he or she can best assist you.
7. Be sure to tell the attorney about standards of practice for your underlying profession (RN, SW, etc.) and the standard for case management practice, policies and procedures, protocols, and other information that were in effect at the time of the occurrence and may be helpful in your defense.
8. Discuss the matter with *only* your attorney and not with your coworkers.
9. Be honest with your attorney. He or she cannot help you without accurate information. Don't tell what you wish happened; rather tell exactly what happened.
10. Don't panic. An allegation is just that, a claim unless and until it is proven. Often, several defendants are eliminated from a lawsuit before the matter ever goes to court.

PRETRIAL

The time between the filing of a complaint (the document that starts a lawsuit by a plaintiff) and the trial itself is the pretrial phase of the case. Discovery is the fact-finding process that occurs in this pretrial phase and permits the attorneys on both sides to prepare their case. Discovery includes investigation, review of documents, and pretrial testimony. There are two methods in which sworn testimony is obtained before trial: interrogatories and depositions.

INTERROGATORIES *Interrogatories* are a formal request for additional information in a case; a series of questions that a party to a case, or witness in a case, must answer. After answering the questions, the individual signs a document that contains answers to the questions, certifying to the truth and accuracy of the information provided. This certification is equivalent to testifying under oath. Later at deposition or at trial the answers that the same individual gives can be compared to the interrogatory answers included in the signed document. Inconsistencies must be explained because these may affect the credibility of the witness. These tools are used to obtain background information and clarify facts surrounding the case.

DEPOSITION A *deposition* is a question-and-answer session conducted in a lawyer's office under oath. The witness, known as the deponent, is sworn in just as if in court. The proceeding is recorded by a court reporter and transcribed into a booklet referred to as the *transcript*. The deposition transcript may be used for further pretrial investigation, or to impeach or challenge a witness's testimony at trial. In certain circumstances a video deposition may also be used. It is an essential method: if during the trial the witness cannot be present in court, the video deposition can then be shared.

STATUTE OF LIMITATIONS

In most states, the statute of limitations for adults in personal injury cases is 2 years. That is the time limit for a person to file a lawsuit. However, Kentucky is an example of a state that permits only a 1-year statute of limitations from the discovery of the alleged injury (Ken. St. Title 36, Chapter 413, § 413.140). Some states measure the time for filing a lawsuit strictly from the date of injury. Other states extend the time to include a period when the patient knew or should have known of the discovery that a certain event caused a newly discovered consequence (illness or injury).

In the case of children, the date for filing may be extended past the first 2 years (or other statutory limit) and up to two or more years after the child reaches the age of maturity. This is one area where there is greater variation from state to state. Each state has its own definition of adulthood; there is no national standard. However, even in those states that would extend the filing date for an injured child, the statute of limitations may remain only 2 years for any out-of-pocket costs or damages claimed by the parents related to their child's claim. For a complete list of state statutes of limitations and access to each state's legislative website, refer to: http://injury.findlaw.com/accident-injury-law/time-limits-to-bring-a-case-the-statute-of-limitations.html

One reason for a statute of limitations is that few people remember intimate and complex details from years past. Another is to limit the time a reasonable practitioner must retain records and be expected to remember complex details from any particular case.

DOCUMENTATION

Courts in general and juries often believe that what is written and properly documented in the normal course of business is more credible than live testimony. Therefore, your documentation as a case manager is critical to your professional practice, no matter the medium, such as electronic medical records (EMRs) or the practice setting. In particular, if you find yourself the defendant in a professional liability/malpractice lawsuit, you want to be confident that your documentation can be relied upon with the passage of time.

Following are four general criteria for documentation, no matter what documentation tools (electronic or manual) are used:

1. *Chart the facts.* Be objective. Subjective complaints are acceptable and must come from the patient (i.e., Mr. Jones stated, "My left abdomen pain is much worse"). On the contrary, subjective statements or those that are judgmental or opinionated in nature, when made by a case manager, should be considered carefully, as they will take on an entirely different meaning out of context. For example, unless the occurrence was actually witnessed, the case manager should write, "patient found on floor" (with details), not "patient fell out of bed." Documentation should be complete and correct. If true, you might even go as far as stating, "when I returned from the Code Blue two rooms away, I found Mr. J on the floor. Immediately I performed an assessment of his condition and especially checked for signs of bleeding, bruising, etc.; I stayed with Mr. J and called for help." Two or more years later, there would be no confusion or alternate interpretation of what happened and why you were not there. Throughout my lengthy nursing history, there have been many schools of thought on charting; too much, too little; signing clearly, scribbling your name so it cannot be identified, etc. In the end, there is no substitute for complete, timely, and accurate documentation. Documentation is the case manager's best friend and protector.

2. *Use The Joint Commission (TJC), Utilization Review Accreditation Commission (URAC), or other approved abbreviations* (e.g., those adopted and enforced by your healthcare organization). This discourages ambiguity and prevents potentially harmful misunderstandings. Refer to your organizational policies for an approved list of abbreviations. These policies are developed on the basis of nationally recognized standards and usually describe where your organization stands in relation to abbreviations. They also explain what is allowed and what is forbidden. If unsure, it is best to spell things out; this prevents confusion, misinterpretation, and miscommunication. A complete narrative note is the only way someone can know what you were thinking on a particular day.

3. *Use legible penmanship.* It would be embarrassing to have your own documentation shown on a giant screen in court and you yourself are unable to decipher it. It may affect your credibility. Increasingly, healthcare organizations (hospitals and other agencies) are switching over to computer-based documentation, both complicating and simplifying this process. Beware of checklist charting, especially charting by omission. This supposed time-saving simplification can lead to error, omission, and an

inability to rely on the record at a later date. The old adage, *if it isn't written it didn't happen*, remains true, even and especially with EMR. For those who practice telephonic case management, the rules are the same. Documentation is essential. On the good side, the use of electronic documentation systems with the increasing availability of EMRs helps reduce the risk of illegible penmanship.

4. *Record your information as promptly as possible* so that details are not lost or forgotten. Use actual times accurately and chart in chronological order. If you must chart information at a later time, because of an emergent situation or simple forgetfulness, DO NOT squeeze it in or backdate the information. Make your note the next entry and state clearly and accurately why you are charting out of order. For example, "1/1/17, 2:10 PM I was called away to a code and failed to chart Mr. Jones' blood sugars this morning; however, they were taken on time and insulin coverage given to the patient immediately." It is only this entry that was delayed. Attorneys later use such time notings to reconstruct a case, as in a play. For example, if you called a physician at 5-minute intervals or gave sublingual nitroglycerine according to protocol, providing the time details will be to your advantage. Honesty remains the best policy.

▶ NEGLIGENT REFERRALS

Negligent referrals are an area that has been growing as a danger point for case manager liability and is closely related to the discharge and transitional planning role. From the lawyer's standpoint, the problem with these cases is proving measurable damages, but this does not limit the potential for liability for case managers. Making a bad referral or recommending a defective product is directly linked to your duty to advocate for your client. If the plaintiff can prove that, because of the case manager's choice or recommendation, he or she chose a particular product or service that resulted in injury, delayed recovery, or worse, the case manager will be defending how and why a particular vendor, facility, or product was selected. The case manager may find himself or herself as a party to a lawsuit containing, among other causes of action, a negligent referral claim. In recent years there have been several cases that have been settled out of court, with facts related to "negligent referral." Following up in a timely fashion is another element of referral; it is not enough to provide a list to be done. Reasonable effort to assure that the patient has the necessary tools for the next level of treatment is part of the case manager's role.

Many health maintenance organizations (HMOs) and preferred provider organizations (PPOs) have large networks of providers (hospitals, healthcare professionals such as physicians, home care agencies, SNFs, and other institutions) who have contracted with the HMO/PPO or other entities to provide products (e.g., durable medical equipment such as wheelchairs, canes, and bedside commodes) and services at reduced rates. With the advent of big mergers and acquisitions in healthcare, dealing with network limitations has become a greater challenge for case managers. In addition, large medical centers across the country have developed extensive integrated healthcare networks, including subacute, long and short-term rehabilitation centers, step-down facilities, and even durable medical supply and medical transport companies. Case managers who work in these environments are often faced with a difficult ethical dilemma. Their employers instruct them (either openly or covertly) to refer patients only "within network" or the client's health insurance limits choice and the case manager has learned through experience that one or more of the network businesses or providers are of lesser quality. One of the goals of medical centers is to keep costs down for themselves and/or for the insurance companies to which they are tied up. Liability exposure for case managers in such cases occurs when there is a poor or harmful outcome from one of the contracted network providers where it can be shown that the case manager knew, or should have known, but ignored the fact that a high-quality, cost-effective (albeit out-of-network) option was geographically and financially viable.

To prevent situations where the case manager participated in the referral process without critically and objectively assessing the provider, or even without performing a cost-benefit analysis comparing different providers, courts in California, New York, Alabama, and elsewhere have stipulated that it is the responsibility of case managers to adhere to the standard of practice. Case managers can minimize risks related to the referral process by considering the following:

▶ Credentialing in any organization is a key safety net and is now required by recognized credentialing bodies, such as the URAC and TJC. A periodic review of the credentials, complaint logs, and certifications of providers of all types is an important task to decrease liability.

▶ Compare costs and ask questions to determine the quality of products and services offered by a provider. Negotiate price for equivalent products even in a network or, more importantly, when you identify a higher-quality choice and successfully negotiate a competitive out-of-network rate. Then advocate, on behalf of your client, to secure payment.

▶ Physicians are becoming increasingly resistant to making direct referrals due to their fear of liability exposure. Patients or families may ask the case manager for recommendations. When making recommendations and referrals, always give the patient, family, and/or caregiver several options to choose from and let them make the ultimate decision. If the patient's plan has a provider network,

AVOID NEGLIGENT REFERRAL

A thorough, accurate, and ongoing credentialing process is the *best prevention* for negligent referral claims.

have the patient choose from among those listed in the reference book once you have assessed their quality. However, make the patient aware that paying privately for a product or service that is out of the network is an alternative, especially if the individual is unhappy with the choices within the plan. When considering a private pay option, you can attempt to negotiate a favorable price for the patient. This possibility may not be financially viable in every case, but it is the client/patient who should make the choice. Your duty as a case manager is to provide fair and honest information.

Cost-benefit analyses are part of the case manager's patient advocacy responsibility. The concept of client- and family-centered case management services implies a responsibility to always act in the best interest of the patient (client)/family. Document that a reasonable process was applied; show the steps taken; demonstrate that you (the case manager) were, in fact, acting in the best interests of the patient and/or family (Display 8-3).

▶ HEALTH INSURANCE PORTABILITY AND ACCOUNTABILITY ACT OF 1996

The Health Insurance Portability and Accountability Act (HIPAA), Public Law 104-191, was enacted on August 21, 1996, and is a significant piece of civil rights legislation.

Since the 1960s there have been two significant pieces of health-related civil rights legislation. The first is the Americans with Disabilities Act (ADA), which many confuse with labor law; the second is the HIPAA of 1996. The HIPAA affects more people than the ADA does, as it affects every person in the United States, rather than a unique and protected group. The HIPAA is intended to improve the portability and continuity of health insurance by protecting individuals against laws regarding preexisting conditions and other restrictions. A preexisting condition is a medical condition diagnosed or treated before an individual changes to a new health plan. In the past, healthcare for a preexisting condition was not covered in a new health insurance plan until after a waiting period. The new law changes the rules. It is called the "portability act" because it protects a person's ability to maintain insurance coverage when changing jobs or insurance plans; in effect, even with preexisting conditions or chronic illnesses, insurance is portable; however, this remains limited when there is a lapse in coverage.

Health insurance providers must offer insurance to individuals who lose coverage for reasons such as a change in employment, a job not offering health insurance, or job termination. To qualify, the individual must first exhaust a full 18 months of Consolidated Omnibus Reconciliation Act of 1985 coverage and be ineligible for other programs such as Medicaid and Medicare.

The Privacy Rule was published on December 28, 2000 (67 C.F.R. § 82462) with the goal of providing consumers with greater rights for protection of individually identifiable health information. Modifications of the Privacy Rule were published in final form on August 14, 2002 (65 C.F.R. § 53182). In the spring of 2003 there were further modifications to the Final Privacy Rule. The HIPAA is here to stay; the key to the HIPAA is demonstrating compliance. Case managers must understand these laws and adhere to them at all times to reduce the risk for, or completely avoid, negligence or malpractice.

The best resource for HIPAA compliance is the primary source from the federal Office of Civil Rights (OCR) (http://www.hhs.gov/ocr/hipaa). There are guidance documents on the OCR website on such topics as government access, business associates, protected health information, incidental uses and disclosures, public health, workers compensation, and others. Other resources include the HIPAA confidentiality and privacy policies and procedures of the healthcare organization to which you belong.

▶ EMPLOYEE RETIREMENT INCOME SECURITY ACT OF 1974

The Employee Retirement Income Security Act (ERISA) is primarily concerned with the regulation of pension plans. The ERISA was originally enacted so that employers who hire employees in multistate areas would not be encumbered by multiple state laws. For example, coordination-of-benefit state laws do not apply to ERISA employers. This means that if a patient has more than one insurance plan, state rules about who is the primary source of insurance and who is the secondary source of insurance do not apply; however, ERISA employer plans must comply with federal laws.

From a case management perspective, those who work with employer plans or self-funded plans must consider the other aspects of this act: the benefit plan becomes the controlling document and establishes coverage, coordination of benefits provisions, claims processes, appeals procedures, and essentially all rules and regulations governing the rights of beneficiaries and plan participants, including the liabilities of the plan administrator (Gammage & Burham, 1997). Case managers must be aware of the specific guarantees and exemptions written into the benefit plans. Managed Care Organizations (MCOs) have successfully used the ERISA as a shield against malpractice lawsuits. Many case managers have heard stories of tremendous loss where no punitive damages were awarded because the ERISA protected the plan administration. Recovery of damages under the ERISA cannot exceed the cost of the benefit that should have been provided; therefore, if a bone marrow transplant was in question, and the patient died, approximately $91,000 would be allowed in damages. In other words, only the denial of benefits can be the focus of an ERISA lawsuit (Robbins, 1998).

In the past several years a number of lawsuits that address ERISA issues have been filed. One bottom-line ERISA issue is whether or not the claim "relates to" the ERISA benefit plan. Essentially, if the court determines that a claim relates to the ERISA, then the patient is not likely to receive any recovery of damages. That is essentially what happened in the case of *Corcoran v. United Healthcare, Inc.* (Mellette & Kurtz, 1993). For safety reasons, Mrs. Corcoran's physician wanted 24-hour fetal monitoring for her last trimester of pregnancy. She was already admitted to the hospital when she was told her health plan would not cover the admission but would cover 10 hours of home nursing services per day. She returned home and, during one of the gaps without monitoring, the fetus went into distress and died. No wrongful death damages were rendered to the mother because ERISA rules preempted other laws. On the other hand, if the court determines that the claim does not relate to the ERISA, damages can be won.

ERISA issues are a complex problem best left to legal experts. This is further complicated by state statutes that challenge the ERISA, and even specific aspects of the HIPAA. Case managers who work with patients under the ERISA may require expert counsel in some predicaments. This situation is a moving target; in fact, because of new laws being considered and being enacted (both federally and statewide), no one is quite sure how several case management/managed care legal situations will play out. Still, the following are a few preventive actions case managers can take:

- ▶ Know the plan documents, including the coverage and payment decisions.
- ▶ Call the plan's consultant for anything that is unsure, whether it is the fine points of a covered service or a nebulous definition such as medical necessity. Be persistent. If consultants are unsure, they often go to their supervisor or legal counsel for the answers.
- ▶ Make sure the utilization management criteria are consistent with the plan's standards and benefits.
- ▶ Do not forget to tell the patient of the right to appeal when a service is not included in the benefits or is deemed not medically necessary by a physician advisor.
- ▶ Keep abreast of changing legislation.
- ▶ Consult with legal experts in your own organization.

Certain health care plans are controlled by federal law under the ERISA of 1974 (29 U. S. C., §§ 1001-1461

(2000). Since the ERISA is a federal law, in most cases where there is a conflict, federal law preempts or supersedes state law. This is true in cases where the administration of the ERISA plan is at issue; however, in 2003 in the case of *Villizon v. PruCare* (843 So.2d 842 [2003]), the Florida Supreme Court held that "Upon an appropriate finding, the trial court may dismiss the estate's direct negligence, corporate liability and implied contract claims for a lack of subject matter jurisdiction [due to federal preemption]. However, in no event may the vicarious liability count be dismissed, as the same does not 'relate to' an employee benefit plan" (*Citing Estate of Frappier, 678 So. 2d at 88, 888, Fla. 4th DCA 1996*). Therefore, the vicarious liability suit was heard in the Florida State Court. In this case there was delay in diagnosis due to the "hoops" that claimants and their HMO physicians had to go through before a specialist could make timely referral to diagnostic testing and evaluation. The primary care physician was found to be liable for delayed diagnosis and PruCare was vicariously liable when a cancer was not appropriately and timely diagnosed.

The Patient Protection and Affordable Care Act of 2010 (PPACA) was enacted to bring accessible healthcare to more Americans. Although federally funded, it is state controlled and varies greatly in applicability from state to state. The PPACA outlawed the concept of preexisting condition and allows adult children (up to age 26) to remain on their parents' health insurance plans. The case manager must remain mindful to changes in this or any other law that relates to the provision and payment for healthcare.

▶ NEGLIGENT UTILIZATION MANAGEMENT/REVIEW

One of the first cases to address potential MCO liability for negligent utilization management and review was *Wickline v. State of California* (29 Cal.Rptr at 818.2). In this landmark decision, the physician was deemed responsible for treatment decisions; however, the court also indicated that in some situations, third-party payors "can be legally accountable when medically inappropriate decisions result from defects in the design or implementation of cost-containment mechanisms as, for example, when appeals made on a patient's behalf for medical or hospital care are arbitrarily ignored or unreasonably disregarded or overridden" (Sturgeon, 1997, p. 68). Ultimately, the California Appellate Court held that the HMO was not liable and that the *Wickline* decision was limited to its unique facts.

Subsequently in *Wilson v. Blue Cross of Southern California*, the court determined that even though a treatment decision and a payment decision are two distinct subjects, if the payment decision is made negligently and is a factor in subsequent harm to the patient, the MCO (and its agents) can be held liable. However, other courts

AVOIDING UTILIZATION REVIEW NEGLIGENCE

When performing utilization management activities, apply utilization review criteria *consistently* to avoid negligent utilization review practices. The utilization review criteria applied must be those that are recommended and used by the health insurance or benefit plan such as InterQual or Milliman Care Guidelines, referred to today as MCG. InterQual is an evidence-based criteria system that provides "appropriateness of care decision support covering medical and behavioral health across all levels of care as well as care planning and complex care management. With an outstanding track record, widespread adoption and continual enhancement, InterQual Criteria are the standard for evidence-based clinical decision support" (McKesson, 2017, p.1). MCG guidelines are also evidence based and apply to various care settings. InteQual criteria tend to be more commonly used in federal benefit programs (e.g., Medicare and Medicaid), whereas MCG guidelines are popular within commercial or private health insurance plans.

do not agree that physicians will be improperly influenced by utilization review systems (Sturgeon, 1997).

When appeals made on a patient's behalf are arbitrarily ignored or unreasonably disregarded or overridden, they are considered negligent utilization review. This type of review (Display 8-4) will be less common as mandatory appeals protocols go into effect (see "Denials and the Appeals" later in this chapter).

In 1995, the New Jersey Supreme Court held in *Dunn v. Praiss* (606 A.2d 862) that an HMO was liable for the contribution toward the malpractice of a physician they hired as an independent contractor. Logically it would follow that a case manager performing telephonic or field case management services for an HMO, who deviates from the "accepted standards of practice," could be held liable for his or her actions. In addition, the HMO could share in that liability. This is known as joint liability.

In 2007, in *Basil v. Wolf* (193 N.J. 38, 67 [2007]) the same New Jersey Supreme Court would not extend liability to a workers' compensation insurance company for the malpractice of a physician who performed an independent medical examination (IME) on its behalf and failed to diagnosis cancer metastasis over a period of 2 years. Such cases are important to case management as the selection of a physician, including IME physicians, is often left to the case manager. One should make a reasonable inquiry into the physician's qualifications and past practices. At a minimum, one should check the state medical board's website to determine if the physician is in good standing or if any board action is pending against the physician. Similar inquiries should be made for pharmacies, pharmacists, home care companies, and other practitioners to whom referrals are considered.

Twenty years ago, in an Alabama case, *Reid v. Aetna Casualty & Surety Co.* (1997), the allegation by a plaintiff/employee, "that the nurse [case manager] was more concerned with saving money than with the employee's recovery," was found to be insufficient to support a claim. In this case, the client was offered a variety of choices for the treatment of pain management and the provider chosen was also the least expensive. In addition, there was an allegation of fraud on the part of the defendant or insurance carrier, in that they had suppressed the following material information (among other things): "that the nurse [case manager] was not acting as a registered nurse with the normal professional obligations toward the worker [client]" (*Reid v. Aetna Casualty & Surety Co.*, 1997). The court held that even if that were true (and made no finding that it was true), there was no evidence that the actions of the case manager caused any harm to the patient. "It is undisputed that Aetna hired [a case management company] to perform medical case management, that the [case manager] was employed as a registered nurse . . . and that she worked on the client's case." Although the patient claimed that the case manager "prevented her from undergoing beneficial treatments," she failed to offer proof of such alternate beneficial treatments, and the case was dismissed (*Reid v. Aetna Casualty & Surety Co.*, 1997). Even with the passage of time, this case stands as a cautionary tale to case managers.

▶ DENIALS AND APPEALS

The courts have mandated that MCOs have a duty to inform patients of their right to appeal insurance denials. In the case of *Sarchett v. Blue Shield of California* (43 Cal.3d 1, 10 [1987]), Blue Shield denied a patient's hospitalization on the grounds that it was not medically necessary and the insurance company did not mention to the patient the right to appeal. The California Supreme Court held that the insurance company breached its covenant of good faith and fair dealing by failing to inform the insured of the right to appeal. Rather, the insurance company's conduct appeared designed to mislead the insured into giving up the right to impartial review (Sturgeon, 1997). Case managers must be familiar with denials, appeals (both expedited and standard appeals), grievances, reconsiderations, and patient rights. It is not up to the case manager to interpret an insurance contract, but there is a duty to be forthcoming with the client.

▶ Grievances, Expedited and Standard Appeals

An *appeal* is a request to reexamine a healthcare decision, usually one in which the patient and the physician believed that the procedure or service was medically necessary, but the authorizing agent denied the procedure or service.

Depending on the state laws and the insurance procedures, the process may vary. However, the appeals process is one with which a case manager must be familiar for several important reasons.

First, the case manager may be asked by the patient/family or the physician to help obtain services for the patient. If the insurance benefits are vague in nature or the services are not authorized, the appeals procedure may be the first line of defense. It may also be that the case manager agrees that this is not only a necessary service, but also one that is inappropriately denied and is a covered benefit. The appeals process exists precisely for such a scenario.

As a patient advocate, see that every opportunity is provided to the patient to receive services that the physician deems necessary and important for the patient's health and well-being. This is not just a nice thing to do, but legally prudent as well. When cases are filed, the case manager, who has walked through the appeals procedure with the patient, family, and physician, will be viewed as an advocate and not as an adversary. This can have important ramifications for the case manager on the court's witness stand.

Common reasons for denial of claims of which case managers must be careful include, but are not limited to, the following:

▶ Errors (incomplete or inaccurate) in the information shared with the funding source, health insurance plan, or payor.
▶ Additional supporting documentation was needed. This may include manufacturer pricing and a description of the item (if equipment is being requested, for example).
▶ The physician failed to supply clear, supporting information or documentation.
▶ Consumer expectations exceed the limitations of their health insurance plan coverage.
▶ Failing to follow agreed-upon utilization review and management procedures such as ignoring to notify an acute care hospital about the health insurance plan related to the patient's admission.

Often, the first part of the appeals process involves a simple reconsideration, which is a request by telephone, e-mail, or fax for an additional review of a utilization review determination not to certify. This is performed by the peer reviewer who reviewed the original decision on the basis of the submission of additional information; sometimes, it is a peer-to-peer discussion. In other words, when a service or procedure is denied, the physician who is providing care to the patient speaks with the physician at the payor/insurer organization who reviewed (and denied) the service and discusses the case. More patient information may be all that is needed. If the service is then approved, the appeals process does not need to go any further. If this does not settle the matter, it will become a formal appeals consideration.

An appeals consideration is a clinical review conducted by appropriate clinical peers, who were not involved in the clinical review, when a decision not to certify a requested admission, procedure, or service has been appealed. There are two types of appeals: expedited and standard.

▶ An *expedited appeal* is a request by telephone or fax for additional review of a determination not to certify imminent or ongoing services, requiring a review conducted by a clinical peer who was not involved in the original decision not to certify.
▶ A *standard appeal* is a request to review a determination not to certify an admission, extension of stay, or other healthcare services conducted by a peer reviewer who was not involved in any previous noncertification pertaining to the same episode of care.

Various credentialing organizations and state and federal laws mandate specific time frames and conditions in which to perform an appeal procedure. The expedited appeal is for "imminent or ongoing services" that must be attended to quickly (usually within 1 business day) for patient safety. The physician (clinical peer) who is allowed to perform the expedited appeal must not be the same physician who made the initial determination to deny the service. A standard appeal is usually for retrospective services that do not require immediate attention (usually within 30 days of receiving the documentation). A physician who was not involved in any other part of the appeals process can perform this level of appeal. Standard appeals are initiated in writing and include examining parts of the medical record. Other requirements may also be expected in appeals (e.g., board certification of a physician who is knowledgeable about the type of case being reviewed).

A *grievance* is a "formal written request by a member for a hearing by the (provider) regarding: (1) a complaint about care or services received from the network or from a network provider, or (2) an appeal of a decision made by the network with regard to the provision of a requested service." This is a complaint that is usually made when no urgency of medical care is needed. It may precede a standard appeal or it may stem from a complaint about an expedited or standard appeal decision (often called a determination).

As more Americans opt for Medicare benefits under the HMO plans (i.e., Medicare Advantage Plans) rather than the traditional fee-for-service design, case managers are increasingly expected to perform utilization review and precertification for services rendered or to be rendered to beneficiaries of Medicare Advantage Plans. As a result, there is an increased chance that some services and procedures will be denied and appeal procedures will be indicated. The Medicare appeals process may vary from private insurance appeals processes (which could also vary from state to state). (For more information, refer to Chapter 5, Utilization Management.)

Medicare expedited appeal reasons are similar to those of commercial insurance providers; they imply that expedited appeals are used for "imminent or ongoing services." The expedited appeal is used when:

▶ The health insurance plan refuses to provide services that the beneficiary believes should be furnished or arranged for by the health plan.

▶ The beneficiary has not received the services outside the health insurance plan and it is believed that the beneficiary requires those services or else an adverse health condition may result.

▶ The health insurance plan discontinues services when the beneficiary believes there is a continuing need for such services.

▶ Exhaustion of benefits occurs and a medical need is still present; depending on the circumstances, this may become an expedited or a standard appeal process.

The standard appeal is used when less emergent services are denied, such as:

▶ Precertification denial when the physician or the beneficiary thinks the service is necessary and is a covered benefit.

▶ Nonpayment of claims for which the physician or the beneficiary believed the care was necessary and was a covered benefit; this nonpayment could be for the total bill or for a part of the bill.

▶ Emergency or urgent services were billed and the health insurance plan did not find they were urgent.

▶ Discontinuation of services, although the physician or the beneficiary feels such services are still needed.

▶ Exhaustion of benefits occurs and a medical need is still present; depending on the circumstances, this may become an expedited or a standard appeal process.

▶ Who May Request an Appeal

▶ A Medicare beneficiary can request an appeal. A beneficiary may request, either orally or in writing, an expedited appeal if he or she believes that health, life, or ability to regain maximum function may be jeopardized by the standard appeal process, which sometimes may take up to 60 days. It is not necessary for the beneficiary to enlist the support of the physician for an expedited appeal (although it may be a wise choice); the health plan cannot require this. It is the health plan's responsibility to decide whether the request for an expedited appeal meets the necessary criteria. If the beneficiary desires a standard appeal, and no expedited appeal has been filed, the standard appeal request is made in writing.

▶ A Medicare beneficiary can request a representative to file an expedited or standard appeal. The beneficiary must provide his or her name, Medicare number, and a statement that appoints the individual as the representative. The beneficiary must also sign and date the form and have the representative sign and date the form.

▶ A physician can request an appeal on behalf of the beneficiary. A physician may provide oral or written support for a beneficiary's request, or a physician may act in the beneficiary's interest by requesting an expedited appeal as the beneficiary's representative. The same paperwork as stated in number 2 must be provided. The expedited appeal can be initiated verbally or in writing by fax. The physician should be very clear that he or she believes the situation is time sensitive and/or the review should be conducted within 72 hours or less as medically necessary or appropriate.

▶ A court-appointed guardian or an agent/representative under a healthcare proxy can request an appeal. This must be in accordance with what is provided by state laws.

▶ If the beneficiary is an inpatient in the hospital and disagrees with the decision to be discharged or transferred to a facility that is of a lesser level of care, the case manager should steer the patient to the use of the hospital-issued notice of noncoverage procedure, rather than an expedited appeal process. The appeal in this case can be done by calling the state's peer review organization/quality improvement organization.

▶ What to Do to Reduce the Need for Appeal Procedures

▶ Check to ensure that the bill/claim was accurately coded. Incorrect coding may lead to denials, and coding may differ between companies; a claim will be denied if it is not found in *the insurance company's* list of covered items or services.

▶ Communicate the patient's condition and the medical necessity of the service or equipment. It is not uncommon for a request or claim to be denied due to lack of some important information. Payors want medical justification for spending medical dollars. Sometimes a claim is denied for not-so-obvious reasons.

▶ Make sure that the insurance company/payor receives the claims and the utilization review information or case management reports. The reports should include the information needed to adjudicate the claims.

▶ Document carefully and fully. Keep the benefits in mind while you are documenting and match the patient's condition with the requested service or equipment. Validate that the service or equipment is medically needed and is the most appropriate for the situation, as well as where it fits into the benefit design. If convenience or preference is conveyed, it will be more difficult to obtain authorization. In most cases this information must be written by a physician. The case manager can assist by understanding and suggesting what must be communicated, including pictures or consumer letters if appropriate.

▶ Speak plainly at the appeals board. Use pictures if it would help. Many people in the appeals process do not have a medical background.

▶ Explain the benefit limitations and the appeals process to the patient and the family. Often it is the case manager's role to explain coverage limitations to patients. Assess if consumer expectation is a contributing factor to the problem. However, it is also the case manager's role to be a patient advocate when medical needs truly exceed benefits.

▶ Use a cost-benefit analysis approach. Occasionally, benefits will be altered if the case manager can prove that the suggested treatment, service, or piece of equipment is the best and most cost-efficient for the patient and the payor. Using this approach before a denial notice may obviate the need for an appeal in the first place. However, an informed analysis requires complete and accurate data. Information that may be needed for such an analysis should include inputs from the patient's multidisciplinary team and also include some or all of the following:

   ▶ Complete history and physical assessment

   ▶ Proposed treatment plan

   ▶ Timing for implementing treatment plan (with estimated length of treatment or equipment need)

   ▶ When and what changes may be made to the treatment plan

   ▶ How will the treatment plan be evaluated and monitored; expected outcomes

   ▶ How often the patient is seen

   ▶ How long the patient was evaluated before developing the treatment plan

▶ Explore product support programs as an option. Many case managers are aware of community support programs for various diseases, and pharmaceutical help for required medications when a patient cannot pay. Less well known is that pharmacies and high-tech medical device companies have case managers who act as representatives for their products. These case managers are highly trained in insurance and reimbursement issues and claims processing; they assist in verifying benefits and answering questions about denials. They conduct a comprehensive funding search, identify trends in reimbursement, and approach the payor to resolve problems.

▶ In some states, very specific language that will help in the appeal process can be found. As a case manager, you should be familiar with the language and the laws in your state.

▶ INTERSTATE/DISTANCE CASE MANAGEMENT PRACTICE

In the United States today, a professional may practice only in the state or states in which he or she is licensed and is in good standing. A nurse, for example, must be licensed in the state where the patient/client is located. Otherwise, the nurse would not be able to provide care to the patient. This appears to be complicated by the move to a global economy where healthcare organizations are securing multistate and offshore sites.

Each nurse's practice is controlled by the law in the states(s) where he or she is licensed and by the Nurse Practice Act of that state(s). The advent of the Nurse Licensure Compact (NLC) places nurses on notice that interstate practice is recognized only in those states that have passed legislation, rules, and regulations adopting the Compact. The Compact permits nurses whose home state participates in the Compact to practice in any other state participating in the Compact. In the absence of such law being adopted by one's home state, a nurse must be licensed in each and every state in which he or she practices, even if the practice is limited to services such as telephonic triage. With half of the states being included in the Compact, and a lesser amount being included in the Advanced Practice Nurse Compact (APRN Compact), the majority of nurses are left having to be licensed in each and every state in which they practice their profession. For a complete list and interactive map of those states that have adopted and readopted the revised NLC, go to: https://www.ncsbn.org/compacts.htm

In December 2005, the Case Management Society of America (CMSA) took an official position on this issue and incorporated its position in the *CMSA's Standards of Practice for Case Management*. The *Standards* were then revised in 2016 and formally and explicitly introduced the "professional" reference to case managers rather than the prior implicit professional nature of the role. The *Standards* currently clearly states that: "The professional case manager shall adhere to all applicable federal, state, and local laws and regulations, which have full force and effect of law, governing all aspects of case management practice including, but not limited to, client privacy and confidentiality rights. It is the responsibility of the professional case manager to work within the scope of his/her license and/or underlying profession." The *Standards* also notes that in the event "the professional case manager's employer policies or those of other entities are in conflict with applicable legal requirements, the case manager should understand that the law prevails. In these situations, case managers should seek clarification of questions or concerns from an appropriate and reliable expert resource, such as a legal counsel, compliance officer, or an appropriate government agency" (CMSA, 2916, p. 27).

- ▶ The CMSA encourages case managers and case manager employers to work aggressively with state Boards of Nursing to encourage compliance and entry into the National Council of State Boards of Nursing as the Compact states so that appropriate multistate nursing licensure might continue appropriately and cost-effectively.
- ▶ Alternatively, the CMSA encourages the enactment of federal legislation mandating the recognition of nurse licensure in all states.
- ▶ The CMSA has added its name to the growing list of those organizations supporting and endorsing the Nurse Compact. A copy of the CMSA Position Paper can be obtained through its website, www.cmsa.org (Powell & Tahan, 2008, pp. 591–593).

The nature of a telephonic conversation may quickly change from being informational to one of nursing practice when it ceases to be about an appointment or about a delivery of a product and becomes caring when the simple question is asked, "How are you doing?" If the nurse case manager uses that information to assess the client's condition, then he or she is said to be practicing nursing. Clients offer symptoms over the phone and in person and nurses are trained to make nursing assessment on the basis of such symptoms. That is called nursing practice and it requires a license to practice in the state where the patient is located.

The question often arises: "But what if the patient is a pilot or sales representative and is traveling?" Although there are no cases to date, the controlling law states two (sometimes conflicting) rules. If a case pertains to workers' compensation, the law that is applicable is the one that is enforceable when the individual was hired. For example, pilots employed by certain airlines are presumed to work where the airline's corporate office is located, even if they receive treatment around the globe. In general health or more traditional employment scenarios, the state of the patient's residency applies. Obtaining an additional license by waiver (entry into another state without examination) is the way in which a professional learns and is kept up-to-date on changes in the law and the legal requirements, such as specific continuing education training. It is reasonable for a case manager to request contribution by the employer for the cost of the additional license while employed in a multistate field for a telephonic case management setting. This is something that can be discussed at the time of interview or after the case manager is hired and learns that the assignment will require case management across state lines.

▶ USE OF COMMUNITY STANDARDS IN THE UTILIZATION MANAGEMENT ROLE

A patient with multiple sclerosis was receiving a standard treatment protocol for the condition but was having side effects that led to at least two hospitalizations. The physician wanted to try a commonly used treatment protocol for multiple sclerosis in Arizona. However, the patient's primary insurance company was in Massachusetts and denied the Arizona treatment because it was not a standard treatment on the east coast. The request to change protocols was reasonable (and medically necessary). The argument was one of the "right to use treatment protocols" according to the standards of the medical community in which the patient resides.

Lawsuits against MCOs can be based on the theory that an MCO did not make a utilization decision in accordance with the standard of medical necessity of the local community. In the case of *Hughes v. Blue Cross of Northern California* (215 Cal.App.3d 832 [1989]), the issue was whether a third-party payor acted in bad faith by using a standard of medical necessity significantly at variance with that of the medical community when making insurance coverage decisions. In a mental health case, the hospital's utilization review department determined that the hospitalizations for the illness were medically necessary; the insurance company denied most of the claims, saying they were not medically necessary. The court held that Blue Cross used a standard of medical necessity that was different from the standard of the community, and that Blue Cross also denied benefits on the basis of a cursory review of incomplete records (Sturgeon, 1997). "Thus, good faith mandates that the reviewer apply a standard of medical necessity consistent with community medical standards" (Sturgeon, 1997, p. 68).

In response to *Hughes* and other similar cases, effective January 1, 2001, the California State Legislature passed new laws, including California Civil Code, § 3428, to protect HMO members. The law established liability for insurance carriers and by extension their employees (including case managers) for any and all harm legally caused by its failure to exercise ordinary care when both of the following apply:

1. The failure to exercise ordinary care resulted in the denial, delay, or modification of the healthcare service recommended for, or furnished to, a subscriber or enrollee; and
2. The subscriber or enrollee suffered substantial harm.

See Display 8-5, California Civil Code, § 3428. The significance of this law, besides the recognition of liability on the part of the insurance provider, is that it lowers the standard from one of professional liability and its prerequisites (discussed earlier in this chapter) to the

CALIFORNIA CIVIL CODE, SECTION 3428 [LIABILITY OF HEALTH CARE SERVICE PLANS]

a. For services rendered on or after January 1, 2001, a health care service plan or managed care entity, as described in subdivision (f) of Section 1345 of the Health and Safety Code, shall have a **duty of ordinary care** to arrange for the provision of medically necessary health care service to its subscribers and enrollees, where the health care service is a benefit provided under the plan, and shall be **liable for any and all harm legally caused by its failure to exercise that ordinary care** when both of the following apply:
   • The failure to exercise ordinary care resulted in the denial, delay, or modification of the health care service recommended for, or furnished to, a subscriber or enrollee.
   • The subscriber or enrollee suffered substantial harm.

b. For purposes of this section:
   • substantial harm means loss of life, loss or significant impairment of limb or bodily function, significant disfigurement, severe and chronic physical pain, or significant financial loss;
   • health care services need not be recommended or furnished by an in-plan provider, but may be recommended or furnished by any health care provider practicing within the scope of his or her practice; and
   • health care services shall be recommended or furnished at any time prior to the inception of the action, and the recommendation need not be made prior to the occurrence of substantial harm.

c. Health care service plans and **managed care entities are not health care providers** under any provision of law, including, but not limited to, Section 6146 of the Business and Professions Code, Sections 3333.1 or 3333.2 of this code, or Sections 340.5, 364, 425.13, 667.7, or 1295 of the Code of Civil Procedure.

d. A health care service plan or managed care entity **shall not seek indemnity**, whether contractual or equitable, from a provider for liability imposed under subdivision (a). Any provision to the contrary in a contract with providers is void and unenforceable.

e. This section shall not create any liability on the part of an employer or an employer group purchasing organization that purchases coverage or assumes risk on behalf

of its employees or on behalf of self-funded employee benefit plans.

f. **Any waiver** by a subscriber or enrollee of the provisions of this section is contrary to public policy and shall be **unenforceable and void**.

g. This section does not create any new or additional liability on the part of a health care service plan or managed care entity for harm caused that is attributable to the medical negligence of a treating physician or other treating health care provider.

h. This section does not abrogate or limit any other theory of liability otherwise available at law.

i. This section shall not apply in instances where subscribers or enrollees receive treatment by prayer, consistent with the provisions of subdivision (a) of Section 1270 of the Health and Safety Code, in lieu of medical treatment.

j. Damages recoverable for a violation of this section include, but are not limited to, those set forth in Section 3333.

k. [Exhaustion of IMR]
   • A person may not maintain a cause of action pursuant to this section against any entity required to comply with any independent medical review system or independent review system required by law unless the person or his or her representative has exhausted the procedures provided by the applicable independent review system.
   • Compliance with paragraph (1) is not required in a case where either of the following applies:
      ○ Substantial harm, as defined in subdivision (b), has occurred prior to the completion of the applicable review.
      ○ Substantial harm, as defined, in subdivision (b), will imminently occur prior to the completion of the applicable review.
   • This subdivision shall become operative only if Senate Bill 189 and Assembly Bill 55 of the 1999–2000 Regular Session are also enacted and enforceable.

l. If any provision of this section or the application thereof to any person or circumstance is held to be unconstitutional or otherwise invalid or unenforceable, the remainder of the section and the application of those provisions to other persons or circumstances shall not be affected thereby.

lesser standard of "ordinary care." Ordinary or simple negligence is far easier to prove and therefore provides greater protection to the public.

Proving a community standard for professional liability was not very difficult in the aforementioned multiple sclerosis case, it was just time-consuming. The neurologist who was a local expert in treating multiple sclerosis had written a letter, as did an Arizona pharmacist. There were also two articles from case management magazines stating that this particular protocol was used. Following the Hughes case, standards are being tested in

many facets of healthcare, including the use of alternate treatments. Thus, case managers may require the perspective of "consistent community standards" in some of their cases. Conversely, case managers who perform interstate utilization management for MCOs should be aware of community standards in other regions. However, as more disease-specific guidelines and protocols become accepted, community-based standards may become a thing of the past.

Two themes repeat throughout any discussion of interactions between case managers and their clients:

documentation and communication. The fact that our society has become more litigious is no secret. However, one should remember that good, culturally sensitive, and effective communication, which includes thoughtful efforts that demonstrate caring when someone is ill or injured, goes a long way to avoiding litigation. Clear, factual, objective, nonjudgmental, and complete documentation and communication make litigation less likely or, more importantly, should a lawsuit occur, make case managers the less likely target. Remember the following:

▶ When making observations either visually or through telephonic communications, the words that you choose can make all the difference.
▶ Describe objectively, rather than characterizing observations; for example:

Do say/write "The client expressed his upset with delays, when he said, 'I've called three times and I simply can't get an MRI appointment.'"
Don't say/write "The client was raving and carrying on about the MRI appointment."
Do say/write "The condition of Ms. X's home made mobility difficult. We discussed a plan to eliminate unnecessary obstacles."
Don't say/write "Ms. X is a slob, her house is a mess; she's going to fall."

A study of lawsuits reveals that the underlying cause of litigation is often lack of information, lack of patient understanding, discourtesy, and other communication failures. Patients with chronic illnesses, for which the medical profession can only temporarily abate the symptoms and distress, are especially prone to frustration. In the 1980s, a study performed nationally with U.S. Postal Service employees revealed that a simple follow-up after an employee went home ill or injured reduced workers' compensation litigation and days lost from work by a great percentage. People need to know that someone cares; that's where communication comes in.

The case manager can be acutely successful by simply calling an injured or ill employee on the day of injury or a few days into the illness to inquire if needed services are set in motion. Have you been able to get an appointment with the physician? Have you been able to get your prescriptions filled? How can we (employer) help you? Sometimes, just asking the question is enough, other times facilitating and coordinating medical services is exactly what case managers do.

In my own experience, I supervised a team of case managers for the sheriff's department in a suburban area. We would receive an accident report via facsimile within 24 hours following a work injury. A courtesy call was made within 24 hours of receiving the report and most times little or nothing but a few well-invested moments of time were needed and the officer returned to work appropriately. By reviewing accident reports from the same facility over and

over again, a pattern of time, location, and type of injury appeared. It turned out that there was a slow-dripping water leak in the ceiling, above a concrete stairwell. Officers on rounds on the night shift were falling and sustaining a variety of sprains, strains, and fractures. I made a site visit, met with the administration, which called building maintenance. The problem was identified and fixed, and the injuries stopped. When you take into consideration that these employees received unlimited full-pay sick time because of the nature of their job, even if the injury was a simple slip and fall, the cost savings were enormous and turnover was greatly reduced. Case management, when effectively implemented, can save time, improve safety, reduce litigation, and save thousands of dollars.

▶ DOCUMENTATION

In any case related to medical treatment, whether within a facility or in the community, the first place where an investigation begins is with the record. The record can be an office or hospital chart or merely case management notes or reports. It is not uncommon for medical records to be incorrect and incomplete. For example, one individual went to the emergency department with severe nausea, vomiting, watery diarrhea, and abdominal pain. During the emergency department admission, he was administered a medication that caused his blood pressure to drop; IV fluids were infused, and he was placed in a Trendelenburg position. The emergency department medical record stated that he came in with complaints of chest pain; no mention was made of the reaction to the medication or the subsequent treatment. Many nurses and case managers have had similar experiences. This particular case did not become a legal issue, but if the same set of facts had occurred today, it very well could have become one. It is critically important that case managers incorporate assessment and document the results of that assessment. Whether you are face to face with people or on the telephone, you are expected to meet the obligations of your professional practice/license.

You might receive a referral of a person with an orthopedic problem, perhaps a fracture. During your initial telephonic assessment of the individual, he mentions that his toes are cold and the small toe used to hurt, but it stopped and he can't feel it anymore. These acute symptoms of impaired circulation could easily be overlooked and go undocumented. Three days later when that small toe is amputated due to a gangrenous state, the lack of documentation could very well be linked causally to the loss of the toe. Would the same standard of liability exist if the case manager was a social worker by education, license, and experience? Probably not! A social worker doesn't receive the same training as it relates to disease processes, nursing assessment, and nursing diagnosis. A nurse must be able to identify deviations in body systems as a cause for emergent medical intervention. Each person does the best he or she can with his or her unique education and training.

It is also very confusing to case managers when they read contradictory statements; one or the other must be wrong. What about missing documentation of drug reactions that is needed for a thorough assessment? Case managers must procure the correct facts (as must all medical professionals) and must document them accurately.

For a long time, The Joint Commission, formerly known as The Joint Commission on Accreditation of Healthcare Organizations, *Accreditation Manual for Hospitals* (1985) gave an excellent overview of the main points to document. Although it was originally written for staff nurses, much of the following quote is important for the case manager:

> Documentation of nursing care shall be pertinent and concise and shall reflect the patient's status. Nursing documentation should address the patient's needs, problems, capabilities and limitations. Nursing intervention and patient response must be noted. When a patient is transferred within or discharged from the hospital, a nurse shall note the patient's status in the medical record. As appropriate, patients who are discharged from the hospital requiring nursing care should receive instructions and individualized counseling prior to discharge, and evidence of the instructions and the patient's or family's understanding of these instructions should be noted in the medical record. Such instructions and counseling must be consistent with the responsible medical practitioner's instructions. (The Joint Commission, 1985, pp. 98–99)

The question that we need to examine in the modern case management setting is, "Has technology changed anything?" The case manager's initial answer is probably "Yes. It's great; we just click on the buttons in the case management program (software application) and no more awful narrative reports." Any abbreviated method of charting is a double-edged sword, however. The time-saving aspects are wonderful and those programs that can provide outcomes, statistical information, and cost-savings can further assist the case manager in many expected functions, but there is a down side.

The law is slow to catch up with technology in medicine as well as other industries. Legal requirements of complete and accurate charting have not changed. If you review the Nurse Practice Act in the state in which you practice, you will find a documentation obligation. In October 2007, the state of Illinois updated its Nurse Practice Law. Title 68, § 1300 states, in the relevant part, that a nurse must take a complete history and do a complete physical assessment, including all body systems, to develop a nursing care plan.

Case management shares the requirement with Illinois' Nurse Practice Act; however, for those case managers who are not also direct caregivers, it translates simply into an obligation for a case manager to perform a complete assessment, including all body systems, in the development of

CASE MANAGEMENT DOCUMENTATION

The key to successful case management documentation is to present a clear and objective picture and to demonstrate that the chronological progression of events was within the standards of care of the documenter's professional scope of practice, based on the underlying professional license and case management standards of practice.

the case management plan. That requisite assessment can be performed at arm's length or telephonically over great distances. The only way to demonstrate compliance with this very common and basic requirement is to document the assessment and resulting interventions and recommendations contained in a Case Management Care Plan. Case management practice tools have changed, but the essential elements of practice have not. Documentation remains a case management obligation and an ally in demonstrating compliance with laws, rules, and regulations, as well as quality case management practice standards.

Documentation in medical records is discoverable, meaning it can be requested for use in court. More documentation recommendations are discussed under specific issues (Display 8-6).

▶ PRIVACY RULES

The *Standards for Privacy of Individually Identifiable Health Information* (Privacy Rule) establishes, for the first time, a set of national standards for the protection of certain health information. The U.S. Department of Health and Human Services (HHS) issued the Privacy Rule to implement the requirement of the HIPAA (Pub. L. 104-191, 1996). The entire rule is available online, along with numerous valuable resources (http://www.hhs.gov/ocr/hipaa).

The Privacy Rule was published on December 28, 2000 (67 C.F.R., § 82462), with the goal of providing consumers with greater rights for protection of individually identifiable health information. Modifications to the Privacy Rule were done on August 14, 2002 (65 C.F.R., § 53182). In the spring of 2003 there were further modifications to the Final Privacy Rule. Now the HIPAA is here and it is here to stay. The key is to have an organized system of demonstrating HIPAA compliance. The HIPAA is a *minimum* mandatory national standard. If you, your state, or your individual practice is stricter than the declared HIPAA requirements, there is no need for you to make changes.

Patient's medical records can legally be used for billing, auditing, utilization review, quality assurance studies, and research. When they are used for these purposes or when a patient makes his or her medical condition the basis for a lawsuit, HIPAA privacy protections are waived by the patient in a limited fashion to allow permitted uses of the information contained in the record. The key to

HIPAA compliance is informing the patient of his or her rights, documenting that you have informed the patient, and taking necessary steps to assure that the patient's expressed wishes are carried out.

In 2013, the HIPAA was modified in response to technological advances and to the advent of EMRs. The Health Information Technology for Economic and Clinical Health (HITECH) Act brought the greatest change in the matter of additional responsibilities to case managers, since 1996. The duty to notify consumers whose protected information was improperly released or potentially viewed by those not involved in their care was strictly regulated and enhanced even further in 2013 with the Omnibus Final Rule, which further enhances Breach Notification obligations. The best source for information on mandates and requirements under these HIPAA regulations remains the HHS.GOV web pages dedicated to these regulations. Updates, alerts, and resources can be found at: https://www.hhs.gov/hipaa/for-professionals/privacy/laws-regulations/combined-regulation-text/omnibus-hipaa-rulemaking/index.html

▶ THE MEDICAL RECORD

The medical record is created through documentation. Whether it is a traditional hospital chart (or EMR), a field case management record, or a telephonic log, the basic goals are the same. The quality and the completeness of the documentation determine the effectiveness of the record.

Today more than ever, hospital case management is becoming the norm rather than the exception. The contents of the medical record must be complete and accurate and contain the necessary documents that the hospital or other healthcare facility requires. In many states, state law (often found in the state's administrative code) specifically mandates the type of medical record used and its contents. Services provided and then submitted for either private insurance payment or a government program such as Medicare or Medicaid must be "clean" if payment is to be forthcoming. It is the role of the case manager to ensure that his or her contribution to the record does not interfere with these requirements. A complete medical record enhances continuity and coordination of patient care by providing interdisciplinary guidance to the entire treatment team. The medical record is more than a medical history and plan of care; it is a legal record and, for the reasons described, the medical record will supply evidence that a standard of care was (or was not) met.

In the case of third-party reimbursement, insurance companies and other payment sources scrutinize patients' charts for several reasons:

▶ *To determine whether services billed for were actually provided.* All orders, tests, and their results, medication administration, supplies, and other procedures will be perused. Insurance companies may not reimburse if the evidence for the billed items is not in the chart.

▶ *To determine whether this hospitalization or procedure was medically necessary.* Nursing and physician documentation should support admitting diagnosis completely and factually, with symptoms, vital signs, and treatments listed. Specific communications with the patient, family, or others, documented accurately, can explain long after discharge the events that might otherwise be vague or confusing with simple entries. Even with computerized charting, narrative notes are still the most valuable tools for professionals to protect themselves and explain events they might otherwise have forgotten.

▶ *Hospitals must establish and defend length of stay.* Any changes in the patient's condition may lend support to an increased length of stay; therefore, it is important for nurses to help identify and document complications and additional problems. Case managers should collaborate with staff nurses and other professionals in emphasizing the importance of accurate charting in this area. The case manager's role may include requesting and justifying additional hospital days; the charting is necessary to aid the case manager when advocating for needed extra days. The present trend is that insurance companies and governmental benefit plans refuse to pay for those aspects of hospitalizations that they determine are due to complications caused by something that the institution could have prevented (hospital-acquired conditions or Never Events). Therefore, complete and accurate documentation is not only a professional duty, but also a legal obligation. The Joint Commission also places great emphasis on evaluating the completeness of patient records when determining whether the agency will attain accreditation status.

Similarly, the URAC scrutinizes medical records, policies, and procedures to determine whether core case management standards are being properly utilized. URAC standards cover several critical operational categories for any quality case management program including:

▶ Staff structure and organization
▶ Staff management and development
▶ Information management
▶ Quality improvement
▶ Oversight of delegated functions
▶ Organizational ethics
▶ Complaints

(For more information, see the URAC website, https://www.urac.org/accreditation-and-measurement/accreditation-programs/).

Who owns the medical record? The actual physical document belongs to the healthcare institution/entity that created it; the entity is the custodian of the hard copy. The hospital owns the patient's hospital medical record; a physician owns his or her office records. The information, however, belongs to the patient. The patient is entitled not only to this information but also to other items, such as actual radiographs, CT scans, pathology slides, gallstones, and others. In most cases, failure to provide a patient with requested records will create a ground for a civil suit. With the advent of the HIPAA, much of this confusion is eliminated; however, the burden remains on patients to request their records, follow through to overcome improper denials of access, and to report HIPAA violations. Entities may require a written request for medical records and reasonable copy costs. For more information about filing a HIPAA complaint, you may visit https://www.hhs.gov/hipaa/filing-a-complaint/patient-safety-confidentiality/index.html. The HIPAA Complaint Form with instructions is available online at https://www.hhs.gov/sites/default/files/ocr/privacy/psa/complaint/pscomplaintform.pdf.

The patient can also authorize the release of medical records to others. Because the entity is responsible for the confidentiality and security of these records, a signed HIPAA Compliant Authorization for the Release of Records Form is required. Under the HIPAA, even family members are not entitled to the records unless the patient has died. Here are some special situations:

- ▶ The parent or legal guardian of a minor may or may not have access to records. A noncustodial parent, following a divorce, may or may not have rights to the medical record. Such access is specifically addressed in Judgments of Divorce and associated agreements. These have the effect of a court order. Consult your entity's attorney or risk management department before initiating the process of releasing records or patient information on the basis of a claim of right under such a document.
- ▶ Since the advent of the HIPAA, a subpoena alone is not sufficient to obtain medical records. The subpoena must be accompanied by an Authorization for Release of Medical Records signed by the patient or another authorized person. If served with a subpoena, immediately contact the entity's attorney or risk management department, as required by policy. A court order may be required to release information.
- ▶ Some records are protected by law. Drug and alcohol records from a drug/alcohol detoxification program and mental health records may need a court order before information is released. It is suggested that case managers be familiar with their own state laws in these instances. Patients have enhanced rights to limit release of these records separately from the medical record.

- ▶ In many states, HIV/AIDS medical records are protected far beyond the HIPAA's minimum standards.

To avoid a trip to the courthouse, in most states custodians of medical records are permitted to certify medical records as being complete, true, and accurate. This is accomplished with an affidavit or certification being attached to the records and signed by the custodian. The HIPAA Compliance Officer in the entity must oversee this function, along with other compliance issues. They must be very aware that computerized charting, although wonderfully efficient, exposes the risk for potential privacy abuses. IT experts should be consulted regarding encryption requirements and risks.

▶ DISCHARGE/TRANSITIONAL PLANNING AND PREMATURE DISCHARGE

Discharge planning, continuity of care, and transitions across the care continuum are among the most important responsibilities of the case manager. A case manager can complement, and be an extremely valuable asset to, a healthcare team; the accuracy of the financial and psychosocial assessment can make or break the discharge plan. The best discharge planning starts on admission. That is true whether we are talking about an acute hospital stay or a referral for an injured employee. The case management assessment should take into consideration all stakeholders, including but not limited to, the client, family, employer, payor(s), and ancillary services that may be needed for short- and long-term outcomes. The important thing to remember is that the assessment is a living document that can be changed and updated as new information is learned or the client's condition changes. The need for client and/or family teaching or support should be considered throughout.

There is a crisis in America today as time-honored systems for safe and efficient continuity of care are being challenged in the name of healthcare cost containment. More than ever, case managers are needed to promote an atmosphere of safe and efficient planning. Cost-efficiency and safe, thoughtful transitions across the care continuum need not be mutually exclusive.

Because of this, there is an increased likelihood of allegations such as abandonment, and unsafe or premature discharge. Premature discharge is often associated with adverse payment decisions by third-party payors and delayed decisions by payors. "Both nurse managers/supervisors and nurses in direct patient care positions are accountable for providing safe nursing care to their patients" (N.J. Board of Nursing Patient Abandonment—Position Statement, 2007). Documentation of your discharge/transitional plan is important and should reflect patient/family awareness and agreement with the plan. Execution of the actual discharge should not happen independent of the physician (Display 8-7).

display 8-7

AN IMPORTANT DOCUMENTATION CONSIDERATION

The physician is the discharging agent. In your case management documentation, *never* make it look like the case manager discharged the patient. A patient's discharge or transfer to another level of care requires an order from a provider who is considered a Licensed Independent Practitioner with prescriptive privileges. Unless you are licensed and credentialed to prescribe, you should not imply in your documentation that you made the decision to discharge a patient.

▶ Adequacy of Discharge/Transitional Planning

The adequacy of discharge planning describes the discharge plan, with the case manager as the link between the patient and community resources. A complete discharge or transition summary report is necessary for the prevention or avoidance of legal and risk management issues. Many outcomes management projects and accreditation mandates include discharge and transitional planning issues (e.g., medications on discharge/transfer, education before discharge, hand-off communication). The questions to be addressed when engaged in discharge and/or transitional planning activities are as follows: Is the plan appropriate and adequate for this individual? Does the plan consider physical, emotional, social, mental health, financial, and safety needs? Is follow-up care addressed? Are health educational needs addressed? Are providers at the next level of care aware of the individual's transition? Are they in agreement and do they have the information they need for safe continuity of care? (Refer to Chapter 6 for more information on transitional planning.)

The following are guidelines to help the case manager with discharge and transitional planning:

1. Before you make any referrals, obtain an informed consent from patient, family/significant other/caregiver, and physician, consistent with HIPAA and state regulations.
2. Document all communications with patient and family/caregiver, including agreement or rejection of recommended services and the postdischarge (or transition) needs. Record the patient's and/or family's/caregiver's direct quotes, if possible.
3. Document the patient's limitations and refusals in an objective manner. Consider the following example:

    Mr. Grant, an 82-year-old unmarried male, refuses an SNF. Your assessment demonstrates that he needs continued care that can be provided in an SNF. The patient states that he lives alone with intermittent visits from one neighbor. You have an obligation to explore available options, even

if they are not your first choice. Physical therapy charts, "Patient can walk 10 feet with front-wheeled walker and maximum assist of two." Now your discharge work begins. This may show that the patient is unsafe for discharge alone at home, but have you asked enough questions to assess the home environment? Maybe Mr. Grant lives in a senior community that is barrier free, with assistive devices already installed in the bathroom, kitchen, and hallways. The options in a home environment will be far different if Mr. Grant lives in an old building with a two-flight walkup. Many times patients later agree to a short SNF stay for the purpose of improving their strength and endurance while home modification, if needed, can be accomplished. Your goal should be a complete, unbiased assessment with reasonable recommendations in a cost-effective manner. Before discharge, an appropriate discharge agreement must be reached and documented, with steps shown to facilitate the plan. Your documentation might be as simple as, "Visiting nurse will do complete home assessment on the morning of discharge and order necessary assistive devices, along with home care, including physical therapy." Documentation can protect you from a lawsuit later on should Mr. Grant fall at home in a manner that could not have been foreseen.

4. If the discharge or transitional plan changes, as is often the case, document the change, including who requested the change, the reasons for the change, and your activities now to make possible necessary changes. Mr. Grant may agree to home healthcare with aides and private duty nursing. Before the actual discharge, he may decide that an SNF is the best alternative temporarily. Sometimes deterioration of the patient's condition or an unexpected improvement deems the plan change appropriate. Document the medical status of the patient to substantiate the necessary change, including the physician's contribution to the discharge plan, such as orders for homecare, including physical therapy, home infusion, etc., or prescriptions for medications.
5. Document all interventions and the patient's responses to them as well as interactions with the treatment team.
6. On the day when a patient is transferred to another facility (a lesser level of care compared to acute, for example) or discharged home, document communication with the family and/or caregiver; this is mandatory. This is especially important when the patient is going home with many discharge needs such as durable medical equipment (DME) and home health services. You want to document who the primary caregiver will be and that you've communicated with that person.

7. Document your contacts with other agencies and institutions, as well as time, dates, with whom you spoke, and what was said and agreed on. Fax or e-mail a confirmation to such agencies to demonstrate your compliance with the plan and that you've properly notified and perhaps transferred responsibility for the patient to another professional. Remember to use encrypted messaging service and one that meets the privacy and confidentiality requirements including related regulations.

8. Documenting patient/family/caregiver education and teaching is extremely important. If anything goes wrong after discharge, documentation can be evidence of proper and adequate teaching. If documentation is inadequate and the patient is readmitted, health insurance companies (payors such as Medicare) may attempt to deny reimbursement on the basis of a supposition that the member was inadequately taught or prepared for discharge/transfer.

9. Chart: If follow-up teaching is necessary, include plans for such teaching and, when completed, add notations. If someone other than you did the teaching, identify the person in your notes.
    ▶ How much time was spent teaching
    ▶ What was taught and methods used (verbal, pictures, resource materials, etc.)
    ▶ To whom the information was given (e.g., caregiver, patient)
    ▶ How well the "student" comprehended the information
    ▶ The outcomes of the teaching

10. **Whenever** possible, provide written as well as verbal instructions and provide demonstrations. Document the teaching tools used and the outcomes of the teaching, applying the teach-back method of evaluation.

11. It is critical to chart confirmation of that not only the patient, but also the patient's caregivers understanding of what is being told—matters such as special diets, treatments, potential complications, follow-up visits with primary or specialty care providers, wound care, medications and side effects, and activity level; most importantly, whom to call in the event of an emergency.

12. It is not enough to explain and document potential side effects and complications of medicines and treatments. Today, there are programs available in hospitals and online providing standardized patient teaching and discharge information. Although these tools are useful, they merely provide a baseline of information. It is important to modify these "cookie cutter" documents, as needed, to properly and completely inform the individual of his or her specific needs.

13. The patient or the caregiver must also know what to do if complications arise (red flags that warrant immediate attention); that is, to seek medical attention. Some people, hearing from a physician about a possible side effect, may wrongly interpret that side effect as being normal and expected and may continue with whatever caused the problem. Document that the patient and the caregiver were told what to do if anything unusual occurs.

14. Many patients go home with DME, such as oxygen, suction machines, bipap ventilators, feeding pumps, and IV fluid and medication delivery systems, including pumps. Without sufficient instruction, this equipment can become more of a hazard than a help. Document what equipment is being used, the teaching that was done (and any follow-up required), and who was taught, along with their comprehension. Documentation of coordination—that the equipment will be available when the patient arrives home—is also important.

15. Educational needs should be addressed as soon as possible; last-minute teaching is typically quick and often inadequate. Begin such activities early on in an acute hospital stay.

16. Document the patient's clinical condition at discharge or transfer, including vital signs and observations made during the assessment. If psychosocial stresses or mental health conditions are present, document the patient's status at discharge/transfer.

17. Medications and discharge planning are often chosen as quality indicators (core measures) to measure. Documentation of these two aspects of care is essential to provide evidence that these expectations were met.

18. Medical stability of patients within 24 hours of discharge from a hospital: Documentation of medical stability may include vital signs (blood pressure, pulse and respiratory rates, and temperature); laboratory and radiology tests, including results, especially if abnormal findings were noted; IV fluid therapy or medication intake (especially last dosage administered); and condition of wounds, incisions, or drainage tubes/catheters. Documentation should also include any abnormalities, notification of physicians of abnormalities, interventions instituted, and patient's response. In addition, documentation should reflect the physician's agreement with the discharge despite the presence of an abnormality.

▶ INFORMED CONSENT

The first thing that any healthcare practitioner needs to understand is that informed consent is a legal requirement that rests with the physician. It is not simply "nice" if the physician gets it signed; it is the physician's legal and ethical responsibility to provide his or her patient with sufficient information to permit the patient to make a knowing and intelligent informed consent or refusal. Further, *Case Management Standards of Practice* say that the client must consent to case management services (CMSA, 2016, p. 19). Ideally, such consent for case management services should be in writing. If for some reason that is impossible, documenting a conversation (ideally with a witness) between the case manager and the client is a viable alternative; include as must detail as possible.

Informed consents are used specifically for treatments and procedures that are invasive or that have potentially dangerous side effects or complications. Depending on the institution's policies and procedures, state laws, and the emergent need of the procedure, a signed informed consent form is required. Implied consent may be appropriate in an emergency situation in which lack of action may cause greater harm than the potential risks of the treatment. The classic example of implied consent to medical intervention is the unconscious patient. In many states there is a legal presumption that an unconscious patient gives tacit or unspoken consent for lifesaving treatment, simply based on the presentation of symptoms and an inability to communicate.

Before a patient is informed of anything, that patient must be capable of comprehending what is being said. It is important to document the patient's ability or inability to understand, particularly in those cases when the information is being given in a language that is not the patient's or family's native language. Capacity versus incapacity is based on a patient's ability to understand the information, to make choices, and to communicate verbally or nonverbally. A patient under chemical sedation may be only temporarily incapacitated, but nevertheless unable to give consent for a period of time. Advance Directives for Healthcare can avoid this problem even in the case of sedation. Only a court of law and a judge's order can find a person legally incompetent. Legally incompetent persons, no matter their age or level of consciousness, cannot sign on their own behalf and a legal guardian is evidenced by a court order naming the guardian. The case manager should never take someone's word for the fact that they are a legal guardian. It is essential to see legal documents that a client, their family, and/or caregiver are relying upon.

There are two basic steps to the informed consent process: the disclosure of information and the signature.

▶ The Disclosure of Information

The following, at the minimum, needs to be discussed with the patient (or surrogate) (Feutz-Harter, 1991):

- The patient's condition or problem
- The nature and purpose of the proposed test, therapy, or procedure
- Any hazards, risks, or potential complications of the proposed test, therapy, or procedure
- Any feasible alternatives to the proposed test, therapy, or procedure
- The benefits and expected outcome of the proposed test, therapy, or procedure
- The risks and prognosis if the proposed test therapy or procedure is not done

Most litigation surrounding disclosure issues address the physician's or healthcare professional's or the failure to reveal "material" risks, dangers, or alternatives. When a complication arises and the patient was unaware of its possibility, liability may attach. Yet there is a delicate balance between disclosing too little and too much. Patients can become so overwhelmed with frightening, potential dangers and risks that they are no longer capable of sifting out the important information and making appropriate choices. The case manager can be helpful to the patent/client and the physician by being able to restate complex issues in simplified terms. Except in those states that acknowledge that Physician's Assistants or Advanced Practice Registered Nurses have a specifically identified statutory duty or ability to obtain informed consent, the responsibility never shifts from the physician to provide the requisite information and obtain the signature.

Complete documentation is essential to demonstrate compliance with the state's requirements for informed consent. Often a patient will claim that he or she was not fully informed, even in those cases where there was complete, truthful, and accurate information provided in a manner that the individual could or should have been able to comprehend. The case manager's notes describing the event can be affirmative proof that all legal requirements were satisfied.

Notations describing obtaining informed consent may include:

- Who informed the patient
- The information discussed—including the above list of topics
- To whom the explanation was given and who else was present
- How long the discussion took
- Teaching materials used, such as videos, flip charts, booklets, or drawings
- Offering the patient the opportunity to ask questions and have them answered
- Indication of comprehension, and whether more thought, time, and discussion are needed before a fully informed decision can be made
- Assessment of the patient's understanding of the topics discussed.

Incomplete or inaccurate information could deem the dispenser of the information liable. Take time to chart comprehensively, objectively, and accurately.

▶ Signing of the Informed Consent

Many times, the case manager is told to present the informed consent form to the patient sometime after the disclosure of information. Often the case manager did not even witness the disclosure. Therefore, the case manager must be skilled in assessing the adequacy of the information and patient comprehension. As a patient advocate, the case manager has a legal and ethical responsibility to protect patients from misinformation, omissions, and errors. If lack of understanding is assessed about the treatment, hazards, alternatives, risks, expected outcomes, or prognosis if therapy is not performed, the case manager can fill in omissions and clarify misunderstandings if he or she feels qualified to do so. Your role as a case manager is really that of a witness to the signature and nothing more. One legal source has the following to say about nurses answering questions regarding procedures and informed consents:

> If the patient doesn't understand the information or wants more information, you can answer any questions that are within the scope of your knowledge. You aren't obligated, however, to answer any of the patient's questions. As a witness, you are not legally responsible for disclosing all relevant information to the patient. The doctor retains this responsibility, and he/she cannot delegate it to you. If you see that a patient is confused, and you can't provide the information he needs, document your observation in the patient's chart and make sure the patient gets the information from his doctor or another appropriate source. (Andrews, Goldberg, & Kaplan, 1996, pp. 73–74)

Forcing a signature is never a good idea.

Notification of the physician regarding problem areas is advised, along with complete documentation of the lack of understanding and of the time and date that you have notified the physician. If you believe that the patient requires more explanation from the physician, communicate that to the physician and document your concerns in the medical record. In today's world of electronic charting, there are always some additional screens for notes or comments, even in those cases where narrative charting is limited.

Where informed consent for minors is concerned, parents and legal guardians must sign consent forms. One rare exception is an emancipated minor, who would be able to show documentation of that fact in the form of a court order. There is great variation from state to state, but as in all things, documentation is your protection. Ask questions, document your questions, and document the answers you relied upon to arrive at a point where you are comfortable obtaining a signature. Questions are as simple as "Which doctor came to discuss this with you and when did this happen? What is your understanding of the procedure that is going to take place?", and so on (Display 8-8).

Once fully informed of the risks and benefits of a procedure, a competent adult may elect to refuse a treatment

---

display 8-8

COURT ORDERS AND LEGAL DOCUMENTS

As a general rule, you must see and should keep a copy of a court order or other documents in the patient's medical record. Never accept a person's word that such documents exist. Refer to these documents as necessary; do not rely on your memory of what the documents are about.

---

or other intervention. Some facilities have a Refusal of Treatment Release Form. It is the patient's right to refuse, and that right must be honored. A patient's refusal of care can be overridden only when:

1. The patient is not mentally or legally competent.
2. There are compelling reasons to overrule the patient's wishes. These may include such issues as: the refusal may endanger the life of another (i.e., if a pregnant woman's refusal threatens the life of her unborn child), it threatens a child's life (for parental refusal), the patient is refusing treatment but also stating that he or she wants to live (i.e., incongruence), and when the public interest outweighs the patient's right, such a patient with tuberculosis or HIV/AIDS who refuses treatment and ignores safety instructions, thereby exposing the public to harm.
3. In large medical or academic centers and in state or county government, there are Offices of Patient Advocacy and Ombudsmen and Protective Services for Adults, Seniors, and Children, all of which can be contacted for guidance and assistance. For example:
   ▶ In New York State [http://pubadvocate.nyc.gov], the public advocacy office of New York City, which serves as a direct link between New Yorkers and their local government, acts as a watchdog over city agencies, and investigates complaints about city services.
   ▶ In New Jersey, The Office of the Ombudsman for the Institutionalized Elderly Health [http://www.state.nj.us/ooie] is a part of a national resident-focused advocacy program that seeks to protect the health, safety, welfare, and civil and human rights of older individuals in institutions.
   ▶ In the United States, the United States Ombudsman Association [http://www.usombudsman.org]) was founded in 1977 to foster the establishment and professional development of public sector ombudsman offices throughout the country and the world.

▶ CONFIDENTIALITY

Both federal and state law control protect confidentiality. The HIPAA is the national minimum mandatory standard;

however, some states have exceeded the federal standard and provided citizens with even greater protection. Statutory mandate gives legal clout to professional relationships. Privilege is the statutory protection of the physician-patient (and in some states nurse-patient) relationship. New York was one of the first states to recognize the nurse-patient relationship as something separate and a distinct and confidential one. Unless state law specifically recognizes the relationship, privilege does not apply.

It is incumbent upon the prudent practitioner to see the document authorizing the sharing of information, such as an "Information Release Form." In case management, you may feel awkward asking for documents, but remember you are not only acting as an advocate for your client by protecting his or her rights under the HIPAA, but also ensuring that his or her wishes are given paramount consideration as you develop the case management plan of care (CMSA, 2016).

Maintaining patient confidentiality is not an easy task. Consider some of the members of the multidisciplinary medical team who may access the patient's medical records: attending physicians, residents, interns, medical students, nurses, nursing students, physical therapists, occupational therapists, speech therapists, social workers, case managers, utilization review personnel, insurance company case managers, hospital utilization reviewers, auditors, coders, billers, quality improvement organization review teams, The Joint Commission accreditation teams, hospital quality assurance, researchers, and many others. As a case manager, you will be collaborating with many people on each case. Care must be taken in each conversation to reveal only what is necessary. Give only that part of the information that the other party requires. Social service needs are different from an insurance company's utilization review requirements. It is important to remember that although persons or entities (such as insurance companies) may be entitled to information contained in the medical record for a specific purpose, such as paying a claim, they are not necessarily entitled to the entire medical record. If a patient is being treated today for a simple fracture of a forearm, the patient's 20-year gynecologic history is irrelevant and may not be released. The HIPAA mandates that only necessary information be released.

Two basic questions to ask yourself are:

1. What patient information needs to be given?
2. What patient information cannot, need not, or should not be given?

If a patient/client makes a written request to access, review, or copy his or her own medical record, do you know how to respond? Patients have the right to access their medical records (45 C.F.R., §164.528). In other words, a person who is the subject matter of the medical record has a legal right to see its contents. However, it is incumbent upon the covered entity to record who, when, what, and why any disclosure is made. Telephonic requests

for confidential information should be rejected; however, you may simply ask the caller to fax or scan and e-mail a signed written request on a letterhead (or an approved form provided by the entity), along with necessary releases. It is far safer for the case manager to follow an established procedure to protect a patient's confidentiality rights than to give instant gratification to an unknown caller. If the case manager is not careful, well-intended calls from family members and friends, simply asking how a patient is doing, can be a confidentiality nightmare. Know your facility's policy and adhere to it; for most hospitals, the policy is to give a general statement of condition (such as "stable") by a nonmedical staff member, rather than exposing the professional staff to potential risk.

Those case managers who work with self-insured employer groups have stronger reasons to be concerned. These case managers often are required by the groups to provide reports on the patients receiving case management services. The HIPAA specifically safeguards employees in such circumstances, requiring "firewalls" to protect employee health information. Health records must be kept separate from employment records and persons with the authority to hire, fire, promote, or demote staff generally have no access to this information, to avoid even an appearance that they might let a medical diagnosis affect their authority and the decisions they make. Failure to keep protected health information (PHI) private can lead to accusations of invasion of privacy, defamation of character, and intentional infliction of emotional distress, and of course, a HIPAA violation.

Case managers, particularly those in the occupational health/workers' compensation arena must take certain actions to protect employee information. For example,

▶ Abide by federal (HIPAA) and state privacy laws.
▶ Abide by federal laws, such as the ADA and the Family Medical Leave Act.
▶ Establish and abide by well-defined policies and the use of "firewalls" to protect employee PHI and limit access to unauthorized persons.

There can be difficulties on both ends of the spectrum. A large employer with a centralized Human Resources (HR) Department can be as problematic as a small family-run business where a limited number of people have access to employee information. In either case, strict adherence to written policies and procedures, acknowledging firewall management, are necessary safeguards.

There are some situations where public safety may outweigh confidentiality; but in each of these cases an agency may not be entitled to the patient's entire medical record. In the case of communicable diseases, for example, public interest outweighs patient privacy and states have reporting requirements for such things as tuberculosis, measles, and other diseases that can spread throughout a population. In some states, failure to report certain situations may result in criminal culpability.

The only exception to the authorization requirement, other than those identified in the Privacy Rule itself (45 C.F.R., §164.512), such as public health and communicable disease reporting, is a court order signed by a judge. If the request is merely for access to medical records and review of information, the HIPAA requires that access be provided within 30 days (45 C.F.R., §164.524). One example of a state where compliance regulations differs is California, which requires the same access to be provided within 10 days.

Confidentiality has become an even bigger issue because disease management programs and outcomes management projects are moving plenty of information to computerized databases. Electronic data are easy to access and patient consents are not always obtained for use in these managed care modalities. It is critical that any case manager involved in such projects or studies either obtain patient-signed consents or ensure that the organization is not using patient identifiers. This could save endless legal trouble in the confidentiality arena.

E-mail and other electronic methods of communication are flooding the healthcare market; each method poses unique legal concerns.

▶ Fax Machines

Nearly every case manager has depended on the convenience of fax machines for both sending and receiving patient-specific information, especially for utilization management and review purposes and between the provider of care and the health insurance company/benefit plan. Such an approach for sharing of information can also apply to discharge/transitional planning from the hospital care setting especially when coordinating the transfer of a patient to another lower level of care facility such as an SNF. Nearly every case manager has wondered if, at some point, confidential patient information may end up at the wrong place. Some fax precautions you may apply to avoid risk include:

- Double-check the number you are to send the fax to before you hit the "start" button; program commonly used numbers into the fax machine to lessen chances of inadvertent misdialing.
- Call the other party advising him or her that you are about to send the fax and then confirm that it has been properly received, including a page count.
- Use a cover sheet that includes a confidentiality statement based on your organization's policy.
- Be sure that nothing is faxed that the recipient does not have a right or a need to know.
- Redact (black out) protected information that is beyond the scope of the recipient's need to know.
- Make sure that appropriate patient releases have been obtained before faxing anything.

Other actions for better management of information and for ensuring privacy include the following:

- Locate fax machines in secure areas with limited access to others.
- Assign a staff member to monitor faxes sent/received to each machine. The staff member's responsibilities should include:
  a. Collecting each document as soon as it arrives.
  b. Checking each document to be sure that it has arrived in its entirety and is legible.
  c. Sealing each document in an envelope and routing it to the intended addressee.
  d. If sending information, remain by the fax machine to ensure completion of the documents transmittal and collect the documents when done; never keep such documents by the fax machine. Additionally, if the fax machine stores information in its memory, delete the information saved as soon as you are done and ensure the machine is password protected.
- Institute a system that ensures that incoming documents are routed to the appropriate people.
- Furnish contingency procedures to follow in the event that a document is misrouted. This information can be included as a part of the confidentiality statement on the fax cover sheet.
- Physician orders should be signed. Orders that are not signed should not be followed until verified with the physician.
- State laws differ; make sure that you are not restricted from faxing patient information about HIV/AIDS or mental health issues. Know what your state requires and adhere to it.

▶ E-Mail

The use of e-mail has become the norm rather than the exception. You must assume that it is simply not secure. Know your facility's policy regarding e-mail and what information may or may not be transmitted in this manner. E-mail policies should cover a broad variety of topics, including but not limited to:

- Encryption is required when PHI is transmitted via e-mail, whether it is in the body of the e-mail or is an attachment.
- Portals giving patients and providers direct, password-protected methods to access personal health records, reports, lab findings, history, and direct communication with patients are appearing across the country. This system greatly improves patient access and assures privacy.
- Permitted and prohibited use of e-mail.

▶ E-mails containing libelous, defamatory, offensive, or other objectionable material that can expose the employer to liability.

▶ Forwarding and/or use of confidential and/or PHI.

▶ Copying messages and other materials without permission.

▶ Annual (at a minimum) Review of E-mail Policies and Procedures with written commentary on maintaining the *status quo*, changes to be implemented and the rationale for either or both.

The same rules that would apply to a written letter, message, or other communication also apply to e-mail. One positive aspect of e-mail is that documentation takes care of itself. Storing e-mails either electronically or as printed hard copies provides documentation of the content, time, date, and parties to a communication. Personal use of company computers should be discouraged, especially on a system containing PHI. Informal personal use of e-mail in an environment containing PHI is an increased security risk, as unintentional disclosures of PHI could occur. Although the HIPAA accepts and tolerates incidental disclosures (i.e., hearing your neighbor's name called out on the pharmacy waiting line or physicians' office), there should be great concern if there are no safeguards in place to protect against PHI getting into personal e-mail. The "minimum necessary" rule (45 C.F.R., §§ 164.502[a][1][iii]) applies, no matter what the method of communication is.

▶ Smart Phones and Tablets

It is common for many people to access and use three or more electronic devices before they even start their business day. What used to require a heavy desktop computer installation can now be held in the palm of one's hand (mobile communication devices). If your hospital, case management company, or other employer issues a smart phone and/or tablet to you, it is for work use and information. Case managers should have their own personal devices and the information contained on either of these devices should not be mixed. Unless your employer has a *written* policy expressly permitting you to use your work-issued phone for personal use, this practice should still be avoided. The employer is the owner of all information contained on a computer, laptop, smartphone, or tablet issued by him or her. No matter how intimate the communication or picture is, the employer can demand to review the contents of a device issued by him or her at any time. For a thorough discussion of the legal and ethical challenges of electronics, see the CMSA Core Curriculum for Case Management, Chapters 19 and 20 (Tahan & Treiger, 2017).

▶ Telehealth/Telemedicine

Telehealth and telemedicine encompass a vast array of platforms, portals, video applications, teleconferencing, and so on. Case managers nationwide are using some or all of the systems available to access clients in remote locations (especially in rural areas) or right in their neighborhoods. Patients with high blood pressure, diabetics, and other diseases are being monitored remotely by healthcare providers, permitting real-time access and accountability. Such devices are issued to patients and monitored by professional staff, cutting down on the need for acute and emergency admissions. Studies have shown that the use of telehealth platforms can lead to increased patient engagement and self-management, accountability, and improved documentation (NORC at the University of Chicago, 2012).

▶ Teleconferencing

Teleconferencing permits education, discussion, and collaboration across the street or around the world. Case managers participating in such meetings should be cautious regarding those present in the room or at the distant location(s) if client PHI is being discussed. If you are uncomfortable disclosing certain information, as there may be those "present" who are not entitled to the PHI, you can always use an alternate method of limited communication for which you are authorized to release PHI.

▶ Retail Clinics

Retail clinics/care settings are opening in a variety of settings. One example is the partnership between Kaiser Permanente, Walmart and Target Stores, and CVS Pharmacies. This practice developed in California and is spreading all over the country. It provides increased access to healthcare for patients, young and old. For a complete discussion of this revolutionary concept (see Jacob, 2016).

▶ ADVANCE DIRECTIVES FOR HEALTHCARE

The right of an individual to direct his or her own destiny is a constitutional one. As a patient advocate, there may not be a more important task than the discussion of end-of-life choices and advance directives, that is, getting a patient's wishes for care and treatment in writing and having them fulfilled. Prolonging life should be the patient's choice. The patient should also participate in choices regarding transitioning to the appropriate level of care affording him/her with as much comfort as possible. The document is the vehicle to accomplish the patient's genuine wishes is the goal.

In compliance with the Patient Self-Determination Act of 1990, hospitals, subacute care facilities, home health agencies, and hospices are federally mandated to counsel patients about their right to accept or refuse treatment and their right to the use of advance directives (Bosek & Fitzpatrick, 1992). Advance directives are legally executed documents, drawn up while the individual is still competent. They can be used only if the individual becomes incapacitated or incompetent. In this situation, patients are directing their own care in advance of the need (before incapacity). Individual autonomy is the end result, because the person is able, without coercion, to make some extremely important decisions for him- or herself.

The two most recognized advance directives are the living will and the medical power of attorney (POA), also called the durable POA for healthcare. A third advance directive is a prehospital medical care directive. This directive focuses on several aspects of a resuscitation event, such as defibrillation, chest compressions, assisted ventilation, intubation, and advanced life support medications (Perin, 1992). The individual can choose all, none, or any number of the above treatments. Case managers today are working with greater numbers of very ill young and older adults. Many may know little about documents such as medical POA, but most have thought a lot about dying and feel very little control over it. Although no one controls the death process, people can sometimes maintain authority over the events surrounding death and can make sure their last wishes are carried out.

Case managers and social workers are often asked to initiate discussions about advance directives; most institutions keep the forms to sign on hand. It is recommended that case managers understand advance directives and feel comfortable discussing the subject with patients and their families, within the scope of practice of their underlying profession. Workshops about advance directives and those addressing death and dying are helpful; another way to learn about advance directives is to choose a medical POA for yourself or become a medical POA for a close family member or friend. The process is enlightening. Because of changing laws and various state mandates, it is an extra protection to attach a state-specific advance directive to the original. These directives are offered free by hospitals, state or city health departments, and the American Bar Association.

Another innovative move in advance directives is one recently launched in several states by a Florida-based nonprofit organization, Aging with Dignity. This do-it-yourself, fill-in-the-blank living will speaks plainly to people about a subject that is not clear to many; the added burden of trying to understand lawyer-speak or doctor-speak is gone. People finally understand the difference between "cure" and "palliative care." The goal of the advance directives document is to prompt discussion about a topic few of us like to discuss. This document addresses five areas, called *five wishes*, and goes beyond feeding tubes and ventilators. Five Wishes is now valid in 40 states and addresses all of a person's needs—medical, personal, emotional, and spiritual—at a time when unable to speak for oneself and suffering a serious and terminal illness. Display 8-9 shares contact information about Aging with Dignity—Five Wishes. This agency is a private, nonprofit organization with a mission to safeguard the human dignity of people

---

display 8-9

▼ AGING WITH DIGNITY

Aging with Dignity—Five Wishes
Mail to: P O Box 1661
Tallahassee FL 32302-1661
Office Location:
3050 Highland Oaks Terrace, Suite 2
Tallahassee FL 32301-3841
Telephone: (888) 5 WISHES/(888) 594-7437
E-mail: fivewishes@agingwithdignity.org
Phone: (850) 681-2010
Fax: (850) 681-2481
Website: www.agingwithdignity.org

---

as they age or face serious illness. This agency has been an advocate for quality care for those near the end of life.

The five wishes, or decisions, in the new living will are:

1. The person I want to make care decisions for me when I cannot is _____. This provides the name of the medical POA/Healthcare Representative.
2. The kind of medical treatment I want/I do not want. Here, a checklist of medical treatments is provided. The checklist may include defibrillation, chest compressions, assisted ventilation, intubation, nutritional support, and advanced life support medications.
3. How comfortable I want to be.
4. How I want people to treat me.
5. What I want my loved ones to know.

[Please Note: There is some risk with the use of checklist Advanced Directives/Living Wills, as they include words and concepts that may not accurately reflect an individual's understanding. Consultation with a lawyer experienced in this area of practice and with a physician/nurse practitioner who is authorized by law to provide end-of-life consultation is also advised].

▶ PROTECTING YOUR LICENSE

Most health professionals fear malpractice lawsuits over anything else. What they fail to understand is that civil liability exposure is only one aspect of risk. Professional Liability or Malpractice insurance is designed to protect you financially from a damaging lawsuit. Professional practice is an area where several areas of law control both at the federal and state levels; civil, criminal, and administrative laws all regulate certain aspects of practice.

▶ State Safeguards to Protect the Public

In 2006, the notorious nurse serial killer, Charles Cullen, was sentenced to 11 consecutive life sentences in New Jersey and 18 in Pennsylvania after pleading guilty to murdering

display 8-10

INFORMATION ON LIVING WILLS AND ADVANCE DIRECTIVES

Helpful information about living wills and advance directors are available from Compassion & Choices, 2017. Patients may find this website helpful as they think through their decisions. The website also supports enhancing the patients' knowledge and understanding of living wills and advance directives. It is also beneficial for health care professionals.

Compassion and Choices
Address: P O Box 101810
Denver, CO 80250
Telephone: (800) 247-7421
Website: www.compassionandchoices.org

at least 35 people between 1998 and 2003; it is suspected that there were many more victims. Cullen, a registered nurse, was labeled the "Angel of Death" when he admitted to administering overdoses of medications to terminal patients or those with fatal diagnoses to "spare them from being coded." New laws have followed this horrific series of deaths at the hands of one individual and placed all nurses and other healthcare providers under a new level of scrutiny.

During the investigation of these deaths and Cullen's behavior, it was revealed that he moved from hospital to hospital without notice because of lax or absent reporting requirements. In response to this case, the New Jersey State Legislature enacted strict laws requiring background checks, including mandatory fingerprinting of all healthcare professionals (Display 8-11). "The Health Care Professional Responsibility and Reporting Enhancement Act ("the Act") (N.J. Stat., § 45:1–33 [2007]) requires that a criminal history background check be conducted for all healthcare professionals licensed or certified by the Division of Consumer Affairs by 2009." In the years, since the passage of the Act, and with the additional reporting requirements enacted in 2017, nurses and other health practitioners who choose to leave one facility, home care company, registry or other healthcare entity to improve their career opportunities are subject to the inquiry contained in the new CN-9 Form, which asks about the circumstances of the change (NJHA, 2017). "The CN-9 form is called the Health Care Facility Inquiry Regarding Health Care Professional. As a Health Care Entity, you are reaching out to another Health Care Entity to find out about someone that you are either hiring, granting privileges, continuing employment, or continuing privileges" (NJHA, 2017, p.3).

▶ Your Signature is Your Bond

After going through the long and arduous task of education, background checks, gaining experience, and certification, it would be dreadful to lose your professional license due to misuse of your signature. On any given day in the acute care and other settings, we are asked to sign a chart or another document. The only time your signature with professional credentials should appear is when you are completing work of your own creation. For example, you work in the acute care setting. There is an experienced Licensed Practice Nurse (LPN) on your unit. You are not the charge nurse or nurse manager, nor have you assumed another leadership role, but you are simply another nurse on that unit. The LPN performs tasks that may or may not be beyond his/her scope of practice and then says, "Would you mind just signing this for me?" or worse, your manager instructs you to "sign-off" for the LPN. This act shifts liability from the LPN to you and there really is no defense for your actions. LPNs lack the in-depth reasoning of "why" we do what we do because their education is task oriented.

You are legally responsible for anything that bears your signature. In the case management environment, historically supervisors have signed reports for case managers they manage. There is no problem with a person reviewing and editing your report; however, the report must then be returned to you for completeness and accuracy and then you add your signature. It is the converse of the concept "if it isn't written it didn't happen." If your signature appears on a note, report, medication chart, or anything else in your professional capacity, you are presumed to have acted with full knowledge and have responsibility for the contents.

Case management reports and hospital charts are legal documents and are used regularly in court cases, agency actions, and hearings. One example comes from a 1996 appeal from a Louisiana trial court decision. In that case, a case manager's determination was used to ascertain whether a claimant's injury was work related. At trial, the employee claimed that the case manager's assessment was not sufficient. On appeal, the court held: the case manager's visit, assessment, and recommendations did constitute "reasonable effort" to ascertain an employee's exact medical condition (Muller, 2008, in Tahan and Treiger, 2017, citing [*Cochennic v. Dillard's, 668 So.2d 1161 {La. App. 5 Cir., 1996}]*).

▶ MANDATORY REPORTING

All states have laws that require mandatory reporting by healthcare professionals of acts of abuse, injury, or violence that they observe. Refer to Display 8-12 for an example of mandatory reporting (New Jersey State Board of Nursing mandatory reporting guidelines). The State of New York provides a complete list of mandated reporters at: http://www.nysmandatedreporter.org/MandatedReporters.aspx. California makes training easily accessible at: http://mandatedreporterca.com/training/generaltraining.htm.

In recent years the scope of this requirement has broadened from reporting suspected child abuse to include protection of the elderly and disabled. Criminal penalties can be imposed if those events are not reported to the

BACKGROUND CHECKS

N.J. ST§ 10:48A-2.1 General standards

a. N.J. S.A. 30:6D-63 to 72 requires that the Department shall not contract with any community agency for the provision of services unless it has first been determined that no criminal history record information exists on file in the Federal Bureau of Investigation Identification Division, or in the State Bureau of Identification in the Division of State Police, which would disqualify the community agency head or the community agency employee from such employment.

b. **Fingerprints** shall be taken electronically through a "live scan" process. The agency staff shall be responsible to call a toll-free number to schedule an appointment to have **fingerprints** taken. The State Bureau of Identification will **check** its own records and forward an inquiry to the Federal Bureau of Investigation.

c. It shall be the responsibility of the community agency head to assure compliance with this chapter.

d. If the criminal history record indicates a conviction for certain criminal or disorderly persons offenses, the employee shall be terminated from employment unless he or she affirmatively demonstrates to the community agency head or the community agency board, if the individual is the community agency head, clear and convincing evidence of his or her rehabilitation.

e. If a prospective employee refuses to consent to or cooperate in securing a **background check,** the person shall not be considered for employment.

f. If a current employee refuses to consent to or cooperate in securing **fingerprints** for the purpose of a **background check,** the person shall be immediately removed from his or her position and the person's employment shall be terminated.

g. 6. A **background check** shall be conducted at least once every two years.

h. The community agency head and all employees who may come in contact with persons served by the agency, shall submit their **fingerprints** upon employment to the Department of Human Services office as directed by the Division.

i. If the **background check** of the community agency head reveals a criminal record as identified below, the community agency board shall determine within 15 working days, if the community agency head has been rehabilitated in accordance with N.J. A.C. 10:48-3.4.

j. 9. The community agency head shall ensure that each employee who may come in contact with persons served by the agency shall be fingerprinted in accordance with the procedures contained in this chapter.

k. All employees shall sign a written consent to the criminal **background check** (refer to chapter Appendix A, incorporated herein by reference) prior to the time the **fingerprints** are taken. This consent shall remain on file in the agency.

l. Individuals shall be disqualified for employment for any of the following crimes or disorderly persons offenses in New Jersey:

  1. Any crime or disorderly person offense (See Note Below) involving danger to the person as set forth in N.J. S.A. 2C:11-1 et seq. through 2C:15-1 et seq., including the following:

    i. Murder;

    ii. Manslaughter;

    iii. Death by auto;

    iv. Simple assault;

    v. Aggravated assault;

    vi. Recklessly endangering another person;

    vii. Terroristic threats;

    viii. Kidnapping;

    ix. Interference with custody of children;

    x. Sexual assault;

    xi. Criminal sexual contact;

    xii. Lewdness; or

    xiii. Robbery.

  2. Any crime against children or incompetents as set forth in NJSA 2C:24-1 et seq., including the following:

    i. Endangering the welfare of a child; or

    ii. Endangering the welfare of an incompetent person;

  3. A crime or offense involving the manufacture, transportation, sale, possession or habitual use of a controlled dangerous substance as defined in N.J. S.A. 24:21-1 et seq.; or

  4. In any other state or jurisdiction, conduct which, if committed in New Jersey, would constitute any of the crimes or disorderly persons offenses described in (l)1 through 3 above.

NOTE: New Jersey does not use the term misdemeanor; a "disorderly person's offense" is one that is punishable with a potential sentence of up to 180 days in jail, or $1000.00 in fines, or both. A crime is a felony offense punishable with more than one (1) year in jail.

proper authorities, because the law recognizes the need to protect the public and the special relationship that health professionals have with the public. When such a report is made on the basis of a reasonable cause and in good faith, most states and federal law provide civil immunity to the reporter for possible repercussion. It is critically important that you document objective information and personal, objective observations, especially in abuse cases. Most states require that health and education

professionals complete a course in identifying abuse and the specifics of the reporting requirements (see Muller & Fink-Samnick, 2015).

Some states require professionals to report coworkers who appear to be under the influence of drugs or alcohol. Teachers are under a similar mandate. Mandatory reporting is required of case managers specifically. The CCMC Code of Professional Conduct (the Code) Standard 7 for Case Managers expressly states that certified case managers

NEW JERSEY BOARD OF NURSING MANDATORY REPORTING GUIDELINES

What should be reported?

LEVEL I—Always requires reporting to the Board of Nursing

▶ Conduct that clearly violates expected standards of care and may result in various degrees of harm
▶ Conduct that demonstrates a pattern of poor judgment or skill

Examples: suspected drug diversion, misappropriation, theft, physical/verbal abuse, sexual abuse or exploitation, falsification of documents, cover-ups, a single serious medication error, repeated medication errors or charting errors, signing out without a physician's order or failing to account for wastage of controlled medication, serious medication errors, arrests, indictments and convictions, intoxication on duty and patient neglect (such as failing to properly assess, treat, monitor, notify or intervene).

LEVEL II—Depending on an analysis of the facts, may require reporting to the Board of Nursing.

▶ There is no list of what should or should not be reported under this category. It is a matter of judgment for the person(s) making the report, based upon a review of all the relevant factors.
▶ Conduct that may be indicative of a more serious problem should be reported.

LEVEL III—Does not require reporting to the Board of Nursing.

▶ Low-level infractions that do not involve patient care, professional judgment or wrongdoing.

Examples: co-worker disputes, personality conflicts, absenteeism, tardiness, labor-management or employer-employee disputes, fee or wage disputes, unanticipated adverse outcomes independent of anyone's fault (such as equipment failures or allergic reactions) and minor policy infractions.

Who should report?

▶ All licensed nurses have an affirmative obligation to report suspected violations of the Nurse Practice Act and the Uniform Enforcement Act to the Board of Nursing.
▶ Generally, in the work setting (e.g., licensed health care facility or agency) the highest nursing officer should take responsibility for reporting to the Board (e.g., Director of Nursing/Vice President of Patient Care) However, it is also appropriate for the Director of Security, the Director of Human Resources or Risk Manager to file a complaint. If the facility or agency's administrators refuse or delay a report, it is appropriate for a staff nurse or nurse manager to take responsibility for reporting to the Board.
▶ The Board also receives complaints from consumers/patients, families of consumers/patients, the Ombudsman

for the Institutionalized Elderly, the Department of Health and Senior Services and the Criminal Authorities.

How should a report be made?

INITIAL REPORTS TO THE BOARD OF NURSING SHOULD:

▶ Be in writing (except for emergent matters involving suspected drug diversion/misappropriation or sexual abuse complaints).
▶ Contain basic information about the "who, what, where, why and how" of the incident.
▶ Contain the name of a contact person and a telephone number and address where he/she can be reached during business hours.

ALL PERSONS MAKING A REPORT TO THE BOARD OF NURSING SHOULD BE PREPARED TO:

▶ Provide legible copies of all relevant records, materials and information as requested by the Board's representative.
▶ Speak with the Board's representative by telephone, in writing or in person, as requested.
▶ Assist the Board's representative in gaining access to all relevant information, witnesses or other persons, as requested.
▶ Follow through and agree to appear before the Board, if necessary.

For purposes of these guidelines, the Board's representative may include any one of the following individuals: The Board's executive director, paralegal, deputy attorneys general or Enforcement Bureau investigators.

Where should a report be made? All letters of complaint should be made to:

Board of Nursing
P.O. Box 45010
124 Halsey Street, Sixth Floor
Newark, New Jersey 07101
Tel. Number: (973) 504-6457

Emergent complaints of drug diversion or sexual abuse may be made by telephone to the Board of Nursing at (973) 504-6457, or to the Deputy Attorney General at (973) 648-7093 or the Enforcement Bureau of the Division of Consumer Affairs at (973) 504-6300.

FOR LINKS TO ALL BOARDS OF NURSING IN THE UNITED STATES, GO TO:

https://www.ncsbn.org/boards.htm

(CCM) possessing knowledge that another CCM has committed a violation of the Code must promptly report that knowledge to CCMC (CCMC Code of Professional Conduct for Case Manager, G-2, G-26) and are required to assist with the enforcement of the Code (CCMC Code, G-27) (CCMC, 2015).

▶ Domestic Violence

Violence in America is not limited to street crime. In 2013, Congress reauthorized the 1994 Violence Against Women Act. The Act clarified and provided funding services for victims, who had been subject to the defined acts committed against women. Stalking was a significant addition to the Act, as it recognized a behavior that, far too often, places women at risk. Domestic violence affects the workplace, the classroom, and the sanctity of the home. Case managers, as health professionals, must be ever vigilant and sensitive to their patient's/client's symptoms and injuries, and listen to what they are saying, recognizing that it is difficult for victims of domestic violence to speak out and ask for help. Domestic violence as a topic has been incorporated in many nursing curricula. In the past decade, domestic abuse was identified as a health problem of epidemic proportion by such organizations as the Institute of Medicine, American Medical Association, American Nurses Association, and the American Association of Colleges of Nursing (AACN). The AACN position statement calls on nurses to "be aware of assessment methods and nursing interventions that will interrupt and prevent the cycle of violence (AACN, 1999)." Case managers should be encouraged to participate in continuing education programs that focus on domestic violence identification and prevention.

Case managers may find themselves dealing with a completely unrelated illness, injury, or topic with their client when the trust that is established between clients and case managers invites a victim to reach out. Learn and maintain a list of area resources so that appropriate referrals can be made on a timely basis. If the present opportunity is lost for a victim to reach out for help, it may be months or years before he or she feels safe enough to tell the story to someone else or to call the police. More information on how one can help victims of domestic violence is available on the National Coalition on Domestic Violence website, accessible at http://www.ncadv.org. A list of sources for information regarding domestic violence is available in Display 8-13. For a case manager's guide to domestic violence and reporting (see Muller, 2014).

▶ Child Abuse

Child abuse is an issue that can produce rage in the most nonjudgmental case manager. Although cultural sensitivities are essential to understanding a family dynamic, child abuse has many variations and is not limited to any ethnic or socioeconomic group. Not only is reporting of suspected child abuse mandatory, but if a classic case is not reported and the child suffers further danger or even death, healthcare professionals involved in caring for the child can be charged criminally, as well as being found to be negligent. It is clear that case managers, nurses, social workers, teachers, and others charged with a duty of care must report acts of child abuse that they either witness or identify the symptoms thereof. In observing the behavior of children, there are signs that must be learned to help in identifying these problems. One classic sign is a child who wears clothing that is not seasonally appropriate. For example, why would a child wear a winter jacket or long-sleeve sweatshirt on a hot summer day?

Definitions of child abuse speak of nonaccidental injuries from mistreatment, sexual abuse, or exploitation; such as child prostitution and deprivation of necessities. The perpetrator can be a parent, legal guardian, uncle or aunt, grandfather or grandmother, baby-sitter, boyfriend, neighbor, or stranger. Many books and articles have been written on how to recognize child abuse. Some classic signs are certain types of bodily harm (especially with radiologic evidence of older, healing fractures); failure to attend to medical, physical, or hygiene problems; sexually transmitted diseases; apprehensiveness or secretiveness; bruising or bleeding near genitalia; overly compliant passive behavior; suicidal attempts or gestures; and failure to thrive (which can also be caused by medical problems; therefore, a medical cause must first be ruled out). When observations don't align with "stories" being told, the case manager should investigate further.

Verbal reports are acceptable initially to a law enforcement officer and state agency (these agencies go by various names, from state to state; for example, Child Protective Services). You should know your state's reporting requirements and keep the hotline number readily available. When you make a report, it is very important that you do not guess or give personal opinions. Report only the facts that you have seen or heard. Providing basic facts will give the agency investigator the necessary information to determine whether there has been an act of child abuse or merely an unfortunate accident or a justifiable series of events. Kids get hurt, but it is not for us to assume or guess and make excuses for what we suspect. Our duty is to factually and properly report accurate information to the state-mandated investigatory agency or police authority. When in doubt, let the police be your first point of contact, and remember you are not an investigator. The police, too, can make appropriate referrals.

▶ Adult/Elder Abuse

Elder abuse has many of the same characteristics as those of child abuse. It is also an event that brings with it mandatory reporting requirements. As with reporting child abuse, if the person reporting elder abuse does it in good

display 8-13

DOMESTIC VIOLENCE RESOURCE LIST

If you, or someone you know, are a victim of domestic violence, please call:

The National Domestic Violence Hotline
Telephone: 1-800-799-7233 (SAFE)
Website: www.ndvh.org

National Dating Abuse Helpline
Telephone: 1-866-331-9474
Website: www.loveisrespect.org

National Resource Center on Domestic Violence
Telephone: 1-800-537-2238
Websites: www.nrcdv.org and www.vawnet.org

Futures Without Violence: The National Health Resource Center on Domestic Violence
Telephone: 1-888-792-2873
Website: www.futureswithoutviolence.org

National Center on Domestic Violence, Trauma & Mental Health
Telephone: 1-312-726-7020 ext. 2011
Website: www.nationalcenterdvtraumamh.org

Americans Overseas Domestic Violence Crisis Center
Telephone: International Toll-Free (24/7) 1-866-USWOMEN (879-6636)
Website: www.866uswomen.org

National Child Abuse Hotline/Childhelp
Telephone: 1-800-4-A-CHILD (1-800-422-4453)
Website: www.childhelp.org

National Sexual Assault Hotline
Telephone: 1-800-656-4673 (HOPE)
Website: www.rainn.org

National Suicide Prevention Lifeline
Telephone: 1-800-273-8255 (TALK)
Website: www.suicidepreventionlifeline.org

National Center for Victims of Crime
Telephone: 1-202-467-8700
Website: www.victimsofcrime.org

National Human Trafficking Resource Center/Polaris Project
Telephone: 1-888-373-7888 | Text: HELP to BeFree (233733)
Website: www.polarisproject.org

National Network for Immigrant and Refugee Rights
Telephone: 1-510-465-1984
Website: www.nnirr.org

National Coalition for the Homeless
Telephone: 1-202-737-6444
Website: www.nationalhomeless.org

If you, or someone you know, are a victim of sexual assault, please call:

▶ Rape, Abuse, and Incest National Network (RAINN) 1-800-656-HOPE (4673)
▶ National Sexual Violence Resource Center (NSVRC) 1-877-739-3895
▶ American Bar Association Commission of Domestic Violence http://www.abanet.org/domviol/home.html
▶ For a complete list of State Domestic Violence Coalitions, visit http://www.ovw.usdoj.gov/statedomestic.htm
▶ Center for Hope and Safety (formerly known as: Shelter Our Sisters (New Jersey) http://www.hopeandsafetynj.org
▶ Pennsylvania Domestic Violence Resources http://www.dvresources.org/
▶ The National Criminal Justice Reference Service http://www.ncjrs.gov/

---

faith and with reasonable cause, he or she enjoys immunity against libel or slander claims in most states. Adult abuse can also take many forms like physical abuse, neglect, exploitation of property or pets, unreasonable confinement, sexual assault, medical neglect, financial imprisonment and neglect, psychological abuse, or failure to thrive not caused by medical conditions. Most definitions include the stipulation that the adult is incapacitated or vulnerable and is helpless to defend himself or herself (Perin, 1992). Just as was discussed for child abuse, the case manager should contact the appropriate state agency to report the situation and document completely the observations made and what was discussed/reported and to whom he or she spoke. The case manager should also include in his or her notes what steps were discussed; in other words, what will happen next?

Some states have an Adult and/or Senior Protective Services for reporting and investigation, including but not limited to the Ombudsman in your county or region. These cases are investigated on a priority basis, taking emergency cases first. These agencies also have an arsenal of resources available to them and make referrals to public health and other services. The case manager can make such referrals; using public services can increase your client's ability to access resources, particularly when finances are at or near the poverty level.

Elder abuse in long-term care or subacute care has gotten much press. It can cost the facility its Medicare and Medicaid income and place their state-issued license at risk; more importantly, it simply should not be a part of the fabric of medical and case management practice. Many families, including those of case managers themselves, find their time and resources divided between multiple generations. With a large aging population and life expectancies greater than they have ever been in history, states have found it necessary to enact laws, rules, and regulations to protect seniors both in medical facilities and in their own homes. The federal Administration on Aging, under HHS, was created in response to these needs. Congress passed the Older Americans Act of 2006 (Display 8-14) with the intent to ensure equal opportunity for all Americans to have access to healthcare, community services, employment opportunity, etc. The term *caregiver* is broadly defined in subparagraph 18(A) of the Act as an "individual who has the responsibility for the care of an older individual, either voluntarily, by contract, by receipt of payment for care, or as a result of the operation of law and means a family member or other individual who provides (on behalf of such individual or of a public or private agency, organization, or institution) compensated or uncompensated care to an older individual" (§ 102[18][B]). It is incumbent on the case manager to be familiar with the Act, which can be found in its entirety at http://www.aoa.gov/oaa2006/Main_Site/index.aspx. In fact, the term *fiduciary*, discussed previously in this chapter, is specifically defined by the Act:

A. means a person or entity with the legal responsibility to make decisions on behalf of and for the benefit of another person; and to act in good faith and with fairness; and

B. includes a trustee, a guardian, a conservator, an executor, an agent under a financial power of attorney or health care power of attorney, or a representative payee.

Therefore, when dealing with this population, this definition is the minimum mandatory national standard, and state laws cannot limit these duties. State laws can, however, provide additional protections to older Americans, and often they do.

With the advent of the HIPAA, many of the protections found in the Omnibus Budget Reconciliation Act of 1987, such as the right to privacy, to receive notice before a room or roommate change, to voice grievances, to meet with other residents, and to participate in the planning of care or treatment, as well as freedom from physical or mental abuse, involuntary seclusion, or the use of physical or chemical restraints for the purposes of (staff) convenience or punishment, are not encompassed in these two very extensive pieces of legislation. Like child abuse, elder abuse cannot be tolerated in any level of care. All medical professionals have an affirmative duty to report elder abuse. Failure to report elder abuse can lead to the same criminal consequences as if the negligent reporter was the actor.

---

display 8-14

OLDER AMERICANS ACT OF 2006

Title I—Declaration of Objectives; Definitions

Declaration of Objectives for Older Americans

Section. 101.

The Congress hereby finds and declares that, in keeping with the traditional American concept of the inherent dignity of the individual in our democratic society, the older people of our Nation are entitled to, and it is the joint and several duty and responsibility of the governments of the United States, of the several States and their political subdivisions, and of Indian tribes to assist our older people to secure equal opportunity to the full and free enjoyment of the following objectives:

1. An adequate income in retirement in accordance with the American standard of living.
2. The best possible physical and mental health which science can make available and without regard to economic status.
3. Obtaining and maintaining suitable housing, independently selected, designed and located with reference to special needs and available at costs which older citizens can afford.
4. Full restorative services for those who require institutional care, and a comprehensive array of community-based, long-term care services adequate to

appropriately sustain older people in their communities and in their homes, including support to family members and other persons providing voluntary care to older individuals needing long-term care services.
5. Opportunity for employment with no discriminatory personnel practices because of age.
6. Retirement in health, honor, dignity—after years of contribution to the economy.
7. Participating in and contributing to meaningful activity within the widest range of civic, cultural, educational and training and recreational opportunities.
8. Efficient community services, including access to low-cost transportation, which provide a choice in supported living arrangements and social assistance in a coordinated manner and which are readily available when needed, with emphasis on maintaining a continuum of care for vulnerable older individuals.
9. Immediate benefit from proven research knowledge, which can sustain and improve health and happiness.
10. Freedom, independence, and the free exercise of individual initiative in planning and managing their own lives, full participation in the planning and operation of community-based services and programs provided for their benefit, and protection against abuse, neglect, and exploitation.

(42 U.S.C. 3001)

SOURCE: OLDER AMERICANS ACT OF 1965 [Public Law 89–73] [As Amended Through P.L. 114–144, Enacted April 19, 2016] [Section 101, (42 U.S.C. 3001)]. Accessed 7/10/2017. Available https://legcounsel.house.gov/Comps/Older%20Americans%20Act%20Of%201965.pdf.

▶ DO NOT RESUSCITATE—NO "CODE BLUE"

In most states a physician's written order is required in addition to an Advanced Directive for Healthcare or Living Will for a Do Not Resuscitate Order. In 1998, Ohio adopted a Do Not Resuscitate (DNR) law. Ohio's DNR law gives individuals the opportunity to exercise their right to limit care received in emergency situations in special circumstances. "Special circumstances" include care received from emergency personnel when 911 is dialed. The law authorizes a physician to write an order letting healthcare personnel know that a patient does not wish to be resuscitated in the event of a cardiac arrest (no palpable pulse) or respiratory arrest (no spontaneous respirations or the presence of labored breathing at end of life). (For more information, refer to Franklin County Probate Court, State of Ohio, 1998.)

The intent of such laws is to provide assurances that patient rights will be respected, even when a 911 call is made. If a patient is competent, the right to choose or refuse resuscitation measures belongs solely to that person. Incapacitated patients need a prior signed advance directive or a Surrogate Decision Maker. DNR orders must be written prior to their need. In other words, in the event of an emergency situation or "code" where there is the cessation of breathing, heartbeat, or both, a physician cannot telephonically give a No Code or DNR order. The order must predate the need, even if it is within a matter of seconds. Without the existence of a DNR order, a full code must commence and continue until successful or a physician determines that death is irreversible.

Historically, "slow codes" and "partial codes" have emerged as legal and ethical quagmires. These codes are illegal in some states and carry liability because of their vagueness. Hospital policy consistent with state law clears up this uncertainty. Rather than fear a conversation regarding end-of-life issues, a case manager can provide individuals and family members with a well-trained and sympathetic ear. A well-drawn Health Care Directive will reference DNR and express the individual's wishes, providing the healthcare representative/proxy and the physician with guidance for end-of-life choices. Caution should be used with menu-like directives, as individuals don't have the medical training and knowledge to distinguish between lifesaving cardiopulmonary resuscitation and life-sustaining interventions, such as intubation and use of a respirator.

Families often are confused about what DNR means, feeling that their loved ones will not get necessary treatment. It must be clearly explained that DNR is not the same as do not treat, that the patient will not be abandoned, and that everything will be done for the patient up to the point where lifesaving is no longer possible.

If that is not complex enough, living wills stating no extraordinary measures are contested in some states. In Georgia, for example, the physician must obtain the patient's permission or other authority to write a DNR order; in the absence of that, the physician must get another physician's concurrence or use the hospital ethics committee as a second vote. Patient's wishes in a living will are not enough. In Georgia, the living will statute applies only to three clinical conditions: if the patient is terminally ill, in a vegetative state, or in an irreversible coma. Alternatively, other states allow unilateral decisions by physicians that do not require any other consent for a DNR order (Banja, 1998). In 2000, New Jersey established additional administrative rules (with full force and effect of law) to protect persons with dementia, including Alzheimer disease, who live in rooming and boarding houses. Even if there is a DNR order, the law requires, "Even if a resident has a 'Do Not Resuscitate' (DNR) order, staff must call 911 for appropriate assistance in the event of an emergency, so that appropriate medical staff can assist the resident and act, if appropriate" (N.J. Stat., §5:27-13.1[f]). In addition, home health agencies or subacute care facilities must include in their medical record of any individual, particularly when there is a transfer in or out of one subacute facility to another, "a notice of the existence of an advance directive and/or Do Not Resuscitate (DNR) order" (N.J. Admin. Code, §8:42-11.2[d][7]). The bottom line is that the case manager must know the patient's wishes, communicate those wishes to the next provider of care or setting, and follow state law and facility policies.

POLST (The Physician Orders for Life-Sustaining Treatment): In simple terms, POLST is the bridge between an Advanced Directive for Healthcare, Medical Power of Attorney or Living Will and the practical application of one's wishes. Even if an Advanced Directive expressly states that the individual does not wish to be resuscitated, a 911 call will initiate a lifesaving response. There is a great difference between lifesaving and life-sustaining treatment and interventions. In those cases, where competent individuals work with their physicians to discuss and decide what end-of-life choices they wish, POLST provides a vehicle to advise emergency medical services. Case managers should check their state(s) law, as official forms may also be required to be in 'official' colors, such as dayglow green in those states that have enacted POLST legislation. For links to all state forms, go to: http://polst.org/programs-in-your-state/.

▶ DEATH, ANATOMICAL GIFTS, AUTOPSY

Most states define death as an irreversible cessation of cardiopulmonary functions or an irreversible cessation of brain function. This is essentially an irreversible loss of consciousness and function (Feutz-Harter, 1991). An example of this would be the persistent vegetative state, in which there is seemingly no awareness of anyone or anything. Such patients live at a primitive reflex level and often have eye-blink reflexes and react to noxious smells, sound, pain, or light. Although their prognosis is poor, diagnosis as a form of death strains the definition.

In most institutions, the physician must "pronounce" the patient, as defined by state law and complete the Death Certificate. As stated in the section on coroner's cases, under certain conditions such as home hospice care, and Advanced Practice (Nurse Practitioners), nurses may pronounce the patient and fill out paperwork. Often the case manager is tending to the family or attempting to contact the family. If the family is in route to the hospital after its loved one has died, every effort should be made to meet the family before it reaches the room.

A thorough review and documentation is warranted in situations when deaths (1) occur during or after elective surgery or procedure, (2) occur after returning to an intensive care unit (ICU) or within 24 hours of being transferred out of an ICU, or (3) occur unexpectedly. Documentation should include, but not be limited to, complete patient assessments, prompt responses to any changes in patient's condition (laboratory test results, vital signs, cardiac rhythms, breathing patterns, pain, bleeding, and drug reactions), timely physician notification, equipment malfunctions, and interventions. If the staff believes that an equipment malfunction played a significant role in the demise of the patient, the case manager may want to strongly suggest that the hospital hold on to the piece of equipment, whether it is a ventilator or a pacemaker. The hospital would like to prove that it was equipment failure and not user failure; the manufacturer would like to prove that it was not equipment failure.

▶ Organ and Tissue Donation

Anatomical gifts can be voluntarily donated by anyone 18 years or older. Driver's licenses and Advanced Directives for healthcare documents are two ways to check a person's wishes about organ and tissue donation. If there are no indications that the person had any objections, the following can approve donations, in order of legal priority: (1) spouse (or parent if the deceased is younger than 18 years), (2) adult child, (3) either legal parent, (4) adult siblings, (5) legal guardian, and (6) the person responsible for burial (Perin, 1992).

With the modernization of technology and medicine, organ and tissue donation and transplantation can mean amazing lifesaving or life-improving results. Organ procurement organizations (OPO) are the state designated and authorized agencies for donation. Some OPOs cover vast regions and others are limited to the boundaries of a single state, even though "one person's organ donation can save 8 lives" (UNOS, 2017, p. 1). In February 2017, the number of people waiting for transplants exceeded 155,555 (United Network for Organ Sharing [UNOS], 2017).

When you, as the case manager, are given an opportunity to answer questions, or if it is part of your job to initiate the discussion, it is important for you to have up-to-date information on organ procurement and transplantation from a reliable source. Myths and misconceptions contribute to the length of the waiting list (see Display 8-15). This is obviously a very sensitive job, and you may, at one time or another, be left with the task amid enormous grief.

▶ Autopsies

Autopsies (postmortem examinations) are usually required in coroner's cases. In other cases, they may not be mandatory. Similar to organ donation, the following can give authorization for autopsy: (1) spouse (or parent if the patient is a minor), (2) adult child, (3) legal guardian, and (4) next of kin. If none of these is found, the person responsible for the burial can give consent (Perin, 1992).

Coroner's cases must be autopsied. Other reasons for autopsies may be for informational purposes or because the results of the autopsy may be required in the future (i.e., for lawsuits). Autopsies should be considered in the following situations:

- ▶ When deaths resulted from high-risk infections or contagious diseases;
- ▶ When the cause of death was not absolutely known, and an autopsy could help explain the circumstances leading to the death and thus ease concerns of the family or the public;
- ▶ Unexpected or unexplained deaths: these may have occurred spontaneously or during/after a diagnostic procedure or therapy;
- ▶ Obstetrical, neonatal, or pediatric deaths;
- ▶ When the autopsy could reveal a suspected illness that might affect survivors;
- ▶ If organ donation is a possibility;
- ▶ When the death was suspected of being the result of environmental or occupational hazards;
- ▶ When the patient underwent experimental or approved clinical trials before his death;
- ▶ When the patient is dead on arrival at the emergency department, the death occurred within 24 hours of admission, or if the patient sustained an injury during hospitalization.

A case manager may be asked about who pays for autopsies. Autopsies are not a covered expense under Medicare/Medicaid (Stoppler, 2016). Many hospitals perform autopsies as a matter of courtesy to the medical staff. Hospitals often perform autopsies at no charge even when the patient had left the hospital previously and subsequently died. There is usually a time limit in this case; 6 months is an average.

Most facilities have an authorization for autopsies form that must be signed. However, this is not always the case, and the issue of autopsies is very personal to some

DONATE LIFE AMERICA

There is a severe organ shortage in this country. Despite continuing efforts at public education, misconceptions and inaccuracies about donation persist. It's a tragedy if even one person decides against donation because he or she doesn't know the truth. Following is a list of the most common myths along with the actual facts:

Myth: If emergency room doctors know you're an organ donor, they won't work as hard to save you.

Fact: If you are sick or injured and admitted to the hospital, the top priority is to save your life. Organ donation can be considered only after brain death has been declared by a physician. Many states have adopted legislation allowing individuals to legally designate their wish to be a donor should brain death occur, although in many states Organ Procurement Organizations also require consent from the donor's family.

Myth: When you're waiting for a transplant, your financial or celebrity status is as important as your medical status.

Fact: When you are on the transplant waiting list for a donor organ, what really counts is the severity of your illness, time spent waiting, blood type, and other important medical information.

Myth: Having "organ donor" noted on your driver's license or carrying a donor card is all you have to do to become a donor.

Fact: While a signed donor card and a driver's license with an "organ donor" designation are legal documents, organ and tissue donation is usually discussed with family members prior to the donation. To ensure that your family understands your wishes, it is important that you tell your family about your decision to donate LIFE.

Myth: Only hearts, livers, and kidneys can be transplanted.

Fact: Needed organs include the heart, kidneys, pancreas, lungs, liver, and intestines. Tissue that can be donated includes the eyes, skin, bone, heart valves, and tendons.

Myth: Your history of medical illness means your organs or tissues are unfit for donation.

Fact: At the time of death, the appropriate medical professionals will review your medical and social histories to determine whether or not you can be a donor. With recent advances in transplantation, an increasing number of people have become donors like never before. It's best to tell your family your wishes and sign up to be an organ and tissue donor on your driver's license or on an official donor document.

Myth: You are too old to be a donor.

Fact: People of all ages and medical histories should consider themselves potential donors. Your medical condition at the time of death will determine what organs and tissue can be donated.

Myth: If you agree to donate your organs, your family will be charged for the costs.

Fact: There is no cost to the donor's family or estate for organ and tissue donation. Funeral costs remain the responsibility of the family.

Myth: Organ donation disfigures the body and changes the way it looks in a casket.

Fact: Donated organs are removed surgically, in a routine operation similar to gallbladder or appendix removal. Donation does not change the appearance of the body for the funeral service.

Myth: Your religion prohibits organ donation.

Fact: All major organized religions approve of organ and tissue donation and consider it an act of charity.

Myth: There is real danger of being heavily drugged and then waking to find you have had one kidney (or both) removed for a black market transplant.

Fact: This tale has been widely circulated over the Internet. There is absolutely no evidence of such activity ever occurring in the United States. While the tale may sound credible, it has no basis in the reality of organ transplantation. Many people who hear the myth probably dismiss it, but it is possible that some believe it and decide against organ donation out of needless fear.

---

people. I will never forget the grief one woman suffered when she discovered that her husband was mistakenly autopsied against his wishes. If this process is within your realm of job responsibilities as a case manager, make sure to document to whom you spoke and the decision made concerning postmortem examination.

▶ TECHNIQUES TO MINIMIZE LIABILITY

There is no guaranteed method of totally eliminating legal risk in today's litigious environment; however, adherence to the Standards of Practice for Case Management (CMSA, 2016) and the Codes of Ethics and Standards of Practice of your underlying profession is always recommended (American Nurses Association, 2015). It is important for social workers to check the specific standard stipulated for their practice area through the NASW, as it promulgates several standards on the basis of practice setting and the level of license; these are available at: http://www.naswpress.org/publications/standards/index.html.

Anyone can file a lawsuit; the question of proof is entirely different. There are some fundamental, common-sense case management tenets that will certainly minimize liability exposure. Remember, trial lawyers will analyze each word of your job description to determine whether you performed all required and expected aspects of your job or if you overextended your role by stepping into the realm of another professional, such as the physician. In addition, participate in the creation, maintenance, and updates of the policies and procedures in your unique work environment. Failure to follow your own protocols may be worse than having no protocols and policies at all.

The most important source of licensure protection is the law of the state(s) in which you are licensed to practice. Practitioners should check the website for their profession in the states(s) in which you are licensed several times each year. Some states, such as Texas, heavily regulate not only nursing, but also case management practice and have taken steps toward title protection for professional case managers (Texas BON, n.d.).

▶ COMMONSENSE SAFEGUARDS

1. Learn where to find state and federal laws; www.findlaw.com and http://www.law.cornell.edu/states/listing.html both provide a good launch point for all states.
2. Know and incorporate the standards of case management practice (CMSA, 2016) into your activities, as well as the standards of the certifying body of the credential you possess (e.g., CCMC for the CCM- www.ccmcertification.org), or the credentialing/accreditation agencies of your program such as URAC (http://www.urac.org), or The Joint Commission (http://www.jointcommission.org), where applicable.
3. Look at the Authorization for Protected Health Information form signed by your client and/or used by your employer or agency. Don't assume you know what it says. Once you've confirmed whether the patient has limited disclosure, which is his or her right, keep your patient, family, and caregiver informed, consistent with their wishes.
4. Do not make decisions for others that they should make for themselves.
5. Offer all known options, whether in or out of network. Private pay is always an option.
6. Remember the 3 "C's"—Communicate, Communicate, Communicate. Communicate your role clearly to the patient/client, family, and caregiver. Advise them truthfully, from your first contact, what will happen to information they share with you.
7. Remember the 3 "D's"—Document, Document, Document! Documentation demonstrates compliance with laws, regulations, and the standard of care and offers evidence of scope of practice.
8. Do not practice medicine: Do not give the impression that the case manager is the medical authority. Refer medical decisions to physicians or those authorized to prescribe and work in a cooperative spirit with physicians to facilitate case management goals. REMEMBER, the obligation to obtain informed consent remains with the physician and cannot be delegated in most states.
9. Understand how risk managers and legal consultants can assist you and use this resource.
10. Know your job description: Make sure your job description accurately describes your role and establishes boundaries of duties; recommend and make changes as your job develops over time.
11. Operate within the scope of your professional license, practice act, and code of professional conduct/ethics standards.
12. Don't just say, "No!" If you must be the bearer of bad news (i.e., a service is not covered), remember you are only the messenger and should not make financial and contractual decisions in your capacity as a case manager. Inform the patient and the family of the right to appeal and help them through the process if appropriate. This is one aspect of the patient advocacy role in action.
13. Use proper consent forms before releasing information to avoid breach of patient confidentiality or HIPAA violation (https://questions.cms.gov/).
14. Purchase your own professional liability insurance, even if your employer tells you that you are covered under its policy. The "employer's policy" is just that and if your employer can find a reason to carve you out of its coverage, it may. This is a low-cost way to avoid high-priced headaches.
15. Check your professional liability insurance policy when you purchase it and renew it to be sure that your current job description is covered. If unsure, provide your current job description to your insurance carrier and ask to see the section of your policy that covers you.
16. Establish, review, and/or revise all policies and procedures, protocols, marketing materials, contracts, consent forms, and case management manuals on a regular basis. REMEMBER,
    a. The HIPAA requires at least annual documented policy review/update.
    b. The HIPAA requires at least annual in-service regarding policies and procedures.
    c. The days of dusty policy and procedure books on the shelf are over.
    d. Policies and procedures become part of the employment contract, so make sure they are up-to-date and relate to the manner in which you are currently practicing.
17. Apply utilization review and quality assurance criteria consistently, objectively, and in a nondiscriminatory manner.
18. Avoid contradictory and inconsistent inclusions in the medical records and case management notes.
19. Listen and be responsive to your patient/client, family, and caregiver. An angry patient/client is a potential plaintiff. It has been reported that the primary reason people file malpractice lawsuits is that they feel neglected and abandoned.

▶ MARRIAGE LAW

On June 26, 2015, the Supreme Court of the United States (SCOTUS) issued its decision in the case of *Obergefell et al v. Hodges, director of the Ohio Department of Health et al* which held in a 5-4 decision that the fundamental right to marry is guaranteed to same-sex couples by both the Due Process Clause and the Equal Protection Clause of the Fourteenth Amendment to the United States Constitution. The amendment requires a "State to license a marriage between two people of the same sex and to recognize a marriage between two people of the same sex when their marriage was lawfully licensed and performed out-of-State" (*Obergefell et al v. Hodges,* 2015, 3-28). Generally, the legal requirements and rules around marriage can differ from state to state. Prior to June 26, 2015, states had been free to either allow or prohibit marriage among same-sex couples. The state issues details on how people can obtain a marriage license and the requirements to do so, as well as big picture issues such as who can marry whom, age of permissible marriage, and circumstances requiring parental approval.

The passing of this marriage equality law brings about some important implications for case managers and case management practice. These pertain to the areas of healthcare disparities (Display 8-16) same-sex couples may have faced prior to the passage of the new law. The issue of disparities is broad; this section is limited to the changes that have occurred on the basis of the new law, and case managers must understand and maintain a practice that adheres to the legal and ethical standards. Muller (2016) describes what has changed and what has not on the basis of this law. Muller explains that:

▶ Two married people (regardless of whether same sex or heterosexual) are entitled under state law to be identified as "next of kin." Case managers must accept the representation all patients and their families make as to marriage status. The next of kin is then able to make medical decisions on behalf of the patient (other party in the marriage or family) who is no longer able to make appropriate decisions for him/herself. Although normally we do not ask people for proof of marriage status, we should remain alert to the impact of misrepresentation of status on care provision and our ability to adhere to the law. For example, misrepresentation of marriage may result in the wrong person deciding about a patient's care plan and preferences. This increases the case manager's (and other healthcare providers') risk for liability. Awareness of how state laws treat such representation or consulting with someone who knows (risk manager or legal counsel) is essential (Muller, 2016, p. 149).

▶ Other laws related to family relationships and healthcare remain unaffected as a result of the marriage equality law. For example, laws that define a parent, adoption, surrogacy, divorce, and child custody remain the same and state-based (Muller, 2016, p. 149).

▶ Refraining from making any assumption about others, or "labeling" them based on sexual orientation and/or identity. These assumptions without a doubt will interfere in the ability to remain nonjudgmental in the patient assessment and care planning which ultimately results in a suboptimal care experience and poor outcomes. In their professional lives, case managers must accept and tolerate everyone whether heterosexual, lesbian, gay, bisexual, transgender, questioning, or

---

display 8-16

HEALTHCARE DISPARITIES

Healthcare disparities refer to differences in access to or availability of healthcare facilities, resources, and services among people, sometimes related to geography/region of residence, age, gender, race and ethnic group, and sexual identity or preference.

▶ Health status disparities refer to the variation in rates of disease occurrence and disabilities between socioeconomic and/or geographically defined population groups.

▶ Funding of healthcare resources impacts the delivery and distribution of these resources, which ultimately explains an individual's access to healthcare services.

▶ Health and public policy, whether executed at the national, state, or local levels, define what services and programs are available, for whom, when, and where. Such policy may result in a disproportionate distribution of resources and therefore impact the health of individuals and communities. For example, the establishment of the Prevention and Public Health Fund has increased investment into community and clinical prevention initiatives, research, and public health infrastructure.

▶ Examination of the issue of social determinants of health, especially based on research in this area, has led to a better understanding of the full range of factors impacting healthcare quality, outcomes and spending, such as genetics, housing, food security, education, finances, and employment. The health of individuals and communities is deeply influenced by socioeconomic factors such as in the case of low-income individuals and communities often facing greater challenges in leading healthy lives.

▶ Some people avoid seeking healthcare services for fear of discrimination, mocking, bulling, or any other form of misjudgment. This is more common among the poor, uninsured, and most importantly among lesbian, gay, bisexual, transgender, questioning, or of queer lifestyle. Delaying access to healthcare services results in health risk behaviors and poor outcomes.

of queer lifestyle (LGBTQ). When feeling judged or uncomfortable with whatever label is used to describe someone, the result is potentially the person avoids seeking medical care and therefore poor health status and outcomes. In contrast, astute and skilled case managers ensure a safe and welcoming environment of care for everyone where they are able to "express their genuine needs, concerns, and fears" (Muller, 2016, p. 150).

▶ Case managers are well positioned to enhance health equity. "Achieving health equity requires valuing everyone equally with focused and ongoing societal efforts to address avoidable inequalities, historical and contemporary injustices, and the elimination of health and healthcare disparities. . . As with most things, honesty is the best policy. Approaching all patients openly and honestly, by asking necessary questions, the case managers can affect a complete and proper assessment. Engaging LGBT[Q] patients should be no different from engaging any patient" (Skehan & Muller, 2016, p. 159).

DISCUSSION QUESTIONS

1. Describe a risk management case you are aware of, whether from published literature or from your own experience. What are the circumstances that made the case a risk management one? Evaluate if the situation meets negligence criteria. Why? Malpractice criteria. Why?

2. Describe a utilization management case that resulted in denial of treatment. Was the denial based on negligent or inappropriate utilization review practice? What could you have done in this case to prevent a negligent utilization review?

3. Share a situation where you were involved in a medical record review where documentation was incomplete or subjective. What could you do to remedy the situation?

4. What can you do to safeguard a patient's privacy and confidentiality? How can you handle a situation where a patient does not want the family to know his or her diagnosis and the family is asking for the diagnosis and the prognosis?

5. You were preparing a patient's discharge and suddenly you got a call from the payor-based case manager denying the transfer of the patient to a subacute care facility. How would you handle the situation?

6. You arrived at work one morning and found during report that one of the patients you were case managing had been intubated despite the fact that it was clear in the patient's living will or advance directives that the patient did not desire such intervention. What would you do? How would you go about disclosing the situation to the patient's healthcare proxy? What are the legal implications of such an act?

7. While you were discussing the surgical procedure with the patient and the family, you found out that the patient had signed the consent without a clear understanding of the procedure, the risks and benefits, or the postsurgical care. What would you do? You informed the surgeon of the situation and the surgeon dismissed it, claiming that he explained everything to the patient already. How would you handle such a response?

▶ REFERENCES

American Association of Colleges of Nursing. (1999). *Position statement: Violence as a public health problem.* Washington, DC: Author.

American Nurses Association. (2015). *Code of Ethics for Nurses with Interpretive Statements.* Silver Spring, MD: American Nurses Association.

Andrews, M., Goldberg, K., & Kaplan, H. (Eds.). (1996). *Nurse's legal handbook* (3rd ed.). Springhouse, PA: Springhouse Corp.

Banja, J. (1998). Advance directives and the do-not-resuscitate order. *The Case Manager, 9*(2), 30–33.

Bosek, M. S. D., & Fitzpatrick, J. (1992). A nursing perspective on advance directives. *Medsurg Nursing, 1*(1), 33–38.

Case Management Society of America. (2016). *Standards of practice for case management.* Little Rock, AR: Author.

Commission for Case Manager Certification. (2015). *Code of professional conduct for case manager with disciplinary rules, procedures and penalties.* Retrieved from http://www.ccmcertification.org/

Compassion & Choices. (2017). *End-of-Life Info Center.* Retrieved from https://www.compassionandchoices.org/

Cornell University Law School. (2017). *Negligence.* Retrieved from Legal Information Institute: https://www.law.cornell.edu/wex/negligence

Employee Retirement Income Security Act. (n.d.). *E-tools, compliance information and a wealth of related links and information.* Retrieved from http://www.dol.gov/compliance/laws/comp-erisa.htm

Feutz-Harter, S. A. (1991). *Nursing and the law.* Eau Claire, WI: Professional Education Systems Inc.

Franklin County Probate Court, State of Ohio. (1998). *Living will declaration, 1998.* [Online]. Retrieved May 2, 2009, from http://www.franklincountyohio.gov/probate/PDF/Living_Will_Only.pdf

Gammage & Burham. (1997). *Legal issues surrounding managed care and case management.* Phoenix, AZ: Author.

Jacob, W. (2016). Retail clinics: Bringing health care to the neighborhood. *Professional Case Management, 21*(5), 260–262.

The Joint Commission on Accreditation of Healthcare Organizations. (1985). *Accreditation manual for hospitals* (pp. 98–99). Oakbrook, IL: Author.

Keeton, W., Dobbs, D., Keeton, R., & Owne, D. (1984). *Prosser and Keeton on torts. Student handbook* (5th ed., §§ 1–4). St. Paul, MN: West Publishing Co.

McKesson. (2017). *InterQual: Evidence-based clinical criteria.* Retrieved from McKesson.com: http://www.mckesson.com/health-plans/decision-management/decision-management-interqual/interqual

Mellette, P., & Kurtz, J. (1993, May). Corcoran v. United Healthcare, Inc., Liability of utilization review companies in light of ERISA. *Journal of Health & Hospitals Law, 26*(5), 129–132, 160.

Muller, L. S. (2008). Power of attorney and guardianship: What we think we know. *Professional Case Management,* 169–172.

Muller, L. S. (2014). A case management briefing on domestic violence. *Professional Case Management, 19*(5), 237–240.

Muller, L. S. (2016). Engaging the LGBT patient: medical/legal landscape. *Professional Case Management, 21*(3), 149–153.

Muller, L. S. (2017). Legal Considerations in Case Management, chapter 20. In Tahan, H. & Treiger, T. (Eds.), *2017, CMSA core curriculum for case management* (3rd ed.). Philadelphia, PA: Wolters Kluwer.

Muller, L. S., & Fink-Samnick, E. (2015). Mandatory reporting: Let's clear up the confusion. *Professional case management, 20*(4), 199–203.

New Jersey Hospital Association. (2017, October). *Health Care Professional Responsibility Reporting Enhancement Act (HCPRREA), Frequently Asked Questions (FAQs).* Retrieved from http://www.njha.com/media/475927/EDU-1786-Cullen-RegsQAOct-2017.pdf

NORC at the University of Chicago. (2012, June). *Case study report: Patient provider Telehealth Network—Using Telehealth to manage chronic disease.* Retrieved from HealthIT.Gov: https://www.healthit.gov/sites/default/files/pdf/RCCHCandPHS_CaseStudy.pdf

Obergefell v. Hodges, 576 U.S. 11. The Supreme Court of the United States (SCOTUS). (2015, June 26). Obergefell et al. v. Hodges, Director, Ohio Department of Health et al. Certiorari to the United States Court of Appeals for the Sixth Circuit, No. 14–556. Argued April 28, 2015—Decided June 26, 2015. Retrieved July 11, 2017, from https://www.supremecourt.gov/opinions/14pdf/14-556_3204.pdf

Ovando, L., & Thies, L. (1997). Emerging liability risks. *Case Review, 3*(3), 68–73.

Perin, R. L. (1992). *Arizona statutes affecting nursing practice.* Eau Claire, WI: Professional Education Systems Inc.

Powell, S., & Tahan, H. (2008). *CMSA's core curriculum for case management* (2nd ed.). Philadelphia, PA: Lippincott Williams & Wilkins.

Robbins, D. (1998). *Integrating manage care and ethics.* New York, NY: McGraw-Hill.

Skehan, J., & Muller, L. S. (2016). Reducing Disparities in the LGBT Community. *Professional Case Management, 21*(3), 156–160.

Stoppler, M. C. (2016, August 30). Autopsy. Retrieved from Web MD: http://www.medicinenet.com/autopsy/page5.htm

Sturgeon, S. (1997). Legal risks in the operation of referral and utilization review systems. *Managed Care Interface, 10*(12), 66–70.

Tahan, H., & Treiger, T. (2017). CMSA Core Curriculum for Case Management (3rd ed.). Philadelphia, PA: Wolters Kluwer.

Texas BON. (n.d.). FAQs Nursing Practice. Retrieved 2017, from Texas State Board of Nursing: https://www.bon.texas.gov/faq_nursing_practice.asp#t15

Transplant Speakers International, Inc. (n.d.). *4.20-27.2008 UNOS.* Retrieved from www.transplant-speakers.org

United Network for Organ Sharing. (2008). *Donate Life America.* [Online]. Retrieved April 27, 2008, from http://www.unos.org/news/myths.asp

United Network for Organ Sharing. (2009). Waiting list conditions. [Online]. Retrieved May 1, 2009, from http://www.unos.org.

CHAPTER 9

Ethical Principles in Case Management Practice

"The pessimist complains about the wind; The optimist expects it to change; The realist adjusts the sails."

WILLIAM ARTHUR WARD

LEARNING OBJECTIVES

Upon completion of this chapter, the reader will be able to:

1. Describe the process of ethical decision making.
2. Recognize ethical dilemmas in case management practice.
3. List four ethical principles important to case management practice.
4. Differentiate between clinical, organizational, personal, and professional ethics.
5. Identify five strategies for the effective management of ethical dilemmas.
6. Explain the role of the case manager in patient advocacy.

ESSENTIAL TERMS

Advance Directives • Advocacy • Assisted Suicide • Bill of Right • Clinical Ethics • Code of Ethics • Code of Professional Conduct for Case Managers • Ethical Decision Making • Ethical Dilemma • Ethics • Ethics Committee • Gag Orders • Gatekeeping • Guide for the Uncertain in Decision-Making Ethics (GUIDE) • Medical Necessity • Organizational Ethics • Patient Advocate • Patient Self-Determination Act of 1990 • Personal Ethics • Professional Ethics • Rationing of Healthcare • Standards of Professional Performance • Unnecessary Treatment • Withdrawing Treatment • Withholding Treatment

Like a fork in the road, managed care intersects with the scarcity of resources, over 25 million uninsured Americans, and 76 million well-informed baby boomers who are on the verge of turning 65 years of age. This is certainly fodder for complexity and ethical dilemmas. Ethical issues shift as society, technology, social media digital tools, and professional practice patterns change. Step back in time to 1950. Few of the prominent ethical issues of today were discussed then: abortion, euthanasia (assisted suicide), genetic experimentation, or rationing of healthcare. At the time, genetic research was not advanced far enough to cause major concern, and healthcare was basic enough—with little high-tech equipment—to be affordable. Healthcare decisions were made almost exclusively by physicians. For example, the 1950 American Nurses Association (ANA) code of ethics stated that a nurse's obligation was to carry out the physician's orders and to protect the physician's reputation (Wright, 1987). This code left little motivation for a nurse to assess an ethical dilemma concerning a physician's poor treatment choices or practice patterns, if it were to come

up. Case managers today cannot run away from dealing with these issues—in fact, addressing ethical issues is part of the case manager's job description and responsibilities. Professional life in olden days appeared more clear-cut than it does now, but not necessarily more ethical.

A relationship between law and ethics clearly exists; however, the relationship is often nebulous. We know there is a relationship, although sometimes it is difficult to say whether an issue is mostly legal or mostly ethical. But what experienced case managers have found out is that the bridge between the two issues is patient advocacy. This is a key element to remember when ethical dilemmas arise. Delivering care (including making decisions about what treatments should be implemented) that is patient-family-centered is the best way to avoid or prevent ethical concerns.

Ethics in healthcare is about choices, morals, and the basic rights of free choice, self-determination, independence, and autonomy. Ethical dilemmas arise in situations where the ethically correct course of action is unclear, such as when one is not certain about which ethical principle to apply or when multiple ethical principles are in conflict. Ethical dilemmas are challenging; one must select a course of action, whereas in most cases there is more than one choice available. Often each choice holds a potential for an undesirable outcome. Case managers are frequently confronted with ethical dilemmas during the course of a day's work. Each such dilemma can present a new twist. Like the turn of a kaleidoscope, each case necessitates a new perspective on the issue. The perspective we see is also influenced by our values, beliefs, and morals, both personal and professional; these are what shape our choices, helping to resolve conflict and come to a point of resolution.

Each case manager has a portfolio of ethical issues and dilemmas. Some are generic, others are similar, and still others are situation specific. A case manager who works in the neonatal intensive care unit grapples with issues that are different from those of a pediatric case manager, an oncology case manager, or a rehabilitation case manager. Following are some classic examples:

▶ A family member will not consent to do not resuscitate status for a patient. The patient has multisystem failure, and a Code Blue (cardio-pulmonary arrest) is imminent. The code occurs, the patient survives, and the rest of the story is a "nightmare." This scenario has been played out in thousands of hospitals.

▶ A patient, mentally competent to make decisions, insists on being discharged home—to a clearly unsafe situation. He has the right to self-determination and you know well that the home environment will jeopardize his health condition.

▶ A woman patient reveals her dread of being discharged because she will return to witness serious abuse perpetrated by her husband on their young daughter. She has told you to keep this secret. What about confidentiality? What about the legal aspect? Isn't child abuse a reportable event? Can you put aside the judgment about a mother failing to protect her child? A choice—to tell or not to tell—must be made in this case.

▶ A husband makes it clear that he does not want to be placed on a respirator. His medical condition destabilizes and he becomes unconscious, but his wife insists on intubation.

▶ A patient with a medical condition incompatible with pregnancy refuses to have an abortion. Her condition deteriorates daily. In the seventh month, the baby dies in utero. Two days later, the mother dies.

▶ A 75-year-old man had cardiac bypass surgery in 1983 that necessitated several blood transfusions. He is admitted with a perplexing diagnosis. Tests show that he is positive for the HIV virus and has full-blown AIDS. He wants to know what is wrong, but his wife insists that no one tell him the diagnosis.

Some ethical dilemmas end up in the courtroom and often are the theme on which future laws are made. Even court decisions may leave more ethical challenges than the original case appeared to have. They may resolve some aspects but do not always solve all the aspects or the original dilemma. Consider the classical case of Nancy Cruzan, whose parents were aware of her wishes about not wanting to remain in a persistent vegetative state. Still, they waited several years, from 1983 to 1990, for her to regain even basic awareness of the world. When the parents finally asked the courts to allow withdrawal of artificial food and hydration, the court ruled that there was no clear and convincing evidence of Nancy's desires (Kolodner, 1992). Nancy *telling* her family and friends that she would never want to be a "vegetable" was not enough. Similar cases arise even today.

Other cases never make it to the courtroom but have overtones that are more ominous. In Chicago, when a father's pleas to have his brain-dead child removed from the ventilator were met with hospital insistence that he obtain a court order, he held the medical staff at gunpoint and discontinued the ventilator himself (Fiesta, 1992).

These two heartbreaking cases did not go by unnoticed and without consequence. The impact of Nancy Cruzan's case resulted in the Patient Self-Determination Act of 1990 (Kolodner, 1992). Every patient in every hospital in America is affected by this. Had Nancy written her own advance directive, no court would have questioned her wishes. The impact in the second case is more subtle, but the message is clear. Should we hold human beings on the threshold of death just because we have the technology to do so? Fewer hospitals are now resisting removal from life support if the family agrees to it when a patient is declared brain dead.

As case managers, we play important roles in helping the patient and the family understand what advance directives are all about and the choices concerning them. We are often privy to verbal statements about "no heroic measures," but without written, signed documents, the patient's wishes may go unfulfilled. Advance directives are about a patient making his or her own life choices. Explaining these important documents and helping to explore feelings about these life-directing decisions and life (or death) goals may be important advocacy roles. Remember that advance directives, including healthcare proxy, are of great help in situations like this. Documenting the individual's wishes when he or she is alert and competent is important in preventing situations similar to Nancy's and her family's.

▶ WITHHOLDING AND WITHDRAWING CARE

Both of the preceding cases brought up the dilemma of withdrawing some treatment that the patient was receiving: food and hydration in one case and respiratory support in the other. Withholding and withdrawing some aspect of care is a recurrent theme in many ethical dilemmas and is the reason for much debate, both ethically and legally.

The public values on withdrawing or withholding treatment have changed throughout the years. From 1976 to 1991, when conflicts over these issues landed in court, almost every family wanted the treatment stopped or not started. Then, partially because of mistrust of the intentions of managed care (and the large amount of negative press about underutilization of services), conflicts arose that turned the attention to fighting for healthcare and demanding "everything be done" for the patient. Medical Ethicist John Banja tells of a case not uncommon during that period. An elderly woman with a long history of chronic obstructive pulmonary disease was admitted to the hospital in critical condition. In the next 2 days, she also suffered two myocardial infarctions and a major stroke; the stroke left her with a silent electroencephalogram. When the family was approached by the pulmonologist, who protested the family's wishes that she be ventilated and kept in the intensive care unit, the son pointed a finger at the physician saying, "If Momma dies, you die" (Banja, 1996, p. 37).

In 1983, the President's Commission for the Study of Ethical Problems in Medicine and Biomedical and Behavioral Research discussed the withdrawing and withholding of treatment as follows:

▶ The distinction between failing to initiate and stopping therapy—that is, withholding versus withdrawing treatment—is not itself of moral importance. A justification that is adequate for not commencing a treatment is also sufficient for ceasing it (President's Commission, 1983).
▶ The last sentence, written in 1983, has caught on. However, these are ethical recommendations—not legal precedents—and they lead to further questions. Is withdrawing or withholding life-saving treatment a form of assisted suicide? Is there a difference between actively causing death (withdrawing) and allowing it to occur by not intervening (withholding)? Asking tough questions can lead to a resolution that lies somewhere between right and wrong, yet it is neither—it is merely a best choice, hopefully made in good faith.

As in the Nancy Cruzan case, withholding or withdrawing nutrition and hydration is still being debated, and people belonging to the legal and medical professions often have differing viewpoints on this issue. Case managers play a pivotal role in helping patients and their families clarify and articulate their views in cases that are difficult to deal with. Many medical conditions lend themselves to an inability to feed a patient orally. Often the placement of a permanent feeding tube is a very difficult decision for a family to make, even if the patient is alert.

One case involved an 84-year-old nursing home resident who came in with pneumonia (probably aspiration pneumonia) and complaints that he was hungry. He was alert but very confused and managed to pull out every line the physicians and nurses could get into him. Because he had a recent history of several bouts of pneumonia, a modified barium swallow was performed to evaluate his swallowing ability. The results showed a high probability for aspiration if fed orally, so the recommendation was for placement of a permanent feeding tube.

The patient's daughter was distressed by this option. Unquestionably caring, she did not want to prolong her father's life "in this state." The case manager discussed with her the fact that although her father was frail, he was not showing signs of impending death. He had no end-stage organ diseases, and his vital signs were stable. In addition, he was communicating to the facility staff that he was hungry. After much deliberation the daughter agreed to the feeding tube. What if this patient had been imminently dying? Would not feeding him be ethically appropriate? What about hydration with IV fluids? Is this a form of withholding life support?

Leah Curtin has stressed the distinction between withdrawal of life support and withdrawal of nutritional support: "It is one thing to decide not to resuscitate a terminally ill patient, it is quite another to starve a person to death whether or not he has some hope for survival" (Curtin, 1994, p. 14). To lump the question of withdrawal of nutritional support under the same classification as the withdrawal of medical life support measures confuses the issue (Curtin, 1994). The aforementioned patient died suddenly and unpredictably soon after the insertion of the feeding tube, but the decision was sound for this set of circumstances.

Suppose death is imminent. Whether to initiate feeding depends on the patient's medical and mental condition as well the cultural values, beliefs, interests, and social support system. Simple hydration may be appropriate in some cases. A more alert patient should be able to choose. Consider this aspect.

In the face of inevitable death from some other source, nutrition is used to provide comfort—not to sustain life. Any means of feeding that produces more discomfort than comfort can be eliminated from an ethical perspective. In some cases, the patient can tell us clearly what he or she wants. In other cases, we must rely on our own assessment and judgments. In all cases, the goal is comfort, not adequate nutrition (Curtin, 1994, p. 15).

▶ ETHICS COMMITTEES

The kaleidoscope turns. Look at another case about nutritional dilemmas, similar to the last case but with a different perspective, which required the assistance of an ethics committee.

Mrs. Norris is a 79-year-old patient most recently hospitalized for pneumonia (probable aspiration pneumonia). Her medical history includes a cholecystectomy, hysterectomy, several surgeries for metastatic intestinal cancer (including resections for small bowel obstructions), multiple strokes, congestive heart failure, end-stage cardiomyopathy, and most recently, frequent bouts of pneumonia. Mrs. Norris was alert and oriented until 1 year ago. At that time she filled out an advance directives form stating her wishes not to be kept alive through artificial measures; this specified and included intubation and mechanical ventilation, food, and hydration as artificial measures that she did not want if her condition became irreversible and her quality of life was poor. After signing her wishes, a series of strokes occurred. Mrs. Norris is now cognitively poorly responsive. She opens her eyes and has reflexes, but does not respond meaningfully. Her present bout of pneumonia is clearing up. Swallowing studies confirmed that Mrs. Norris has severe esophageal reflux and is a fit candidate for further aspiration pneumonia if fed orally. Nasal feeding tubes have been unsuccessful because they have been coughed up or repeatedly pulled out. Because of multiple intestinal resections, complicated by severe esophageal reflux, a permanent feeding tube could be a rather tricky procedure requiring general anesthesia. The medical team is leaning toward comfort care measures only. Mrs. Norris is an extremely poor surgical risk, but attempts at feeding her without an intestinal feeding tube could lead to further aspiration pneumonia, which could also cause her demise.

Mrs. Norris's daughter Marion is furious with the doctors' suggestions of comfort care and states, "If you let my mother starve to death, I'll sue you!" No other family member voiced an opinion.

▶ Case Discussion

This case leaves several options open for the medical team:

- ▶ Opt for comfort care only on the guidance of the family's own judgment and Mrs. Norris's advance directives.
- ▶ Call for a family (case) conference with the interdisciplinary healthcare team, including the case manager, social worker, and perhaps a patient advocate.
- ▶ Attempt a feeding tube.
- ▶ Ask for judicial intervention.
- ▶ Ask the institution's ethics committee for assistance.

For the purposes of illustration, let us say that the last option was chosen, that is, calling the ethics committee for assistance. Almost all institutions today have organized ethics committees to guide them and their healthcare professionals (including case managers) through the quandary of ethical decision making and problem resolution. The core membership of these committees may include physicians, nurses, administrators, clergy/pastoral care,

an attorney, a case manager, a social worker, an ethicist, and a patient advocate. Today, case managers and social workers are common active participants—in fact, they often coordinate the ethics committee meeting when one is needed. At times, these committees appear to have some kind of magical ethical compass.

First, the ethics committee needs the medical facts, including a medical history, the present status of the patient, the plan of care (case plan), the psychosocial support situation, and a realistic prognosis. All possible treatment options and alternatives are then explored, including the possible outcomes for each modality. Brainstorming for unthought-of treatment alternatives may occur in the hopes that another answer may relieve the ethical dilemma. A psychosocial assessment is also pertinent. Often conflicting morals and values of family members are a main cause of ethical problems. In the case of Mrs. Norris, the patient's directions were challenged by the daughter, and the physician's attempts at explanations did not seem to clarify the medical problems and concerns. Mrs. Norris was not in a condition that would allow her to speak for herself.

When dealing with ethical dilemmas, it is important to distill any legal issues. In Mrs. Norris's case, the advance directives form was an important document to consider. Nevertheless, judicial resolution has its consequences: it is expensive; it is time-consuming, which can disrupt patient care; it can cause a strained relationship between the medical team and the surrogate decision makers; and it can turn a private matter into a media circus. Treading carefully is wise when dealing with sensitive and ethical issues. Fortunately, today copies of healthcare proxies and/or advance directives are being kept in the patients' medical records for ease of access in various settings across the continuum of care and over time than traditionally has been the case. Often these documents are scanned and stored electronically in the electronic medical records.

Next, the ethics committee may apply various ethical decision-making "tools." The following are six examples case managers must become familiar with and use when needed.

1. Use of various schools and theories of ethical thought, which may help bring the case to a point of resolution. (Although this chapter will not analyze the various theories, several excellent books have been written on the subject. Additional resources are available on the Internet.)
2. Some feel it is important to use humor to gain or maintain a sense of perspective. Care must be taken not to "make fun" of the situation at the expense of anyone, especially the patient and/or the family. However, a moment of shared laughter did occur when one of Marion's sisters quipped, "That Marion, even as a child she had trouble following Mom's directions!"
3. Consider contemporary thought on a particular issue. Expert opinions about withholding, or

withdrawing, artificial food and hydration are as follows:

▶ *Unconscious, imminently dying patient (progressive and rapid deterioration)*: The dying process will (most likely) not be reversed, and therefore, nutrition and hydration are an unreasonable burden.

▶ *Conscious, imminently dying patient*: The patient is conscious and can make the decision, but artificial nutrition and hydration may be an unreasonable burden.

▶ *Conscious, irreversibly ill, not imminently dying patient*: Again, the patient can ultimately decide because he or she is conscious. The disease process may not be reversible or curable, but nutrition and hydration to sustain life are useful. As long as the patient wants it and does not feel it is an unreasonable burden, then it has use.

▶ *Unconscious, nondying patient*: Nutrition and hydration should be supplied to this type of patient. In this case, if no provisions were made to feed and hydrate the patient, the physician could be a party to starving the patient to death. Unless there are other indications to the contrary, nutrition and hydration are not an unreasonable burden and are justifiable.

4. Use effective communication skills. The art of listening and well-placed questioning punctuated with a caring and empathetic attitude can often defuse difficult situations.

5. Use honesty. It has been said that, "Ethics is honesty in action." This basic human value is especially important in the final stage—deciding on recommendations. These recommendations will be born out of all the tools, personal values and morals, and judgments of the committee.

6. Balance the various opinions and perspectives associated with the ethical situation being dealt with. Know your own values. Know the patient's/family's values. Know your organization's policies and any laws that apply to the situation. Balance the three. Always remember, it is not about your values and belief system, it is about the patient and the family. Maintain your professional presence and nonjudgmental attitude at all times.

▶ Patient, Personal, Professional, Clinical, or Organizational Ethical Dilemmas

Case managers increasingly face ethical issues that are either clinical in nature, encompassing the medical and treatment needs of patients (e.g., dealing with end-of-life concerns such as in the case of Mrs. Morris); financial (e.g., concerns of the uninsured who also require an expensive treatment, or denials of services by health insurance companies); conflict

between the patient and the family regarding the desired course of action; or conflict between patient/family and the healthcare team about the best treatment option. When faced with any of these issues, it is best for case managers to understand the facts and views of the various parties involved; gather all necessary and relevant information; identify the key dilemma(s); and seek the advice of supervisors and/or the ethicist in the organization regarding the course of action. It is customary today for healthcare organizations to have a designated individual ethics expert or an ethics committee the case manager can defer to for assistance in resolving an ethical dilemma.

Oftentimes, case managers are dealing with ethical dilemmas that involve a challenge of balancing the needs and interests of patients and their families and those imposed by the healthcare organization and the insurance company (i.e., the payor). These situations contribute to organizational ethical dilemmas. When case managers communicate to patients and/or their families the decisions of insurance companies denying certain services and treatments (e.g., an extended length of hospital stay, surgical procedure not requiring inpatient stay, postdischarge services such as home care, or transfer to an acute rehabilitation facility), case managers are perceived by the patients and/or families to be taking the side of the organization or the payor. As a result, case managers may be perceived as being more concerned with cost than the quality of care and therefore no longer are viewed as patient advocates. Issues of distrust and lack of confidence arise and complicate the situation. Such issues have led to a new type of ethical dilemma that was absent when managed care organizations were unpopular or uncommon. Ethical issues today are no longer limited to those that are clinical or medical in nature; therefore, healthcare organizations have implemented the use of organizational ethics committees in addition to the traditional clinical ethics committees.

Case managers must be aware of the difference between a clinical and an organizational ethical issue. They should also know when to seek advice from a clinical ethics committee and when it is necessary to involve the organizational ethics committee (Display 9-1). To clarify the difference, generally speaking, one may describe the main focus of clinical ethics committees as dealing with decisions regarding treatment options or the patient's right to withdrawing treatment such as in the case of terminal/end-of-life care. Organizational ethics committees, however, focus on utilization management issues, including resource allocation, delays in care (or system variance management), and appropriateness of the level of care. Other organizational ethics issues may deal with things that are not specific to an individual patient care situation such as false advertisement of outcomes of a certain treatment modality, public disclosure of errors, and business practices concerning vendors of pharmaceuticals and medical device companies.

MAIN DIFFERENCE BETWEEN CLINICAL AND ORGANIZATIONAL ETHICS

One main difference between clinical and organizational ethics committees relates to the type of experts needed as members.

▶ Clinical ethics committees include members who are experts in clinical care issues including end-of-life care.

▶ Organizational ethics committees include members who are experts in utilization review and management, reimbursement methods, codes of professional conduct, and corporate compliance.

Personal and professional ethics relate to the case manager's professional conduct and representation of personal experience to others, including the recipients of healthcare services. Personal ethics refers to the motivation and innate nature of the case manager to act in an ethical manner—a way that demonstrates adherence to all the common ethical principles, particularly veracity, fidelity, and justice. Often personal ethical dilemmas arise when the personal belief and the value system of the case manager supersede those of the patient/family or fellow healthcare professionals. The case manager must always approach any situation when caring for a patient or interacting with fellow healthcare professionals with respect, transparency, authenticity, and acceptance of others. Such context is usually free of judgment and places the others involved at ease and feeling content.

Professional ethics, on the other hand, is acting according to the expectations of one's profession (e.g., knowledge, skills, competencies, and standards) and maintaining acceptable professional conduct (e.g., ensuring active license to practice and behaving within the authority granted on the basis of the scope of practice). Case managers must demonstrate consistent professional conduct, adhere to corporate compliance standards, and uphold the patient's interest as the priority of care delivery and decision making, especially when ethical dilemmas arise. Case managers may refer to the codes of professional conduct defined by their employers (i.e., place of work through human resource policies), professional associations (e.g., the ANA or National Association of Social Workers [NASWs]), and health discipline (e.g., pharmacy, physical therapy) for more information about such codes and the expectations of professional conduct.

▶ ETHICAL DECISION MAKING

Ethical decision making is an essential skill every case manager must have and be comfortable with. It is the process of evaluating and choosing among alternate solutions about how best to deal with a situation in a manner that respects and adheres to ethical principles, professional conduct, and ethical practice. As a rule of thumb, approach the issue at hand with *patient (and family or caregiver) advocacy* as the top priority. An effective strategy you may apply to help ensure the effectiveness of your approach to ethical conduct and patient advocacy is *always start with eliminating from the potential actions what seems to you as unethical options and select the best ethical alternative(s)*. This approach builds a trusting relationship between the patient/family and the case manager. It also demonstrates the values of successful relationships including respect, responsibility, accountability, patient-centeredness, fairness, equity, compassion, caring, empathy, and acceptance.

The process of making ethical decisions requires four core behaviors of the case manager. These are:

1. *Patient- (and family)-focus*: the deliberate acts of placing the patient (and the patient's family) at the center of the process, accepting the patient as a unique individual (who the patient is including culture, values, beliefs, preferences, and care goals), and ensuring the patient makes informed decisions.
2. *Commitment*: the desire to do the right thing regardless of the complexity or uniqueness of the situation, the intensity of the potentially required resources, and the cost implications, if any.
3. *Consciousness*: awareness and intentionality to apply moral convictions, act in a consistent manner daily, and exhibit behaviors that are free of doubt, concern, or suspicion.
4. *Competency*: the ability to gather and evaluate essential information; develop alternatives, foresee potential advantages, consequences, and risks; and act in a manner that is void of judgment and establishes trusting relationships.

It is also important for case managers to think about the choices they make, or assist their patients to make, in terms of the impact of these decisions on meeting the desired goals; that is, in terms of the ability of these choices to accomplish expectations, contribute to the drawing of distinctions between competing options, and to effect desirable patient care outcomes (Display 9-2).

The case manager can also use the aspects of the case management process to further examine a situation; these are: assessment and problem identification, planning, implementation, and evaluation.

1. Assessment and Problem Identification
   ▶ Gather all the facts, opinions, and perceptions about the situation.
   ▶ Identify key players and their roles, responsibilities, and decision-making abilities.
   ▶ Identify available resources: ethics committees, chaplain, clergy, rabbi, policies, laws, patient advocates, and so on.
   ▶ Identify the problem(s), conflict(s), disagreement(s), or issue(s) to be addressed.

STRATEGIES FOR EFFECTIVE ETHICAL DECISION MAKING

Strategies	Highlights

Pause and think	▶ Help ground the decisions in the context of the patient preference: what is most important for the patient/family.
	▶ A thoughtful and patient-centered approach:
	  ● Prevents rushed decisions,
	  ● Prepares those involved for thoughtful discernment of the issue and possible solutions,
	  ● Facilitates the making of informed decisions, and
	  ● Allows for the deliberate mobilization of resources on the basis of a well-thought-out course of action.

Identify the top priority and goal	▶ Before you brainstorm options and alternate solutions, take the time first and seek to clarify what seems to be the top priority for the patient/family and the desired outcome. ▶ The patient's priority may not be exactly one the healthcare team identified. Reconcile the differences. ▶ Determine how a present gap affects the situation of concern including the care goals and preferences. ▶ Remember that one of the great risks is that the decision you make may fulfill immediate desires or needs, but may not be appropriate for long-term goals. ▶ Seek inputs from the patient, family, and healthcare team.
Gather relevant information	▶ Gather the facts. ▶ Be sure you have adequate information to support each choice; what is most relevant to the situation and important for patient/family. ▶ To access the necessary information and determine the relevant facts, focus on what you need to know first, then move on and secure other relevant information. ▶ Organize the order of the information needed and when to seek the various needed information. This helps you move smoother through the decision-making process. ▶ Be prepared for additional information and to verify assumptions and seek clarification of other uncertain information. ▶ As you move in a systematic manner in information gathering, consider the reliability and credibility of the people providing the information. Honesty, transparency, and accuracy are essential.
Brainstorm options and potential solutions	▶ Once you are sure of the desired purpose, outcomes, and potential course of action, affirm what you want to achieve, and use your best judgment to decide on the relevant necessary facts. ▶ Make a list of actions you can take to accomplish your goal. Talk to someone you trust so you can broaden your perspective and think of new choices; for example, an ethicist. ▶ Remember, if you can think of only one or two choices and potential solutions, you're probably not thinking hard enough. ▶ Engage in divergent thinking at this stage; this brings about more alternate solutions than probably warranted. ▶ Identify options that will treat everyone equally and adhere to the core ethical principles. ▶ Seek inputs from the patient, family, and healthcare team.
Consider the consequences and the likelihood of resolution	▶ Screen your choices to determine if any of the options may potentially violate any core ethical values; eliminate any unethical options. ▶ Identify who will be affected by the decision and how the decision is likely to affect them. ▶ Examine each brainstormed solution and determine its potential benefits, disadvantages, associated risk or harm, and feasibility of execution. ▶ Choose the potential solutions with the least disadvantages and risks, best opportunity for accomplishing the desired outcomes, and increased ease of execution (feasibility). ▶ Remember to always confer with the patient and the family, not just with the healthcare team.
Choose priority actions	▶ Take the time and rank-order the solutions starting with the one most likely to resolve the situation first. ▶ Make decisions; take actions. ▶ If you are uncomfortable about a choice or feel unclear about something, discuss with those whose judgment you respect, such as an ethicist. ▶ Think about your degree of comfort with each of the choices. ▶ Seek inputs from the patient, family, and the healthcare team.

display 9-2

STRATEGIES FOR EFFECTIVE ETHICAL DECISION MAKING (continued)

Strategies	Highlights
Apply the ethics "rule of thumb"	▶ Keep your promises. ▶ Maintain the rule of thumb: "patient advocacy above all" as you work through the situation. ▶ Ensure your actions advance what is in the best interest of the patient and the family; ensure they meet the patient/family needs and preferences. ▶ Execute with the greatest care and attention to the concerns of all stakeholders.
Seek feedback	▶ Seek inputs from the patient, family, and the healthcare team. ▶ Seek the opinion of an expert ethicist.
Monitor outcomes and modify approach as necessary	▶ As an ethical decision maker, monitor the effects of your choices and actions. ▶ Examine the ethical implications of your actions; ensure they adhere to the core ethical principles. ▶ Modify your approach or actions if your choices are not producing the intended results, meeting the goals, and achieving the purpose. ▶ Modify your approach or actions if your choices are causing unintended and undesirable consequences. ▶ Reassess the situation and progress. ▶ Determine when it is appropriate to conclude your efforts and put things to closure.

▶ Be a patient advocate. Assist decision makers in a clarification of their own values and what constitutes quality of life, priorities, freedom, and dignity.

▶ Determine the patient's/family's interests, preferences, desires, and care goals. Incorporate these in the plan of care, treatments, and interventions.

2. Planning

▶ Identify the types of moral dilemmas that are involved, such as autonomy, self-determination, impartiality, justice, confidentiality, or veracity.

▶ Identify possible courses of action, along with their potential risks and benefits. Be proactive and have more than one plan/approach for consideration.

▶ List goals and objectives of the people involved in the situation; then assign priorities to the list.

▶ Determine the ethical obligations of those involved and the ultimate goal(s).

3. Implementation

▶ Develop an ethical goal that maximizes the most benefits and good in the situation. Do this collaboratively with the key people involved and ethics experts.

▶ Determine the course of action that will produce results most like the ethical ideal.

▶ Determine if that course of action violates legal or ethical principles. If it does, change or modify the actions.

▶ Implement the plan.

4. Evaluation

▶ Do the results bring the situation closer to the ethical ideal?

▶ Do the outcomes satisfy the parties involved, especially the patient and the family?

▶ If not, have any new moral dilemmas been created?

▶ If necessary, go back to the assessment phase, revise your plan, and attempt again to resolve additional moral dilemmas.

▶ Conduct regular reassessments of the patient/family and the situation. Modify plans according to the assessment findings and changing needs.

Resolving ethical dilemmas requires a shared decision-making approach. This is even more so because the context of the case manager's role is an interdependent one and case management outcomes are best realized in a team-based approach to care planning and management. The traditional approach of individualistic ethical decision making, therefore, no longer achieves the best possible outcomes. As stated earlier, with increased availability of managed care health plans, the ethical dilemmas case managers commonly encounter in their practice are of an "organizational ethics" nature. Those are best resolved applying a deliberative framework that focuses on two main components (Jansen, 2003):

1. Shared decision making is necessary to arrive at decisions that satisfy all parties directly or indirectly involved in the ethical dilemma being addressed (patient/family, provider, organization, and payor). It emphasizes that all affected parties are given the opportunity to express their views and interests and ultimately participate in making the final decision. Participants must also view each other as equal deliberative partners and avoid thinking

in hierarchical terms or use the influence of their positions in the organization. For example, case managers should not always defer to the administrators for the ultimate say about the situation; they should be active and equal contributors to the discussion and decision.

2. The nature and purpose of the deliberation which, as a rule of thumb, should always be the need to reach ethically responsible decisions or solutions that are, and are seen to be, legitimate by the parties involved. This means that participants in the deliberative process should keep open minds, believe it is possible that they will learn something new during deliberations, and anticipate that they may change their minds about the issue at hand.

▶ GUIDE FOR THE UNCERTAIN IN DECISION-MAKING ETHICS

Our present ability to sustain life or to prolong dying process almost indefinitely is the basis for many painful ethical situations. Medical personnel know that a fairly healthy heart plus a ventilator—maybe with the addition of hemodialysis treatments—can keep a human body alive for a long time, even if the brain is fatally damaged. But an increasingly less number of people are seeing the possibility of sustaining life in this manner in a positive light, and today Americans are changing their ideas about issues like prolonging death. In quick succession, both Jacqueline Onassis and Richard Nixon said "no" to futile care that merely postponed the inevitable. Several articles about technology, death, and dying followed. A landmark study found that most dying patients or their families now decide against resuscitation efforts (Knox, 1994) and extreme measures. Even with more public awareness and new attitudes, medical professionals—especially physicians and case managers—are often asked to referee disagreements between the patient/family and the healthcare team. This is a difficult task. Some believe the Guide for the Uncertain in Decision-Making Ethics (GUIDE) (Display 9-3) to be concrete help, especially when an ethics committee is not readily available.

The GUIDE, along with its companion algorithm, takes into consideration advance directives, healthcare

---

display 9-3

GUIDE FOR THE UNCERTAIN IN DECISION-MAKING ETHICS

Scenario	Guidelines
1. Healthcare team favors treatment, patient/family opposed to treatment	▶ Review options carefully to ensure that the patient has a complete understanding of prognosis and treatment options; a competent adult patient has the right to decline medical treatment if he or she has an adequate understanding of information and the risks of not pursuing the recommended treatment. ▶ If the patient has executed an advance directive, it should be reviewed. In Virginia (and in almost all states today) the Health Care Decisions Act provides an optional formal advance directive procedure that can be written or oral and that applies when the patient's death is imminent or the patient is in a persistent vegetative state. ▶ Discussions and patient's decision(s) should be completely documented in a chart in a manner that is objective and free of judgment.

2. Healthcare team favors treatment/patient not competent, family opposed	▶ Need to identify primary decision maker among involved family/significant others.*
	▶ Review information carefully to ensure that family/significant others have a full understanding of the patient's prognosis, condition, and options, and that they can make informed decisions. This should include any advance directives made by the patient.
	▶ If the other family member disagrees with the primary decision maker, see Scenario 5.
	▶ May consult ethics committee.
	• Surrogate decision maker: Virginia law (similar laws are available in other states) recognizes the authority of a surrogate decision maker to make treatment decisions for an individual who is incompetent or incapable of making an informed decision. If the patient previously made an advance directive appointing someone as "agent to make healthcare decisions" for him or her, that individual is empowered as the proxy (equivalent to durable power of attorney for healthcare). In the absence of any advance directive, Virginia law establishes the following order of priority for proxies:
	  a. A legal guardian, if one already had been appointed
	  b. The spouse
	  c. An adult son or daughter
	  d. A parent
	  e. An adult brother or sister
	  f. Any other relative in descending order of blood relationship

GUIDE FOR THE UNCERTAIN IN DECISION-MAKING ETHICS (continued)

Scenario	Guidelines
3. Patient and family in disagreement concerning treatment decisions	▶ An adult patient has the right to refuse or consent to any intervention if he or she has an adequate understanding of all information and is competent to make an informed decision. ▶ The family should be included in all discussions, but the final decision about resuscitation and other interventions is made by the competent adult patient. ▶ Patient should consider an advance directive. ▶ Provision for family support may be needed.
4. Healthcare team does not favor treatment/patient (or family if incompetent patient) does favor treatment.	▶ The healthcare team is not required to undertake interventions that cannot improve the patient's condition. Engage in further conversation with patient/family; ensure that they have received adequate information about the futility of treatment. Reinforce that intervention(s) in question is not being offered because no benefit (either cure or comfort) will accrue. ▶ Encourage or arrange for a second opinion. ▶ Give the patient/family an option to transfer the patient's care to another physician/hospital. ▶ May consult hospital ethics committee and patient advocate.
5. Patient is incompetent/family in disagreement concerning treatment	▶ Attempt to identify primary decision maker (see Scenario 2 for statutory priority). Under Virginia law, if two or more persons of same priority level (e.g., adult children of patient) disagree, the physician may rely on the authorization of a majority. ▶ Every effort should be made to bring the family to agreement. Attempt to have family/significant others focus on what the patient's wishes would be. Ask questions such as: "What would the patient tell us himself if he could speak?" and "Has he ever discussed what he would want if this happened?" Any advance directive made by the patient should be reviewed with the family. ▶ May consult ethics committee and patient advocate.
6. Healthcare team in disagreement concerning treatment (i.e., physician vs. nurse, attending physician vs. medical director)	▶ Attempt to reconcile through discussion and justification of viewpoint. ▶ Seek guidance from chief of service or nurse manager, or follow other appropriate administrative pathways such as chain of command. ▶ If the patient favors treatment, seek second opinion about the appropriateness of treatment. If the treatment is judged to be futile (offering no benefit), see Scenario 4.
7. Healthcare team and family favor treatment/incompetent patient not objecting	▶ See Scenario 2 for guidance. Should identify the primary decision maker, but parties essentially in agreement in this scenario.
8. Healthcare team and family favor treatment/incompetent patient objecting to treatment	▶ Under Virginia law, if an incompetent patient actively refuses treatment, a surrogate decision maker cannot be used without judicial review. This may take the form of seeking the appointment of a legal guardian, or a judicial order allowing involuntary medical treatment. ▶ Contact hospital superintendent, legal advisor, and/or ethics committee.
9. Not clear if (a) the patient is competent and/or (b) the patient is in favor of or opposed to treatment.	▶ Reassessment of the patient's capacity for decision making and/or of patient's preferences by the primary physician. If possible, the source of the patient's ambivalence should be identified. ▶ Psychiatric consultation if competence still unclear or if patient continues to express contradictory preferences. ▶ If still unresolved, consult ethics committee and/or patient advocate.

proxy decision makers, and healthcare teams' preferences in their recommendations (Levenson & Pettrey, 1994). These guidelines contain nine controversial scenarios, each defining key issues and conflicts between the patient/family and the medical team. The recommendations use logically sequenced questions about the patient's competency, advance directives, treatment options, benefits and burdens of the treatment options, patient and family preferences, and patient prognosis. The case manager should be cautioned that this GUIDE and algorithm are not intended to take the place of legal or risk management advisement, nor that of an ethics committee or an ethicist consult. However, it is consistent with applicable laws and good risk management. It should also be noted that it was written in Virginia with its legislation in mind. Similar laws and guidelines are available in other states. Case managers should be knowledgeable of such laws in their own state of practice. As stated in Chapter 8, case managers should also know the statutory regulations pertinent to healthcare in their state, not just those with ethical implications. Finally, the GUIDE is essentially for adult patients and perhaps for legally emancipated adolescents. It remains applicable in today's environment of healthcare delivery.

▶ CODES OF ETHICS

Codes of ethics are established to protect the public interest by guiding professionals about what constitutes ethical conduct and how one can ensure acceptable behavior. Case managers may be held accountable by one (or more) of several codes of ethics depending on the professional background discipline of the case manager (e.g., nursing, social work, medicine, and pharmacy). Examples include the following:

- Nurse case managers (NCMs) must adhere to the *ANA's Code of Ethics* and the *Standards of Professional Performance.*
- Vocational rehabilitation case managers who also hold a Certified Rehabilitation Counselor credential are accountable to the *Commission on Rehabilitation Counselor Certification's Code of Professional Ethics.*
- Every case manager who holds the certified case manager (CCM) credential must also comply with the *Code of Professional Conduct for Case Managers* promulgated by the Commission for Case Manager Certification (CCMC).
- Case managers certified by the American Case Management Association (ACMA) must abide by its *Accredited Case Manager (ACM) Code of Conduct.*
- Social work case managers must adhere to the *NASWs Code of Ethics.*

▶ Statement of Ethical Case Management Practice

The *Statement of Ethical Case Management Practice* is an umbrella statement under which all case managers fall. Although not all case managers have the comfort of an ethics committee to call on when needed, more institutions today are forming these important links to quality healthcare. All case managers have their pet list of ethical doubts and difficulties. The names and faces change, as do some of the medical and psychosocial details, but often the dilemmas have common roots. Realizing the need for ethical support for case managers, the Case Management

Society of America (CMSA) formed an ethics taskforce and created the *Statement of Ethical Case Management Practice* which was published in 1996. This document provides a basis for identifying ethical decision making while maintaining quality of care for patients. Case managers should obtain, read, understand, and apply this document. The document is available at the CMSA's website at http://www.cmsa.org.

The CMSA intended its *statement* to guide the individual case manager "in the development and maintenance of an environment in which case management practice is conducted ethically . . . morality prevails . . . and there is support for right (good) decisions and actions" (CMSA, 1996, p. 1). The CMSA notes that ethics is inherently intertwined with morality. It also explains that because case managers come from diverse health disciplines, they are required to adhere to the code of ethics of their original profession; that is, nursing, social work, and so on. Additionally, the CMSA states that there are five ethical principles that guide the practice of case management (Display 9-4).

Although it never updated its 1996 Statement of Ethical Case Management Practice, the CMSA has continued to promote the importance of ethical conduct of case managers. Ethics as a standard has been included in the CMSA's Standards of Practice for Case Management since their inception, including the most recent 2016 revision. The CMSA emphasizes that the "professional case manager should behave and practice ethically, and adhere to the tenets of the code of ethics that underlie her/his professional credentials (e.g., nursing, social work, and rehabilitation counseling)" (CMSA, 2016, p. 28). The CMSA also explains that case managers demonstrate this standard by adhering to the five basic ethical principles and applying them in their daily practice. Case managers can demonstrate these principles in their practice through the following activities:

- Recognize that the primary obligation is to the patients cared for and their families.
- Engage in and maintain respectful relationships with patients and their families, coworkers, employers, and other professionals.
- Address conflicts that may arise to the best of abilities and/or seek appropriate consultation from experts.
- Treat patients as unique individuals and engage each patient without regard to gender identity or expression; race or ethnicity; national origin and migration background; sex and marital status; age, religion, and political belief; physical, mental, or cognitive disability; other cultural preferences or socioeconomic status.
- Maintain policies that are universally respectful of the integrity and worth of each person.
- Advocate for the patient and the family or the caregiver. Focus on expanding existing or establishing

ETHICAL PRINCIPLES RELEVANT TO CASE MANAGEMENT PRACTICE

Principle	Description	Application in Case Management
Autonomy	Respecting an individual's personal liberty of action (to respect individuals' rights to make their own decisions).	Case managers: ▶ Collaborate with the patient as an autonomous consumer of healthcare services. ▶ Foster and encourage patient's independence and self-determination. ▶ Respect the need for the patient to determine his or her own course of action. ▶ Enhance the patient's ability to choose his or her own plan of care and treatments through informed decisions. ▶ Promote the patient's self-advocacy and self-direction. ▶ Preserve the patient's dignity and worth.
Beneficence	Promoting good for the consumer of healthcare (to do good).	Case managers: ▶ Actively prevent or remove harm. ▶ Further the patient's interests, desires, and preferences for care. ▶ Do not discriminate on the basis of the patient's social or economic status, personal attributes, or the nature of the health problems faced.
Nonmaleficence	Refraining from harming the consumer of healthcare services (to do no harm).	Case managers: ▶ Focus on prevention of medical errors and delays in care. ▶ Ensure patient safety and delivery of quality care and services. ▶ Promote optimal care experience.
Justice	Maintaining a fair approach to care delivery for all (to treat others fairly).	Case managers: ▶ Advocate for appropriate allocation of resources and for the patient's timely access to healthcare services and treatments. ▶ Secure resources for those in need and who perhaps cannot afford these services either because of lack of (or limited) health insurance, or inability to pay; ultimately to prevent harm for lack of intervention. ▶ Allocate and promote access to resources on the basis of the patient's needs. ▶ Optimize the patient's ability to assume self-management.
Veracity	Telling the truth (to follow through and keep one's promises).	Case managers: ▶ Build trusting and respectful relationships with patients and their families. ▶ Treat the patient with authenticity and honesty.

Adapted from Case Management Society of America. (1996, February). *CMSA's statement regarding ethical case management practice.* Retrieved July 14, 2017, from http://www.cmsa.org/LinkClick.aspx?link=PDF/MemberOnly/EthicalCMPracticeStatement.pdf.

new services and for patient-centered changes in organizational and governmental policy.
▶ Improve the patient's access to quality, safe, and cost-effective services. Facilitate the patient's access to necessary and appropriate services while educating the patient and the family about the resources available.
▶ Promote the patient's self-determination, informed and shared decision making, autonomy, growth, and self-advocacy.
▶ Respect the patient's needs, strengths, and care goals.
▶ Recognize, prevent, and eliminate disparities in accessing high-quality care and in experiencing optimal patient healthcare outcomes.

▶ Ensure a culture of safety by engagement in quality improvement initiatives in the workplace.
▶ Encourage the establishment of client, family, and/or family caregiver advisory councils to improve client-centered care standards within the organization.
▶ Join relevant professional organizations in call to action campaigns, whenever possible, to improve the quality of care and reduce health disparities.
▶ Weigh decisions with the intent to uphold client advocacy, whenever possible, especially when advocacy can sometimes conflict with the need to balance cost constraints and limited resources (CMSA, 2016, pp. 28–29).

▶ ANA's Code of Ethics/Standards of Professional Performance

Nurses are held liable to perform nursing duties responsibly, legally, and ethically. In addition to adhering to the *Statement of Ethical Case Management Practice*, NCMs must adhere to both the *ANA Code of Ethics for Nurses with Interpretive Statements* and the *Standards of Professional Performance*. The *Standards of Professional Performance* states that the nurse is guided by the Code of Ethics for Nurses; the nurse maintains client confidentiality; acts as a client advocate; delivers care in a nonjudgmental, nondiscriminatory manner that is sensitive to cultural diversity; delivers care in a manner that preserves and protects client autonomy, dignity, and rights; and seeks available resources to help formulate ethical decisions. The *ANA Code of Ethics* is one of the oldest codes developed for healthcare professionals and has undergone several revisions since it was established; it was most recently revised in 2015.

The code is accessible at the ANA website (http://www.nursingworld.org/MainMenuCategories/EthicsStandards/CodeofEthicsforNurses).

1. The nurse, in all professional relationships, practices with compassion and respect for the inherent dignity, worth, and uniqueness of every individual, unrestricted by considerations of social or economic status, personal attributes, or the nature of health problems.
2. The nurse's primary commitment is to the patient, whether an individual, family, group, community, or population.
3. The nurse promotes, advocates for, and strives to protect the rights, health, and safety of the patient.
4. The nurse has authority, accountability, and responsibility for nursing practice; makes decisions; and takes action consistent with the obligation to promote health and to provide optimal patient care.
5. The nurse owes the same duties to self as to others, including the responsibility to promote health and safety, preserve wholeness of character and integrity, maintain competence, and continue personal and professional growth.
6. The nurse, through individual and collective effort, establishes, maintains, and improves the ethical environment of the work setting and conditions of employment that are conducive to safe, quality healthcare.
7. The nurse, in all roles and settings, advances the profession through research and scholarly inquiry, professional standards development, and the generation of both nursing and health policy.
8. The nurse collaborates with other health professionals and the public to protect human rights, promote health diplomacy, and reduce health disparity.
9. The profession of nursing, collectively through its professional organizations, represented by associations and their members, must articulate nursing values, maintain the integrity of the profession, and integrate principles of social justice into nursing and health policy (ANA, 2015).

▶ The Code of Professional Conduct for Case Managers

All case managers who possess the CCM credential must adhere to the *Code of Professional Conduct for Case Managers* and the professional code of ethics for their specific profession (such as nursing, social work, pharmacy, and so on). One of the underlying principles in the *Scope of Practice for Case Managers*, developed by the CCMC, is that board-CCMs are guided by the principles of autonomy, beneficence, nonmaleficence, justice, and fidelity (CCMC, 2015). Although the CCMC does not include veracity as one of its ethical principles, it does include this principle in the list of definitions available as part of the Code. The definitions of these principles are not everyday language, so here they are further explained on the basis of the CCMC's *Code of Professional Conduct for Case Managers*:

- *Autonomy*: "Agreement to respect another's right to self-determine a course of action; support of independent decision making" (CCMC, 2015, p. 5). It is a form of personal liberty whereby the individual possesses sufficient mental capacity to determine his or her course of action in accordance with a plan chosen and developed by himself or herself.
- *Beneficence*: "Compassion; taking positive action to help others; desire to do good; core principle of client advocacy" (CCMC, 2015, p. 5). It is the obligation or duty to promote good, to further another's legitimate interests, and to actively prevent harm or diminish its impact as much as possible.
- *Fidelity*: "The ethical principle that directs people to keep commitment or promises" (CCMC, 2015, p. 5).
- *Nonmaleficence*: The CCMC does not define this principle in its Code. It is, however, the act of refraining from harming others, or if harm is inevitable, ensuring that as little harm occurs as possible.
- *Justice*: "The ethical principle that involves the idea of fairness and equality in terms of access to resources and treatment by others" (CCMC, 2015, p. 6). It is achieving a fair distribution of benefits and burdens.
- *Veracity*: "Principle that states that a health professional should be honest and give full disclosure; abstain from misrepresentation or deceit; report known lapses of the standards of care to the appropriate agencies" (CCMC, 2015, p. 6). It is simply being honest and truthful.

The *Code of Professional Conduct for Case Managers* was first published in 1996 and has gone through multiple revisions, most recently in 2015. In addition to the ethical principles described in the Code, the CCMC requires board-CCMs to adhere to six standards of professional conduct (CCMC, 2015). The 2015 version of the Code promulgates the Code as a requirement for board-CCMs who possess the CCM credential. This characterization was not as specific in prior versions of the Code. The standards are described as follows:

1. *Advocacy*, which focuses on the role of the case manager as a client advocate, performing comprehensive client assessments, explaining to the client their options for necessary treatments, and facilitating access to needed services.
2. *Professional responsibility*, especially in the areas of representation of practice, competence (defined by educational preparation, work experience, and ongoing professional development), representation of qualifications, legal and benefit systems requirements, use of CCM designation, conflict of interest, reporting of misconduct, and compliance with proceedings.
3. *Case manager/client relationship*, which emphasizes description of services to clients, relationships with clients, termination of services, objectivity, and maintaining professional relationships.
4. *Confidentiality, privacy, security, and record keeping*, which describe the role of the case manager in legal compliance (adherence to local, state, and federal laws), disclosure, client identity, records (including maintenance, storage, and disposal), protection of client's personal health information, electronic recordings, and reports.
5. *Professional relationships*, which address testimony, dual relationships, unprofessional behaviors, fees, advertising, and solicitation. This standard also addresses legal compliance in the conduct of research (cultural competence and sensitivity, scientific research procedures, and adherence to applicable federal and state laws) and research subject privacy.

The CCMC takes ethical complaints against case managers very seriously, and the review process is extensive. For accessing or obtaining copies of the *Scope of Practice for Case Managers*, the *Code of Professional Conduct for Case Managers*, or information about case management certification, refer to the CCMC's website (http://www.ccmcertification.org). Although the CCMC's *Code of Professional Conduct* is written specifically for case managers who are certified by the Commission (i.e., those who hold the CCM credential), over time, the application of the *Code* has expanded to those who are not certified as well. When a legal or ethical issue is being addressed, authorities (including legal, ethical, employers, and others) have used the *Code* as a standard against which they examined the issue. As a result, case managers are better off adhering to the *Code*, regardless of certification status. Therefore, they should be familiar with the *Code* and abide by it in their practice at all times.

▶ Code of Conduct of the American Case Management Association

The National Board for Case Management (NBCM) and the ACMA expect both those already certified and those applying for certification to adhere to the ACMA Code of Conduct referred to as the *ACM Code of Conduct*. The Code guides ACMs in the ethical practice of case management and defines ethical behavior. It states that the primary obligation of ACMs is to provide quality care and ensure the best outcomes possible for the patients, clients, and communities served (ACMA, 2017). The Code consists of 13 principles and expects ACMs and applicants for the ACM credential to:

1. Be in continuous compliance with all NBCM standards, policies, and procedures. This includes maintaining a current professional credential as required by the jurisdiction of practice.
2. Be accurate, truthful, and complete in any and all communications, direct or indirect, with any client, employer, regulatory agency, or other parties as relates to their professional work, education, professional credentials, research, and contributions to the field of case management.
3. Report to the NBCM and/or ACMA anyone who steals, shares, colludes, or otherwise compromises the ACM certification program integrity.
4. Provide accurate and truthful representations to both the NBCM and the ACMA concerning all information related to aspects of the certification program, including, but not limited to, the submission of information when applying for certification or renewal, changes to licenses, criminal charges, disciplinary action situation; test security violations, misrepresentations of credentials and/or education, and the unauthorized use of the NBCM's or the ACMA's intellectual property.
5. Cooperate with the NBCM and the ACMA concerning investigations of violations of the Code of Conduct.
6. Comply with state and/or federal laws, regulations, and statutes governing the practice of their discipline and case management.
7. Maintain good standing, avoid conviction of a crime, and engage in the safe practice of case management or the original discipline.
8. Refrain from engaging in behavior or conduct, lawful or otherwise, that causes a threat or potential threat to the health, well-being, or safety of recipients or potential recipients of case management services or services related to the discipline of practice.

9. Not electronically post personal health information or anything, including photos, that may reveal a patient's/client's identity or personal or patient relationship, thus violating the state and/or federal law (i.e., Health Insurance Portability and Accountability Act [HIPAA]).

10. Not engage in the practice of case management while impaired due to chemical (i.e., legal and/or illegal) drug or alcohol abuse.

11. Assure that a real or perceived conflict of interest does not compromise legitimate interests of a patient or an employer, and does not influence or interfere with work-related judgments.

12. Respect appropriate professional boundaries in the interactions with patients and others.

13. Provide professional services in a reasonably prompt and thorough manner, including the proper planning for, and supervision of, the rendering of proper and professional services (ACMA, 2017).

▶ National Association of Social Workers' Code of Ethics

According to the NASW, social workers promote social justice and social change with and on behalf of *clients* (a term generically used to refer to individuals, families, groups, organizations, and communities). The association also believes that professional ethics is the core of social work. The *NASW Code of Ethics* offers a set of values, principles, and standards to guide decision making and everyday professional conduct of social workers. The *Code* was approved by the NASW Delegate Assembly in 1996 and then revised in 1999, and most recently in 2008. It is currently used by most social work licensing boards. The *Code* sets forth the values, principles, and standards that guide social workers' conduct. It serves six purposes (NASW, 2008):

1. To identify core values on which social work's mission is based.

2. To summarize broad ethical principles that reflect the profession's core values and establish a set of specific ethical standards that should be used to guide social work practice.

3. To help social workers identify relevant considerations when professional obligations conflict or ethical uncertainties arise.

4. To provide ethical standards to which the general public can hold the social work profession accountable.

5. To raise awareness of social workers, who are new to the field, to social work's mission, values, ethical principles, and ethical standards.

6. To articulate standards that the social work profession itself can use to assess whether social workers have engaged in unethical conduct.

The NASW emphasizes six ethical principles that are listed in the following paragraph. Case managers who are social workers must be familiar with and adhere to these principles at all times to ensure ethical practice. For more information on the *NASW's Code of Ethics*, refer to the association's website (http://www.socialworkers.org). The six principles are:

1. *Service*: Social workers' primary goal is to help people in need and to address social problems. They promote services to others putting aside professional or personal self-interest.

2. *Social Justice*: Social workers challenge social injustice and pursue social change, particularly with and on behalf of vulnerable and oppressed individuals and populations. They provide services in a culturally and linguistically appropriate manner and ensure patients' access to needed information for effective decision making.

3. *Dignity and Worth of the Person*: Social workers respect the inherent dignity and worth of the person and treat each person in a caring and respectful fashion, mindful of individual differences and cultural and ethnic diversities. Social workers also promote clients' self-determination. Social workers seek to enhance patients' capacity and opportunity to change and to address their own needs.

4. *Importance of Human Relationships*: Social workers recognize the central importance of human relationships and understand that relationships between and among people are important vehicles for change. Social workers engage people as partners in the helping process. They seek to strengthen relationships among people in a purposeful effort to promote, restore, maintain, and enhance the well-being of individuals, families, social groups, organizations, populations, and communities.

5. *Integrity*: Social workers behave in a trustworthy manner. They are continually aware of their profession's mission, values, ethical principles, and ethical standards, and practice in a manner that is consistent with these. Social workers also act honestly and responsibly and promote ethical practices on the part of the organizations with which they are affiliated.

6. *Competence*: Social workers practice within their areas of competence and develop and enhance their professional expertise. They continually strive to enhance their professional knowledge and skills and to apply them in practice.

The NASW Code of Ethics also articulates six main standards that are relevant to the professional activities of all social workers. These include the social workers' ethical responsibilities to clients, colleagues, social work profession, broader society, in practice settings, and as professionals. Some of the standards are enforceable guidelines for professional conduct, and some are aspirational. The extent to which each standard is enforceable is a matter of professional judgment to be exercised by those responsible for reviewing alleged violations of ethical standards (NASW, 2008).

The NASW, in its standards for social work case management, states that social work case managers must advocate for patients' right to self-determination, confidentiality, and access to supportive services and resources they need on the basis of the patients' health condition and social situation. The standards also emphasize the appropriate inclusion of patients in decision making concerning their well-being, and participation in the development and refinement of public policy at the local, state, and federal levels (NASW, 2013).

The social work case manager shall also adhere to and promote the ethics and values of the social work profession using the NASW Code of Ethics as a guide to ethical decision making in case management practice. The primary mission of the social work profession is to enhance a person's health and well-being and to help meet the basic needs of all people, especially the vulnerable. The core values that constitute the foundation of social work also underlie social work case management. As listed here, they build on the professional social work values, however with a case management context:

1. *Service*: The social work case manager applies her or his knowledge and skills to support the biopsychosocial well-being of patients and to address the challenges they face.
2. *Social justice*: The social work case manager pursues change to reduce poverty, discrimination, oppression, and other forms of social injustice experienced by patients.
3. *Human dignity and worth*: The social work case manager treats clients in a caring and respectful manner and enhances their capacity to improve their condition and achieve their health goals.
4. *Importance of human relationships*: The social work case manager promotes the role of human relationships in the change process and cultivates a therapeutic relationship with each patient as a partner in care goal identification, service planning and implementation, and practice evaluation.
5. *Integrity*: The social work case manager acts in an ethical manner and uses the power inherent in the professional social work role responsibly in presenting resource options and providing services to patients.
6. *Competence*: The social work case manager practices within her or his area of competence and continually strives to enhance knowledge and skills related to case management and the population served (NASW, 2013).

Additionally, social work case managers promote patient self-determination and involvement in goal identification and decision making about care options throughout the case management process. Nonetheless, when a patient's ability for informed decision making is limited, the social work case manager collaborates with the individual who is legally authorized to represent the patient (e.g., guardian, next of kin, healthcare proxy) while continuing to promote the patient's participation in case management. The social work case manager must also be aware of and demonstrate adherence to federal, state, local, and tribal laws, regulations, and policies, addressing issues of guardianship, parental rights, advance directives and reporting requirements for abuse, neglect, suicide, threat of harm to others, confidentiality and privacy of client information (i.e., HIPAA), and use of health information technology (NASW, 2013).

With the continuing demands for effective allocation of resources, and in some instances where a lack of organizational or community resources may be found, patients' options for healthcare services may also sometimes be limited. The social work case manager in such cases is responsible for informing the patients and their families of the existing choices so that they may decide which services will best meet their needs. In situations of conflict, the social work case manager may seek the assistance of ethics committees or expert consultants to resolve such dilemmas (NASW, 2013). Other ethical responsibilities of social work case managers include ensuring patients have the necessary information to engage in informed consents; terminating services when they are no longer helpful to patients; notifying patients when services are being interrupted temporarily or permanently discontinued by a service provider or payor; and completion of safe transition of care activities to maintain patients' continuity of care (NASW, 2013).

▮ Consumer Bill of Rights and Responsibilities/Patient Bill of Rights

In November 1997, the Presidential Advisory Commission on Consumer Protection and Quality in the Health Care Industry released its *Consumer Bill of Rights and Responsibilities* in healthcare; because this is not in the form of law, it has been included in the chapter on ethics. This bill is an effort to give back to patients some empowerment in their healthcare. Many states have similar clauses, and the Centers for Medicare & Medicaid Services (CMS) has had a Patient Bill of Rights for Medicare beneficiaries for many years. Various levels of care have *Patient Bills of Rights*: hospitals, hospices, skilled nursing facilities (SNFs), and long-term care facilities. The Patient Bill of Rights also applies to the health insurance plans offered to federal

display 9-5

CONSUMER BILL OF RIGHTS AND RESPONSIBILITIES

Free copies of the Consumer Bill of Rights and Responsibilities are available from:

White House website (http://www.whitehouse.gov) or the Commission's website (http://www.hcqualitycommission.gov).
Copies can also be obtained from
Consumer Bill of Rights
P.O. Box 2429
Columbia, MD 21045-1429
Telephone: (800) 732-8200

employees. Additionally, many other health insurance plans have also adopted these values.

The bills of rights issued by healthcare institutions are not legally binding unless there are state laws to back them up; however, federal funding for those who are regulated by the CMS or those accredited by The Joint Commission may be jeopardized if the bills of rights are not enforced.

When reading the bill of rights (and patient responsibilities), keep in mind that these are the types of issues case managers have always been dealing with. The stated goals of the *Consumer Bill of Rights and Responsibilities* (Display 9-5) include:

▶ To strengthen consumer confidence by ensuring that the healthcare system is fair and responsive to consumers' needs, providing consumers with credible and effective mechanisms to address their concerns, and encouraging them to take an active role in improving and ensuring their health.

▶ To reaffirm the importance of a strong relationship between patients and their healthcare professionals.

▶ To reaffirm the critical role consumers play in safeguarding their own health by establishing both rights and responsibilities for all participants in improving health status (Commission on Consumer Protection and Quality in Health Care, 1998).

The *Consumer Bill of Rights and Responsibilities* includes eight areas (President's Advisory Commission on Consumer Protection and Quality in the Health Care Industry, available at https://archive.ahrq.gov/hcqual/press/cbor.html) (Commission on Consumer Protection and Quality in Health Care, 1998):

1. Information Disclosure

Consumers have the right to receive accurate, easily understood information to make informed healthcare decisions about their health plans, professionals, and facilities. Such information includes:

▶ *Health plan information*: Covered benefits, cost-sharing, and procedures for resolving complaints; licensure, certification, and accreditation

status; comparable measures of quality and consumer satisfaction; provider network composition; the procedures that govern access to specialists and emergency services; and care management information.

▶ *Health professional information*: Education, board certification, and recertification; years of practice; experience in performing certain procedures; and comparable measures of quality and consumer satisfaction.

▶ *Healthcare facility information*: Experience in performing certain procedures and services; accreditation status; comparable measures of quality and worker and consumer satisfaction; and procedures for resolving complaints.

▶ *Information about consumer assistance programs*: Programs must be carefully structured to promote consumer confidence and to work cooperatively with health plans, providers, payors, and regulators. Sponsorship that ensures accountability to the interests of consumers and stable, adequate funding are desirable characteristics of such programs.

2. Choice of Providers and Plans

Consumers have the right to a choice of healthcare providers that is sufficient to ensure access to appropriate high-quality healthcare. To ensure such choice, the Commission recommends the following:

▶ *Provider network adequacy*: All health plan networks should provide access to sufficient numbers and types of providers to ensure that all covered services will be accessible without unreasonable delay. This includes access to emergency services 24 hours a day, 7 days a week. If a health plan has an insufficient number or type of providers to provide a covered benefit with the appropriate degree of specialization, the plan should ensure that the consumer obtains the benefit outside the network at no greater cost than if the benefit were obtained from participating providers.

▶ *Women's health services*: Women should be able to choose a qualified provider offered by a plan (such as gynecologists, certified nurse midwives, and other qualified healthcare providers) for the provision of covered care necessary to provide routine and preventive women's healthcare services.

▶ *Access to specialists*: Consumers with complex or serious medical conditions who require frequent specialty care should have direct access to a qualified specialist of their choice within a plan's network of providers. Authorizations, when required, should be for an adequate number of direct access visits under an approved treatment plan.

▶ *Transitional care*: Consumers who are undergoing a course of treatment for a chronic or disabling condition (or who are in the second or third trimester of a pregnancy) at the time they involuntarily change health plans, or at a time when a provider is terminated by a plan for other than a just cause, should be able to continue seeing their current specialty providers for up to 90 days (or through completion of postpartum care) to allow for transition of care.

▶ *Choice of health plans*: Public and private group purchasers should, wherever feasible, offer consumers a choice of high-quality health insurance plans.

3. Access to Emergency Services

Consumers have the right to access emergency healthcare services when and where the need arises. Health plans should provide payment when a consumer presents to an emergency department with acute symptoms of sufficient severity—including severe pain—such that a "prudent layperson" could reasonably expect the absence of medical attention to result in placing that consumer's health in serious jeopardy, serious impairment to bodily functions, or serious dysfunction of any bodily organ or part.

4. Participation in Treatment Decisions

Consumers have the right and responsibility to participate fully in all decisions related to their healthcare. Those who are unable to participate fully in treatment decisions have the right to be represented by parents, guardians, family members, or other conservators.

Physicians and other health professionals should:

▶ Provide patients with sufficient information and opportunity to decide among treatment options consistent with the informed consent process.

▶ Discuss all treatment options with a patient in a culturally competent manner, including the option of no treatment at all.

▶ Ensure that persons with disabilities have effective communication with members of the health system in making such decisions.

▶ Discuss all current treatments a consumer may be undergoing.

▶ Discuss all risks, benefits, and consequences to treatment or nontreatment.

▶ Give patients the opportunity to refuse treatment and to express preferences about future treatment decisions.

▶ Discuss the use of advance directives, both living wills and durable powers of attorney for healthcare, with patients and their designated family members.

▶ Abide by the decisions made by their patients and/or their designated representatives consistent with the informed consent process.

Health plans, providers, and facilities should:

▶ Disclose to consumers factors—such as methods of compensation, ownership of or interest in healthcare facilities, or matters of conscience—that could influence advice or treatment decisions.

▶ Ensure that provider contracts do not contain any so-called "gag clauses" or other contractual mechanisms that restrict healthcare providers' ability to communicate with and advise patients about medically necessary treatment options.

▶ Be prohibited from penalizing or seeking retribution against healthcare professionals or other health workers for advocating on behalf of their patients.

5. Respect and Nondiscrimination

Consumers have the right to considerate, respectful care from all members of the healthcare industry at all times and under all circumstances. An environment of mutual respect is essential to maintain a quality healthcare system. To ensure that right, the Commission recommends the following:

▶ Consumers must not be discriminated against in the delivery of healthcare services consistent with the benefits covered in their policy, or as required by law, on the basis of race, ethnicity, national origin, religion, sex, age, mental or physical disability, sexual orientation, genetic information, or source of payment.

▶ Consumers eligible for coverage under the terms and conditions of a health plan or program, or as required by law, must not be discriminated against in marketing and enrollment practices on the basis of race, ethnicity, national origin, religion, sex, age, mental or physical disability, sexual orientation, genetic information, or source of payment.

6. Confidentiality of Health Information

Consumers have the right to communicate with healthcare providers in confidence and to have the confidentiality of their individually identifiable healthcare information protected. Consumers also have the right to review and copy their own medical records and request amendments to their records.

7. Complaints and Appeals

Consumers have the right to a fair and efficient process for resolving differences with their health plans, healthcare providers, and the institutions that serve them, including a rigorous system of internal review and an independent system of external review.

8. Consumer Responsibilities

In a healthcare system that protects consumers' rights, it is reasonable to expect and encourage consumers to assume reasonable responsibilities. Greater individual involvement by consumers in their care increases the likelihood of achieving the best outcomes and helps support a quality improvement, cost-conscious environment. Such responsibilities include:

▶ Take responsibility for maximizing healthy habits, such as exercising, not smoking, and eating a healthy diet.

▶ Work collaboratively with healthcare providers in developing and carrying out treatment plans.

▶ Disclose relevant information and clearly communicate wants and needs.

▶ Use the health plan's internal complaint and appeal processes to address concerns that may arise.

▶ Avoid knowingly spreading disease.

▶ Recognize the reality of risks and limits of the science of medical care and the human fallibility of the healthcare professional.

▶ Be aware of a healthcare provider's obligation to be reasonably efficient and equitable in providing care to other patients and the community.

▶ Become knowledgeable about their health plan coverage and health plan options (when available) including all covered benefits, limitations, and exclusions; rules regarding the use of network providers; coverage and referral rules; appropriate processes to secure additional information; and the process to appeal coverage decisions.

▶ Show respect for other patients and health workers.

▶ Make a good-faith effort to meet financial obligations.

▶ Abide by administrative and operational procedures of health plans, healthcare providers, and government health benefit programs.

▶ Report wrongdoing and fraud to appropriate resources or legal authorities.

On June 22, 2010, then President Obama announced new interim final regulations, the Patient's Bill of Rights, which included a set of protections that apply to health insurance coverage of consumers from private insurance agencies. These regulations took effect on or after September 23, 2010, as part of the Patients Protection and Affordable Care Act of 2010. The U.S. Departments of Health and Human Services, Labor and Treasury collaborated on this Patient's Bill of Rights which intended to help children and eventually all Americans with preexisting health conditions to be able to receive health insurance coverage. The regulation is referred to today as the "preexisting condition insurance plan (PCIP)" coverage entitlement for Americans. It, therefore, protects Americans' choice of healthcare providers and has ended the lifetime limits on the care consumers may receive. The new protections create an important foundation of patients' rights in the private health insurance market (CMS, 2017a). In 2017, and at the time of writing this textbook, the future of these regulations was unknown as the "appeal and replace" efforts of the Patient Protection and Affordable Care Act were still underway.

The PCIP program was intended to provide health insurance coverage to eligible uninsured individuals with preexisting conditions until 2014. Beginning in 2014, most health insurance agencies were required to offer coverage to all individuals, regardless of preexisting conditions, pursuant to the Public Health Service Act. Eligible individuals were able to obtain health insurance coverage either by enrolling in a qualified health insurance plan offered through the Health Insurance Exchanges or Marketplaces established under the Patient Protection and Affordable Care Act or by enrolling in health insurance coverage offered in the individual or group market outside of the Exchanges (U.S. Department of Health and Human Services, 45 CFR Part 152, 2013).

▶ ETHICAL DILEMMAS IN CASE MANAGEMENT

▶ Balancing Advocacy versus Cost-Containment Roles

Ethical dilemmas are a consequence of our contemporary healthcare climate, and they continue to haunt us. The issues are not static, and more will be revealed as healthcare reform unfolds. As case managers, we may be subject to ethical discomfort from the very roles we must perform: as gatekeepers of resources versus patient advocates and as coordinators-facilitators of multidisciplinary teams. One common thread that appears over and over, sometimes in subtle disguises, is the issue of healthcare rationing. The role of the case manager in balancing the patients' demand for healthcare services with the pressure to lower costs through more effective allocation of resources will undoubtedly face ethical challenges.

The very idea of rationing healthcare is extremely distasteful to many Americans. However, like any other sector's budget, healthcare's is finite—and it continues to spiral out of control. Healthcare spending reached $2.3 trillion in 2007. It grew to $3.4 trillion in 2016 and is expected to reach $5.5 trillion by 2025 (Keehan et al., 2017). To better understand the importance of the case manager's patient advocacy role, let us consider the following statistics on the national health expenditure reported by the CMS in 2015. These data underline how necessary advocacy is and the need to maintain a patient- and family-centered approach to care delivery and the distribution of healthcare services and resources.

▶ The national health expenditure grew by 5.8% compared with the previous year, to $3.2 trillion or $9,990 per person, and the expenditure accounted for 17.8% of GDP.

▶ Medicare spending during the same year grew by 4.5%, to $646.2 billion or 20% of the total national health expenditure. Medicaid spending grew by

9.7%, to $545.1 billion or 17% of the total national health expenditure. These expenses constituted the largest share of the total health spending in 2015 (28.7%), whereas the expenses incurred by state and local governments accounted for 17.1%.

▶ Private (or commercial) health insurance spending grew by 7.2%, to $1,072.1 billion or 33% of the total national health expenditure. This private health insurance spending accounted for 19.9% of total national healthcare spending in 2015.

▶ Personal out-of-pocket spending grew by 2.6%, to $338.1 billion or 11% of the total national health expenditure. Household expenses accounted for 27.7% of the national spending.

▶ Hospital expenditures grew by 5.6% to $1,036.1 billion compared with the 4.6% growth in 2014.

▶ Physician and clinical services expenditures grew by 6.3% to $634.9 billion compared with the 4.8% in 2014.

▶ Prescription drug spending increased by 9.0% to $324.6 billion; however, this was slower than the 12.4% growth noted in 2014 (CMS, 2017b).

When one considers the national healthcare spending for 2016 to 2025, the national spending is projected to grow at an average rate of 5.6% per year for 2016 to 2025 and 4.7% per year on a per capita basis. Such a dynamic is expected to result in a projected growth that is 1.2% points faster than the GDP growth per year over the same period; the healthcare share of the GDP is expected to rise from the 17.8% noted in 2015 to 19.9% by 2025 (CMS, 2017b).

When most people think of rationing healthcare, they have visions of cutting off life-saving, high-cost procedures to a defined population. Perhaps people older than 80 years of age will not be allowed coronary bypasses; or anyone older than 65 years would not be allowed organ transplants or hemodialysis; or heroic measures would not be started on premature babies younger than 22 weeks' gestational age. The truth is that America already rations healthcare. The present discussions on newer, more stringent sets of criteria are for the purpose of rationing it further. Some feel that this is in order to serve a larger population (i.e., the currently uninsured). Others believe it is for reasons of financial benefit to the payor agency. The rationing fire is also being fueled by the media (Internet, print, broadcast, etc.), Congressional debates on healthcare reform (Medicare and Medicaid, and the Patient Protection and Affordable Care Act reform), and presidential debates.

Americans are grappling with the question of whether healthcare is a right or a commodity, which is another subtle way to evaluate whether healthcare should be rationed. Many of today's questions cross-examine whether healthcare is a right and how far the rights of individuals should go. Should noncompliant people who engage in unhealthy lifestyles be covered? Should those who are uninsured and cannot afford healthcare be mandated to pay for it regardless? Some question whether rationing

or limiting of healthcare should be imposed on noncompliant persons. Should ceilings be placed on their medical care dollars? Should those who can afford to pay have higher premiums? Should those with preexisting health conditions be scrutinized differently than those who do not? What is legal and what is ethical?

Even the definition of noncompliance does not consider all the ethical ramifications. Noncompliance is a failure of the patient to cooperate with the medical and health plan by not carrying out needed procedures or lifestyle changes (e.g., healthy behaviors). The very concept of noncompliance betrays the professional's concern about patient autonomy and self-determination; in other words, that patients are free to make life-directing decisions. Care must be taken not to label all those who do not follow a prescribed medical or health plan of treatment as noncompliant. Cultural beliefs are deeply ingrained in people's psyche. Food, health, and religious rituals will not be changed simply because a Western health practitioner dictated a prescription. Also, children and incapacitated adults who are in the care of noncompliant guardians may be penalized if society rations healthcare to noncompliant people. The kaleidoscope turns and the perspective changes. What is the role of healthcare professionals, including case managers, in patient/family engagement and ability to self-manage own health condition? Case managers may employ the tools and skills of motivational interviewing to understand where the patient and/or the family stand vis-à-vis self-management and to ultimately enhance adherence and care outcomes including patient quality of life and well-being.

Case managers deal with rationing daily. For example, two women have breast cancer. Both could die. Both have families and young children. One woman is allowed a bone marrow transplant by her insurance carrier; the other is not. Health insurance companies ration their healthcare dollars through the allocation of benefits to enrollees/insured persons all the time: who is allowed benefits such as organ transplants, bone marrow transplants, extended care benefits, or experimental treatments. Subtle rationing of benefits takes many forms, and the case manager must be alert to a denial of services on the basis of an interpretation of benefits that may be erroneous.

One case involved a cancer patient with stomach, esophageal, and intestinal tumor involvement. Surgically, there was little to be done for the patient and her prognosis was poor, although death was not imminent. She was alert and oriented and chose hospice care, as she was no longer trying to cure the cancer with medical treatment. She was receiving total parenteral nutrition (TPN) as her only possible source of nutrition and was receiving radiation for palliative, not for curative, purposes. Her case manager was told that the TPN was disallowed because hospice does not cover services that are merely for prolonging life. Not agreeing that basic nutrition falls under the "not prolonging life" umbrella in this case, any more than eating food would in a lung cancer hospice patient, the case manager argued. The patient received hospice and TPN. The bottom line is that TPN is an expensive treatment option and difficult to budget for, so it is not routinely considered a covered service.

Some insurance companies cloak their rationing under terms such as medical necessity, appropriateness of the level of care, or unnecessary treatments. These vague terms must be treated carefully, as they are arbitrary and prone to personal judgments when used as a measuring stick for health insurance guidelines. Clarifying the implications and the use of medical necessity sometimes requires semantic analysis, but it is not merely a semantic exercise. Confusion, conflict, and refractory dilemmas inevitably emerge when the intertwined layers of meaning(s) inherent in the concept remain hidden. The case manager—as a patient advocate—must be alert to vague interpretations of benefits. In addition, a payor inappropriately interpreting benefit language to cut its losses to the detriment of the claimant is courting malpractice and possibly litigation.

In a positive sense, case managers help to ration healthcare. Through astute care planning and attention to detail, case managers avoid duplication, fragmentation, and overutilization of finite resources. This is done through their gatekeeper role. As a gatekeeper, the case manager's job responsibilities may include monitoring resources, allocating and authorizing resources, and introducing incentives to improve the quality of care provided. In essence, the gatekeeper controls and rations limited resources in a world where there appears to be unlimited need. When the case manager superimposes the role of patient advocate on that of the gatekeeper, role conflict and ethical dilemmas may result. Many feel that the combined patient advocate-gatekeeper role of a case manager is an impossible marriage. A gatekeeper controls entry to services and uses them economically; an advocate strives to gain all the services the patient needs for a safe, efficient, and effective care plan. Is it possible for one person to be both a patient advocate and a gatekeeper of healthcare resources? Can the case manager maintain quality and safety while cutting costs? It is a challenge. There are factors that play into how effectively a fine balance between quality and cost cutting can be achieved.

The type and definition of the individual case management position may weight one role more heavily than another. A case manager for a Medicaid plan may feel that allocation of resources for her population of many thousands of patients (the whole) supersedes the needs of the individual (the part); therefore, her gatekeeping role may be stressed. A case manager on an oncology unit may feel that her patient's needs are the most important factor; this case manager may practice 75% patient advocacy and 25% gatekeeping. Potentially serious conflicts of interest are possible when the agencies that provide services send their case managers to complete the assessment of need and develop the care plans. If the company's objective is to increase business, overutilization may be practiced; if the company's objective is to control utilization of services, underutilization may be the result. The case manager may be placed in the unfavorable position of asking, "How can I really advocate for this patient when it means fighting with the person paying my salary?" A preferred approach is the conscientious use of healthcare resources that meet the patient's needs, in the most appropriate care setting and by the right healthcare providers.

The answer to how this can be effectively accomplished lies in your own personal style and your ability to balance the roles of patient advocacy and gatekeeping so that everyone wins. Although this is not always possible, you should strive for it. Whenever it is not possible, err on the side of patient advocacy. A case manager misinterpreting his or her role to be primarily that of a provider or payor *employee* and secondarily that of a *patient advocate* will truly cause divisiveness regarding case management. Consumers of healthcare services will perceive the case manager as an "unethical" person.

▶ The Coordinator/Facilitator Role

Another case management role that at times is the cause of ethical discomfort is that of a coordinator/facilitator of care and services. Case managers are often asked to facilitate consensus of a large interdisciplinary care team, especially when a case is spiraling out of control. A forum such as a case conference is held for this purpose. It may include any, or all, of the following: the patient, the family, the attending physician, physician specialists, residents or interns, respiratory therapists, speech therapists, occupational therapists, physical therapists, staff nurses, hospital administrators, risk management specialists, social workers, health insurance company liaisons, insurance utilization review nurses or case managers, nutritionists, finance officers, patient advocates, or anyone else essential to that individual's case. Depending on the main issue at hand, the team may also include an expert ethicist. Case managers deal with so many people making decisions on each complex case that it is perhaps dizzying to think about it. Ethicist John Banja likens this facilitator role to an air traffic controller who must coordinate flight patterns so that everyone is not crashing into one another (Boling, 1991) and ultimately everyone is kept safe.

At times, it feels as though some team members are on a collision course. Most case managers have been in situations in which the payor (insurance company) was found to have an agenda that was different from that of the physician. The payor felt that the patient could be safely provided for at a lesser level of care. The physician felt that the patient was not stable enough for a change to a lesser level of care. The payor felt that it must make wise and strict use of resources, because it has a very large population to manage and must ration the funds carefully. The physician was focused on the best care for this patient at this time.

Sometimes biases result from opposing viewpoints about the best treatment for a particular patient. One physician believes that a patient needs a lower extremity amputation; another believes that care should be "comfort only" at this point. The physical therapist believes it is unsafe for the patient to go home alone; the patient insists that he will go home. A patient refuses care for a gangrenous foot; the family threatens to sue if the patient dies of a gangrenous foot. As the air traffic controller/case manager gathers a meeting and allows each dissenting opinion time on the runway to air views on the best way to handle this situation, he or she should not forget to state the heart of the case management agenda—that of patient advocacy.

▌ Gag Clauses

This section is for the purpose of "case manager—beware." Gag clauses are provisions in managed care contracts that prevent physicians (and potentially other healthcare professionals) from being fully open with their patients. This issue is so potent that it is even addressed in the *Consumer Bill of Rights and Responsibilities*. Issues that have been under gag clauses are the following:

- ▌ Discussing with patients their treatment options that are not covered by the managed care plan.
- ▌ Referring a patient to specialists outside the plan, even if the physician feels it is in the patient's best interests to see a particular specialist.
- ▌ Discussing financial relationships between the physician and the managed care plan with the patient, especially if there are financial incentives for the physician to earn more by providing less care.
- ▌ Most beneficiaries have the periodic opportunity to choose their health plans. As part of that selection process, many consult with their physician to determine which plans the physician accepts and how a certain plan's payment practices compare with other plans. Gag orders interfere with this decision-making process.
- ▌ Gag orders prevent physicians from informing patients about any decision to terminate a physician's contract with a plan. Plans, on the other hand, often retain the authority not only to communicate such changes, but to arbitrarily assign a new physician to a patient.
- ▌ Arguing with a health plan on behalf of a patient's medical needs is time-consuming and frustrating. The result of such disputes is often interpreted as damaging to a health plan's reputation. Gag orders effectively limit a physician's freedom of speech, while making the physician appear unsympathetic to the patient.

The American Medical Association took a strong stand against these gag clauses several years ago. Although many managed care companies have, one by one, removed them from contracts, they still exist, and case managers need to be aware of the implications. Of all the ethical issues these clauses attack, none is more important than the issue of trust between a patient and the healthcare team. Healthcare professionals are obliged to discuss treatment alternatives with patients so that patients cannot be subject to making decisions with inadequate information, as this would be a violation of informed consent requirements.

Pressures to soften these clauses also have been surfacing. The *Consumer Bill of Rights and Responsibilities* mentions accreditation as one possible method of ensuring consumer protection in the healthcare system; for example, certain accreditations require that financial incentives be revealed. Others, although for good intentions, place physicians between two differing paradigms. On the one hand, physicians have to deal with gag clauses. On the other hand, CMS bars physicians who work with Medicare and Medicaid patients from withholding information on treatment options.

State legislation has been very active. For example, Massachusetts enacted the Patient Confidentiality Bill that would bar health maintenance organizations (HMOs) from including gag orders in their provider contracts. In California, legislation has been enacted that prevents retaliation against physicians who advocate on behalf of patients despite contractual prohibitions. Laws in Arizona and Indiana require organizations to disclose financial incentives or penalties that are intended to encourage the minimalization of services provided. Likewise, similar bills have been considered in all other states.

▌ Organ Donation

Effective from late 1999, CMS-certified facilities are required to report all deaths to the organ procurement organization in their city, county, or state. The intent of this is to increase the availability of organs for people who cannot live without them. There are at least two ethical dilemmas with regard to organ donation:

1. Who gets the scarce organs?
2. What is legal and ethical when harvesting suitable organs?

Perhaps someday organs will not be scarce; humans appear to have the ability to clone living things at will, and certainly they will clone human organs. This may bring up additional ethical problems. For the purposes of case management at this time, let us assume that organs will remain scarce for a few more years. For example, in 2007 about 26,400 transplants were performed, but more than 96,600 people were waiting for transplantation of a single organ or of multiple organs; more than 7% died before transplantation occurred (Organ Procurement and Transplantation Network, 2008). In 2016, 33,606 organ transplants were performed, a 19.8% increase since 2012;

117,089 were on the transplant waiting list; and today on an average 20 people die every day waiting for organ transplant (United Network for Organ Sharing, 2017). Then the question arises: Who will get the first chance at scarce resources?

The government has ordered that life-saving organs be given to the sickest first. Under the previous system, organs went to the patients living closest to the donor, even if there was someone more critical elsewhere. In March 1998, Donna Shalala, Secretary of United States Department of Health and Human Services, declared that people are dying simply because of where they live. A regulation was issued governing the United Network for Organ Sharing that included a mandate that the network devise a new allocation scheme for organ distribution. The network and the government have had more than a few problems ever since. As with many of life's events, no answer will make everyone happy. As case managers, many of us have watched our patients die while awaiting an organ; have we not wondered who could have needed it more?

The ruling stated at the beginning of this section may increase the chances of more successful organ transplantations. However, there are other, less ethically clear-cut, methods being examined to increase the organ pool. Organ cloning or "personal pigs" are the lesser of the dilemmas. Prisoners are being targeted as a potential answer to organ scarcity. In 1996, Arizona rejected the Death Row Inmate Organ Donor Bill (HB 2271) (Johns, 1996). This would have effectively harvested the organs of inmates. One major problem is how a prisoner can be executed and still have usable organs. A lethal injection of a fatal chemical is not conducive to organ recycling. Who knows what electricity does to livers or cardiac tissue? One entrepreneurial legislator in Georgia introduced a bill to use the guillotine method; this would not harm the organs and therefore facilitate organ extraction.

Arizona's bill would have allowed the prisoner to have his choice between lethal injection or dying on the operating table. This leaves one more "quirky medical ethical issue" (Johns, 1996). Can a physician take a person's organs before that individual is brain-dead? What about first causing no harm?

▶ Assisted Death and the Right to Die

Assisted suicide, doctor-assisted suicide, euthanasia, mercy killing, legalized killing, managed death, terminal sedation, end-of-life care, murder—assisted death has been called by many names. Case managers may continue to be affected by its ethical and legal implications. Withholding or withdrawing life support or food/fluids is the tip of the iceberg, as that is more like passively assisting death. What physician-assisted suicide does is actually end life at a given moment in time and through intentional actions. In November 1998, the first "euthanasia" was broadcasted publicly on national television.

Regardless of what the process is called, the result is the same: a patient's death. The difference between assisted suicide and euthanasia appears to be the degree to which assistance is provided. Consider this: the American Hospital Association states that approximately 70% of the deaths in hospitals happen after a decision has been made to withhold treatment, another degree to which assistance for the dying is provided. Other patients die when pain medications depress their breathing, or medications to maintain blood pressure are discontinued. Nurses have witnessed these events for decades. Less information is known about SNF deaths and those in private homes.

Like many healthcare issues, it is difficult to separate the legal issues from the ethical ones pertaining to assisted death. Like abortion, the debate will go on for decades, the difference being that one ends life at the beginning, whereas the other focuses on the end of life. Those who want physician-assisted suicide state that it allows terminally ill people, who so desire, the ability to die peacefully and with dignity. Those against it feel it is a radical departure from existing medical and legal tradition and risks fallible judgments and irreversible errors; needless to say, opposition is strong on many fronts. It is also clear that there are no absolutes in life. Einstein did not intend for atomic energy to be used as a weapon of mass destruction. Assisted suicide laws should not be used for anything except for relief from suffering. There are no answers at the back of a book on ethics. There are no assurances that the choice one makes is the best one. However, for decisions to be truly ethical ones, they must be uncontaminated by personal gain, fear of reprisal, or other ulterior motives. The kaleidoscope changes colors and shapes again, but only history will tell what is (or should have been) the right thing to do.

Although the Patient Protection and Affordable Care Act of 2010 has addressed some aspects of end-of-life care, the Act falls short of making services for the dying a priority. Palliative care remains an expense that is not universally reimbursable—a concern that presents a great challenge for case managers coordinating a patient's plan of care and facilitating access to necessary services and resources. Palliative and hospice care are considered valuable and sustainable services that hospitals provide to patients with chronic illnesses, while these services are viewed as a cost-saving approach in an environment of increased concern for healthcare expenditure. Although the Affordable Care Act did not specifically address palliative care as a distinct service from hospice care, there is a need to develop practice guidelines and methods of quality improvement at the end of life, as well as explore nontraditional reimbursement options.

Despite these continued challenges in patient care at the end of life, the Patient Protection and Affordable Care Act of 2010 expanded access to high-quality end-of-life care to Americans with serious and terminal illnesses including cancer. Provisions in the Act demonstrate the opportunity to improve care in three specific areas of end-of-life care (Parikh & Wright, 2017):

1. Expansion of concurrent oncologic and palliative care which requires that programs for children enrolled in state Medicaid programs or Children's Health Insurance Programs (CHIPs) must allow patients to receive hospice care with disease-modifying treatment. This provision applies to children who are younger than 21 years, terminally ill (defined as having a prognosis of less than 6 months to live), and eligible for the state's Medicaid programs or CHIPs. This provision expanded through demonstration projects to adult patients with a life expectancy of 6 months or less.

2. Payment reform at the end of life which mandated hospice service payment reform with the goal of reducing barriers to access to high-quality hospice care. This provision also called for the testing of a value-based purchasing program for hospice employing advanced care planning and care coordination services and their impact on the patient experience and other quality measures such as admission to hospice at least 3 days prior to death. Coordination of care includes sharing with the patient information about prognosis, treatment goals, and expected response to treatment, and advanced care plans, including advanced directives and other legal documents.

3. Quality improvement of end-of-life care to enhance patient's access to services regardless of race, geographical region, or hospice care provider. This also includes mandatory public reporting of hospice quality data under the Hospice Quality Reporting program. Under this provision, failure to submit quality data results in a 2% reduction in hospice reimbursements for the following year (Parikh & Wright, 2017).

▶ ADVOCACY

Case managers advocate for patients and their families all the time, every time they care for a patient, and in every action they implement or decision they make. Ethical case managers demonstrate advocacy during their involvement in care coordination, transitions of care, interdisciplinary collaboration, and provision of timely access to care for patient and families. Advocacy is at the heart of the case manager's role and the relationship with the patient, patient's family, and support system (Tahan, 2016a).

Tahan defines advocacy as a "moral and ethical obligation that can be evident in the decisions and actions of case managers when managing, coordinating, and facilitating health care delivery; deciding on the appropriate use of resources; and enhancing quality and safety outcomes for their clients[patients]/support systems[families]. Moreover, advocacy is an essential element of interdisciplinary collaboration, communication, and cooperation for the purpose of meeting and respecting clients' needs, desires, interests, and preferences" (Tahan, 2016a, p. 164). He adds that advocacy is most effective when it entails the following actions:

- ▶ Open communication
- ▶ Transparency
- ▶ Connection with others who are involved
- ▶ Honesty
- ▶ Respect, especially for different perspectives and opinions
- ▶ Truth-telling
- ▶ Trust
- ▶ Listening
- ▶ Supporting
- ▶ Empowering
- ▶ Engaging
- ▶ Patience
- ▶ Guidance
- ▶ Sharing of information

Case managers advocate for those they care for during every phase of the case management process (Display 9-6). They also engage in advocacy at four different levels: the individual patient (e.g., making referrals to specialty care providers or community-based resources); the healthcare organization (e.g., changing processes of care to improve patient's timely access to services); the community (e.g., offering outreach programs such as health risk screening); and the global level (e.g., effecting a change in health law or public policy that results in reducing the number of the uninsured) (Tahan, 2016a).

Patient advocacy is a critical function of case managers. For example, case managers assist their patients/families to speak for themselves and express their opinions about healthcare services and care options, advocate for their own rights, become knowledgeable about their health insurance benefits, and demonstrate accountability and empowerment about their health status and well-being (Tahan, 2016b). Advocacy is included in the various codes of ethics and professional conduct of case management–related associations or agencies including ANA, ACMA, CCMC, CMSA, and NASW. These bodies emphasize the advocacy role of case managers by highlighting the following role responsibilities:

- ▶ Protecting client's autonomy, right to choice, and self-determination;
- ▶ Keeping the client as the central focus (i.e., provision of client-centered and culturally competent care) and promoting what is in the client's best interest;
- ▶ Ensuring client's engagement in informed and shared decision making;

display 9-6

EXAMPLES OF CASE MANAGER'S ACTIONS OF ADVOCACY

▶ Assessing clients' needs and those of their support systems.

▶ Planning, facilitating, coordinating, managing, and integrating required healthcare services and support resources.

▶ Monitoring and evaluating the delivery of services and clients' responses.

▶ Transitioning the clients from one level of care/setting or provider to another.

▶ Educating clients about and engaging them in their treatment plans, tests, procedures, and healthcare regimens, building self-care and self-management skills, and understanding how to navigate the complex healthcare system.

▶ Monitoring and addressing patient care delays, whether related to tests and procedures or responding to their results in an effort to progress care.

▶ Communicating with payors (e.g., insurance companies such as managed care organizations) regarding the clients' conditions and treatment and transitional plans.

▶ Obtaining authorizations for treatments and services necessary for providing care to clients.

▶ Facilitating shared and informed decision making concerning care options.

▶ Being transparent with the client and the support system regarding care progression, quality and safety concerns, and cost of services.

From Tahan, H. (2016). Essentials of advocacy in case management. Part I: Ethical underpinnings of advocacy—Theories, principles, and concepts. *Professional Case Management*, *21*(4), 163–179, used with permission.

▶ Enhancing client's access to equitable, timely, and appropriate healthcare services and resources;

▶ Safeguarding client's right to privacy and confidentiality;

▶ Improving client's health outcomes, safety, and quality of life; and

▶ Engaging in social justice, and health and public policy change efforts (Tahan, 2016a, p. 176).

▶ SUMMARY

Regardless of the ethical issues faced, if case managers act on the basis of ethical principles and professional codes of conduct, keeping the patient/family interests above all others, they can ensure the achievement of desired outcome(s)—those that please all parties: patients and their family members, providers of care, healthcare organizations they work for, payors, and regulatory or accreditation agencies. Ethically competent case managers

protect their patients and advance what is in the patients' best interest (patient advocacy); do the right thing when coordinating care and services and ensure patient safety and quality of care especially during vulnerable times such as transitions of care; are accountable for their own practice; effectively mediate ethical conflicts when they arise; and abide by their professional code of conduct and related ethical principles.

DISCUSSION QUESTIONS

1. What do ethics mean to you? What constitutes an ethical dilemma? What constitutes ethical case management practice?

2. Would Nancy Cruzan's case be resolved differently today than in the 1980s? Why?

3. Recall and discuss an ethical dilemma that occurred with one of your cases.

4. For each of the nine scenarios in the GUIDE presented in Display 9-1:
   • Discuss a real case that matches the scenario.
   • Discuss the recommendations given for the case scenario.

5. If an ethics committee has ever been consulted on one of your cases, discuss the case, the ethical dilemma, and the committee's recommendations. Were the issues organizational, clinical, personal, or professional in nature? How did you go about organizing an ethics committee meeting to deliberate the issue? Discuss what worked and what did not. Could you have done anything differently?

6. In your opinion, is there an ethical difference between withholding and withdrawing life-sustaining treatment? Describe cases from your own practice that are examples of these issues.

7. When does ordinary treatment become extraordinary? Provide one or more examples from your practice where ordinary treatment became extraordinary. How did it change? Who was involved? How could you have avoided or prevented the situation?

8. Is withholding or withdrawing nutritional support from a person ethically justifiable? When, if ever? What criteria could be used? What about hydration?

9. Are nutritional support and hydration different from other forms of life support? If so, how are they different? Is discontinuing nutritional support active euthanasia? Is it passive euthanasia?

10. Discuss differences between a patient who is terminally ill and one who is imminently dying. Would the case plans differ? What are the ethical implications for the care of each patient?

11. Discuss your views on the points mentioned in the Delphi poll.

12. Discuss a case that you felt had an ethical twist to it concerning rationing healthcare. How did you address the situation? What ethical principles did you apply?

13. Discuss a case in which you felt your patient advocate role was compromised by your gatekeeper role. How did you deal with that? What actions did you find to work?

14. Discuss a case in which your gatekeeper role was influenced by your patient advocate role.

15. Discuss a case in which you felt medical necessity was misused. Explain the ethical decision-making process you pursued to handle the issue.

▶ REFERENCES

American Case Management Association. (2017). *Accredited case manager code of conduct.* Retrieved July 14, 2017, from http://www.acmaweb.org/section.aspx?sid=132

American Nurses Association. (2015). *Code of ethics for nurses with interpretive statements.* Silver Spring, MD: Author.

Banja, J. (1996). If Momma dies, you die. *The Case Manager, 16*(1), 37–39.

Boling, J. (1991). Profile—John Banja. *The Case Manager, 11*(4), 76–81.

Case Management Society of America. (1996). *CMSA's statement regarding ethical case management practice.* Little Rock, AR: Author.

Case Management Society of America. (2016). *Standards of practice for case management.* Little Rock, AR: Author.

Centers for Medicare & Medicaid Services. (2017a). *The center for consumer information & insurance oversight, patient's bill of rights.* Retrieved July 14, 2017, from https://www.cms.gov/CCIIO/Programs-and-Initiatives/Health-Insurance-Market-Reforms/Patients-Bill-of-Rights.html

Centers for Medicare & Medicaid Services. (2017b, June 14). *National health expenditure, fact sheet.* Retrieved July 14, 2017, from https://www.cms.gov/research-statistics-data-and-systems/statistics-trends-and-reports/nationalhealthexpenddata/nhe-fact-sheet.html

Commission of Case Manager Certification. (2015). *Code of professional conduct for case managers with standards, rules, procedures, and penalties.* Retrieved from https://ccmcertification.org/sites/default/files/docs/2017/code_of_professional_conduct.pdf

Commission on Consumer Protection and Quality in Health Care. (1998). *President's advisory commission releases consumer bill of rights and responsibilities.* Retrieved from www.hcquality-commission.gov

Curtin, L. (1994). Ethical concerns of nutritional life support. *Nursing Management, 25*(1), 14–16.

Fiesta, J. (1992). Refusal of treatment. *Nursing Management, 23*(11), 14–18.

Jansen, L. (2003). Ethical Decision making in case management. In T. Cesta & A. Tahan (Eds.), *The case manager's survival guide: winning strategies for clinical practice* (2nd ed., pp. 324–335). St. Louis, MO: Mosby.

Johns, C. (1996, February, 18). Should prisons be organ farms: "harvesting" bills raise scary implications. *The Arizona Republic,* H3.

Keehan, S. P., Stone, D. A., Poisal, J. A., Cuckler, G. A., Sisko, A. M., Smith, S. D., ... Lizonitz, J. M. (2017). National health expenditure projections, 2016–25: price increases, aging push sector to 20 percent of economy. *Health Affairs, 36*(3), 553–563.

Knox, R. (1994, May 27). Noted deaths reflect attitude shift: Most patients and families oppose resuscitation efforts, study finds. *The Phoenix Gazette,* A26.

Kolodner, D. (1992). Advance medical directives after Cruzan. *Medsurg Nursing, 1*(1), 56–59.

Levenson, J., & Pettrey, L. (1994). Controversial decisions regarding treatment and DNR: an algorithmic guide for the uncertain in decision-making ethics (GUIDE). *American Journal of Critical Care, 3*(2), 87–91.

National Association of Social Workers. (2008). *Code of ethics.* Washington, DC: Author. Retrieved July 14, 2017, from http://www.socialworkers.org/pubs/Code/code.asp

National Association of Social Workers. (2013). *NASW standards of social work case management.* Washington, DC: Author. Retrieved July 14, 2017, from https://www.socialworkers.org/practice/naswstandards/casemanagementstandards2013.pdf

Organ Procurement and Transplantation Network. (2008). *Data reports.* Retrieved September 18, 2008, from http://optn.org

Parikh, R., & Wright, A. (2017). The affordable care act and end-of-life care for patients with cancer. *The Cancer Journal, 23*(3), 190–193.

President's Commission for the Study of Ethics Problems in Medicine and Biomedical and Behavioral Research. (1983). *Deciding to forego life-sustaining treatment.* Washington, DC: U.S. Government Printing Office.

Tahan, H. (2016a). Essentials of advocacy in case management. Part I: Ethical underpinnings of advocacy—Theories, principles, and concepts. *Professional Case Management, 21*(4), 163–179.

Tahan, H. (2016b). Essentials of advocacy in case management. Part II: Client advocacy model and case manager's advocacy strategies and competencies. *Professional Case Management, 21*(5), 217–232.

United Network of Organ Sharing. (2017, January 9). *2016 annual report.* Retrieved July 15, 2017, from https://www.unos.org/about/annual-report/2016-annual-report/

United States Department of Health and Human Services. (2013, May 22). Pre-existing conditions insurance plan program. *Federal Register, 78*(99). Retrieved July 14, 2017, from https://www.gpo.gov/fdsys/pkg/FR-2013-05-22/pdf/2013-12145.pdf

Wright, R. A. (1987). *Human values in health care: The practice of ethics.* New York: McGraw-Hill.

PART 4

Practical Applications

"To laugh often and much; to win the respect of intelligent people and the affection of children; to earn the appreciation of honest critics and endure the betrayal of false friends; to appreciate beauty; to find the best in others; to leave the world a bit better, whether by a healthy child, a garden patch or a redeemed social condition; to know even one life has breathed easier because you lived. This is to have succeeded"

RALPH WALDO EMERSON

CHAPTER 10

Case Management Standards and Professional Organizations

LEARNING OBJECTIVES

Upon completion of this chapter, the reader will be able to:

1. Identify professional organizations or societies that are important to case management practice.
2. Describe accreditation and accreditation agencies impacting case management responsibilities and processes.
3. Identify the various case management credentials and certifications.
4. List the eligibility criteria and examination content for organizations and agencies that provide case management certification and credentialing services.
5. Describe case management standards of practice, guidelines, and protocols.
6. Define accreditation and certification.

ESSENTIAL TERMS

Accreditation • American Case Management Association (ACMA) • American Nurses Association (ANA) • American Nurses Credentialing Center (ANCC) • Case Management Adherence Guidelines • Case Management Practice Guidelines • Case Management Society of America (CMSA) • Case Management Standards • Certification • Commission for Case Manager Certification (CCMC) • Credentialing • Healthcare Effectiveness Data and Information Set (HEDIS) • National Association of Healthcare Quality (NAHQ) • National Association of Social Workers (NASW) • National Committee for Quality Assurance (NCQA) • National Transitions of Care Coalition (NTOCC) • Standards of Practice for Case Managers • The Joint Commission (TJC) • The Joint Commission International (JCI) • URAC (formerly Utilization Review Accreditation Commission)

As the healthcare industry strives to monitor and demonstrate accountability to the population it serves, professional specialty certifications, standards, and accreditations have become an important part of the overall picture. Case management is no exception. Further, the certifications and accreditations are no longer just medals on a uniform, but are considered by some employers, businesses, and governmental agencies to be mandatory. The Joint Commission's (TJC) seal of approval has been mandatory for many years for facilities that provide care to Medicare beneficiaries. Now, regulatory agencies and quality improvement organizations are weaving outcomes management into the mix. Outcomes are being addressed by a number of accountability-oriented initiatives, including the National Committee for Quality Assurance (NCQA) utilizing the Healthcare Effectiveness Data and Information Set (HEDIS); TJC utilizing the core measures program (previously known as ORYX); and the Centers for Medicare & Medicaid Services (CMS) using core measures for specific diagnoses such as heart failure and pneumonia in the value-based purchasing (VBP) Program.

Many of these different quality initiatives appear to be duplicative. In some respects, this is true. Nevertheless, they are also complementary and are providing a service that cannot be fully realized yet. Managed care quality assessments have been evolving. A challenge lies in the fact that unmanaged care is more difficult to assess. Further, a comparison of managed care and unmanaged care plans has not yet been completely worked out, and remains a challenge today. Assessing the quality and outcomes of healthcare services has been evolving for the past two decades; and until recently such assessment focused on volume as a driver for quality. Today, however, with the advent of the VBP and other similar programs the definition of quality has shifted to be one of value to the consumer or recipient of healthcare services. One thing is clear: case managers contribute to quality care and safety (i.e., value) in more ways than perhaps any other single strategy. Case managers are more than an asset to any organization; during these times of regulatory monitoring and accountability, they are critical.

This chapter will discuss the following:

▶ Professional organizations or societies important to case management practice and case managers;

▶ Guidelines, protocols, and case management standards;

▶ Credentials germane to case management practice, utilization management, and quality management; and

▶ Regulatory and accreditation agencies influencing case management responsibilities and processes.

▶ ORGANIZATIONS

▶ The Case Management Society of America

The Case Management Society of America (CMSA) is an international nonprofit organization that was founded in 1990 to promote and support the development of professional case management through educational forums, networking opportunities, and legislative and health policy involvement. It collaborates with other organizations across the healthcare continuum to advocate for patients' well-being and improved healthcare outcomes. It promotes these efforts through fostering case management growth and development, healthcare policy activities, and evidence-based tools and resources. The CMSA's membership has grown to more than 35,000 individuals and companies who belong to over 75 chapters which are based in the United States (CMSA, 2017a).

The CMSA describes its vision on the basis of the role case managers play in the delivery of healthcare services and caring for the recipients of care. It states, "Case managers are recognized experts and vital participants in the care coordination team who empower people to understand and access quality, efficient health care" (CMSA, 2017b) services. The CMSA has also articulated its mission with special focus on its membership and improving health outcomes. Its mission states that the CMSA "is the leading membership association providing professional collaboration across the health care continuum to advocate for patients" well-being and improved health outcomes through:

1. Fostering case management growth and development;
2. Impacting health care policy; and
3. Providing evidence-based tools and resources (CMSA, 2017b).

Care managers, according to the CMSA, are "advocates who help patients understand their current health status, what they can do about it and why those treatments are important. In this way, care (and case) managers are catalysts by guiding patients and providing cohesion to other professionals in the health care delivery team, enabling their clients to achieve goals more effectively and efficiently" (CMSA, 2008). The CMSA envisions case managers as pioneers of healthcare change, as key initiators of and participants in the healthcare team who create new areas of thought, research, and development, and as those leading the way toward the day when every American will know what a case/care manager does and will know how to access case and care management services. To execute on its vision and mission, the CMSA has based its efforts on the following three ideologies:

1. To inform consumers about the services case and care managers provide;
2. To educate providers, including physicians, and health policy advocates about improved patient outcomes through the services case and care managers provide; and
3. To educate payors and regulators about improved patient outcomes that case and care management services can provide (CMSA, 2008).

The CMSA sponsors annual conferences and educational forums, promotes international networking among case managers, and participates in legislative and health policy activities. It has developed the *Standards of Practice for Case Management* and the *Ethics Statement on Case Management Practice*, both released in 1995. The CMSA has revised its standards in 2010 and most recently in 2016. In addition, it has organized several critical taskforces to enhance research and knowledge pertinent to the case management profession. These include the Career and Knowledge Pathways (CKP) educational program, which offers a diverse list of educational courses with continuing education credits; the Council for Case Management Accountability (CCMA), which aims to research and develop case management outcomes, evidence-based guidelines, and accountability; and the public policy committee, which focuses on government affairs, advocacy, and legislative and public policy issues relevant to case management practice and healthcare delivery. The CMSA provides its members information about accreditation programs and certifications in case management. It has also established special interest groups to serve its diverse membership, and is currently working on title protection for the case manager (CMSA, 2017c).

With healthcare costs rising around the world, case management has become the focus of international attention. Countries around the world were curious to know how the United States was containing costs and sustaining quality of care and turned to the CMSA for leadership and collaboration. The next logical step for the CMSA was to expand and form international chapters. Today, CMSA members live in Australia, New Zealand, Canada, the United Kingdom, Puerto Rico, South Africa, and Germany. Interested groups have also formed in China, Japan, Singapore, and Spain. Australia has formed CMS Australia; Singapore has formed Case Management Society of Singapore; and Canada has formed its National Case Management Network.

The CMSA has members from various health disciplines and with a diversity of professional licenses. This diversity is responsible for much of its success. Given the complexity of the healthcare system, each profession adds a different, yet complimentary, perspective. Only by looking at the magnitude of the challenges from a 360-degree perspective can case managers exercise influence on healthcare to the degree that has been accomplished thus far.

CMSA members are offered two publications. The first is *Professional Case Management: Leading Evidence-Based Practice Across Transitions of Care.* This peer-reviewed journal is published by Wolters Kluwer, formerly Lippincott Williams & Wilkins, and features best practices and industry benchmarks for the professional case manager. It focuses on coordination of patient care, efficient use of resources, improving the quality of care, data and outcomes analysis, research in case management, ethical and legal practices, and patient advocacy, among many other topics.

The second publication is *CMSA Today*, a magazine established in 2011 and published by the CMSA with support from Naylor Association Solutions. It is a contemporary, nationally focused magazine designed to meet the professional, personal, and lifestyle needs of today's case managers. The magazine offers cutting-edge clinical information to address challenges that confront healthcare professionals and covers the latest issues, resources, trends, tools, technology, and news in healthcare, enabling case managers to stay up-to-date and promoting professional growth and development. *CMSA Today* also provides CMSA members with the latest news and information from the association by including the CMSA president's message and other relevant society activities.

Both publications offer a wealth of case management information to keep case managers and other readers on the cutting edge of the profession. The CMSA website is an updated source of information, healthcare links, and communication forums. Although the CMSA strongly supports the concept of credentialing case managers, it is not the credentialing body (Display 10-1).

The CMSA's CKP educational program provides experienced and new case managers with practical instruction of the basic concepts of case management which complements the available theoretical knowledge and supports the employer-based training efforts. The CMSA relies on case management thought leaders in the development of CKP content. The first course CKP has featured is the *CMSA Standards of Practice: The Foundation for Professional Excellence in Coordination of Care Across the Continuum*; it has contributed to the basic understanding of the standards that govern case management practice.

On the basis of the CMSA's Standards of Practice for Case Management, CKP educational program is viewed as a self-paced learning tool that features content about each of the Standards of Practice. It also allows the case manager to learn at own choice. Moreover, the CKP applies a multimodal learning delivery method that consists of videos, simulations, and case studies. Such an approach is known to encourage a collaborative and flexible learning experience for the case manager.

▶ The Care Continuum Alliance

The Care Continuum Alliance was established in March 1999 as the Disease Management Association of America. It is an organization that represents more than 200 corporate and individual stakeholders, including wellness, disease, and care management organizations; pharmaceutical manufacturers and pharmacy benefits managers; health information technology innovators; biotechnology innovators; employers; physicians, nurses, and other healthcare professionals; researchers; and academicians. Its primary goal is population health improvement through health and wellness promotion, disease and condition (chronic care) management, care coordination, complex case management, and patient advocacy. Through alignment of the diverse stakeholders, the Care Continuum Alliance (Display 10-2) promotes the role of population health improvement in raising the quality of care, improving health outcomes, and reducing preventable healthcare costs for individuals with chronic conditions and those at risk of developing chronic conditions. The Alliance's activities in support of these efforts include advocacy, research, and the promotion of best practices in care management (The Care Continuum Alliance, 2017a).

display 10-1

CMSA CONTACT INFORMATION

For information on the Case Management Society of America (CMSA), contact:

Case Management Society of America
6301 Ranch Drive
Little Rock, AR 72223
Telephone: (501) 225-2229
Fax: (501) 221-9068
E-mail: cmsa@cmsa.org
Website: http://www.cmsa.org

display 10-2

THE CARE CONTINUUM ALLIANCE CONTACT INFORMATION

For information on the Care Continuum Alliance, contact:

Care Continuum Alliance
701 Pennsylvania Avenue NW, Suite 700
Washington, DC 20004-2694
Telephone: (202) 737-5980
Fax: (202) 478-5113
E-mail: info@carecontinuum.org
Website: http://www.carecontinuum.org

The mission of the Care Continuum Alliance focuses on the following key activities and aims:

▶ Promoting a proactive, patient-centric focus across the care continuum;
▶ Convening healthcare professionals to share and integrate care models;
▶ Emphasizing the importance of both healthful behaviors and evidence-based care in preventing and managing chronic health conditions;
▶ Promoting high-quality standards that address wellness, disease, and, where appropriate, case management and care coordination programs, as well as support services and materials;
▶ Identifying, researching, sharing, and encouraging innovative approaches and best practices in care delivery and reimbursement models;
▶ Establishing consensus-based outcomes measures and demonstrating health, satisfaction with the care experience, and financial improvements. These can be achieved by wellness, disease prevention, care coordination, and case management programs.
▶ Supporting healthcare delivery system and models that ensure appropriate care for chronic conditions and coordination among all healthcare providers. This may include strategies such as the Chronic Care Model, the physician-led medical home concept, and the disease management model.
▶ Encouraging the widespread adoption and interoperability of health information technologies;
▶ Advocating the principles and benefits of population health improvement to public health officials, including state and federal government entities;
▶ Underscoring the level of commitment to population health improvement and the time frames necessary to realize the full benefits (The Care Continuum Alliance, 2017b).

The Care Continuum Alliance emphasizes the importance of a proactive, accountable, patient-centric population health improvement model of care that promotes a physician-guided healthcare delivery system. It states that such a model should develop and engage informed and activated patients over time to address both illness and the individual's long-term health. The Alliance and its members also believe that managing health requires a fully connected healthcare system where care coordination efforts must be proactive and integrate the various healthcare professionals, besides physicians, and the active involvement of patients and their families/caregivers. The population health improvement model consists of three main components that ensure higher levels of quality and experience of care:

1. The central care delivery and leadership roles of the primary care physician;
2. The critical importance of patient activation, involvement, and personal responsibility; and

3. The patient focus and capacity expansion of care coordination provided through wellness, disease, and chronic care management programs (The Care Continuum Alliance, 2017b).

The Care Continuum Alliance believes that the highest health status is attained through the promotion and alignment of population health improvement through the following activities (The Care Continuum Alliance, 2017c):

▶ Strategies and processes for the identification of the patient population to benefit from care coordination and management;
▶ Conduct of comprehensive needs assessments that identify the physical, psychological, economic, and environmental needs of the patient population;
▶ Provision of proactive health promotion and wellness programs that increase individual's awareness of the health risks associated with certain personal behaviors and lifestyles;
▶ Patient-centric health management goals and education: These may include primary prevention, health behavior modification programs, and support for concordance between the patient and the primary care provider.
▶ Implementation of self-management interventions that aim to influence healthy lifestyle and behavior in the target population;
▶ Evaluation of care outcomes on an ongoing basis with the goal of improving overall population health. Outcome measures address the following.
  ▶ Clinical indicators, including process and outcome measures;
  ▶ Functional status and quality of life;
  ▶ Economic and healthcare utilization indicators;
  ▶ Assessment of patient satisfaction with the healthcare experience; and
  ▶ Impact on known population health disparities.
▶ Regular reporting of outcomes and provision of feedback: These may include ongoing communications with patients, physicians, health insurance plans, and ancillary service providers.

The Care Continuum Alliance provides healthcare professionals with vehicles for information sharing that help them in population health management under which are included the development, implementation, assessment, and improvement of disease prevention and management strategies. It also provides its members with information on current research, partnerships, processes, and best practices that underscore the delivery of cost-effective, quality care. *Population Health Management*, the official journal of the Alliance, is a member benefit, peer-reviewed international journal published on a bimonthly basis. It comprehensively covers the clinical and business aspects of the field of population health management. The journal features peer-reviewed clinical research and case studies, papers on the practical aspects involved in implementing population health management initiatives, and perspectives and insights from professionals involved in population health, disease, and care management (The Care Continuum Alliance, 2017d).

▌ The American Case Management Association

The American Case Management Association (ACMA) was initially launched to primarily address the needs of the hospital-based case manager. Today, the ACMA aspires "to be the association for healthcare delivery system case management and transitions of care professionals" (ACMA, 2013). With broadening its focus, it now provides professional services to those other than case managers, including physician advisors, medical directors and chief medical officers, chief nursing officers, case management program leaders, transitions of care leaders, and other healthcare administrators. The ACMA consists of 30 chapters located throughout the United States. These chapters provide enhanced networking and educational opportunities to members and other case management professionals. They also enhance members' ability to network among peers at the local, regional, or national level, and host educational events periodically.

The objectives of the ACMA are: (1) to provide its constituencies with innovative professional development services, including mentoring, educational forums, and resource information; (2) create new opportunities for networking; and (3) influence the policies, laws, and other issues related to the practice of case management. It defines case management in the context of hospitals and healthcare systems as "a collaborative practice model including patients, nurses, social workers, physicians, other practitioners, caregivers and the community." It also describes the case management process as one that "encompasses communication and facilitates care along a continuum through effective resource coordination." Additionally, it articulates the goals of case management in care provision to patients and their families to include "the achievement of optimal health, access to care and appropriate utilization of resources, balanced with the patient's right to self-determination" (ACMA, 2017a).

The ACMA (Display 10-3) offers its members and other case management professionals opportunities for the exchange of best practices and innovations through educational forums including the following:

- ▌ An annual conference that focuses on case management and transitions of care practices. This event offers case management professionals continuing education credits/hours that meet the needs of nurses, social workers, and physicians.
- ▌ Live webinars series sessions;
- ▌ On-demand continuing education programs;

- ▌ Leadership conference sessions;
- ▌ Specialty-based information or education such as utilization review, denials management, reimbursement, ethics, and end-of-life care.

One of the hallmarks of the ACMA is its online continuing education program known as *Compass*. This program is available to case management professionals and other stakeholders. *Compass* as a training system is a comprehensive program designed to provide standardized training for case management staff. It is not intended to be a preparatory course for the Accredited Case Manager (ACM) Exam or a stand-alone preparatory resource. This online learning system focuses on teaching and testing case management professionals about their foundational knowledge in case management and physician advisory practices. The *Compass* platform consists of two comprehensive course libraries; one targets the needs of case managers, whereas the second addresses the needs of physician advisors. The content of this system is developed and maintained by an interdisciplinary taskforce of case management and physician advisor leaders. The learning courses are professionally presented by experts in the field and include interactive case studies and competency-based examinations. Courses in the library of online continuing education are tailored for the needs of the nurse and social work case managers, physician advisors, and physician advising faculty. The courses consist of cognitive knowledge content, case studies, competency testing, and an electronic manual for case management professionals to download or print. The library content is presented in four sections:

1. Scope of practice,
2. Care coordination and resource management,
3. Transitions of care and advocacy, and
4. Regulatory requirements (ACMA, 2017b).

Collaborative Case Management is the official journal of the ACMA. It is a peer-reviewed quarterly publication for hospital and healthcare system case management professionals. It aims to enhance the practice by featuring solutions to current case management issues. These may include successful strategies, innovative interventions,

---

display 10-3

AMERICAN CASE MANAGEMENT ASSOCIATION CONTACT INFORMATION

For more information about the American Case Management Association, contact:

American Case Management Association
11701 West 36th Street
Little Rock, AR 72211
Telephone: (501) 907-2262
Fax: (501) 227-4247
E-mail: theacma@acmaweb.org
Website: www.acmaweb.org

and best practices, the use of effective tools, and the educational needs of hospital case managers and physician advisors. Through this publication, the ACMA continues its commitment to supporting the evolving practice of the acute care and hospital-based case managers.

▶ Case Management Practice Guidelines

Early on, case managers realized that the quality of life improved, patient and family satisfaction increased, and the costs of healthcare decreased, on a case-by-case basis. Evaluation of case management outcomes began with measuring details specific to the individual patient. Next, case managers pooled total caseloads and disease-specific populations to assess factors across larger groups of patients. With the assistance of the CCMA, these pooled outcomes will grow in statistical significance (power in numbers) and can eventually become the core ingredients of which guidelines are made. Guidelines are not static entities; they are dynamic statements that must change when improved methods of care delivery and practice are discovered.

Aetna Health Plans and the Individual Case Management Association (ICMA) collaborated on the development of *The Case Management Practice Guidelines* (Coeur, 1996). The ICMA has since merged with the CMSA, and the name CMSA is used. The guidelines were published in 1996 as an effort to move case management from a predominately intuitive model to one of a more concrete nature (i.e., one in which chronic disease management and case management could originate, and outcomes measurement studies could be initiated).

Several disease-specific guidelines are outlined, including those dealing with AIDS/HIV, brain injury, high-risk neonate/pregnancy, low back injury, oncology, pediatrics, workers' compensation, spinal cord injury, transplants, amputations, asthma, cystic fibrosis, renal failure, substance abuse, and gerontology. Within each guideline the following attributes are discussed: primary diagnosis, referral triggers, goals, medical considerations, special considerations, long-term care/life-care planning, patient/family teaching, psychosocial issues, vocational issues, patient and family issues, resources/support groups, barriers to effective outcomes, and the effectiveness of case management outcomes (Coeur, 1996). One important consideration with any disease-specific condition is that the knowledge and the treatment options of the disease are dynamic. All guidelines, even those of the Agency for Healthcare Research and Quality guidelines, they must be periodically updated or they may become less useful. The case manager must be aware of changes and check current, credible information.

CASE MANAGEMENT ADHERENCE GUIDELINES

An example of practice guidelines is the CMSA's medication and treatment adherence tool, known as a *Case Management Adherence Guideline* (CMAG). Launched in 2004, it was developed on the basis of key concepts including patient information, motivation, and behavior skill needs. This guideline has received positive feedback and ratings from the case management community. The CMAG is now recognized as the "best standard" and set of tools ever developed to assist case managers in working effectively with their patients to improve their adherence to taking prescription medications. Specifically, the purpose of the CMAG is to help case managers from diverse care settings (e.g., managed care organizations and acute care hospitals) in the assessment, planning, facilitation, and advocacy of patient adherence to ultimately achieve better health and financial outcomes, and optimal well-being. The guidelines include an interaction and management algorithm for use in the assessment and improvement of the patient's knowledge and his or her motivation to take medications as they are prescribed. They are flexible enough to allow case managers to incorporate a patient's individual needs. The guidelines also extend to specific disease states including breast cancer, chronic obstructive pulmonary disease, depression, diabetes, and pain (CMSA, 2017d). For more information on the CMAG, refer to the CMSA's website (http://solutions.cmsa.org/acton/fs/blocks/showLandingPage/a/10442/p/p-0025/t/page/fm/3).

INTEGRATED CASE MANAGEMENT

The CMSA provides case managers with the knowledge and skills necessary for the delivery of integrated care to patients and their families. Through its publication, *Integrated Case Management (ICM) Manual*, the CMSA equips case managers with the knowledge, skills, and tools to effectively care for patients suffering from complex and multimorbid conditions, although this manual is not a traditional practice guideline. The ICM Manual offers case managers practical information about new evidence-based assessment tools and application guides. It also supports case managers in advocating for improved quality and safe care for all patients. This manual encourages case managers to assess patients with both medical and mental health barriers to health improvement and to coordinate appropriate and integrated health (medical and mental) interventions and treatment plans (CMSA, 2017e).

Built upon the goals and values of the CMSA, the ICM Manual guides case managers through the process of developing new and important interdisciplinary skills, which will allow them to alter the health trajectory of some of the neediest patients in our healthcare system. Key features of the ICM Manual include:

- ▶ Tools and resources about the application of an integrated healthcare delivery model to the care of patients with complex conditions. Information about the development and implementation of comprehensive, coordinated, and integrated plans of care (physical and mental health treatments and interventions) is also provided.
- ▶ Evidence-based complexity assessment grids: a color-coded tool for tracking patient progress and

outcomes throughout the trajectory of the patient's illness/health condition. The manual offers the case managers essential information on how to perform a systematic complexity assessment.

▶ Strategies for building collaborative partnerships among interdisciplinary healthcare teams involved in patient care delivery.

▶ Use of ICM approaches to improve efficiency, effectiveness, accountability, and positive outcomes in clinical care settings.

▶ Guidance on building collaborations and partnerships among members of interdisciplinary healthcare teams to assist with the management of the patient's various health issues and needs, biologic, psychological, and social domains, and to overcome treatment resistance, reduce complications, enhance adherence, and reduce the cost of care (CMSA, 2017e).

The CMSA also provides case managers with training on the use of the ICM Manual, which is offered on a regular basis throughout the year. The training is an advanced educational program designed to provide case managers coming from either medical or mental health backgrounds with the content and skills needed to implement the recommended ICM guidelines available in the ICM Manual. Topics addressed include: principles of integrated care management for physical and mental health conditions, health system basics, cross-disciplinary team collaboration, ICM assessment process and complexity tools that focus on the biologic, physical, social, psychological, and health system domains, care planning, evaluation, and documentation of the patient's progress. The training also addresses the development of an alliance between the case manager and patient/family using motivational interviewing skills and techniques, while disentangling physical, psychological, social, and health system barriers to improvement. During the training, managers learn how to alter barriers in each of these domains without the need to transfer patients/clients to other managers (CMSA, 2017e).

CMSA CORE CURRICULUM FOR CASE MANAGEMENT

The CMSA has sponsored the development and publication of the only core curriculum in case management for use by case managers and other health professionals who are directly or indirectly involved in case management practice. This Core Curriculum was first published in 2001, revised in 2008, and again revised most recently in 2016. It is written by experts in the case management field as a comprehensive guide that follows a quick reference and a detailed outline format and provides essential knowledge for practice that is both theoretical and practical in nature. The Core shares important information about best practices, descriptions of key terms and concepts, essential skills, tools, and helpful references that fulfill the CMSA's

current standards and requirements. Additionally, the Core addresses the full spectrum of healthcare professional roles, care settings, and practice environments. Moreover, it has been found helpful in academic programs as a textbook for teaching case management, in employer-based orientation curricula, and as a crucial specialty certification study guide. The Core has been used as a vital clinical resource for case management professionals in virtually every specialty area of practice, from students to veteran case managers.

The CMSA core curriculum for Case Management features a wide range of topics of which are the following:

▶ Highlights from the CMSA Standards of Practice for Case Management
▶ Transitional planning and transitions of care
▶ Utilization management and resource management
▶ Case management roles, functions, tools, and processes
▶ Plans, clinical pathways, and use of technology
▶ Care coordination
▶ VBP
▶ Use of health information systems and digital technology
▶ Accreditation and certifications in case management
▶ Leadership skills and concepts
▶ Quality and outcomes management
▶ Legal issues in case management practice
▶ Ethical standards and principles, including ethics and social media
▶ Healthcare insurance, benefits, and reimbursement systems
▶ Practice settings: hospitals, community clinics, private practice, acute care, home care, long-term care and rehab settings, palliative care, and hospice settings
▶ Case management specialty practices: nursing, life-care planning, workers' compensation, disability management, care of the elderly, behavioral health, subacute and long-term care, and primary care and medical/health home
▶ Case management models design and performance or program evaluation.

▶ Standards of Practice for Case Management

The literature often cautions professions against writing standards of care that are too idealistic—this would put an impossible burden on the one who must perform under those standards. It is recommended that standards represent the safe, minimum level that the profession must follow; therefore, it is expected that, at this level, the standards must be followed explicitly. Standards can and do end up in courts of law. To this end, it is essential that case managers know the recommended standards that pertain to case management practice.

The *Standards of Practice for Case Management* were developed and released by the CMSA in 1995. They were revised in 2002; again in 2010, and most recently in 2016. The standards are generic and provide a framework for case managers in a variety of settings and specialties. They can be translated into working tools for preparation, management, and evaluation of case managers. Case management experts assisted the CMSA in the development of its standards which are meant as guidelines for practice excellence. They have been the forerunner for establishing formal guidelines from a variety of settings.

Some have questioned whether these standards have put an impossible burden on case managers. The burden, if any, is not so much due to the way they are written; rather, case management is a tremendously pervasive specialty with multiple roles and responsibilities, and involving professionals from diverse health disciplines and educational backgrounds. Not all case managers are required to perform every case management role or responsibility addressed in the CMSA's case management practice standards. However, it is important that case managers follow those portions that correspond to their job descriptions.

The CMSA *Standards of Practice for Case Management* is divided into 10 parts as described herewith (CMSA, 2016).

I. *Introduction*: This section describes the concept of case management with its purpose and goals. It shares the CMSA's vision and mission of case management, provides a brief history, highlights the impact of key related regulations, and explains who is the professional case manager. Additionally, this section describes the continuum of healthcare and professional case management, and select key terms with their intended use in the standards.

II. *Evolution of the Standards of Case Management*: This section explains the history of the standards with their development and publication in 1995 and how they evolved overtime until the most recent revision in 2016.

III. *Definitions of Case Management*: This section shows the evolution of the CMSA's definition of case management over the years.

IV. *Philosophy and Guiding Principles*: This section features the philosophy of case management practice and lists 13 guiding principles with their intended use and benefit.

V. *Case Management Practice Settings*: This section of the standards explains the diverse care settings across the continuum of health and human services where case managers are found to practice. These include traditional (e.g., acute care/hospital) and nontraditional (e.g., retail pharmacy) settings.

VI. *Professional Case Managers' Roles and Responsibilities*: This section differentiates the use of the terms role, function, and activity. It also highlights 18 primary responsibilities of case managers.

VII. *Components of the Case Management Process*: This section notes that the process is cyclical and recurrent rather than linear. It also explains each of the six steps in the process, and these are: client identification, selection, and engagement in case management services; assessment and opportunity identification; the development of the case management plan of care; the implementation and coordination of the case management plan of care; the monitoring and evaluation of the case management plan of care; and the closure of the professional case management services. As each step is described, the relevant standards of care required for safe and effective case management services are defined.

VIII. *Standards of Professional Case Management Practice*: This section describes 16 standards, including expectations of how case managers demonstrate each of these standards. Examples of these standards are: client selection process for case management services; client assessment; facilitation, coordination, and collaboration; qualifications for professional case managers; legal which includes confidentiality and client privacy, and client's consent for case management services; ethics; advocacy; cultural competency; resource management and stewardship; and professional responsibilities and scholarship.

IX. *Acknowledgments*: This section expresses gratitude for the volunteers, expert case managers, and CMSA board of directors who contributed to the standards and their revision.

X. *Glossary*: This section describes several pertinent definitions such as evidence-based criteria, case management plan of care, predictive modeling, risk stratification, VBP, transitional care, stewardship, and patient activation.

The full text of the CMSA's *Standards of Practice for Case Management* can be obtained from the CMSA (see previous section on the CMSA in this chapter). It is available online for download at http://www.cmsa.org/LinkClick.aspx?fileticket=BwBCDTjuj3k%3d&tabid=36.

▶ American Case Management Association Scope of Services and Standards of Practice

Another professional organization that offers standards of practice for case managers is the ACMA. It has convened a taskforce for the sole purpose of developing standards of practice for the hospital- and healthcare system–based case manager. Most recently, in 2013, the ACMA published the *Standards of Practice and Scope of Services for Health Care Delivery System and Transitions of Care (TOC) Professionals* (Display 10-4). These are a revision of a prior version and provide case management professionals in the acute care setting and those involved in TOC with guidance on their role expectations in the form of scope of services and standards of practice.

display 10-4

ACMA'S SCOPE OF SERVICES AND STANDARDS OF PRACTICE

Scope of Services

▶ *Education*: provide education relevant to the effective progression of care, appropriate level of care, and safe patient transition.

▶ *Care Coordination*: apply a defined method for screening/identification and assessment of patients in need of case management services. Also follow defined standards for ongoing monitoring and interventions that advance the progression of care and must include the clinical, psychosocial, financial, and operational aspects of care.

▶ *Compliance*: knowledge of and adherence to federal, state, local hospital, and accreditation requirements that impact the case manager's scope of services.

▶ *Transition Management*: based on assessment findings, patient choice, and available resources, develop and coordinate a successful patient's transition plan, keeping in mind that transition management planning begins at the time of case management's initial patient encounter and continues throughout the patient's hospital stay.

▶ *Utilization Management*: advocate for the patient while balancing the responsibility of stewardship for their organization and in general, the judicial management of resources.

Standards of Practice

▶ *Accountability*: claiming ownership for the achievement of optimal outcomes within their standards of practice.

▶ *Professionalism*: emulating the standards of practice of case managers, their professional disciplines, and the mission vision and values of their organization.

▶ *Collaboration*: working with patients/families/caregivers and the healthcare team to jointly communicate, problem–solve, and share accountability for optimal outcomes that must respect patient preferences and available resources.

▶ *Care Coordination*: facilitating the progression of care by advancing the care plan to achieve desired outcomes and integration of the work of the healthcare team by coordinating resources and services necessary to accomplish agreed-upon goals.

▶ *Advocacy*: supporting or recommending on behalf of patients/family/caregivers and the hospital for service access or creation and for the protection of the patient's health, safety, and rights.

▶ *Resource Management*: prudently utilizing resources (fiscal, human, environmental, equipment, and services) by evaluating the resources available to the patient and balancing cost and quality to ensure the optimal clinical and financial outcomes.

▶ *Certification*: achieving certification as it validates a case manager's knowledge, competency, and skills.

Compiled from American Case Management Association. (2013). *Standards of Practice and Scope of Services for Health Care Delivery System and Transitions of Care (TOC) Professionals*. Little Rock, AR: Author.

▶ National Transitions of Care Coalition

The National Transitions of Care Coalition (NTOCC) was formed in 2006 by the CMSA and Sanofi-Aventis as an independent not-for-profit organization. It brought together thought leaders, patient advocates, and healthcare providers from various care settings across the continuum for the main purpose of improving the quality of care coordination, TOC, and communication when patients are transferred from one level of care or provider to another. The original work of the NTOCC was developed by an Advisory Task Force that consisted of an invited group of leading healthcare organizations. In 2013, the NTOCC established the National Transitions of Care Foundation, which supports the technical analysis, educational work, and consultative efforts that the NTOCC provides to the healthcare industry. Today, the NTOCC has an Advisors Council of more than 30 organizations representing industry professionals (i.e., healthcare professional associations and medical societies), standards designing bodies, patients, caregivers, thought leaders, policy makers, and regulators. All share a common goal: "to raise awareness about transitions of care among healthcare professionals, government leaders, patients and caregivers to increase the quality of care, reduce medication errors and enhance clinical outcomes." The NTOCC addresses the critical issues and challenges surrounding TOC by developing solutions and providing essential information for the improvement of patients' transitions with the support of its national governing board and councils (NTOCC, 2017a).

Since the NTOCC's inception, the Advisors Council has sought to develop significant tools and resources that all participants in healthcare (i.e., patients, caregivers, employers, professionals, and policy makers) can use to improve patient safety and decrease errors associated with poor transitions (NTOCC, 2017b). The NTOCC also has a Partners Council that consists of a select group of companies that represent various sectors of healthcare and support industries such as pharmaceuticals, acute care delivery, managed care organizations, retail pharmacy, medical device manufacturing agencies, healthcare support services, and information technology companies (NTOCC, 2017c).

The NTOCC views TOC as a major challenge to healthcare delivery and acknowledges that this concern can be addressed only by breaking down the existing silos and barriers between the various healthcare settings. As a result, the NTOCC is working collaboratively for the good of the patient to provide key information and tools to patients, caregivers, healthcare professionals, policy makers, and media representatives to assist them to better understand and improve TOC challenges (NTOCC, 2017d).

TOC, as described by the NTOCC, are the movements of patients from one care setting or provider to another. During these transitions, poor communication and coordination between professionals, patients, and caregivers can lead to unsafe and serious events, wastage of healthcare resources, or frustration of healthcare consumers and providers. The NTOCC was formed to define solutions addressing these gaps that impact the safety and quality of care for transitioning patients.

The NTOCC Advisors Council has created four work groups to address key areas associated with TOC. Various organizations on the Advisors and Partners Councils collaborate within each work group to discuss solutions and create resources for use by the entire healthcare industry, patients, and caregivers. The Advisors Council includes representatives from leading organizations who discuss ways to create and implement solutions and resources to benefit patients during TOC. These two councils are joined by associate members, that is, organizations that wish to support this important work and are able to raise awareness to transitional care concerns and advance solutions. The work groups are as follows:

1. *Education and Resources Workgroup*—which addresses awareness and general knowledge about the problems associated with TOC and to provide the necessary information to various stakeholders—patients, caregivers, healthcare professionals, and government officials. In order to do this, the NTOCC focuses on identifying practical tools and resources for use by healthcare professionals, patients, and caregivers to improve communication and enhance consistency between care settings, and to reduce risk associated with care transitions.

2. *Policy and Advocacy Workgroup*—which assesses ways to improve care through enhanced communication tools, collaborative partnerships, and improved reimbursement methods for transitional care support and technical medical information shared between care settings. This work group also provides advice and recommendations to healthcare policy makers.

3. *Measures Workgroup*—which assesses and defines appropriate performance measurement frameworks to demonstrate the impact of interventions on reducing risk associated with transitional care, improving outcomes, and reducing costs.

4. *Health Information Technology Workgroup*—which determines gaps in the available healthcare information technology that create barriers to effective and safe transitions. This work group also suggests technology solutions that incorporate the NTOCC's recommendations for transitions safety (NTOCC, 2017e).

On its website, the NTOCC (Display 10-5) shares key information and several tools that healthcare providers, including case managers, patients, and families, can access,

download, and use for free. These tools are useful for case managers to incorporate in their work with patients, especially to encourage adherence to medications intake and to educate regarding safety and self-care. The tools include the following:

▶ My Medicine List (consumer-focused in three languages: English, French, and Spanish);
▶ Taking Care of My Health Care (consumer-focused in three languages: English, French, and Spanish);
▶ TOC Checklist;
▶ Patient Bill of Rights during TOC;
▶ Medication Reconciliation and Essential Data Specifications;
▶ Informational brochure about TOC;
▶ Information slides that describe the issue of TOC and the NTOCC's work in this regard;
▶ Improving TOC with Health Information technology;
▶ Cultural Competence: Essential Ingredient for Successful TOC;
▶ Policy paper (a white paper) that describes the state of TOC and recommended actions that can be taken to improve transitions;
▶ Framework for Measuring Outcomes of TOC;
▶ Improving on TOC: How to Implement and Evaluate a Plan. This tool also includes a guidebook and two modules that apply the plan: a hospital to home and an emergency department to home modules; and
▶ A set of Issue Briefs on improving TOC.

The NTOCC has developed the TOC bundle which consists of seven key elements as described in the next paragraph. These are essential care-transition intervention strategies that any healthcare provider (including the case manager) may implement to improve care transitions. This bundle is applicable to any type of care-transition "exchange/hand-off" and is categorized into main topics that are important for any care transition with descriptive language and examples to aid the healthcare provider in adopting these strategies (NTOCC, 2011). It is important for case managers to apply the bundle in their own practice and to ensure safe and quality transitions of care.

1. *Medications Management*: Ensures the safe use of medications by patients and their families and is based on patients' plans of care. This element focuses on (a) the assessment of the patient's

medications intake; (b) the conduct of patient and family education and counseling about medications use; and (c) the development and implementation of a plan for medications management as part of the patient's overall plan of care.

2. *Transitional Planning*: A formal process that facilitates the safe and effective transition of patients from one level of care or provider (or practitioner) to another including home. This element focuses on: (a) a clearly identified practitioner (or team dependent on care setting) to facilitate and coordinate the patient's transition plan; (b) the management of the patient's and family's transition needs; (c) the use of formal transitional planning tools; and (d) the completion of a transition summary to be shared with the next level of care.

3. *Patient and Family Engagement and Education*: Education and counseling of patients and families to enhance their active participation in their own care including informed decision making. This element focuses on: (a) ensuring that patients and families or caregivers are knowledgeable about the condition and plan of care; (b) having a patient and family-centered transition communication; and (c) supporting the patient and family in developing self-care management skills.

4. *Information Transfer*: Sharing of important care-related information among patient, family, caregiver, and healthcare providers in a timely and effective manner. This element focuses on (a) the implementation of clearly defined communication models for use during the transition process; (b) the use of formal communication tools; and (c) having a clearly identified practitioner to establish accountability and facilitate timely transfer of important information among those involved.

5. *Follow-up Care*: Facilitating the safe transition of patients from one level of care or provider to another through effective follow-up care activities. This element focuses on: (a) ensuring that patients and families have timely access to key healthcare providers for follow-up care after an episode of care as required by the patient's condition and needs and (b) communicating with patients and/or families and other healthcare providers post transition from an episode of care to ensure continuity of care.

6. *Healthcare Provider Engagement*: Healthcare providers demonstrating ownership, responsibility, and accountability for the care of the patient and family/caregiver at all times. This element focuses on: (a) a clearly identified personal physician (primary care provider) of the patient; (b) the use of nationally recognized evidence-based practice guidelines; (c) the identification of the healthcare provider as the hub of case management (and care coordination) activities; (d) the provision of patient and family health education and counseling activities; and (e)

the ensuring of an open and timely communication among healthcare providers, patients, and families.

7. *Shared Accountability across Healthcare Providers and Organizations*: Enhancing the transition of care process through accountability for care of the patient by both the healthcare provider (or organization) transitioning and the one receiving the patient. This element focuses on: (a) clear and timely communication of the patient's plan of care among providers; (b) ensuring that a healthcare provider is responsible for the care of the patient at all times; and (c) assuming responsibility for the outcomes of the care-transition process by both the provider (or organization) sending and the one receiving the patient.

▶ CASE MANAGEMENT CREDENTIALS

▶ The Certified Case Manager

The Certified Case Manager (CCM) is one of the premiere and oldest case management certifications. Since the first CCM examination in 1993, an estimated 60,000 case managers have earned the CCM credential. To take the examination, an applicant must meet acceptable standards with regard to work experience and hold a recognized license or certification in a field that promotes client physical, psychological, or vocational well-being. The Commission for Case Manager Certification (CCMC) is an independent credentialing agency that sponsors and oversees the CCM credentialing process. The CCMC is accredited by the National Commission for Certifying Agencies (NCCA).

While researching the necessity of this credential in 1991, the National Case Management Task Force realized that no single profession could "own" case management; rather, it was the coordinating and advocacy approach to healthcare that case managers brought to the table. Therefore, the CCM is not a primary credential. It is a secondary credential as an adjunct to a licensed professional in a recognized health and human services field (i.e., RN, LCSW, RPT, MD, etc.).

According to its vision statement, the CCMC aspires to "be the global leader committed to the advancement and evolution of case management." Its mission is "to advocate for professional case management excellence through certification and interrelated programs and services." The CCMC promotes the importance of the case management certification credential and ongoing education to meet the dynamic practice of case management. It also communicates that "board certification" is essential for quality and effective practice. Through the development and management of a comprehensive professional certification for qualified case managers, the CCMC promotes, advances, and advocates for consumer protection, quality case management practice, ethical standards and behavior, and scientific knowledge development and dissemination (CCMC, 2017a).

A major strength of the CCMC is its research-based approach for the development of the CCM certification examination. The CCMC conducts a role and functions study, referred to as practice analysis. Findings of the study are then used to develop the blueprint for the certification examination. Such research captures the breadth of the knowledge, skills, and activities case managers perform in the field. The role and functions study is completed every 5 years, using a large sample of case managers from across the United States, to validate and improve the CCM credential. This approach ensures that the certification examination remains valid and reflects current case management practice (CCMC, 2017b).

The CCMC (2017c) defines case management as "a collaborative process that assesses, plans, implements, coordinates, monitors, and evaluates the options and services required to meet the client's health and human service needs. It is characterized by advocacy, communication, and resource management and promotes quality and cost-effective interventions and outcomes." The CCMC promotes the value of board certification stating that it demonstrates that the case manager possesses the education, skills, knowledge, and experience required to render appropriate services delivered according to sound principles of practice. It also articulates in its philosophy that case management:

- Is an area of specialty practice within the health and human services profession.
- Benefits everyone: the clients reaching their optimum level of wellness, self-management, and functional capability; the stakeholders include the clients being served; their support systems; the healthcare delivery systems, including the providers of care; the employers; and the various payor sources.
- Facilitates the achievement of client wellness and autonomy through advocacy, assessment, planning, communication, education, resource management, and service facilitation.
- Involves the role of case managers who, on the basis of the needs and values of the client, and in collaboration with all service providers, link clients with appropriate providers and resources throughout the continuum of health and human services and care settings, while ensuring that the care provided is safe, effective, client-centered, timely, efficient, and equitable.
- Includes the provision of services that are optimized best if offered in a climate that allows direct communication among the case manager, the client, the payor, the primary care provider, and other service delivery professionals. Case managers enhance the provision of these services by maintaining the client's privacy, confidentiality, health, and safety through advocacy and adherence to ethical, legal, accreditation, certification, and regulatory standards or guidelines (CCMC, 2017c).

The CCM certification examination focuses on five core domains of case management knowledge. These core domains evolved from a large survey of case managers, both CCM and non-CCM credential holders, and represent an aggregate view of the most important roles, responsibilities, and spheres of knowledge required for case managers to perform their case management functions. It is an extensive list; however, the CCMC is testing for case management knowledge, skills, and experience—a broad and comprehensive set of responsibilities. (Note: Details of the core domains are from *The CCM Certification Guide*, published by the CCMC, and available for free on the CCMC's website.) The domains covered on the certification examination are described in Display 10-6 (CCMC, 2017d).

These five domains are further clarified through the following attributes:

- The case manager must perform according to all of the eight essential activities with direct contact with the patient, including assessment, planning, implementation, coordination, monitoring, evaluation, outcomes, and general (e.g., privacy, advocacy, and adherence to ethical, legal, and accreditation standards).
- The case management practice reflects the application of at least four of the five core domains of knowledge described in Display 10-6.
- At least 30% of the case manager's qualified work time must focus primarily on case management practice.
- Case management services are provided across the continuum of care, beyond a single episode, and address the ongoing needs of the patient.
- The core domains require that the case manager interact with other relevant professionals and parties within the patient's healthcare system.
- The case manager maintains a moral character.

The CCM is a voluntary credential. However, its influence in case management should not be underestimated; every year, more advertised case management positions require this credential. Those interested in applying for the case management certification, requesting *The CCM Certification Guide*, or in need of information on continuing education credits for recertification should contact the CCMC (Display 10-7).

▌ The American Nurses Association: Nursing Case Management Credential

The Nursing Case Management (RN, CM) credential is provided by the American Nurses Credentialing Center (ANCC), the credentialing arm of the American Nurses Association (ANA). The ANA established its certification program in 1973 to offer professional achievement recognition in various clinical areas of nursing practice. Later in 1991, it incorporated its certification programs as a subsidiary of the ANA, the ANCC. The ANCC's certification programs provide national and international recognition

COMMISSION FOR CASE MANAGER CERTIFICATION—FIVE KEY DOMAINS (CCMC, 2017d)

Care Delivery and Reimbursement Methods

▶ Adherence to care regimen
▶ Alternate care facilities (e.g., assisted living, group homes, residential treatment facilities)
▶ Case management process and tools
▶ Coding methodologies (e.g., Diagnosis-related group [DRG], Diagnostic and Statistical Manual of
▶ Mental Disorders [DSM], International Classification of Diseases [ICD], Current Procedural
▶ Terminology [CPT])
▶ Continuum of care/continuum of health and human services
▶ Cost containment principles
▶ Factors used to identify client's acuity or severity levels
▶ Financial resources (e.g., waiver programs, special needs trusts, viatical settlements)
▶ Goals and objectives of case management practice
▶ Healthcare delivery systems
▶ Healthcare providers including behavioral health and community vendors
▶ Hospice, palliative, and end-of-life care
▶ Insurance principles (e.g., health, disability, workers' compensation, long-term care)
▶ Interdisciplinary care team (ICT)
▶ Levels of care and care settings
▶ Managed care concepts
▶ Management of acute and chronic illness and disability
▶ Management of clients with multiple chronic illnesses
▶ Medication therapy management and reconciliation
▶ Military benefit programs (e.g., TRICARE, VA, CHAMPVA, TRICARE for Life)
▶ Models of care (e.g., patient-centered medical home [PCMH], accountable care organization, health home, special needs plan [SNPs], chronic care model)
▶ Negotiation techniques
▶ Physical functioning and behavioral health assessment
▶ Private benefit programs (e.g., pharmacy benefits management, indemnity, employer-sponsored health coverage, individual-purchased insurance, home care benefits, COBRA)
▶ Public benefit programs (e.g., SSI, SSDI, Medicare, Medicaid)
▶ Reimbursement and payment methodologies (e.g., bundled, case rate, prospective payment systems, value-based purchasing)
▶ Roles and functions of case managers in various settings
▶ Roles and functions of other providers in various settings
▶ Transitions of care/transitional care
▶ Utilization management principles and guidelines

Psychosocial Concepts and Support Systems

▶ Abuse and neglect (e.g., emotional, psychological, physical, financial)
▶ Behavioral change theories and stages
▶ Behavioral health concepts (e.g., dual diagnoses; substance use, abuse, and addiction)
▶ Client activation
▶ Client empowerment
▶ Client engagement
▶ Client self-care management (e.g., self-advocacy, self-directed care, informed decision making, shared decision making, health education)
▶ Community resources (e.g., elder care services, fraternal/religious organizations, government programs, meal delivery services, pharmacy assistance programs)
▶ Conflict resolution strategies
▶ Crisis intervention strategies
▶ End-of-life issues (e.g., hospice, palliative care, withdrawal of care, Do Not Resuscitate)
▶ Family dynamics
▶ Health coaching
▶ Health literacy assessment
▶ Interpersonal communication (e.g., group dynamics, relationship building)
▶ Interview techniques
▶ Multicultural, spiritual, and religious factors that may affect the client's health status
▶ Psychological and neuropsychological assessment
▶ Psychosocial aspects of chronic illness and disability
▶ Resources for the uninsured or underinsured

display 10-6

COMMISSION FOR CASE MANAGER CERTIFICATION—FIVE KEY DOMAINS (CCMC, 2017d) *(continued)*

▮ Spirituality as it relates to health behavior
▮ Support programs (e.g., support groups, pastoral counseling, disease-based organizations, bereavement counseling)
▮ Wellness and illness prevention programs, concepts, and strategies.

Quality and Outcomes Evaluation and Measurements

▮ Accreditation standards and requirements
▮ Case load calculation
▮ Cost-benefit analysis
▮ Data interpretation and reporting
▮ Healthcare analytics (e.g., health risk assessment, predictive modeling, Adjusted Clinical Group [ACG])
▮ Program evaluation and research methods
▮ Quality and performance improvement concepts
▮ Quality indicators techniques and applications
▮ Sources of quality indicators (e.g., Centers for Medicare and Medicaid Services [CMS], Utilization
▮ Review Accreditation Commission [URAC], National Committee for Quality Assurance [NCQA],
▮ National Quality Forum [NQF], Agency for Healthcare Research and Quality [AHRQ])
▮ Types of quality indicators (e.g., clinical, financial, productivity, utilization, quality, client experience)

Rehabilitation Concepts and Strategies

▮ Assistive devices (e.g., prosthetics, text telephone device [TTD], teletypewriter [TTY], telecommunication device for the deaf, orientation, and mobility services)
▮ Functional capacity evaluation
▮ Rehabilitation post an injury, including work related
▮ Rehabilitation post hospitalization or acute health condition
▮ Vocational and rehabilitation service delivery systems
▮ Vocational aspects of chronic illness and disability

Ethical, Legal, and Practice Standards

▮ Affordable Care Act (ACA)
▮ Case recording and documentation
▮ Critical pathways, standards of care, practice guidelines, and treatment guidelines
▮ Ethics related to care delivery (e.g., advocacy, experimental treatments and protocols, end of life, refusal of treatment/services)
▮ Ethics related to professional practice (e.g., code of conduct, veracity)
▮ Healthcare and disability related legislation (e.g., Americans with Disabilities Act [ADA], Occupational Safety and Health Administration [OSHA] regulations, Health Insurance Portability and Accountability Act [HIPAA])
▮ Legal and regulatory requirements
▮ Meaningful use (e.g., electronic exchanges of summary of care, reporting specific cases to specialized client registries, structured electronic transmission of laboratory test results, use of electronic discharge prescriptions)
▮ Privacy and confidentiality
▮ Risk management
▮ Self-care and well-being as a professional
▮ Standards of practice

display 10-7

INFORMATION ABOUT THE COMMISSION FOR CASE MANAGER CERTIFICATION

For more information about the Commission for Case Manager Certification, contact:

Commission for Case Manager Certification
1120 Route 73
Suite 200
Mount Laurel, NJ 08054
Email: ccmchq@ccmcertification.org
Telephone: (856) 380-6836
Fax: (856) 439-0525
Website: http://www.ccmcertification.org

for nurses who have proven themselves through education, experience, knowledge, testing, and professional conduct. The program consists of 25 certifications including the RN, CM credential for nurse case managers.

The nursing case management board certification applies a competency-based examination that provides a valid and reliable assessment of the entry-level clinical knowledge and skills of registered nurses in the nursing case management specialty after initial RN licensure. Candidates for the RN, CM credential must meet the following criteria to qualify for the certification exam:

▮ Hold a current, active, and unrestricted RN license.
▮ Have practiced the equivalent of 2 years full time as a registered nurse.

▶ Have a minimum of 2,000 hours of clinical practice in case management within the last 3 years.

▶ Have completed 30 hours of continuing education in case management within the last 3 years (ANCC, 2017a).

The ANCC also offers the RN, CM credential by reciprocity. Registered nurses who hold the CCM certification offered by the CCMC are eligible for the RN, CM certification through reciprocity by the ANCC. These nurses do not need to complete the ANCC's case management certification examination. These nurses must hold a current, active unrestricted RN license within a state or territory of the United States or the professional, legally recognized equivalent in another country.

Both the ANCC (Display 10-8) and the CCMC offer well-respected certifications in case management. The difference, however, is that the CCMC certification is multidisciplinary compared with that of the ANCC, which has been developed for registered nurses, by nurses, and focused specifically on nursing case management and the role nurse case managers play in today's healthcare system. Various healthcare professionals may be eligible for the CCMC certification, including registered nurses, social workers, physical and occupational therapists, physicians, rehabilitation counselors, and others.

The framework for the Nursing Case Management credential includes five domains of practice, each of which also includes essential knowledge and skills. The domains are: fundamentals, resource management, quality management, legal and ethics, and education and health promotion. Display 10-9 includes the RN, CM examination specifications on the basis of the test content outline available on the ANCC website, which went into effect in February 2015 (ANCC, 2017b).

---

display 10-8

INFORMATION ABOUT THE AMERICAN NURSES CREDENTIALING CENTER

For information about the RN, CM credential, contact:

American Nurses Credentialing Center
8515 Georgia Avenue, Suite 400
Silver Spring, MD 20910-3492
Telephone: (800) 284-4378 or (301) 628-5000
Fax: (301) 628-5004
Website: http://www.nursecredentialing.org

---

display 10-9

TEST SPECIFICATIONS FOR THE ANCC NURSING CASE MANAGEMENT CERTIFICATION (ANCC, 2017b)

Domain of Practice	Practice Element	Knowledge Of	Skills In
Fundamentals	Concepts, standards, and tools	1. Nursing case management concepts (e.g., functions, principles, roles) 2. Standards of practice for case management 3. Clinical guidelines and pathways 4. Tools (e.g., assessment, evaluation, screening)	
	Processes	1. Biopsychosocial health 2. Evidence-based practice	1. Conducting screenings and assessments 2. Identifying and managing risk factors and barriers 3. Developing a client-focused plan of care using evidence-based practice 4. Verifying interventions are consistent with the client's needs and goals 5. Linking the client to available resources 8. Implementing a client-focused plan of care using evidence-based practice 6. Modifying the plan and services on the basis of the evaluation of outcomes 7. Synthesizing pertinent data from multiple sources 8. Communicating the plan, interventions, and outcomes to stakeholders 9. Collaborating with stakeholders 10. Facilitating communication, problem-solving, and conflict resolution with stakeholders

TEST SPECIFICATIONS FOR THE ANCC NURSING CASE MANAGEMENT CERTIFICATION (ANCC, 2017b) *(continued)*

Domain of Practice	Practice Element	Knowledge Of	Skills In
Resource management	Healthcare utilization	1. Utilization of management concepts (e.g., authorizations, benefits, contract management, criteria, denials and appeals, discharge planning) 2. Payor and reimbursement methodology (e.g., forms of payment, government, private, disability, worker's compensation, uninsured)	1. Determining level of care using utilization review criteria 2. Negotiating benefits for clients 3. Planning for transition of care 4. Facilitating resolution of denials and appeals
	Support services	1. Community and support resources 2. Medical supplies and durable medical equipment 3. Benefit and payment options for support services (e.g., insured, uninsured, charity)	1. Negotiating for support services (e.g., medical supplies, durable medical equipment, pharmaceuticals)
	Provider services	1. Scope of services for providers (e.g., primary care, specialty providers, ancillary services)	1. Identifying providers (e.g., contracted, nonparticipating, preferred, participating) 2. Negotiating with providers to facilitate care services
Quality management	Quality and performance improvement	1. Quality and performance improvement processes and concepts 2. Quality indicators (e.g., core measures, outcome measures) 3. Risk management concepts 4. Benchmarking principles and concepts	1. Identifying potential risks and liabilities (e.g., client, facility, financial, safety) 2. Collecting data (e.g., variance tracking, benchmarking) 3. Conducting a cost-benefit analysis
	Outcomes evaluation	1. Outcome evaluation tools 2. Data management (e.g., individual, aggregate)	1. Synthesizing data to improve services (e.g., client, program)
Legal and ethics	Legal and regulatory	1. Accreditation and licensure 2. Scope of practice 3. Governmental regulations and policies that affect healthcare delivery 4. Legal responsibilities (e.g., abandonment, abuse and neglect, malpractice, guardianship)	1. Documenting the case management process
	Ethics	1. Nursing code of ethics 2. Professional code of conduct for case managers 3. Standards of practice for case management	1. Identifying potential conflicts of interests 2. Facilitating resolution of ethical issues
	Patient advocacy and rights	1. Patient's bill of rights 2. Advanced directives and living wills 3. Informed consent	1. Collaborating with multiple providers to facilitate access to care 2. Advocating for the client throughout the continuum of care
Education and health promotion	Education and learning	1. Change theories and concepts (e.g., motivational interviewing, behavioral change) 2. Interpreter services and materials	1. Assessing readiness for change 2. Selecting educational materials for specific learner needs 3. Providing client-focused instruction 4. Evaluating educational outcomes
	Population health management	1. Disease management 2. Wellness promotion and disease prevention 3. Biopsychosocial characteristics of wellness 4. Cultural perspectives of wellness 5. Predictive modeling concepts and principles	1. Identifying at-risk populations 2. Conducting population screenings 3. Referring clients for interventions (e.g., health maintenance, symptom management, wellness promotion)

▶ National Association for Healthcare Quality and Certified Professional in Healthcare Quality

The National Association for Healthcare Quality (NAHQ) was founded in 1976 and is one of the largest and leading organizations for healthcare quality management professionals. Its mission is to empower healthcare quality professionals from every specialty by providing vital research, education, networking, certification, and professional practice resources, as well as acting as the strong voice for healthcare quality. Its goal is to promote the continuous improvement of quality in healthcare by providing educational and development opportunities for professionals at all management levels and within all healthcare settings (NAHQ, 2008). The NAHQ is the parent organization of the Healthcare Quality Certification Commission (HQCC), previously referred to as the Healthcare Quality Certification Board (Display 10-10). The HQCC oversees the Certified Professional in Healthcare Quality (CPHQ) examination program and establishes policies, procedures, and standards for certification in healthcare quality management. The NAHQ also provides an educational foundation through the Healthcare Quality Educational Foundation (HQEF) (NAHQ, 2017).

The Journal for Healthcare Quality (JHQ) is the bimonthly official journal of the NAHQ. The journal is peer-reviewed; it promotes the art and science of healthcare quality practice to improve health outcomes and advance the practice in changing environments. The journal serves as the premier resource for scientific solutions in the pursuit of healthcare quality. Additionally, it addresses professionals who are responsible for promoting and monitoring quality, safe, cost-effective healthcare, and provides practical applications and tools for its delivery. The journal covers topics that span the continuum of care, including quality improvement, risk management, case/utilization review,

and the latest regulations from TJC, quality improvement and peer-review organizations, and payment systems. More information about the *JHQ* is available at http://nahq.org/education/journal-healthcare-quality.

The CPHQ is a voluntary credential that recognizes professional and academic achievement of individuals in healthcare quality management. The examination's focus is on performance improvement and includes quality improvement, case and population health management, utilization management, and risk management at all employment levels and in the various healthcare settings. More than 10,000 professionals have taken the examination, which was first introduced in 1984. The CPHQ examination is accredited by the NCCA.

The 1998 CPHQ examination was changed to include more emphasis on case management activities. This change occurred after test writers and research reviews showed that hospitals were using case managers more than ever, regardless of their level of managed care penetration. Resource case management is listed separately from clinical case management. Resource case management emphasizes cost-effective ways to deliver care, financial issues, and the identification of available resources for patients; this may include home health versus skilled nursing facility settings, or hospice versus home health choices. Clinical case management focuses on patient treatment, particularly in terms of pre- and postoperative care, preventive teaching, and posthospital follow-up. Questions about risk management, quality management, and utilization management are also included in the examination.

The HQCC recognizes that to survive, institutions must be data-driven; therefore, information management comprises one-fourth of the examination. Case managers taking this examination will need to understand data management; what constitutes valid, reliable data; data analysis; continuous quality improvement principles, tools, and techniques; and cross-functional teams.

INFORMATION ABOUT THE NATIONAL ASSOCIATION OF HEALTHCARE QUALITY AND THE HEALTHCARE QUALITY CERTIFICATION COMMISSION

display 10-10

For more information about the National Association for Healthcare Quality (NAHQ), for general inquiries about the Certified Professional in Healthcare Quality (CPHQ) certification and recertification, or for information about the Healthcare Quality Certification Commission (HQCC), contact:

National Association for Healthcare Quality
Healthcare Quality Certification Commission Headquarters
8735 W. Higgins Road Suite 300
Chicago, IL 60631
Telephone: (800) 966-9392
Fax: (847) 375-6320
E-mail: info@cphq.org.
Website: http://www.nahq.org
Candidates can register for the CPHQ certification examination online at www.cphq.org

For questions related to the CPHQ certification examination, refer to:

PSI/AMP
CPHQ Examination
18000 W. 105th Street
Olathe, KS 66061-7543
Telephone: (913) 895-4600
Fax: (913) 895-4650
Email: info@goAMP.com
Website: www.goAMP.com

In 2003, more changes to the certification exam took place. The HQCC (the HCQB at the time) Board of Directors voted to eliminate the minimum education and experience criteria previously required to apply for and take the CPHQ examination. The decision, effective January 1, 2004, removed perceived subjective barriers to certification. However, with elimination of the previous minimum education and experience requirements, each candidate must now take the time to assess and judge his or her own readiness to apply to take the CPHQ examination, particularly if the candidate has not worked in the field for at least 2 years. A careful review of all available information

about the tasks covered in the CPHQ examination content outline, the sample examination questions, reference list, and any other available data is essential before one makes the decision to apply for the examination. Display 10-11 outlines the CPHQ certification examination (NAHQ, 2017).

▶ American Board of Quality Assurance and Utilization Review Physicians

The American Board of Quality Assurance and Utilization Review Physicians (ABQAURP) was established in 1977 and has evolved to become one of the largest organizations

---

display 10-11

CONTENT OUTLINE FOR THE CERTIFIED PROFESSIONAL IN HEALTHCARE QUALITY EXAMINATION (NAHQ, 2017)

Quality Leadership and Structure

A. Leadership
1. Support organizational commitment to quality
2. Align quality and safety activities with strategic goals
3. Engage stakeholders
4. Provide consultative support to the governing body and medical staff regarding their roles and responsibilities (e.g., credentialing, privileging, quality oversight)
5. Participate in the integration of environmental safety programs within the organization (e.g., air quality, infection control practices, building, hazardous waste)
6. Assist with survey or accreditation readiness
7. Evaluate and integrate external quality innovations (e.g., resources from IHI, WHO, AHRQ, NQF)
8. Promote population health and continuum of care (e.g., handoffs, transitions of care, episode of care, utilization)

B. Structure
1. Assist in developing organizational measures (e.g., balanced scorecards, dashboards)
2. Assist the organization in maintaining awareness of statutory and regulatory requirements (e.g., OSHA, HIPAA, PPACA)
3. Assist in selecting and using performance improvement approaches (e.g., P'CA, Six Sigma, Lean thinking)
4. Facilitate development of the quality structure (e.g., councils and committees)
5. Communicate the impact of health information management on quality (e.g., ICD10, coding, electronic health record, meaningful use)
6. Ensure effective grievance and complaint management
7. Facilitate selection of and preparation for quality recognition programs and accreditation and certification options (e.g., Magnet, Baldrige, TJC, DNV, ARF, ISO, NCQA)
8. Communicate the financial benefits of a quality program
9. Recognize quality initiatives impacting reimbursement (e.g., capitation, pay-for-performance)

Information Management

A. Design and Data Collection
1. Maintain confidentiality of performance/quality improvement records and reports
2. Apply sampling methodology for data collection
3. Coordinate data collection
4. Assess customer needs/expectations (e.g., surveys, focus groups, teams)
5. Participate in activities like development of data definitions, goals, triggers, and thresholds
6. Identify or select measures (e.g., structure, process, outcome)
7. Assist in evaluating quality management information systems
8. Identify external data sources for comparison (e.g., benchmarking)
9. Validate data integrity

B. Measurement and Analysis
1. Use tools to display data or evaluate a process (e.g., fishbone, Pareto chart, run chart, scattergram, control chart)
2. Use statistics to describe data (e.g., mean, standard deviation)
3. Use statistical process controls (e.g., common and special cause variation, random variation, trend analysis)
4. Interpret data to support decision making
5. Compare data sources to establish benchmarks
6. Participate in external reporting (e.g., core measures, patient safety indicators)

(continued)

CONTENT OUTLINE FOR THE CERTIFIED PROFESSIONAL IN HEALTHCARE
QUALITY EXAMINATION (NAHQ, 2017) (continued)

Performance Measurement and Process Improvement

A. Planning
1. Assist with establishing priorities
2. Facilitate development of action plans or projects
3. Participate in selection of evidence-based practice guidelines
4. Identify opportunities for participating in collaboratives
5. Identify process champions

B. Implementation and Evaluation
1. Establish teams and roles
2. Participate in monitoring of project timelines and deliverables
3. Evaluate team effectiveness (e.g., dynamics, outcomes)
4. Participate in the process for evaluating compliance with internal and external requirements for: clinical practice (e.g., medication use, infection prevention), service quality, and documentation, practitioner performance evaluation (i.e., peer review)
5. Perform or coordinate risk management activities (e.g., identification, analysis, prevention)

C. Education and Training
1. Design organizational performance/quality improvement training (e g., quality, patient safety)
2. Provide training on performance/quality improvement, program development, and evaluation concepts
3. Evaluate the effectiveness of performance/quality improvement training
4. Develop/provide survey preparation training (e.g., accreditation, licensure, or equivalent)

D. Communication
1. Facilitate conversations with staff regarding quality issues
2. Compile and write performance/quality improvement reports
3. Disseminate performance/quality improvement information within the organization
4. Facilitate communication with accrediting and regulatory bodies
5. Lead and facilitate change (e.g., change theories, diffusion, spread)
6. Organize meeting materials (e.g., agendas, reports, minutes)

Patient Safety

A. Assessment and Planning
1. Assess the organization's patient safety culture
2. Determine how technology can enhance the patient safety program (e.g., computerized physician order entering (CPOE), barcode medication administration (BCMA), electronic medical record, abduction/elopement security systems, human factors engineering)

B. Implementation and Evaluation
1. Assist with the implementation of patient safety activities
2. Facilitate the ongoing evaluation of patient safety activities
3. Participate in these patient safety activities: incident report review, sentinel/unexpected event review, root cause analysis, failure mode and effects analysis (proactive risk assessment), patient safety goals review, and the identification of reportable events for accreditation and regulatory bodies
4. Integrate patient safety concepts throughout the organization
5. Educate staff regarding patient safety issues

of interdisciplinary healthcare professionals in the United States. Through its goal to improve the overall quality of healthcare that is provided to the consuming public, it offers healthcare education and certification for physicians, nurses, and other professionals. The ABQAURP is the only healthcare quality and management organization to offer a certification examination that is developed, administered, and evaluated through the testing expertise of the National Board of Medical Examiners'. This credential is referred to as the Certification in Health Care Quality and Management (HCQM). An eligible candidate must be a licensed physician (MD, DO, DDS, DMD, DPM), RN, or other licensed healthcare professional. The certification is recommended for individuals dedicated to the principles

of quality improvement, utilization management, managed care, risk management, case management, and workers' compensation. The certification is based on work experience and work-related activities in the area of healthcare quality and patient safety.

The eligibility criteria for the HCQM credential are:

▶ A current, nonrestricted license in each state or territory of the United States in which the candidate is licensed (as applicable to the candidate's profession);
▶ Documentation of active involvement in Health Care Quality within the past 5 years, a minimum of 208 hours (2 hours per week for 2 years) in any of the following exam categories: Quality Improvement,

Utilization Management, Risk Management, Case Management/Disease Management, Managed Health Care Systems, TOC, or Government (listed on Application and Verification);

▶ References from two colleagues or supervisors;
▶ Evidence of a minimum of 20 hours of ABQAURP-approved continuing education (pertinent to at least one of the exam categories), or completion of the ABQAURP Core Body of Knowledge online course; and
▶ Professional, working knowledge of the English language (ABQAURP, 2017a).

ABQAURP certifications have been given to more than 10,000 diplomates to date, making it one of the largest interdisciplinary healthcare professional credentials. The HCQM certification demonstrates that the healthcare professional has the practical knowledge and the tools to ensure patient safety and reduce medical errors, eliminate waste and unnecessary services, while avoiding potentially harmful delays in care. These professionals demonstrate to stakeholders that they are accountable for safer care environments and more efficient and cost-effective systems of care that satisfy the needs of patients, providers, purchasers, and payors. They also exhibit a deep commitment to safety, quality, and effective care. Additionally, they show ability to critically evaluate industry literature, identify evidence-based best practices, and make recommendations that balance the appropriateness of healthcare services with cost and quality (ABQAURP, 2017b).

The ABQAURP offers subspecialty certifications in the following categories:

▶ Physician Advisor,
▶ TOC,
▶ Managed Care,
▶ Patient Safety and Risk Management,
▶ Case Management, and
▶ Workers' Compensation (ABQAURP, 2017b).

The examination contains factual material, application of concepts, and realistic vignettes. Key concepts covered in the examination include those listed in Display 10-12 (ABQAURP, 2017c).

---

display 10-12

TOPICS INCLUDED IN THE HEALTH CARE QUALITY AND MANAGEMENT (HCQM) CERTIFICATION EXAMINATION (ABQAURP, 2017c)

Accreditation Organizations

▶ American Board of Quality Assurance and Utilization Review Physicians (ABQAURP)
▶ National Committee for Quality Assurance (NCQA)
▶ Healthcare Effectiveness Data and Information Set (HEDIS)
▶ The Joint Commission
▶ ISO (International Organization for Standardization)
▶ NQF

Transitions of Care (TOC)

▶ Transitions of Care Models
▶ Patient Protection & Affordable Care Act (PPACA)
▶ American Recovery & Reinvestment Act (ARRA)
▶ Seven Essential Elements
▶ Readmission Avoidance

Credentialing and Privileging

▶ Core Competencies
▶ The Data Bank
▶ Medical Staff Credentialing / Recredentialing
▶ Institutional Bylaws
▶ Economic Credentialing

Pay-for-Performance

▶ Meaningful Use
▶ Leapfrog Group
▶ Provider Performance
▶ Value-Based Purchasing

Insurance and Managed Care

▶ Accountable Care Organizations
▶ Health Maintenance Organizations (HMOs)
▶ Medicare
▶ Medicaid
▶ Preferred Provider Organizations (PPOs)

Workers' Compensation (WC)

▶ Compensability
▶ Independent Medical Exams (IME)
▶ Disability Protocols
▶ Regulations

Physician Advisor Medical Specialty

▶ Defining the Physician Advisor's Role
▶ Two-Midnight Rule
▶ Management of Observation Services
▶ Medicare Audits, Denials, and Appeals
▶ Transition to ICD-10

Quality Improvement, Management, and Assurance

▶ Theoretical Concepts
▶ Quality Improvement Organizations (QIOs)
▶ Peer Review
▶ Continuous Quality Improvement (CQI)
▶ Total Quality Management (TQM)
▶ Physician Quality Reporting System (PQRS)

Clinical Resource Management

▶ Utilization Review
▶ Medicare Audits
▶ Demand & Disease Management

Case Management

▶ Case Management Components
▶ Legal and Ethical Principles
▶ Informed Consent

(continued)

display 10-12

TOPICS INCLUDED IN THE HEALTH CARE QUALITY AND MANAGEMENT (HCQM) CERTIFICATION EXAMINATION (ABQAURP, 2017c) (continued)

Risk Management/Patient Safety

▶ Stark Laws
▶ Anti-Kickback Statutes/Safe Harbor
▶ Patient Self Determination Act (PSDA)
▶ Informed Consent
▶ Patient Safety Initiatives
▶ Computerized Physician Order Entry (CPOE)

Regulatory Environment

▶ Health Insurance Portability and Accountability Act (HIPAA)
▶ Centers for Medicare & Medicaid Services (CMS)
▶ Employee Retirement Income Security Act (ERISA)
▶ Consolidated Omnibus Budget Reconciliation Act (COBRA)
▶ Affordable Care Act (ACA)
▶ Health Care Quality Improvement Act (HCQIA)

The ABQAURP (Display 10-13) certification examination includes case management scenarios and questions relating to case management such as history and philosophy, case manager profile, and elements of a case management plan.

▶ Certified Social Work Case Manager and Certified Advanced Social Work Case Manager

Established in 1955, the National Association of Social Workers (NASW) consists of 132,000 members which makes it the largest membership organization of professional social workers in the world. The NASW aims to enhance the professional status, growth, and development of its members; create and maintain professional standards; advance sound social policies; and protect its members (NASW, 2017a). It launched its specialty certification program in early 2000 to help its members attain enhanced professional and public recognition and increased visibility as specialized, professional social workers. It also facilitates the association of social workers with a group of specialized professionals who have achieved national distinction. The NASW specialty certifications provide a vehicle for recognizing social workers who have met national standards and possess specialized knowledge, skills, and experience. The NASW is committed to assisting in the process of certifying social workers and is working to

emphasize the importance of employing social workers who have specialized training and experience. The NASW's specialty certifications and other professional credentials provide recognition to those who have met national standards for higher levels of experience and knowledge and are not considered by the association as a substitute for required state licenses or certifications (NASW, 2008).

The NASW offers eligible social workers two case management–related certifications. These are the Certified Social Work Case Manager (C-SWCM) and the Certified Advanced Social Work Case Manager (C-ASWCM) (Display 10-14). Additionally in 2017, the NASW established a formal collaboration with the CCMC to offer eligible social workers with the opportunity to pursue board certification in case management through the CCMC's credential which is the CCM. The NASW considers this affiliation as an important

display 10-13

INFORMATION ABOUT THE AMERICAN BOARD OF QUALITY ASSURANCE AND UTILIZATION REVIEW PHYSICIANS

For more information about the American Board of Quality Assurance and Utilization Review Physicians (ABQAURP), Inc, contact:

ABQAURP
6640 Congress Street
New Port Richey, FL 34653
Telephone: (800) 998-6030
Fax: (727) 569-0195
Website: http://www.abqaurp.org

display 10-14

INFORMATION ABOUT THE NATIONAL ASSOCIATION OF SOCIAL WORKERS AND CASE MANAGEMENT CERTIFICATION PROGRAMS

For Information about the National Social Workers Association (NASW) or the Certified Social Work Case Manager (C-SWCM and C-ASWCM), refer to the NASW:

National Association of Social Workers
750 First Street, NE
Suite 800
Washington, DC 20002
Telephone: (800) 742-4089 (NASW Member Services)
E-mail: membership@socialworkers.org

For the Certified Social Work Case Manager, contact:

National Association of Social Workers
750 First Street, NE
Suite 800
Washington, DC 20002
Telephone: (202) 4638-8799, extension 447 or (202) 408-8600, extension 447
E-mail: credentialing@socialworkers.org
Website: http://www.naswdc.org/credentials/specialty/c-aswcm.asp

step to meet the needs of the evolving social work professional landscape. Upon applying to and receiving approval from the NASW, social workers who meet the eligibility criteria for the C-SWCM or the C-ASWCM certification are also considered eligible to sit for the CCM certification examination at no additional cost (NASW, 2017b).

The NASW's specialty certifications in case management examination are based on the seven core functions of case management delineated by the association. These are listed herewith with examples (NASW, 2017b).

1. *Engagement*: Outreach, working alliance, screening, consent (release) forms, initial intake, and referral receiving.
2. *Assessment*: Needs (functional and/or psychosocial), strengths, challenges, opportunities, biopsychosocial, comprehensive intake, sociocultural, and resource/financial.
3. *Planning*: Service, intervention, treatment, care, direction, rehabilitation, strategic, support, and crisis prevention.
4. *Implementation and coordination*: Resource/service brokering, service delivery monitoring, service provision, project implementation, client support, and crisis management.
5. *Advocacy*: Working for systems improvement, promoting client well-being and/or client functioning, liaison, and mediation.
6. *Reassessment and evaluation*: Monitoring, efficacy, effectiveness, appropriateness, efficiency, review/revision, planning, data collection, and analysis.
7. *Disengagement*: Termination, transfer, and discharge planning.

The NASW's case management certifications also reflect its views on the practice of case management. It states that the primary goal of social work case management is to optimize client functioning by providing quality services in the most efficient and effective manner to individuals and families with multiple complex needs. It also notes that social work case managers practice in a variety of settings, including, but not limited to, acute care hospitals, nursing homes and skilled nursing facilities, rehabilitation facilities, hospice agencies, managed care organizations, community-based mental health agencies, schools, and the military. More specifically, the NASW emphasizes that social work case management practice:

▶ Applies the social work methods and rests on a solid foundation of professional training, values, knowledge, theory, and skills.
▶ Focuses on the biopsychosocial model that uses a Person-in Environment perspective to assess strengths and challenges within a systems framework.
▶ Not only considers the biologic needs in a patient's (client's) life, but also assesses the familial, social, environmental, and other systems needs affecting the patient's life.

▶ Is based on social work training in the micro and macro practice levels, and acts as advocates and brokers for patient's care and services. In this regard, social workers are uniquely skilled in identifying needs for resources, assessing the appropriateness of resources, and managing the use of these resources in both cost-effective and clinically sound ways.
▶ Can vary depending on the case management or social work program and/or care setting (NASW, 2017b).

Eligibility criteria for the C-SWCM are a Bachelor's of Social Work (BSW) degree from an institution accredited by the Council on Social Work Education; 3 years and 4,500 hours of paid, supervised, post-BSW work experience, exclusive of administrative duties or tasks; and an evaluation from an approved supervisor that should also reflect the work experience requirements. The supervisor's evaluation must address the applicant's case management skills, knowledge, and abilities across the seven case management core functions. Other criteria are: a reference from a BSW or Master's in Social Work (MSW) colleague; and licensure or credentials that may consist of either NASW/ACBSW (Academy of Certified Baccalaureate Social Workers) credential, current state BSW-level license, or a passing score on the ASWB Basic exam (NASW, 2017b).

The eligibility criteria for the C-ASWCM are the same as those of the C-SWCM except for the requirement of a MSW degree; 3,000 work experience hours instead of 4,500; supervision evaluation reflective of 3,000 hours of work experience; the reference from an MSW colleague; and the licensure or credentials to practice social work reflective of MSW level rather than BSW. Candidates must also agree to adhere to the NASW Code of Ethics, the NASW Standards for Social Work Case Management, the NASW Standards for Continuing Professional Education, and the CCMC Code of Professional Conduct. Although NASW membership is not a requirement, such membership makes one eligible to receive a discount on the certification fees as long as one maintains good standing (NASW, 2017b).

▶ The Accredited Case Manager

The ACMA offers the ACM certification to both the nursing and social work case managers. Upon successful completion of the certification, nurse case managers use the credential ACM-RN, whereas social work case managers use ACM-SW. The purpose of the ACM certification process is to measure entry-level competence of healthcare delivery system case managers and to promote professional practice standards. The selection of case managers in these settings is not regulated by states or national authorities; thus, achievement of the credential allows for case managers to voluntarily demonstrate their knowledge and competence. ACM credentials indicate successful completion of the specialty specific certification examination in Health Care Delivery System Case Management and ongoing competency in the practice.

The ACM certification is governed by the National Board for Case Management (NBCM) and managed by the ACMA (Display 10-15). The content of the ACM certification examination is defined through a national job analysis study which involves surveying case management practitioners in the field to identify routine tasks considered important to competent practice. These practitioners are selected from a wide variety of practice environments, healthcare settings, and geographical regions. The certification examination is developed and maintained through a combined effort of qualified subject-matter experts and testing professionals who construct the examination in accordance with the ACM certification examination content outline (ACMA, 2017c).

The eligibility criteria for the ACM certification examination include a combination of education, paid work experience, and professional practice (ACMA, 2017c):

- ▶ For RN case managers, a valid and current nursing license.
- ▶ For SW case managers, a bachelor's or master's degree from an accredited school of social work or a valid social work license.
- ▶ At least 1 year, or 2,080 hours, of full-time, supervised, paid work experience as a case manager, or in a role that falls within the ACMA's scope of services and the standards of practice.
- ▶ Candidates with less than 2 years of experience are expected to provide supervisor contact information and an attestation that they have at least 1 year of supervised case management experience.
- ▶ If a candidate meets the eligibility requirements of both an RN and SW, the candidate must indicate on the application whether he or she is interested in the RN or SW certification examination and provide the applicable eligibility documentation (ACMA, 2017c).

The NBCM and the ACMA do not produce or endorse any preparatory courses or study materials for the certification examination. It, however, suggests that those interested in pursuing the exam can make use of the ACM certification examination review content outlines and other materials available within the ACM Candidate Handbook. Display 10-16 lists the content outline addressed in the certification examination and Display 10-17 includes the content for the specialty simulation component (ACMA, 2017c).

---

display 10-15

ACCREDITED CASE MANAGER CERTIFICATION CONTACT INFORMATION

For questions and requests for information about the ACM certification, contact:

The National Board for Case Management (NBCM)
11701 W. 36th Street
Little Rock, AR 72211
Telephone: (501) 907-2262
Fax: (501) 227-4247
E-mail: certification@acmaweb.org
Website: www.acmaweb.org

For questions and requests for information about the ACM certification examinations, contact:

PSI/AMP Candidate Services
18000 W. 105th Street
Olathe, KS 66061-7543
Telephone: (913) 895-4600
Fax: (913) 895-4650
E-mail: info@goAMP.com
Website: www.goAMP.com

---

display 10-16

CORE CONTENT OUTLINE FOR THE ACM CERTIFICATION EXAMINATION (ACMA, 2017c)

1. *Screening and Assessment:* conduct screening and assessment activities for the purpose of preadmission, admission, or following admission to an inpatient or bed placement in an outpatient setting.
   - Obtain relevant, comprehensive information and data required for client assessment from the client, family, and significant others (and/or legal guardians), primary care physician or attending physician, consulting physician(s)/specialist(s), other members of the interdisciplinary team, and community providers
   - Assess and gather information regarding the client's health behaviors, health literacy, response to illness, belief or value system (e.g., cultural influences), medical history psychosocial history, financial situation, environment, functional status, support system, developmental level, readmission risk, decisional capacity/designated decision maker, current medical status, and level of care.
   - Formulate and communicate assessment findings.
   - Educate clients about the importance of advanced directives.
2. *Planning:* apply assessment findings to prepare a client-centered plan of care
   - Identify healthcare system services and resources to meet client needs
   - Identify continuum of care needs
   - Collaborate with the team to develop a plan of care
   - Educate the client about options for care

CORE CONTENT OUTLINE FOR THE ACM CERTIFICATION EXAMINATION (ACMA, 2017c) *(continued)*

- Obtain client choice regarding the aspects of care plan
- Coordinate client care conferences
- Establish goals and anticipated outcomes
- Evaluate alternative treatment and therapeutic plans on the basis of efficacy, cost, safety, and potential
- Ensure compliance and anticipated outcomes
- Integrate client choice, resources, and team recommendations into a plan of care
- Ensure client is educated about the plan of care
- Identify contingencies to the plan
- Identify resources for emerging client populations where resources are scarce.

3. *Care Coordination, Intervention, and Transition Management:* facilitate effective management of client care throughout the identified continuum of care
   - Establish linkages with internal systems to provide resources, services, and opportunities
   - Establish linkages with external systems to provide resources, services, and opportunities
   - Assist clients lacking in comprehensive coverage in pursuing entitlement programs (e.g., Medicaid, Medicare, and Veterans Administration)
   - Apply regulatory/accrediting requirements to practice inclusive of: state licensing, Health Insurance Portability and Accountability Act (HIPAA), Centers for Medicare and Medicaid Services (CMS), The Joint Commission (TJC), National Integrated Accreditation of Healthcare Organizations program, Emergency Medical Treatment and Active Labor Act, and Patient Protection and Affordable Care Act (PPACA)
   - Apply legal requirements to practice (e.g., mandated abuse reporting)
   - Apply ethical guidelines to practice (e.g., honoring client's right to choose, self-determination)
   - Coordinate timely and effective service delivery: facilitate diagnostic and treatment services (e.g., tests, consultations, procedures); ensure appropriate sequencing of diagnostic and treatment services; identify and manage operational, clinical, and/or client/family barriers; facilitate referral to continuum services (e.g., patient-centered medical home, medication payment assistance, skilled nursing facility, DME, home health, community agencies); provide/reinforce appropriate client education
   - Review admissions and level of care with respect to medical necessity of care, quality of care concerns, appropriateness of care, and payor authorization
   - Integrate cultural competence into the plan of care
   - Communicate potential payor issues to client, healthcare team, and other internal services orally
   - Communicate potential payor issues to client, healthcare team, and other internal services in writing
   - Facilitate clinical and therapeutic interventions across the care continuum throughout the life span
   - Record variances and avoidable delays in order to advance the plan of care
   - Analyze variances and avoidable delays in order to advance the plan of care
   - Mitigate variances and avoidable delays in order to advance the plan of care
   - Negotiate with service providers, payors, and members of the healthcare team to meet client care needs
   - Advocate on behalf of the client and/or facility for needed client resources and services
   - Provide education to other healthcare providers (e.g., infection control, healthcare economics, payor methods, discharge options, documentation, service utilization)
   - Document changes in the plan and responses to interventions
   - Communicate changes in the plan and responses to interventions
   - Conduct ongoing reassessment of all aspects of care
   - Communicate client status and needs to the next level of care
   - Assist clients in navigating the healthcare system
   - Serve as a resource for the issues of outcomes management, transition planning, and the development of improved strategies to benefit high-risk patients.

4. *Evaluation:* utilize outcome management and process improvement strategies to measure and improve the quality and effectiveness of care and processes
   - Systematically collect timely and accurate data to evaluate interventions
   - Participate in process improvement: identify opportunities for improvement; collaborate with the interdisciplinary team to create solutions and take corrective action to address issues; and evaluate the efficacy and effectiveness of the interventions
   - Establish relationships with external organizations related to service delivery utilization and contracting issues including payors, providers (e.g., primary care medical homes, skilled nursing facilities, home health agencies), and regulatory/governmental agencies
   - Identify patient safety and risk management issues
   - Resolve or refer patient safety and risk management issues for corrective action
   - Participate in activities that promote team cohesiveness and effective performance
   - Lead activities to promote team cohesiveness and effective performance.

display 10-17

CONTENT OUTLINE FOR THE ACM CERTIFICATION EXAMINATION—
SPECIALTY SIMULATION COMPONENT

Specialty Assessment, Care Coordination and Intervention—facilitate effective management of client care throughout the identified continuum of care as applied to social work/nursing practice in case management

▶ Perform client screening
▶ Assess and gather information from the client and all relevant sources
▶ Obtain relevant, comprehensive information and data required for client assessment from all sources of information
▶ Coordinate timely and effective service delivery: facilitate diagnostic and treatment services (e.g., tests, consultations, procedures) and client education; and identify and manage operational, clinical, and/or client/family barriers
▶ Facilitate clinical and therapeutic interventions across the care continuum throughout the life span
▶ Monitor delivery of service against the plan of care
▶ Continuously reassess client and family response to care

▶ Enhance client capacities (e.g., developmental, health literacy, problem-solving, coping, self-care)
▶ Conduct ongoing reassessment of the integration/interaction of all aspects of care
▶ Review admissions and level of care with respect to the medical necessity, quality, appropriateness of care, and readmission risk
▶ Verify payor authorization for services
▶ Review, process, and issue notices of noncoverage to client/responsible party following regulatory guidelines and facility protocols by informing client/responsible party of right of appeal and appeal process
▶ Establish relationships with external organizations related to service delivery utilization and contracting issues with payors, providers (e.g., patient-centered medical homes, skilled nursing facilities, home health agencies), and regulatory/government agencies
▶ Provide education to clients (e.g., safety, disease process, compliance, medication management, plan of care).

▶ The Case Management Administrator Certification

The case management administrator certification (CMAC) is sponsored by The Center for Case Management (CFCM). The Center was established in 1986 to provide leadership in case management to the healthcare industry. In its philosophy statement, the CFCM states that every patient and patient's family requires continuity of a plan of care and continuity of a healthcare team to create a three-way balance of clinical, financial, and satisfaction (i.e., optimal care experience) outcomes. The CFCM also emphasizes that the classic case management and/or care coordination processes serve as the glue that creates the needed continuity of care and healthcare providers/professionals. One of the CFCM's services is the CMAC (CFCM, 2017a). The Credentialing Advisory Board for the CMAC initiated the certification in 1997 and the CFCM has been supporting the offering of this credential ever since. The CMAC is offered to individuals who have responsibility for the leadership or administration function of case management services in any venue of practice. Holding the CMAC certification demonstrates professional recognition of the knowledge required to be a case/care management administrator, director, manager, educator, or supervisor of any case management service or independent practice throughout the continuum of healthcare (CFCM, 2017b).

CMAC certification is designed for individuals who are not the frontline case managers providing direct case management services to patients and their families; it is rather for those who are responsible and accountable for meeting the fundamental goals of case management services

through leadership and supervision of others. Case management administrators (leaders) and academic faculty lead organizations in the development and implementation of strategies to achieve clinical quality, financial, and satisfaction outcomes. Their activities may include education, program design and collaboration, direct supervision, consultation, and evaluation. These are potentially eligible for the CMAC credential. The CFCM identifies case management administrators as those who supervise case management personnel (including case managers and case manager associates) in various areas of the healthcare continuum and environments (payors, providers, private practice, or community) with the understanding that these professionals perform the functions specified in Display 10-18 (CFCM, 2017b).

Those individuals who meet any one of the three broad categories listed herewith (CFCM, 2017b) are eligible to take the examination for the CMAC (Display 10-19):

1. General criteria
   ▶ Master's degree and 1-year experience in case management administration, or
   ▶ Bachelor's degree and 3 years' experience in case management administration, or
   ▶ Master's degree and 3 years' experience as a case manager, or
   ▶ Bachelor's degree and 5 years' experience as a case manager.
2. Equivalent certification criteria
   Active certification in one or more of the following organizations (evidence of certification must be supplied upon application):
   ▶ A-CCC from the National Board of Certification in Continuity of Care.

display 10-18

CONTENT OUTLINE OF THE CASE MANAGEMENT ADMINISTRATOR CERTIFICATION EXAMINATION (CFCM, 2017b)

The Case Management Administrator-Certified certification examination reflects the roles and responsibilities of the case management leader and is categorized into five content areas:

I. Management and Leadership
- Collaboration with the executive team
- Human resource management
- Change management

II. Healthcare Laws and Regulations
- Compliance, laws, and regulatory organizations
- CMS Conditions of Participation
- Legal considerations for patient care related to case management

III. Development of a Continuum of Care
- Service gap analysis
- Risk-based contracting/bundled payment
- Assessment of at-risk populations
- Improvement of population health programs of care
- Accountable Care Organizations
- Functions of emergency department case management
- Medical Homes and Medical Specialty "Neighborhoods"
- Skilled nursing facilities—short- and long-term
- Homecare and hospice

- Outpatient services of physical and mental health
- Community services and resources
- Roles to manage patients across the continuum
- Care plans and paths to manage patients across the continuum
- Skills needed by professionals in the continuum
- Trends toward consumerism

IV. Tools of Clinical Case Management Practice
- Case management–related software
- Information technology
- Assessment and intervention tools

V. Using Data to Create Information, Understanding, and Improvement
- Data that is publicly available
- Payor mix data
- Quality data
- Satisfaction data
- Financial data
- Physician utilization data/Practice profiles and feedback methods
- Visual data displays
- Using dashboards for case management services
- Principles of performance improvement and continuous quality improvement

- ACM from the American Case Management Association.
- CRRN from the Rehabilitation Nursing Certification Board.
- CCM from the CCMC.
- Certified Disability Management Specialist (CDMS) from the Certification of Disability Management Specialists Commission.
- C-SWCM and C-ASWCM from the NASW.
- RN, C (Certification in Nursing Case Management) from the ANCC.

3. Faculty criteria

Faculty in academic settings teaching graduate-level courses in case management and/or case management—related content will be admitted to the certification examination. The length of experience in teaching case management and/or case management content must be:
- A minimum of two consecutive academic semesters within a 24-month period, or
- Two academic semesters within a 24-month period.

4. Physician involved in case management administration

There are other agencies that offer certification in case management or a related field. Case managers interested in becoming certified must review what is available before they choose a certification. This review may focus on the following:
- Identifying the certification most relevant to the case manager's practice setting or the patient population served.
- Examining the foundation (e.g., the evidence base for the certification examination) and the reputation (e.g., the certifying agency is accredited by the NCCA) of the certification.
- Determining which certification facilitates the case manager's career progression and advancement.
- Eligibility requirements: for example, matching the requirements to the case manager's current experience, educational background, and licensure.
- Affordability: for example, initial cost, renewal cost, and retest cost.

display 10-19

INFORMATION ABOUT THE CASE MANAGEMENT ADMINISTRATOR-CERTIFIED CREDENTIAL

For information about the Case Management Administration Certification, refer to:

The Center for Case Management
386 Washington St. 2nd floor
Wellesley, MA 02481
Telephone: (781) 446-6980
Fax: (781) 446-6984
E-mail: info@cfcm.com
Website: http://cfcm.com/resources/certification.asp

▶ Time frame: for example, certification examination cycles per calendar year and the number of years the certification is valid before it is up for renewal.

Examples of other certifications available to case managers are, but not limited to, the following:

▶ Continuity of Care Certification—Advanced (A-CCC); sponsored by the National Board for Certification in Continuity of Care. The target professionals are registered nurses, social workers, therapists, dietitians, and physicians involved in continuity of care and case management.
▶ Case Manager Certified (CMC), Utilization Management Certified, Clinical Audit Professional Certified; sponsored by the American Institute of Outcomes Healthcare Management. These national certifications focus on outcomes-case management and utilization management, as well as claims processing and management. Target professionals are those who practice in these specialties.
▶ CDMS, formerly known as the Certified Insurance Rehabilitation Specialist; sponsored by the Commission for Disability Management Specialists and currently the CCMC has the oversight responsibility for this certification. The target professionals are any health discipline practicing with individuals with disabilities.
▶ Certified Managed Care Nurse; sponsored by the American Board of Managed Care Medicine and targets health professionals involved in the health insurance industry including managed care organizations.
▶ CMC; sponsored by the National Academy of Certified Care Managers. This certification targets those directly involved in care management or in a field related to care management such as mental health counseling, psychology, social work, and rehabilitation.

▶ REGULATORY AND ACCREDITATION AGENCIES

Accreditation is a process of verifying that an organization meets a certain set of nationally recognized standards. It is a voluntary and formal review process to certify that an organization has the necessary structures and processes to provide quality healthcare services and preserve the rights of patients and providers. According to TJC, standards for accreditation are statements of expectation set by a competent authority concerning a degree or level of requirement, excellence, or attainment in quality or performance.

Whether in a hospital setting, a health maintenance organization, or a community-based healthcare facility, accreditation standards enhance quality, safety, and

consistency. More specifically, accreditation efforts provide the following benefits:

▶ Quality benchmarks
▶ Accountability
▶ Reliability
▶ National standards
▶ Cost reduction
▶ Enhancement of the healthcare consumer's experience of care
▶ More specialized reviews
▶ A demonstration to the public that an organization is concerned about the public's safety
▶ Identification of the next generation of improvements
▶ Enhancement of an organization's reputation and credibility.

An ever-growing challenge to all those who provide healthcare services is that all regulatory and accreditation agencies require different measures using various time frames and their own brand of measurement.

▶ Centers for Medicare & Medicaid Services and Quality Improvement System for Managed Care

The Centers for Medicare & Medicaid Services (CMS) is the regulatory agency responsible for overseeing and monitoring all health plans that provide care to Medicare and Medicaid beneficiaries (Display 10-20). As the nation's largest purchaser of healthcare services, the CMS developed in the early 2000s an approach to the measurement an improvement of quality of care in the Medicare/Medicaid population. The Quality Improvement System for Managed Care (QISMC) initiative is a part of the CMS's Quality Assessment and Performance Improvement (QAPI) program, a system created for managed care organizations contracting with Medicare and Medicaid. The QAPI program requires healthcare organizations to engage in quality assurance and improvement activities as a priority to demonstrably improve their performance. The CMS recognizes that organizations' capabilities may vary in terms of sophistication, information systems, personnel, and other resources. Nevertheless, these healthcare organizations must be committed to the common goal of *assuring a consistently high-quality and cost-effective standard of*

---

display 10-20

THE CENTERS FOR MEDICARE & MEDICAID SERVICES (CMS)

The Centers for Medicare & Medicaid Services (CMS)
7500 Security Boulevard
Baltimore, MD 21244
Telephone: (410) 786-3000 or (877) 267-2323
Web site: http://www.cms.hhs.gov

care through the development of mechanisms for measuring improved outcomes of healthcare and the services provided to Medicare and Medicaid beneficiaries.

Audits on performance of these health insurance plans determine if a managed care organization is eligible to enter into a Medicare or Medicaid contract. The ultimate goal of the QISMC is to establish objective and measurable standards that will improve the health and satisfaction of the Medicare/Medicaid population enrolled in a managed care plan (advantage plan). The QISMC looks beyond whether an organization's infrastructure has the capacity to improve care, to whether an organization actually improves such care and services. In this initiative the CMS has defined, in advance for health plans, what is acceptable, demonstrable, and measurable improvement. One thing is certain: The *QISMC is another managed care component that pushes case management into the limelight.*

QISMC standards consist of four domains:

1. QAPI
2. Enrollee rights
3. Health services management
4. Delegation.

The basic requirements of health plans are:

▶ Plans must operate an internal QAPI program with demonstrable improvements in enrollee health, functional status, or satisfaction.

▶ Plans must collect and report data of standardized measures of health outcomes and enrollee satisfaction, and meet minimum performance levels.

▶ Plans must comply with administrative structures and process requirements.

The QISMC system for Medicare uses the CMS as the oversight organization, and compliance with the QISMC is mandatory for managed care organizations covering Medicare beneficiaries. The Medicaid-related system uses the Medicaid state agencies as the oversight organization; managed Medicaid compliance with the QISMC is currently determined by the Medicaid state agencies and may vary statewise.

This regulatory accreditation is important for any case manager who works with Medicare or Medicaid beneficiaries covered under a managed care plan; the requirements will impact case management activities. Furthermore, case management is important to those who provide services to managed Medicare or managed Medicaid patients. The four domains of the QISMC standards include multiple case management interventions and processes:

I. QAPI

This domain includes three distinct but related strategies:

a. Performance levels; case managers are key players when addressing:
- How well the care provided by an organization meets established standards for

preventive care or the care and treatment of certain health conditions.
- How well an organization ensures access and appropriate utilization of services.
- Measures of beneficiaries' satisfaction with the care provided.

b. Performance improvement projects; case managers are key players when addressing:
- Any component of a quality improvement project that is also chosen to comply with QISMC regulatory requirements.
- Both clinical and nonclinical conditions must be addressed in QISMC quality improvement projects. Clinical conditions are primary, secondary, and tertiary prevention of acute and chronic conditions; care of acute and chronic conditions; high-volume and high-risk services; and continuity and coordination of care. Nonclinical focus areas are availability, accessibility, and cultural competency of services. This almost sounds like a case management job description.
- Other areas that can be addressed in QISMC projects include "the management of social and psychological interaction between client and practitioner" and projects relating to appeals, grievances, and complaints.

c. Attributes of performance improvement projects; case managers are key players when addressing many of the interventions that can be chosen to improve the quality of care.

II. Enrollee Rights

Case managers are key players when addressing:

a. Communication with beneficiaries related to policies, procedures, appeals, grievances, submitting complaints, changing primary care physicians (PCPs), enrollment issues, billing issues, how to obtain services, federal and state laws affecting beneficiary rights.

b. The implementation of patient confidentiality policy and procedures.

c. Assurance that the beneficiaries receive services that are meaningful to them. Services must be accessible to those with limited English proficiency or reading skills, those with diverse cultural and ethnic backgrounds, the homeless, and those with physical and mental disabilities.

d. Patient autonomy: The QISMC requires that patients participate in decision making regarding their healthcare, treatment decisions and options, and advance directive decisions. Patients must receive information on accessibility of their medical records.

III. Health Services Management

Case managers are key players when addressing:

a. Availability and accessibility of
services for beneficiaries, without impedance
from cultural barriers, geographical
barriers, or undue waiting periods for
obtaining care.

b. Identifying patients with complex needs,
thoroughly assessing these patients, and
providing and monitoring appropriate medical
treatment. This includes access to specialists
when needed. The QISMC expects that within
90 days of a patient becoming a new enrollee,
an attempt at an initial assessment will be
made; the assessment is not mandatory (thus,
the word "attempt" because of possible patient
variables/resistance that may preclude the
assessment from taking place).

c. Continuity and coordination of care, which
emphasize the role of the primary care provider
as a gatekeeper and the case manager as
coordinator and facilitator of care for enrollees
with complex health conditions.

   • That mechanisms are in place to ensure
   consistent application of review criteria (the
   utilization management part of the case
   management-hybrid role).

d. The appeals process (all phases) and the
specific time frames that must be honored.

e. Completeness of the medical record,
which must include identifying information
about the enrollee; identifying all providers
involved in the enrollee's care and
information on the services they provided;
a problem list; presenting complaints,
diagnoses, and treatment plans; prescribed
medications, including dosages, dates, refills;
information on allergies and adverse reactions;
information on advance directives; medical
history; physical examination results; and risk
factors.

f. The confidential exchange of information among
those treating the patient; this includes the
standard that, when an enrollee changes PCPs,
his or her medical record must transfer as well.

IV. Delegation

The fourth domain addresses the oversight of "carve
outs" and "carve ins."

Case management skills are interwoven into
every aspect of the QISMC standards. It is clear
from this brief overview that case managers are of
critical value to monitoring and improving care to
Medicare and Medicaid beneficiaries.

The Patient Protection and Affordable Care Act
(PPACA) of 2010 includes a provision that requires
health insurance plans to report annually on their efforts
for quality improvements; and on how these efforts
demonstrate healthcare quality, and apply incentives in
the benefit design and provider reimbursement structures.
Reporting includes how these health insurance plans
improve health outcomes, prevent hospital readmissions,
ensure patient safety and reduce medical errors, and
implement wellness and health promotion activities.
Reporting is also required from employer group health
insurance plans, self-insured plans, individual market
plans, and qualified health plans available through the
health insurance exchanges (Hoo, Lansky, Roski, &
Simpson, 2012).

Reporting on quality improvement activities is also
a requirement of health insurance plans that contract
with the CMS to offer managed healthcare insurance
(advantage plans) for the Medicare and Medicaid beneficiaries. The CMS's VBP and hospital readmission
reduction programs have accelerated the adoption of
quality and outcomes-based risk contracts with health
insurance plans with payments (reimbursement) linked to
performance, public reporting, health insurance market
exchanges, and participation in regional or multistate
collaboratives. The reporting requirements outlined in
the PPACA align with the National Quality Strategy
(NQS) in pursuit of achieving the Institute for Healthcare
Improvement's triple aim: improving population health,
improving consumers' care experience, and controlling
per capita costs of affordable care. Common domains
across the quality improvement initiatives and the
NQS priorities reflect an important focus on quality
as described subsequently. Case managers are essential
professionals who assist health insurance plans and
providers to improve their outcomes demonstrative
of these domains and the application of effective care
approaches.

▶ Making care safer by reducing harm and medical
errors;

▶ Engaging patients and their families/caregivers as
partners in their care (provision of patient-centered
care);

▶ Promoting effective communication across providers and care setting, including a special focus
on care coordination;

▶ Promoting the most effective prevention and treatment practices applying evidence-based standards
and guidelines;

▶ Working with communities to enable healthy living;
and

▶ Making care more affordable through new healthcare delivery models (Hoo, Lansky, Roski, & Simpson,
2012).

Today, the performance of health insurance plans is measured through an array of standardized performance measures that assess the following:

1. Preventive care such as screening for illness or health risk assessments;
2. Clinical care processes such as access to healthcare providers;
3. Intermediate health outcomes such as blood pressure or cholesterol levels;
4. Care experiences of enrollees such as the consumer assessment of healthcare providers and systems (CAHPS) survey; and
5. Health outcomes of enrollees such as functional status or quality of life (Hoo et al., 2012).

The CMS requires health plans participating in Medicare Advantage to report on many such performance measures. In addition, the state Medicaid managed care programs also require such reporting, sometimes under regulatory requirements promulgated through states' health departments or insurance commissioners. These advance the use of case management strategies and therefore case managers and care coordinators. As a result, many health insurance plans attempt to improve their performance by rewarding and reimbursing healthcare providers for a range of activities, including case management, care coordination, medication management, patient adherence, and the use of primary care medical homes. In addition, health insurance plans have sought to improve value through insurance benefit designs that provide incentives for members to choose evidence-based treatments (e.g., by waiving copayments) or select providers with higher performance ratings.

▶ Utilization Review Accreditation Commission (URAC)

URAC, formerly known as the Commission, is an independent, not-for-profit organization, founded in 1990, and is known as a leader in promoting healthcare quality through accreditation. When originally launched, the URAC was known as the Utilization Review Accreditation Commission (URAC) and focused primarily on utilization review activities. The URAC has since expanded its accreditation activities to include other aspects of managed care organizations, health insurance plans and networks, and preferred provider organizations. It has changed its name to the URAC. The URAC's mission is to promote continuous improvement in the quality and efficiency of healthcare management through the processes of accreditation and education, and measurement (URAC, 2017a).

The URAC uses a modular approach to accrediting organizations. What this means is that organizations can seek accreditation through several interlocking and complementary sets of standards; each addresses a different component of managed care operations. The modular approach allows flexibility, so that an organization can tailor its accreditation process to the specific services it offers healthcare consumers. The URAC provides accreditation and certification programs in over 30 areas across the continuum of healthcare: health and dental plans, healthcare management, healthcare operations, pharmacy quality management, and provider integration and coordination. Some of these programs are related to case management practice, such as those listed herewith (URAC, 2017b).

- ▶ Accountable care
- ▶ Healthcare utilization management and claims processing
- ▶ Health insurance plans and networks
- ▶ Patient-centered Medical Home
- ▶ Worker's compensation utilization management
- ▶ Healthcare practitioner credentialing
- ▶ Credentials verification organizations
- ▶ Disease management
- ▶ Medicare Advantage
- ▶ Case management
- ▶ Pharmacy benefit management
- ▶ Telehealth

The URAC's health insurance plan accreditation is nationally recognized and signifies a distinguished status of excellence. The healthcare industry, as well as federal and state governments, views this accreditation as an assurance that the health plan has met rigorous standards and measures of quality and operational integrity, health consumer protection, and consumer empowerment. Such accreditation also demonstrates a clear commitment to quality and continuous improvement. More specifically, the URAC-accredited health insurance plan:

- ▶ Provides accurate and clear communication to members;
- ▶ Documents the makeup of its enrollee and maintains the confidentiality of his or her personal health information;
- ▶ Creates healthcare provider networks accessible to the communities it serves, and ensures that these providers are credentialed and meet nationally recognized standards;
- ▶ Continuously reviews and improves its quality of care and safety;
- ▶ Ensures the availability of healthcare providers and applies policies for accessing providers during emergencies and for out-of-network coverage;
- ▶ Engages qualified healthcare professionals in making medical necessity decisions that are based on the latest clinical guidelines;

▶ Provides guidance and educational support for obtaining plan services in a language that respects members' diverse backgrounds;

▶ Collects enrollees' opinions on their experience of care and level of service; uses this information for quality improvement purposes;

▶ Gives members access to complaint and appeal processes; and

▶ Offers mental and physical health services on an equal basis (URAC, 2017b).

The URAC's health plan accreditation standards emphasize their focus on quality improvement activities to promote patient safety across the continuum of care. Measures integral to the quality program are closely aligned with the domains of the NQS that are adopted by the United States Department of Health and Human Services. Efforts of quality improvement and measures that are of special interest to the URAC's health insurance plan accreditation program focus on the following:

▶ Wellness and health promotion
▶ Care coordination
▶ Medication safety and care adherence
▶ Reward of quality performance
▶ Care delivery through a Patient-Centered Health Care Home Network
▶ Mental health parity
▶ Health Insurance Portability and Accountability Act (HIPAA) breach requirements
▶ Quality and Outcomes Measures inclusive of patient-centeredness, communication and care coordination, patient safety, population health management, public health, efficiency of services, cost reduction, and effectiveness of clinical care
▶ Enrollee experience of care using the consumer assessment of healthcare providers and systems (CAHPS) survey (URAC, 2017b).

The URAC has adopted the Quality Rating Measure Set in its health insurance plan accreditation program. This approach aligns the measure set with the current industry standard and reduces the administrative burden of submission. Within each set of standards, the URAC monitors several organizational processes. The different accreditation and certification programs have different monitoring expectations; however, Display 10-21 lists the quality domains that the URAC applies (URAC, 2017c).

The URAC has identified specific measures that it expects the health insurance plans to report on annually. These measures are incorporated into select URAC accreditation programs. The programs include case management, disease management, pharmacy, drug therapy management, and comprehensive wellness. Display 10-22 lists examples of these measures.

display 10-21

URAC DOMAINS OF QUALITY (URAC, 2017c)

1. *Engagement and Experience of Care:* Measures the degree of patient and family member engagement, their experience with the healthcare organization, and how well the organization meets patient and family expectations.

2. *Communication and Care Coordination:* Measures the effectiveness of communications and service coordination between providers and between providers and their patients.

3. *Access and Affordable Care:* Measures the degree of success in making quality healthcare more affordable and available to those that need it.

4. *Prevention and Treatment:* Measures the degree of success in preventing disease and the effectiveness of treatments once a diseased state is present.

5. *Healthy Living:* Measures the provision of preventive services for children and adults and the adoption of evidence-based behavioral interventions to improve health.

6. *Safe Care:* Measures medical and health care–related errors and infections that account for a significant amount of harm and death.

7. *System/Health Information Technology Integration:* Measures the degree to which the organizational systems integrate health information technology into its daily workflow.

8. *Healthcare Management:* Measures the efficiency and effectiveness of the management of services provided by the organization.

9. *Healthcare Disparities:* Measures racial or ethnic differences in the quality of healthcare other than access-related factors or clinical needs, preferences, and appropriateness of intervention.

The URAC established its health utilization management accreditation program in 1990—the first accreditation program to be available in this area. This program is widely recognized at the state and federal level, and applies to both stand-alone (independent) utilization management organizations and programs within health insurance benefit plans. The URAC (Display 10-23) designed the standards of this program to ensure that healthcare organizations involved in utilization management apply a process that is clinically sound, demonstrates fair and impartial medical necessity determination or peer review, and respects the rights of both patients and healthcare providers. The utilization management accreditation program also assures the adequacy and quality of the utilization management processes available in the accredited organizations. The URAC uses broadly recognized standards and measures in the evaluation of an organization's practices and determination of accreditation. The standards address the use of evidence-based practice guidelines, incorporation of adherence guidelines, and evaluation of utilization rates

display 10-22

URAC QUALITY MEASURES EMBEDDED IN THE CASE MANAGEMENT AND DISEASE MANAGEMENT ACCREDITATION PROGRAMS (URAC, 2016a,b)

Case Management Program:

1. Communication and care coordination
   - Medical readmissions (excludes behavioral health, disability, and workers' compensation populations)
   - Percentage of individuals that refused case management services
   - Three-item care transitions measure*
2. Prevention and treatment
   - Percentage of participants that were medically released to return to work (disability and workers' compensation only)
3. Engagement and experience of care
   - Complaint response timeliness
   - Overall consumer satisfaction (excludes disability and workers' compensation)
   - Patient activation measure*

Disease Management Program:

4. Prevention and treatment
   - Unhealthy alcohol use: screening and brief counseling
   - Prevention and management of obesity for adults
   - Screening for clinical depression and follow-up plan
   - Screening and cessation counseling for tobacco use
   - Medication therapy for persons with asthma
5. Access and affordable care
   - Pediatric asthma event rate
   - Chronic obstructive pulmonary disease or asthma in older adults event rate
   - Hypertension event rate
   - Heart failure event rate
   - Diabetes short-term complications event rate
6. Engagement and experience of care
   - Patient activation measure*
   - Proportion of days covered (PDC)*
   - Adherence to nonwarfarin oral anticoagulants*
7. Safe care
   - Drug–drug interactions*

*Exploratory measures.

of healthcare services. Health organizations may apply these standards to establish consistency, improve quality of services, and maintain the highest confidentiality in the utilization management processes they have in place (URAC, 2017d).

The URAC-accredited healthcare utilization management program:

▶ Provides an independent, unbiased determination of medical necessity beginning with an initial clinical review, then moving to a peer clinical review if needed;

▶ Uses evidence-based treatment guidelines to enhance the quality and effectiveness of patient care, while eliminating excessive treatment and expense;

display 10-23

URAC CONTACT INFORMATION

For more information about URAC's accreditation programs in utilizations management, disease management, or case management, refer to:

URAC
1220 L Street NW—Suite 400
Washington, DC 20005
Telephone: (202) 216-9010
Fax: (202) 216-9006
E-mail: businessdevelopment@urac.org
Website: http://www.urac.org

▶ Adheres to time frames outlined in the standards for urgent and nonurgent review determinations;

▶ Understands and adheres to applicable state and federal regulations;

▶ Employs drug utilization management mechanisms to address therapeutic appropriateness, over- and underutilization, dosage, duration of treatment, duplication, drug allergies; and

▶ Is prepared to address any risk to patient safety, such as contraindicated treatments, adverse drug interactions, or inappropriate treatment, during the review process (URAC, 2017d).

The URAC's accreditation and certification programs examine written policies and procedures and ensure that these policies have actually been implemented during the on-site review portion of the accreditation process. This is a rigorous survey process, and an organization must demonstrate compliance with the applicable accreditation standards.

▶ Network or organizational structure
▶ Policies and procedures
▶ Regulatory compliance
▶ Consumer empowerment, education, and engagement
▶ Program design and components
▶ Interdepartmental coordination
▶ Healthcare system coordination
▶ Oversight of delegated functions
▶ Quality management

- ▶ Utilization management services
- ▶ Licenses, credentialing, and certification
- ▶ Information management including confidentiality, privacy, patient protection procedures and practices including management of complaints
- ▶ Continuing education and training activities
- ▶ Corporate/managerial leadership
- ▶ Appropriate clinical oversight
- ▶ Job descriptions and performance appraisals
- ▶ Performance measures (URAC, 2017e).

▶ Case Management Organization Standards

In the spring of 1998, the URAC and the CMSA formed a partnership to develop accreditation standards for case management. A Case Management Advisory Committee was developed to address the multiple challenges a new accreditation program must face. One of the biggest challenges was to create standards that addressed the range of case management practice patterns in use in those years. This was one reason that the initial accreditation reviews were focused primarily on utilization management organizations, networks, and managed care organizations. The Case Management Advisory Committee included case management experts and representatives from the CMSA, the CCMC, the ANCC, and the American Medical Association. The case management accreditation standards were then developed through collaborative efforts by major constituents impacted by managed care. In addition to the broad-based advisory committee, the standards were circulated for public comment and in draft format. Since then they have undergone multiple revisions; the public forum gave interested parties an opportunity to present their ideas for targeting these national benchmark standards. The standards were revised multiple times; most recently in 2015.

According to the URAC, important benefits can be obtained for managed care and other organizations that undergo the case management accreditation process. Case management program accreditation may:

- ▶ Assist companies in transitioning from the utilization management model to the case management model.
- ▶ Establish a system to measure and assess services provided by case managers with appropriate feedback loops.
- ▶ Require high performance standards and public accountability.
- ▶ Provide an educational forum to help accredited companies keep pace with best practices.
- ▶ Mitigate the need for state-specific case management regulations (utilization management regulations are enforced on a state-by-state basis).
- ▶ Highlight the benefits of case management services to many types of healthcare stakeholders.
- ▶ Create a forum to identify future improvements in the case management profession.

The URAC's case management accreditation standards require managed care and other organizations to establish processes to assess, plan, and implement case management interventions. They also address approaches for ensuring that appropriate patient protection has been established, such as policies for confidentiality of patient information, informed consent, dispute resolution, and other issues. Case management processes and functions considered in the accreditation standards include several critical operational categories as described herewith (URAC, 2017e):

1. *Case management program components*: program description; identification criteria; evidence-based guidelines; collaborative communications; description of the case manager's role; TOC; shared decision making; performance monitoring; use of information support systems to improve efficiency; and the establishment of outcome measures.
2. *Consumer education and engagement*: patient-centered care; disclosure; application of motivational principles; support for patient self-management; engagement of the patient, family, and caregiver; patient accountability; use of health education tools; cultural and linguistic learning needs; case management disclosure; and promotion of optimal levels of wellness.
3. *Staff qualifications and training*: staff composition; qualifications; commitment to excellence; promotion of case manager expertise and proficiency; use of qualified case managers; enforcement of competencies; and role of case management support staff.
4. *Case management assessment and plan of care*: identification of critical assessment categories; patient input; medication safety assessment (medications adherence and reconciliation); patient-centered case management plans; patient safety; cultural relevance.
5. *Care coordination*: alignment with healthcare reform goals for better coordinated care; fostering of improved coordinated care; support for integrated care delivery; social services and supports; patient-identified issues; and enhanced quality and cost-effectiveness.
6. *Measurement reporting to URAC*: reporting on predetermined mandatory and exploratory performance measures.

The URAC offers healthcare organizations an option for TOC accreditation designation when reviewing case management, disease management, or other programs. The TOC standards focus on planning for TOC across settings, developing individualized and comprehensive care plans, providing care-transition information transfer requirements, ensuring timely follow-up interventions for postacute care, and following a coordinated approach to ensure the reduction of hospital readmissions.

The URAC makes the standards of its accreditation programs available in "at a glance" format on its website, accessible at: https://www.urac.org/resource-center/research-publications/standards-and-measures-at-a-glance/#cm.

▶ The Joint Commission and the ORYX/Performance Measures Initiative

TJC, formerly known as the Joint Commission on Accreditation of Health Care Organizations, was founded in 1951 and is the oldest and largest accrediting agency in healthcare. Its mission is to "continuously improve health care for the public, in collaboration with other stakeholders, by evaluating health care organizations and inspiring them to excel in providing safe and effective care of the highest quality and value." TJC has evaluated and accredited nearly 21,000 facilities and programs in the United States (TJC, 2017a). It has also certified a variety of programs, that is, clinical specialties.

- ▶ TJC's accreditation programs include hospitals, critical access hospitals, home health agencies, laboratories, skilled nursing facilities, long-term care facilities, behavioral health facilities, health plans, ambulatory care, and integrated delivery networks.
- ▶ TJC's certification programs include comprehensive cardiac center, disease-specific care (e.g., transplant, orthopedic, acute stroke, or gastrointestinal), integrated care, healthcare staffing services, medications compounding, palliative care, perinatal care, primary care medical home, and patient blood management programs.

Generally, TJC accreditation standards measure the following functional areas:

- ▶ Ethics, rights, and responsibilities
- ▶ Provision of care, treatments, and services
- ▶ Medication management and safety
- ▶ Surveillance, prevention, and control of infections
- ▶ Improvement of organizational performance
- ▶ Leadership
- ▶ Management of the environment of care
- ▶ Human resource management
- ▶ Management of information
- ▶ Medical staff including credentialing and privileging
- ▶ Nursing
- ▶ Sentinel events
- ▶ National Patient Safety Goals
- ▶ Performance measurement and the ORYX initiative/performance measures/core measures.

TJC has been developing performance measures since the mid-1980s. It also has been recognized as a national leader in this area. TJC completes this work through its Division of Healthcare Quality Evaluation which has extensive experience in the identification, development, specification, and the testing and implementation of standardized performance measures. This development methodology is considered the "gold standard" in healthcare today. For example, TJC has successfully developed and nationally implemented many sets of standardized performance measures for hospitals (TJC, 2017b), some of which have been adopted by the National Quality Forum and the CMS.

The ORYX initiative was launched by TJC in 1997 to integrate a healthcare organization's outcomes with accreditation requirements. Organizations are required to collect and report performance data on specific core measure sets to TJC as part of the accreditation process. These are heart failure, acute myocardial infarction, pneumonia, pregnancy and related conditions, surgical infection prevention, immunizations, emergence department, children's asthma, hospital-based inpatient psychiatric services, hospital-based outpatient departments, perinatal care, stroke, substance use, tobacco treatment, and venous thrombosis (TJC, 2017c). Performance measures on these aspects of care are in the form of either chart abstraction or electronic clinical quality. These performance measures have varied over time. TJC may decide to introduce new measures, or retire or temporarily inactivate existing measures. For example, in 2017 TJC retired the surgical care improvement project measures, temporarily inactivated the tobacco use measure, and introduced a new electronic clinical quality measure for stroke: discharged on antithrombotic therapy.

The goals for ORYX include the following:

- ▶ To increase the relevance and value of TJC accreditation.
- ▶ To serve as a support system for quality improvement efforts in accredited organizations.
- ▶ To allow the comparison of patient outcomes between organizations.

Healthcare organizations have been applying the ORYX initiative (Display 10-24) in their preparation for TJC accreditation. It is important that case managers who are in TJC-accredited healthcare organizations understand the quality indicators/performance measures/ORYX/core measures. Often, these indicators pertain to case management roles and responsibilities. Case managers are critical for gaining accreditation in their organizations. TJC believes that its ORYX performance measures apply evidence-based care processes and promote accountability of healthcare organizations; thus, these measures are closely associated with positive patient care outcomes.

CONTACT INFORMATION FOR TJC AND ORYX

Information on TJC and ORYX can be found on the same website.

The Joint Commission (TJC)
One Renaissance Boulevard
Oakbrook Terrace, IL 60181
Telephone: (630) 792-5800
Fax: (630) 792-5005
Website: http://www.jointcommission.org
Washington DC Office
The Joint Commission (TJC)
601 13th Street, NW
Suite 560 South
Washington, DC 20005

▶ The Joint Commission International

The Joint Commission International (JCI) is a subsidiary of TJC and was founded in 1994 as a division of the Joint Commission Resources, Inc., as a private, not-for-profit entity to extend TJC's mission globally. The JCI recognized that commitment to improve healthcare must occur worldwide. Since 1994, the JCI (Display 10-25) has provided consultation services to governments, hospitals, and other healthcare organizations in numerous countries in Western Europe, the Middle East, Africa, Latin America, the Caribbean, Central and Eastern Europe, Asia and the Pacific Rim. It also has accredited various healthcare organizations across the continuum of care in over 90 countries. International standards and principles were developed by an international task force composed of physicians, nurses, administrators, and public policy makers. This task force ensured that the standards apply worldwide, and that they accommodate cultural differences. The mission of the JCI is "to improve the safety and quality of care in the international community through the provision of education, publications, consultation, and evaluation services" (JCI, 2017a).

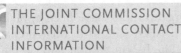

THE JOINT COMMISSION INTERNATIONAL CONTACT INFORMATION

For questions or information about the Joint Commission International, contact:

The Joint Commission International (JCI)
1515 22nd Street, Suite 1300W
Oakbrook, IL 60523
Telephone, customer services: (630) 268-7400
Telephone, accreditation services: (630) 268-4800
Fax: (630) 268-7405
E-mail, customer services: jcicustomerservcie@pbd.org
E-mail, accreditation services: jciaccreditation@jcrinc.com
Website: http://www.jointcommissioninternational.org/

The JCI offers accreditation services for hospitals and academic medical centers globally. It also offers accreditation for nonhospital-based programs including ambulatory care, home care, laboratory, medical transport organizations, long-term care, and primary care centers. To date, the JCI has accredited over 800 healthcare organizations. The manual of the JCI Accreditation Standards for Hospitals is available in its sixth edition. These standards went into effect in July 2017. The standards provide the basis for accreditation of hospitals throughout the world. They define the performance expectations, structures, and functions that must be in place for a hospital to be accredited by the JCI. The hospital accreditation manual consists of the following (JCI, 2017b) features:

▶ The standards are organized into two main sections: (1) patient-centered care and (2) healthcare organization management.
▶ There are two additional chapters specific to academic medical center accreditation. These address research requirements (e.g., human subjects protection) and education of medical professionals.
▶ Each standard includes (1) an intent statement and rationale, and (2) measurable elements that list the related specific requirements.
▶ The accreditation manual also includes an introduction to accreditation, eligibility requirements, summary of key accreditation policies, a glossary, and an index.
▶ The JCI makes its standards accreditation manual available in Spanish, Portuguese, Chinese, Italian, and Hebrew.

▶ National Committee for Quality Assurance and Healthcare Effectiveness Data and Information Set

The NCQA, founded in 1990, is a private, nonprofit accreditation agency, widely recognized as the leader in the effort to assess, measure, and report on the quality of care provided by managed care organizations. The NCQA's original accreditation efforts focused on Health Maintenance Organizations (HMOs). It has since expanded to include the accreditation of behavioral health organizations, physician credential verification organizations, and physician organizations. The NCQA's accreditation is voluntary; however, a growing list of large corporate employers requires contracted health insurance plans to be NCQA accredited. Organizations that achieve NCQA accreditation use it as a symbol of quality; accreditation signifies that these organizations: (1) have passed a rigorous, comprehensive review process; (2) are annually reporting on their performance; (3) demonstrate they are well managed; and (4) deliver high-quality care and service to consumers.

As part of its quality mission and strategy, the NCQA has helped build consensus around important healthcare quality issues by collaborating with employers, policy makers, physicians and other healthcare professionals, patients, and health insurance plans to decide on important measures and to promote improvement opportunities in the delivery of healthcare services. The outcome of these efforts is a rigorous set of more than 60 accreditation standards and 40 areas of performance health insurance plans are expected to report on as part of the NCQA accreditation program. The NCQA believes that these standards and requirements will promote the adoption of strategies, improve care, enhance service, and reduce costs (NCQA, 2017a).

Like TJC, the NCQA (Display 10-26) offers accreditation and certification services. It also offers recognition programs. These services are available either for the whole organization or for a program within the organization. Accreditation programs include health insurance plans, case management, disease management, health promotion and wellness, managed behavioral health, credentialing, utilization management, and provider network. Certification programs consist of disease management, health information products, credentials verification organizations, multicultural healthcare, physician and hospital quality, wellness and health promotion, and Patient-Centered Medical Home content experts. Recognition programs include Patient-Centered Medical Home, Patient-Centered Specialty Practice, Oncology Medical Home, Heart and Stroke, Diabetes, and Patient-Centered Connected Care.

The accreditation standards fall into several broad categories. Except for physician credentials, case managers have responsibilities that directly impact each segment of the NCQA testing grounds.

- *Quality improvement*: Does the plan examine the quality of care it provides to its members? What is done to improve quality?
- *Physician credentials*: Does the plan meet the requirements for investigating and educating physicians?
- *Member rights and responsibilities*: Are members educated on how to access healthcare, choose or change physicians, or make a complaint?
- *Preventive health services*: Does the plan educate and encourage members to have preventive tests and immunizations?
- *Utilization management*: Does the plan have reasonable and consistent processes for utilization management, denials, and appeals?
- *Medical records*: Are physician office medical records in compliance with the standards? Do they demonstrate follow-up for abnormal results?

CASE MANAGEMENT

The NCQA developed its case management accreditation program drawing on its existing expertise in evaluating health insurance plans and from other accreditation programs. It convened a panel of experts and reviewed the latest evidence on the performance of case management programs.

display 10-26

NATIONAL COMMITTEE FOR QUALITY ASSURANCE (NCQA) CONTACT INFORMATION

For questions or information about the NCQA and health insurance plan Healthcare Effectiveness Data and Information Set (HEDIS), contact:

NCQA Corporate Offices
1100 13th Street, NW, Suite 1000
Washington, DC 20005
Telephone: (202) 955-3500
Fax: (202) 955-3599
Submit questions at: https://my.ncqa.org/
Website: http://www.ncqa.org

The result was evidence-based accreditation standards that focus on guiding organizations toward improving their case management and care coordination systems and processes. The NCQA believes that the core of the case management accreditation program is care coordination, patient-centeredness, and quality of care. It also encourages organizations interested in pursuing accreditation to evaluate their case management programs by examining how they:

1. Identify individuals in need of and to benefit from case management services;
2. Target the right services to these individuals and monitor their care and needs over time;
3. Develop personalized, patient-centered care plans;
4. Monitor the conditions of those served to ensure care plan goals are reached and to adjust the goals as needed;
5. Manage communication among healthcare providers and share information effectively as the individuals cared for transition between healthcare settings, especially when there are transitions from institutional settings;
6. Build in consumer protections to ensure people have access to knowledgeable and well-qualified case management staff;
7. Keep personal health information safe, private, and secure; and
8. Ensure that the program reflects the latest evidence and case management practices (NCQA, 2012).

The NCQA realized that although the day-to-day care rendered to patients was administrated by the health insurance plans, it was provided primarily in physician offices and healthcare institutional settings. To measure the quality of care effectively, physicians and provider organizations who participate in health plans must be evaluated. For utilization management accreditation, organizations are expected to demonstrate that they meet the requirements of the following 15 standards (NCQA, 2017b):

1. Internal Quality Improvement Process
2. Agreement and Collaboration with Clients

3. Privacy and Confidentiality
4. Program Structure
5. Clinical Criteria for Utilization Management Decisions
6. Communication Services
7. Appropriate Professionals
8. Timeliness of Utilization Management Decisions
9. Clinical Information
10. Denial Notices
11. Policies for Appeals
12. Appropriate Handling of Appeals
13. Experience with the Utilization Management Process
14. Triage and Referral for Behavioral Healthcare
15. Delegation of Utilization Management

HEALTHCARE EFFECTIVENESS DATA AND INFORMATION SET

The NCQA is also the accreditation agency that administers the HEDIS, which is one of the most widely used sets of healthcare performance measures in the United States. Although the HEDIS measurement system originated in the late 1980s, the NCQA assumed its oversight responsibility in the early 1990s. The NCQA measurement development process has expanded the size and scope of the HEDIS to include measures for physicians, preferred provider organizations (PPOs), and other organizations. It consists of over 90 performance measures today. The HEDIS (Display 10-26) is a set of standardized performance measures designed to assist purchasers of healthcare and consumers to select managed care or other types of health insurance plans on the basis of proven performance, rather than solely on cost. Today the measures also apply to Medicare and Medicaid health benefit plans. The measures were also developed with the intent of holding managed care plans accountable for the competent care of their enrollees. Each indicator outlines the data collection methodologies to enhance comparability and consistency across the health plans.

The HEDIS measures address a range of health issues. Prevention and early detection (i.e., immunizations and mammograms) are emphasized for various age groups (children, adolescents, adults, and seniors). Acute and chronic care evaluate conditions such as AIDS, breast cancer, tobacco use, heart disease, and diabetes.

The seven HEDIS evaluation categories and example performance measures are (NCQA, 2017c):

1. *Effectiveness of Care*: Does the health plan meet the needs of sick enrollees and prevent illness in well members? Examples of performance measures are:
   ▶ Childhood immunizations
   ▶ Comprehensive diabetes care
   ▶ Advising smokers to quit
   ▶ Lead screening
   ▶ Cervical cancer screening
   ▶ Beta blocker treatment after myocardial infarction
   ▶ Medications management for people with asthma.
2. *Access/Availability of Care*: Can the member obtain services in a timely manner and without unnecessary burden? Examples of performance measures are:
   ▶ Availability of PCPs
   ▶ Annual dental visit
   ▶ Adult's access to preventive/ambulatory health services
   ▶ Prenatal and postpartum care.
3. *Experience of Care*: What do the enrollees think about the healthcare services and the HMO? Examples of performance measures are:
   ▶ Member satisfaction survey
   ▶ CAHPS health plan survey, adult version
   ▶ CAHPS health plan survey, children version.
4. *Utilization and Risk Adjusted Utilization*: This category evaluates the resource utilization and charges to an enrollee: coinsurance, deductibles, premiums, etc. Examples of performance measures are:
   ▶ Rate trends, especially for chronic illnesses
   ▶ Relative resources use by illness
   ▶ Well-child visits in the first 15 months of life
   ▶ Inpatient utilization, general hospital/acute care
   ▶ Emergency department utilization
   ▶ Antibiotic utilization
   ▶ Standardized healthcare-associated infection ratio.
5. *Relative Resource Use*: This category documents enrollees' rates of use of healthcare services. Examples of performance measures are:
   ▶ Relative resource use for people with diabetes
   ▶ Relative resource use for people with asthma
   ▶ Relative resource use for people with cardiovascular disease.
6. *Health Plan Descriptive Information*: This category evaluates the structure and strategies of the health plan: networks, utilization management strategies (case management strategies), physician compensation/incentives, and quality improvement processes. Examples of performance measures are:
   ▶ Board certification and compensation of providers
   ▶ Recredentialing
   ▶ Enrollment by product line
   ▶ Race and ethnicity diversity of membership.
7. *Measures Collected Using Electronic Data Systems*: This category describes the performance measures that require electronic reporting. It also explains the data management protocol for data with multiple sources. Examples of performance measures are:
   ▶ Depression screening and follow-up for adolescents and adults
   ▶ Unhealthy alcohol use screening and follow-up
   ▶ Pneumococcal vaccination coverage for older adults.

The HEDIS is a dynamic set of performance standards. For those case managers who practice in health plans, this tool should be used as a guide for the assessment of the enrollee experience of care. More specifically, health plans using the HEDIS are required to submit results on the following measures on the basis of consumer surveys. Case management is a key to success in managed care and other health insurance plans.

▶ Access to needed care
▶ Getting care quickly
▶ Physician's ability to communicate
▶ Courteous and helpful office staff
▶ Ease in locating a physician or nurse
▶ Claims processing
▶ Customer service
▶ Rating of personal physician, nurse, and specialist
▶ Rating of care provided
▶ Overall rating of health plan.

Future versions of the HEDIS standards will continue to focus on outcomes and other measures of clinical quality; however, the effectiveness of care—not merely the provision of care—will continue to be targeted.

PATIENT-CENTERED MEDICAL HOME

The Patient-Centered Medical Home concept is not new to healthcare delivery and the care of vulnerable populations or those with chronic and complex medical conditions. The American Academy of Pediatrics introduced the medical home concept in 1967. In 2004, family medicine as a clinical specialty called for all patients to have a "personal medical home." In 2003, the NCQA launched the Physician Practice Connections, a program that later evolved to become the patient-centered medical home (PCMH). In 2007, leading primary care associations released the Joint PCMH Principles, and in 2008, the NCQA launched the first PCMH recognition program. The NCQA's PCMH program has recognized over 12,000 care sites as of March 2017. The PCMH recognition program requires healthcare practices and ambulatory or community-based care sites to a set of meet rigorous standards (NCQA, 2017c).

In 2015, the NCQA convened a 27-member advisory committee to review the PCMH standards and recommend modifications accordingly. The committee consisted of representatives from physician practices, medical associations, physician groups, health insurance plans, and consumer and employer groups. The NCQA also involved its Clinical Programs Committee in the review. The result was updated PCMH recognition program standards that would drive to achieve the IHI's triple aim; focus on outcomes instead of care process; accommodate a spectrum of practices; and identify practice transformation and innovation. The PCMH 2017 standards reflect the collaboration of these two committees and all involved (NCQA, 2017c).

The standards address six main concepts that are relevant to primary care practices. Each concept consists of a title and brief description; a statement of competency (a set of criteria subgroup that is organized within the broader concept); specific criteria (a set of scorable performance expectations); guidance (information about the intent of the criterion and how it relates to quality and practice transformation); and evidence (the documentation that demonstrates performance against the criterion) (NCQA, 2017d). Practices may use the PCMH recognition program standards to evaluate their care structures, processes, and performance, and to implement action plans for improvement. The six main concepts are:

1. *Team-based care and practice organization*: the practice provides continuity of care; communicates roles and responsibilities of the medical home to patients, families, and caregivers; designs the practice's structure; designates a lead clinician; organizes and trains staff to work to the top of their license and provide effective team-based care; collaborates with external entities; and uses health information technology and electronic health records.

2. *Knowing and managing patients*: the practice uses information about the patients and community it serves to deliver evidence-based care that supports the population health needs and provision of culturally and linguistically appropriate services. It maintains up-to-date problem lists for patients; conducts comprehensive health assessments; screens patients for depression; identifies the predominant conditions and health concerns; understands social determinants of health, monitors at the population level, and implements interventions to address them; educates patients and their families about care and conditions; and maintains an up-to-date list of medication for patients and reconciles these medications.

3. *Patient-centered access and continuity of care*: the practice provides patients with access to clinical advice and appropriate care on a "24 hours a day, 7 days a week basis;" provides same-day appointments and outside routine business hours; provides appointments by phone or other technology-supported mechanism; uses secure electronic systems for scheduling of appointments and two-way communication with patients; assists patients in selecting or changing clinicians; and reviews and manages patient panel size per clinician. These are facilitated by the practice's designated clinician or care team. This concept also considers the needs and preferences of the patient population when modeling standards for access.

4. *Care management and support*: the practice identifies patient needs at the individual and population

levels to effectively plan, manage, and coordinate patient care in partnership with patients, families, and caregivers. It also places emphasis on supporting patients at highest risk; applies a comprehensive risk stratification process for its patient population; establishes a patient-centered plan for care management; shares the plan of care with the patient and family; identifies and manages potential barriers for meeting individual care goals; designs a self-management plan of care; and maintains access to the plan of care across settings and providers.

5. *Care coordination and care transitions*: the practice systematically coordinates care across specialty services and providers; and tracks laboratory and imaging tests, referrals, and care transitions to achieve high-quality care coordination, lower costs, improve patient safety, and ensure effective communication with specialists and other providers in the medical neighborhood. The practice also shares important patient information during referrals to facilitate care; applies clinical protocols for tests and referrals; collaborates and integrates care with behavioral health; tracks admissions to acute care and exchange information with acute care clinicians; and communicates with patient and family or caregiver for follow-up care.

6. *Performance measurement and quality improvement*: the practice establishes a culture of data-driven performance improvement on clinical quality, efficiency, and patient experience, and engages staff and patients, families, and caregivers in quality improvement activities. The practice monitors outcomes in specific performance domains (e.g., immunizations, preventive care, chronic or acute clinical care, behavioral health, care coordination, cost, and experience of care), availability of appointments, and health disparities; establishes performance goals, benchmarks the results, and establishes improvement plans; and reports performance internally and publicly, including Medicare and/or Medicaid benefit program (NCQA, 2017c).

The NCQA requires the primary care practices/PCMHs that have achieved recognition to submit an annual report regarding their performance and ongoing improvements. Every year, the practice submits key data and documentation that cover the six PCMH concept

areas and any other special topics to show how its ongoing activities are consistent with the PCMH model of care. The NCQA reviews the annual status and evidence report submission, and on the basis of the practice's overall performance, it determines and notifies the practice whether it has met the requirements for sustained PCMH recognition (NCQA, 2017d).

DISCUSSION QUESTIONS

1. Do you hold a certification in case management? What type? How does it differ from the others available?

2. What is the difference between accreditation and certification? Give examples of each.

3. Describe a situation where you were engaged in a case management program accreditation survey. What was your experience? What did you learn? What went well? What were the things that need improvement?

4. What preparation activities can one perform to get ready for a case management certification exam? Why do you consider them valuable?

5. What preparation activities can an organization perform to be ready for case management accreditation? Why do you consider them valuable?

6. Does the practice environment of case management matter when it comes to accreditation? Certification? Why?

7. Choose a case management individual certification and discuss its eligibility criteria and topical outline of its certification examination.

8. Choose a case management–related accreditation and discuss its standards and performance measurement requirements.

9. Discuss the commonalities between the PCMH recognition program and the accreditation or certification programs offered by the URAC.

▶ REFERENCES

American Board of Quality Assurance and Utilization Review Physicians. (2017a). *HCQM exam eligibility*. [Online]. Retrieved July 28, 2017, from https://www.abqaurp.org/ABQMain/Certification/The_Exam_Process/Eligibility_Requirements/ABQMain/Exam_Eligibility.aspx?hkey=14c34974-2ff8-4ca1-bc3a-7e4399bf2696

American Board of Quality Assurance and Utilization Review Physicians. (2017b). *Health Care Quality and Management*

(HCQM) certification. [Online]. Retrieved July 28, 2017, from https://www.abqaurp.org/ABQMain/Certification/Overview_of_HCQM_Certification/ABQMain/Certification.aspx?hkey=b6edc3b2-6da9-49d0-a824-3399badf629e

American Board of Quality Assurance and Utilization Review Physicians. (2017c). *HCQM exam topics*. [Online]. Retrieved July 28, 2017, from http://www.abqaurp.org/ABQMain/Certification/

The_Exam_Process/HCQM_Exam_Topics/ABQMain/Exam_
Topics.aspx?hkey=a685bb0e-433b-4dae-b8d1-fbb44acc9515

American Case Management Association. (2013, April 11). *Mission.*
[Online]. Retrieved August 3, 2017, from http://www.acmaweb
.org/section.aspx?sID=4

American Case Management Association. (2017a). *Goals and definition of case management.* [Online]. Retrieved August 3, 2008,
from http://www.acmaweb.org/section.aspx?sID=4

American Case Management Association. (2017b). *About Compass.*
[Online]. Retrieved August 3, 2017, from https://www.acmaweb
.org/compass/compass_main.aspx

American Case Management Association (ACMA). (2017c).
Accredited Case Manager Candidate Handbook. [online]. Re-
trieved July 26, 2017, from https://www.acmaweb.org/forms
/ACMA_ACMhandbook.pdf

American Nurses Credentialing Center. (2017a). *Accredited Case
Manager™ Candidate Handbook: ACM™ Certification For
Health Care Delivery System Case Management.* [Online]. Re-
trieved July 28, 2017, from http://www.acmaweb.org/forms/
ACMA_ACMhandbook.pdf

American Nurses Credentialing Center. (2017b). *Nursing Case
Management Board Certification, Test Content Outline, Effective
Date 2/6/2015.* [Online]. Retrieved July 28, 2017, from http://
nursecredentialing.org/NursingCaseMgmt-TCO2015

Case Management Society of America. (2008). *CMSA's strategic vision.*
[Online]. Retrieved September 18, 2008, from http://www.cmsa.org

Case Management Society of America. (2016). *Standards of practice
for case management.* Little Rock, AR: Author.

Case Management Society of America. (2017a). *Our history.*
[Online]. Retrieved July 26, 2017, from http://www.cmsa.org/
Home/CMSA/OurHistory/tabid/225/Default.aspx

Case Management Society of America. (2017b). *CMSA's mission &
vision.* [Online]. Retrieved July 26, 2017, from http://www.cmsa
.org/Home/CMSA/OurMissionVision/tabid/226/Default.aspx

Case Management Society of America. (2017c). *Case Management
Model Act Supporting Case Management Programs.* [Online].
Retrieved July 12, 2017, from http://solutions.cmsa.org/acton/
attachment/10442/f-0464/1/-/-/-/-/2017%20Model%20Care%20
Act_Final%209.27.pdf

Case Management Society of America. (2017d). *Case Management
Adherence Guide (CMAG)—disease specific resources.* [Online].
Retrieved July 26, 2017, from http://solutions.cmsa.org/acton/fs/
blocks/showLandingPage/a/10442/p/p-0025/t/page/fm/3

Case Management Society of America. (2017e). *Integrated case management manual.* [Online]. Retrieved July 26, 2017, from http://
www.cmsa.org/Individual/Education/IntegratedCMTraining/
IntegratedCaseManagementManual/tabid/443/Default.aspx

Coeur, M. (Ed.). (1996). *Case management practice guidelines.*
St. Louis: Mosby.

Commission for Case Manager Certification. (2017a). *Mission,
vision, values.* [Online]. Retrieved July 28, 2017, from https://
ccmcertification.org/about-ccmc/ccmc/vision-mission-values

Commission for Case Manager Certification. (2017b). *Researchers.*
[Online]. Retrieved July 28, 2017, from https://ccmcertification
.org/about-ccmc/role-function/researchers

Commission for Case Manager Certification. (2017c). *Definition and
Philosophy of Case Management.* [Online]. Retrieved July 28,
2017, from https://ccmcertification.org/about-ccmc/about-
case-management/definition-and-philosophy-case-management

Commission for Case Manager Certification. (2017d). *Certification
Guide to the CCM® Examination.* [Online]. Retrieved July 28, 2017,
from https://ccmcertification.org/get-certified/certification/guides

The Care Continuum Alliance. (2017a). *About us.* [Online].
Retrieved July 26, 2017, from http://www.carecontinuum.org/
about_us.asp

The Care Continuum Alliance. (2017b). *Our mission.* [Online].
Retrieved July 26, 2017, from http://www.carecontinuum.org/
about_our_mission.asp

The Care Continuum Alliance. (2017c). *Advancing the population
health improvement model.* [Online]. Retrieved July 26, 2008,
from http://www.carecontinuum.org/phi_definition.asp

The Care Continuum Alliance. (2017d). *Publications.* [Online].
Retrieved July 26, 2017, from http://www.carecontinuum.org/
pub_journal.asp

Hoo, E., Lansky, D., Roski, J, & Simpson, L. (2012, April 6). *Health
plan quality improvement Strategy reporting under the Affordable
Care Act: Implementation considerations.* [Online]. Retrieved
August 3, 2017, from http://www.commonwealthfund.org/
publications/fund-reports/2012/apr/health-plan-quality-
improvement-strategy

National Association for Healthcare Quality. (2008). *Certified professional in health care quality.* [Online]. Retrieved September 28,
2008, from http://www.nahq.org

National Association for Healthcare Quality. (2017). *Certified professional in healthcare quality: 2017 domestic candidate examination handbook.* [Online]. Retrieved July 28, 2017, from http://
nahq.org/UPLOADS/certification/US_Handbook.pdf

National Association of Social Workers. (2008). *Certified social work
case manager.* [Online]. Retrieved September 28, 2008, from
http://www.socialworkers.org/credentials/specialty/c-swcm.asp

National Association of Social Workers. (2017a). *About NASW.*
[Online]. Retrieved August 1, 2017, from http://www.naswdc.org/
nasw/default.asp

National Association of Social Workers. (2017b). *Information booklet with application and reference forms.* [Online]. Retrieved
August 1, 2017, from http://www.naswdc.org/credentials/
applications/C-ASWCM.FullApplication.pdf

National Committee for Quality Assurance. (2012). *NCQA case
management accreditation.* [Online]. Retrieved from http://www
.ncqa.org/Portals/0/Programs/Accreditation/case%20
mgmt-5_8.2.12.pdf

National Committee for Quality Assurance. (2017a). *About NCQA.*
[Online]. Retrieved August 3, 2017, from http://www.ncqa.org/
about-ncqa

National Committee for Quality Assurance. (2017b). *Utilization
management accreditation evaluation options.* [Online].
Retrieved from http://www.ncqa.org/programs/accreditation/
utilization-management-accreditation/utilization-management-
accreditation-evaluation-options

National Committee for Quality Assurance. (2017c). *HEDIS
measures.* [Online]. Retrieved from http://www.ncqa.org/
hedis-quality-measurement/hedis-measures

National Committee for Quality Assurance. (2017d). *NCQA
patient-centered medical home (PCMH) standards and guidelines,
2017 edition, Version 1 (effective April 3, 2017).* Washington,
DC: Author.

National Transitions of Care Coalition. (2011, February 7). *Care
transition bundle: Seven essential intervention categories.*
[Online]. Retrieved July 26, 2017, from http://www.ntocc
.org/Portals/0/PDF/Compendium/SevenEssentialElements_
NTOCC%20logo.pdf

National Transitions of Care Coalition. (2017a). *About us: The national transitions of care coalition.* [Online]. Retrieved July 26,
2017, from http://www.ntocc.org/AboutUs/tabid/57/Default.aspx

National Transitions of Care Coalition. (2017b). *Advisors council.*
[Online]. Retrieved July 26, 2017, from http://www.ntocc.org/
AboutUs/AdvisorsCouncil/tabid/86/Default.aspx

National Transitions of Care Coalition. (2017c). *Partners council.*
[Online]. Retrieved July 26, 2017, from http://www.ntocc.org/
AboutUs/PartnersCouncil/tabid/87/Default.aspx

National Transitions of Care Coalition. (2017d). *Healthcare professionals.* [Online]. Retrieved July 26, 2017, from http://www.ntocc
.org/WhoWeServe/HealthCareProfessionals/tabid/89/Default.aspx

National Transitions of Care Coalition. (2017e). *Workgroups.*
[Online]. Retrieved July 26, 2017, from http://www.ntocc.org/
AboutUs/Workgroups/tabid/103/Default.aspx

The Joint Commission. (2017a). *History of The Joint Commission.*
[Online]. Retrieved August 3, 2017, from https://www
.jointcommission.org/about_us/history.aspx.

The Joint Commission. (2017b). *Measure development initiative.*
[Online]. Retrieved August 3, 2017, from https://www
.jointcommission.org/measure_development_initiatives.aspx

The Joint Commission. (2017c). *Measures.* [Online]. Retrieved August 3, 2017, from https://www.jointcommission.org/core_measure_sets.aspx

The Joint Commission International. (2017a). *Who is JCI.* [Online]. Retrieved August 4, 2017, from http://www.jointcommission international.org/about-jci/who-is-jci/

The Joint Commission International. (2017b). *Achieve accreditation.* [Online]. Retrieved August 4, 2017, from http://www.joint commissioninternational.org/achieve-accreditation/

The Center for Case Management (CFCM). (2017a). *About the center for case management.* [Online]. Retrieved August 1, 2017, from https://www.cfcm.com/aboutccm/

The Center for Case Management (CFCM). (2017b). *Case management administrator-certified.* [Online]. Retrieved August 1, 2017, from https://www.cfcm.com/cmac/

Utilization Review Accreditation Commission (URAC). (2017a). *About: Mission.* [Online]. Retrieved August 3, 2017, from https://www.urac.org/

Utilization Review Accreditation Commission (URAC). (2017b). *Health plan accreditation.* [Online]. Retrieved August 3, 2017, from https://www.urac.org/accreditation-and-measurement/accreditation-programs/all-programs/health-plan/

Utilization Review Accreditation Commission (URAC). (2017c). *URAC quality domains.* [Online]. Retrieved August 3, 2017, from https://www.urac.org/accreditation-and-measurement/measurement/urac-quality-domains/

Utilization Review Accreditation Commission (URAC). (2017d). *Health utilization management.* [Online]. Retrieved August 3, 2017, from https://www.urac.org/accreditation-and-measurement/accreditation-programs/case-management-programs/health-utilization-management/

Utilization Review Accreditation Commission (URAC). (2017e). *URAC case management accreditation, version 5.1.* [Online]. Retrieved August 3, 2017, from https://www.urac.org/wp-content/uploads/CaseMgmt-Standards-At-A-Glance-10-9-2013.pdf

A-CCC—CONTINUITY OF CARE CERTIFICATION—ADVANCED

Sponsor: National Board for Certification in Continuity of Care
(Continuity of Care and Case Management Professionals)
Target professionals: Nurses, Social Workers, Therapists, Dietitians & Physicians
638 Prospect Ave.
Hartford, CT 06015-4250
860-586-7525
241 Dunlap Court
Jacksonville, IL 60650
TEL: 217-245-7811
FAX: 217-243-7912

AIOCM—AMERICAN INSTITUTE OF OUTCOMES-CASE MANAGEMENT

Providers of Case Management Certification
CMC AIOCM provides national certification of outcomes-case managers as Case Manager Certified (CMC), along with guidance and education to its members on the lines of case management, JCAHO Accreditation, Outcomes Management, and Utilization Management.
12519 Lambert Road
Whittier, California 90606
TEL: 562.945.9990

CDMS—CERTIFIED DISABILITY MANAGEMENT SPECIALIST FORMERLY CERTIFIED INSURANCE REHABILITATION SPECIALIST.

The Commission for Disability Management Specialists
Target professionals: any discipline working with individuals with disabilities
1835 Rohlwing Road, Suite E
Rolling Meadows, IL 60008
TEL: 847-818-0292

CMCN—CERTIFIED MANAGED CARE NURSE

American Board of Managed Care Medicine
4435 Waterford Drive, Suite 101
Glen Allen, VA 23050
TEL: 804-527-1905
FAX: 804-747-5316
See www.CEUs4ManagedCareNurses.com for Exam Prep courses and continuing ed.

CMC—CARE MANAGER CERTIFIED

Sponsor: National Academy of Certified Care Managers
Target professionals: Social Workers, Nurses, Mental Health Counselors, and Psychologists.
3389 Sheridan St, Suite 170
Hollywood, FL 33201
TEL: 1-800-962-2260

NACCM—NATIONAL ACADEMY OF CERTIFIED CASE MANAGERS (LONG-TERM CARE MANAGERS)

3389 Sheridan St. Suite 170
Hollywood, FL 33021
TEL: 847-394-2106

11

Preparation for the Case Manager Role

"Tell me and I forget . . . Teach me and I remember . . . Involve me and I will learn."

BENJAMIN FRANKLIN

LEARNING OBJECTIVES

Upon completion of this chapter, the reader will be able to:

1. List four approaches to preparing case managers for their roles.
2. Define competence and competencies.
3. Design a competency statement that includes the key elements of knowledge, skill, and attitude.
4. Identify the characteristics of successful competency programs.
5. Recognize the importance of orientation programs for case managers.
6. Describe experiential learning and its value for case management practice.
7. Define reflective practice.
8. List the core elements of reflection.
9. Describe the simulation learning method and its role in training case managers.
10. List key topics of case management training programs.
11. Describe the problem-based learning approach to practicing case management by proxy.
12. Demonstrate the ability to apply the problem-based learning method to the practice of case management.

ESSENTIAL TERMS

Academic Preparation • Active Learning • Case Study • Case-Based Scenario • Collaborative Practice • Competence • Competencies • Educator • Experiential Learning • Facilitator of Learning • Hire Competencies • Initial Competencies • Interprofessional Practice • Issue-Centered Instruction • Knowledge • Learning • Learning Group • Mentor • Ongoing Competencies • Orientation • Performance • Problem-Based Learning • Professional Development • Professional Development Specialist • Reflective Practice • Reflective Thinking • Simulation • Skills • Team-Based Care • Transitional Competencies

Case management practice has existed for over a century and has evolved over time. It has gained increased recognition for its contribution to patient care and organizational outcomes during the past three decades. Most importantly, however, since the implementation of the Value-based Purchasing Program and the enactment of the Protection and Affordable Care Act (PPACA) of 2010, reliance on the case manager for the achievement of optimal outcomes has increased, resulting in special focus on the case manager's knowledge, skills, competencies, and overall practice. Despite this evolution, the preparation of case managers for their important roles continues to be primarily in the form of "on-the-job" training (Tahan, Watson, & Sminkey, 2015).

This chapter discusses methods for the effective training of case managers, describes competence and ways of developing realistic case management competencies, and shares examples of learning methods that case managers and their leaders can use for ongoing professional development and advancement of the practice.

▶ CASE MANAGEMENT PREPARATION

In the early days, especially in the 1980s and early 1990s, the only way to learn case management was "trial by fire." For better or worse, many case managers developed and performed the case management role with little (or poor) training. The trend now is, for case managers, to develop or acquire case management knowledge, skills, and competencies in many ways. First, a few professional journals, magazines, and textbooks have moved the educational level up a bit. On-the-job training has helped provide case managers with knowledge of organization-specific responsibilities and mentoring by those who are known experts in the role or have been practicing case management for several years. Next, peer-reviewed journals, magazines, textbooks, and seminars have proliferated over time; major accreditation bodies have added case management to their portfolio of programs, and since 1998, the NCLEX examination that licenses registered nurses (RNs) has begun to include questions about case management. Today, case management is an important topic in other professional licensing examinations for several health disciplines such as social work, vocational rehabilitation counseling, physical therapy, and pharmacy. College courses and university-based programs (degree- and nondegree granting) are now ubiquitous. Some are even available online as distant learning programs.

▶ Levels of Case Manager Education

Essentially, there are four levels of education or training for case managers.

1. *On-the-job training programs.* These are employer-based, offered on the basis of the case manager's job description, required skills, and related competencies. They can be provided within a specific practice setting. They also are useful for training new case managers, and those with experience, because they can be tailored to specific needs of the healthcare organization employing case managers. Generally, these programs are taught by case management experts who are also trained as educators or professional development specialists. The on-the-job training programs address two main objectives: orientation of new hires and ongoing development of case managers for the purpose of professional advancement.

2. *Continuing education programs.* These include local, regional, national, or international conferences specializing in or specifically designated for case management practice. Often these programs are offered on the basis of different tracks to meet the needs of those new to the practice or already experienced; these tracks can also be differentiated on the basis of practice or care setting such as acute, rehabilitation, and community-based or patient-centered medical home. Additionally, these training programs often offer continuing education credits that participants may use toward licensure or certification renewal; examples include the annual Case Management Society of America's (CMSA) conference and the annual Commission for Case Manager Certification's (CCMC) New World Symposium. Continuing education offerings vary in length from 1 day to week-long programs. At the conclusion of these programs, an educational certificate of attendance is usually granted, often indicating the number of continuing education credits, hours, or units.

3. *School-based, nondegree granting programs.* These consist of either a single case management course or a few courses about case management within another program. They focus on the importance of case management as a strategy for providing quality, safe, and cost-conscious healthcare delivery. They may include topics such as what is case management, roles and responsibilities of case managers, and the basic strategies and issues necessary to function in a case management role. Some academic programs may offer a certificate in case management, usually a postgraduate or postbaccalaureate certificate, combining theory and practical courses for the preparation of those interested in becoming case managers but prefer not to pursue a full academic degree program.

4. *Graduate-level academic degree granting programs.* These are full case management programs for professionals who are already licensed and possess an educational background related to a health discipline such as nursing (RNs) or social work (licensed social workers). A total package of theory, leadership, and practical skills is taught. These are full degree programs (i.e., master's degree) at the graduate education level. These programs adhere to accreditation standards of academic programs and offer both core and noncore courses relevant to healthcare delivery systems and case management practice.

▶ Importance of Case Manager Training

Everyone agrees that a solid training for case managers is imperative. Without training, many potentially talented case managers may quickly become discouraged. At what level should a nurse (as an example of a professional case manager) have case management training—with an associate, a baccalaureate, or a master's degree? Certainly, a good debate can be made for each of these educational backgrounds; for example, employers prefer to hire those with advanced practice degrees in nursing for the disease-specific case manager role. However, the truth is that case management skills are needed well before the graduate education level. Staff nurses in hospitals, home health agencies, and skilled nursing facilities (SNFs) require the skills of a case manager, whether they are an RN with an associate or a doctoral degree. The same applies for social workers as case managers or other professionals in this role.

▶ Core Knowledge for Case Management Training

Areas of core knowledge for case management training have been occupying several speech slots at national case management seminars. They also have been discussed and debated in the case management literature. Display 11-1 shows some of the current thinking on what is important for inclusion in case management training, whether this training is on-the-job, a single course, or a university degree. The details in each core knowledge area will change as new case management models are designed and as chronic care/disease management and outcomes management discover the best practices of case management.

CORE AREAS OF CASE MANAGEMENT KNOWLEDGE

Core Areas of Knowledge	On-the-Job Training	Continuing Education/ Graduate Course	Graduate Level—Full Case Management Program
Case management: introduction, history, and characteristics	✓	✓	✓
Case management process	✓	✓	✓
Case management roles and functions: case managers, healthcare team members, and other stakeholders	✓	✓	✓
Case manager skills and competencies	☆	✓	✓
Case manager leadership characteristics and personality traits	☆	✓	✓
Case management standards and scope of services	✓	✓	✓
Case management models		☆	✓
Utilization review and management	✓	✓	✓
Transitional and discharge planning, including transitions of care	✓	✓	✓
Reimbursement methods (government and private), managed care, and other health insurance lines	✓	✓	✓
Legal issues in case management practice	✓	✓	✓
Ethical issues in case management practice	✓	✓	✓
Chronic care and disease management: strategies, processes, and outcomes	☆	✓	✓
Assessment of high-risk populations	✓	✓	✓
Levels of care/continuum of care/continuum of health and human services	✓	✓	✓
Social services/community resources	✓	✓	✓
Life care planning	✳	☆	✓
Quality management and risk management	☆	✓	✓
Case management–related accreditation and certification	☆	☆	✓
Outcomes measurement/variance management	✳	☆	✓
Use of evidence-based care guidelines/clinical pathways/case management plans of care	☆	☆	✓
Case manager's role stress and coping	☆	☆	✓
Case management by proxy	✳	✓	
Case management internship	✳		✓

CORE AREAS OF CASE MANAGEMENT KNOWLEDGE (continued)

Core Areas of Knowledge	On-the-Job Training	Continuing Education/ Graduate Course	Graduate Level—Full Case Management Program
Cost-benefit analysis and return on investment/return on resources	✶	☆	✓
Negotiation skills	☆	☆	✓
Communication/collaboration/interprofessional practice/team-based care	☆	☆	✓
Information systems, electronic health records, telehealth, and digital communication tools and technologies	✶	☆	✓
Case management research, evidence-based practice, and performance improvement		☆	✓
Theoretical frameworks		☆	✓
Health policy, legislation, and case management regulatory trends		☆	✓

✓, Recommended; ☆, at least some discussion recommended; ✶, depends on the needs of the organization.

The following breaks down the core knowledge areas into more detail. These are not listed in any priority order. Some of these topics can also be used in the development of case management competencies.

CASE MANAGEMENT: INTRODUCTION, HISTORY, AND CHARACTERISTICS

▶ Professional organizations such as the CMSA, American Case Management Association (ACMA), National Committee for Quality Assurance (NCQA), and Utilization Review Accreditation Commission (URAC);
▶ First attempts at case management guidelines, The Certified Case Manager, and other accreditations;
▶ Definitions, history, and trends in case management, such as the historical Individual Case Management Association;
▶ In advanced courses, use theories and conceptual frameworks that guide case management practice.

THE CASE MANAGEMENT PROCESS

▶ Steps of the case management process: patient identification and selection, assessment and problem/opportunity identification, development of the case management plan of care, implementation and coordination of care activities and interventions, monitoring and evaluation of the case management plan of care and services, closure (termination) of the case management relationship and services, communication with the patient/family post conclusion of the case management relationship and services;
▶ Use of tools for client screening, assessment, reassessment, and evaluation;

▶ If a single case management course, use case management by proxy as an adjunctive exercise;
▶ If advanced and on-the-job training courses, clinical practicum with an actual caseload of patients and a coach/preceptor/mentor.

CASE MANAGEMENT ROLES/FUNCTIONS

▶ Evolution of the case manager's role in the United States and globally;
▶ Case manager's roles, functions, and responsibilities;
▶ Case manager's skills and personality traits;
▶ Assessment of various job descriptions;
▶ Qualifications for the case manager's role;
▶ Roles of the various members of the interdisciplinary or interprofessional healthcare team;
▶ Variation of the roles by care setting or case management practice environment across the continuum of care.

CASE MANAGEMENT MODELS

▶ Case management models of care: nursing, medical, social services, vocational rehabilitation;
▶ Case management models of care based on practice setting: health insurance organization; acute; subacute; health promotion, wellness, and prevention; chronic care management; patient-centered medical home; and so on;
▶ Descriptions of an organization, including its case management program, like the one the student works in;
▶ The whole case management picture in advanced training and education courses.

UTILIZATION REVIEW AND MANAGEMENT

For this large and important aspect of case management, examine

- ▶ Different utilization review and management modalities, such as InterQual and MCG guidelines, and length-of-stay benchmarks. Look at the pros and cons of each;
- ▶ Utilization review and management procedures based on health insurance plan contractual agreement;
- ▶ Process of authorization or certification of services such as precertification, notification of services, and so on;
- ▶ Denials, reconsiderations, expedited/standard appeals;
- ▶ Types of utilization review: precertification, concurrent review, retrospective review, and so on;
- ▶ Roles of physician advisors and health insurance plan or payor specialists;
- ▶ Utilization management–related accreditations.

REIMBURSEMENT METHODS INCLUDING MANAGED CARE AND OTHER INSURANCE LINES

- ▶ Reimbursement methods and their differences (This is the foundation within which a case manager must function. The student cannot case-manage without a good working knowledge of reimbursement methods and the managed care world; health insurance provides the game rules and the starting parameters of each case.);
- ▶ Indemnity, managed indemnity, HMOs, PPOs, DRGs, capitation, coinsurance, Medicare and Medicaid (managed versus fee-for-service, new Medicare product lines), bundled payment methods, and all other types of contracts and risk-sharing methods of managed care;
- ▶ Value-based purchasing, pay-for-performance, accountable care organizations;
- ▶ Who the insurance players are (e.g., utilization managers, claims payors, claims adjustors, reinsurance carriers, etc.);
- ▶ Use of strategies of different insurance types. (Practice and role play can be valuable; focus on the student's ability to use effective strategies and tactics.)

LEGAL ISSUES RELATED TO CASE MANAGEMENT PRACTICE

- ▶ Liability and malpractice
- ▶ Compensation for errors and significant events
- ▶ Documentation and medical records
- ▶ HIPAA, privacy, confidentiality
- ▶ Fraud, abuse, and waste
- ▶ Special mental health/HIV issues, medical directives, medical power of attorney, Americans with Disabilities Act issues, regulatory issues, surrogates and guardians, do-not-resuscitate orders, autopsy, informed consent
- ▶ Patient Bill of Rights, Patient Self-Determination Act
- ▶ Patient Protection and Affordable Care Act
- ▶ Medicare Conditions of Participation
- ▶ Utilization management grievance and appeals laws
- ▶ Anything from birth injuries to liability from negligent physician care or case management recommendations.

ETHICAL ISSUES RELATED TO CASE MANAGEMENT PRACTICE

- ▶ Ethical principles: autonomy, beneficence, nonmaleficence, justice, veracity, and fidelity;
- ▶ Confidentiality, especially with increased use of technology (health information systems, electronic medical and health records, digital communication tools, and social media);
- ▶ End-of-life issues: withholding versus withdrawal of life support, nutrition, and fluids, physician-assisted suicide, and right to die;
- ▶ Rationing of healthcare;
- ▶ Advocacy;
- ▶ Conflicting roles (e.g., the case manager as gatekeeper vs. patient advocate);
- ▶ Ethical theories and tools; helping students evaluate their own ethical compasses;
- ▶ Use of the CMSA's *Ethics Statement on Case Management Practice* and the CCMC's *Code of Professional Conduct for Case Managers* as the basic foundations from which to apply ethical principles to the practice of case management;
- ▶ Codes of Ethics for other organizations such as the National Association of Social Workers, American Association of Nurses (ANA), and ACMA;
- ▶ Ethical decision making: theories, models, and tools; consulting with ethicists and other experts;
- ▶ Cultural sensitivity and competence;
- ▶ Health disparities.

CHRONIC CARE AND DISEASE MANAGEMENT: STRATEGIES AND PROCESS

- ▶ Chronic care management
- ▶ Population health
- ▶ The disease management process
- ▶ The chronic care model
- ▶ Integrated and holistic case management
- ▶ Clinical indicators for various disease processes
- ▶ Wellness and empowerment through education—a key component in disease management
- ▶ Patient activation, engagement, and self-management
- ▶ Social determinants of health
- ▶ Patient or disease registries (chronic illnesses)
- ▶ Clinical expertise (can be extensive in more advanced courses).

ASSESSMENT OF HIGH-RISK POPULATIONS

Assessment of high-risk or vulnerable populations is another important area! Students must be taught the following:

- How to perform thorough, accurate assessments of all details of medical, psychosocial, financial, and health insurance benefits
- How to avoid being task oriented
- How to look at the whole "universe of the patient"
- How to identify a high-risk population
- Health risk screening and assessment
- Use of electronic tools for the identification of at-risk patients
- Risk stratification models and tools.

TRANSITIONAL AND DISCHARGE PLANNING/ LEVELS OF CARE

- The continuum of care/continuum of health and human services
- Assessing patient needs: different needs for acute care versus through-the-continuum of care
- Understanding levels of care: what is paid for or not paid for; matching level to patient needs
- Transitional planning and transitions-of-care models
- Communication and handoff for continuity of care
- Understanding the relationships between transitional planning and utilization management
- Use of technology and health information systems.

SOCIAL SERVICES, COMMUNITY RESOURCES, AND SUPPORT

- Types of community resources and services including charity care
- Referrals to community resources and services
- Complete psychosocial assessment of the patient/ family
- Conducting a community analysis for a specific population to determine if the community resources can meet the needs of the community (advanced practice)
- Social systems theories
- Assessment of social support systems
- Coping with chronic illness(s).

LIFE CARE PLANNING

- Define life care planning
- Models of life care planning
- Role of the life care planner
- The life care plan
- Patient populations to benefit most from life care planning
- Ability to project the physical, financial, and medical needs of the patient in years to come.

QUALITY MANAGEMENT AND RISK MANAGEMENT

- Differentiating quality management from evidence-based practice and research
- Indicators to look for when completing quality reviews
- Documentation
- Models of quality management: CQI/total quality management (TQM)
- Quality management schools of thought: Deming, Crosby, Juran
- Accreditations and quality credentials (e.g., NCQA, TJC)
- Risk management: triggers, peer review, medical record review
- Medical errors: transparency with patient and family, disclosure.

OUTCOMES MANAGEMENT AND VARIANCES

- Outcomes management: assessment/measurement, monitoring, management;
- Outcomes classification and types: clinical, financial, functional, experience of care, quality of life, and well-being;
- How to measure and assess outcomes; processes of evaluation; tools for process and performance improvement (pareto charts, statistical process control charts, flowcharts, etc.);
- Transparency and public reporting;
- Requirements of the Centers for Medicare & Medicaid Services (CMS);
- Accreditations- or regulatory-related data; for example, the *Health Effectiveness Data and Information Set*, in which health insurance plans are compared using the same set of indicators (comparing apples to apples), value-based purchasing;
- Definition and types of variances (delays in care), early identification and management, variance data reporting and management, improvement of systems, and processes of care.

EVIDENCE-BASED PRACTICE GUIDELINES AND CLINICAL PATHWAYS

- Definitions and descriptions: guidelines, clinical pathways, case management plans;
- Development and use of evidence-based guidelines;
- Standards of practice: for example, the CMSA's *Standards of Practice for Case Management*;
- Use and application of software programs to track and trend data;
- Practice patterns and standardization of care;
- Evaluation of the effectiveness of case management plans, pathways, and guidelines.

CASE MANAGER'S ROLE CLARITY, STRESS AND COPING

▶ Role clarity, confusion, and conflict
▶ Reasons for stress
▶ Coping mechanisms and strategies
▶ Conflict resolution and problem-solving methods
▶ Theories: loss and grief, change theories, change management
▶ Self-care concept, empowerment
▶ Roles: role conflict, role confusion, and role overload; strategies on how to prevent them from happening
▶ Dealing with uncertainty
▶ Role coaching, support, and mentoring.

CASE MANAGEMENT BY PROXY

This is a form of simulation and role-playing using problem-based learning and sample case studies. This can be used:

▶ in a single case management class.
▶ before giving actual cases to a novice case management student.
▶ in evaluating and brainstorming an unusually challenging patient situation.
▶ in assessing knowledge, skills, and competencies as well as improving them.

CASE MANAGEMENT INTERNSHIP

▶ Application of knowledge into practice; clinical experiences, especially in advanced courses. (Offer a variety of practice settings that may help students identify a preferred case management niche area/practice setting.)

COST-BENEFIT ANALYSIS AND RETURN ON INVESTMENT OR RESOURCES

▶ Healthcare system in the United States and its implication for financial management
▶ Budget basics
▶ Budgeting and budget management: salaries of personnel, supplies and equipment, capital budget, operational budget
▶ Fiscal management: how to figure out true case management savings
▶ What constitutes hard versus soft savings
▶ Report writing
▶ Return on investment (or resources) methods and calculation
▶ Cost-benefit analysis methods
▶ Cost or expense reduction strategies.

LEADERSHIP AND NEGOTIATION SKILLS

▶ Leadership versus management; qualities of a leader are needed for performing case management
▶ Leadership styles: authentic, collaborative/participatory, autocratic, servant, transformational
▶ Emotional intelligence

▶ Teamwork
▶ Assertiveness skills
▶ Brokerage of services
▶ Negotiation concepts, principles, processes
▶ Conflict resolution and problem-solving
▶ Accurate assessment of what is available to the patient.

COMMUNICATION/COLLABORATION/ INTERPROFESSIONAL PRACTICE/ TEAM-BASED CARE

▶ Interprofessional teams and practice: members, roles, common purpose, and care processes
▶ Teams: interdisciplinary, multidisciplinary, transdisciplinary, interprofessional
▶ Team management, teamwork, team building, delegation, conflict resolution, problem-solving
▶ Collaboration and role accountability
▶ Models of team-based care and related outcomes
▶ Engagement and role satisfaction.

HEALTH INFORMATION SYSTEMS

▶ Health information systems and technologies in case management
▶ Social media and digital communication tools
▶ Security and safety
▶ Computer literacy: familiarity with software systems, literature searches, word processing, project planning, data entry, graphics, and flowcharts
▶ Necessity for outcomes management projects
▶ Telehealth and telecase management, care provision, and patient monitoring in the virtual or digital health environment using remote care technologies.

CASE MANAGEMENT RESEARCH AND EVIDENCE-BASED PRACTICE

▶ The research/scientific process
▶ Advanced critical thinking using the research process
▶ Evidence-based practice
▶ Research utilization and dissemination
▶ Transforming patient care using evidence and innovation.

THEORETICAL FRAMEWORKS

▶ Philosophical and theoretical foundations of case management practice
▶ Nursing theories, quality management theories, change theories, systems theories, behavioral theory
▶ Social systems theories.

HEALTH POLICY, LEGISLATION, AND CASE MANAGEMENT REGULATORY TRENDS

▶ United States healthcare delivery system and its rapid changes, crisis in Medicare and Medicaid budgets and expenses, changing healthcare policy, universal coverage issues, global impact of case management

▶ Patient Protection and Affordable Care Act
▶ Regulatory implications: utilization review and management, transitional/discharge planning, value-based purchasing
▶ Future of case management
▶ Health and public policy
▶ Institute of Healthcare Improvement
▶ Institute of Patient Safety.

Teaching case management involves an immense amount of understanding and experience. Few who have only taught, without having been on the front lines of practice, can understand the total commitment necessary for this enormous job. Some further suggestions include:

▶ Keep the lessons fun, realistic, and useful.
▶ Plan assignments that can be tailored by the students to the diverse areas of the practice (specialty patient population or healthcare setting) in which they are interested; help the students find their niche.
▶ Facilitate creativity in every class; students will need it in the real case management world.
▶ Apply problem-based learning or case-based scenario strategies; these make the learning experiential and realistic.
▶ Engage students in reflective practice and thinking exercises; ask them to share their clinical experiences.

▶ ORIENTATION PROGRAMS FOR CASE MANAGERS

Orientation of case managers to their case management roles and responsibilities, the practice and care environment, and organizational culture is essential for their success, especially when they are newly employed in a healthcare organization, or are new to the role. It is common practice that case managers undergo an orientation process to socialize them into the organization's culture and the case management department's practice environment. Often, case management leaders establish formal orientation programs and processes that focus on the sharing of important information, review of essential knowledge and skills, and discussion of the competencies required for success in the role. These programs aim to make the transition smooth, effective, manageable, motivating, and engaging. Orienting case managers (and other employees) to the workplace/practice environment and roles is one of the most neglected functions in many healthcare organizations. Having a new case manager learn the role and/or the organizational environment applying an "on-the-job" approach alone is a suboptimal orientation method. Employee handbooks, orientation checklists, and associated paperwork also are insufficient tools when it comes to welcoming new case managers to an organization. When not conducted in a thoughtful and meaningful manner, orientation of new case managers is found to be overwhelming, boring, stressful, frustrating, unhelpful, and disengaging. These case managers

may perceive the organization as being more interested in checking off that a task is done rather than focusing on the quality and outcomes of the task. They may also feel that the organization has dumped too much information on them which they are supposed to understand, apply, and implement in much too short of a time period, without the support of other experienced and knowledgeable case managers to guide this valuable transition phase. When left to sink or swim on their own, the retention and engagement of these new case managers suffers, often resulting in attrition, turnover, and wasted resources.

Inappropriate and ineffective orientation programs contribute to unproductive and confused case managers and result in unnecessary expenses. Attrition is costly to both the employer and the case manager alike. As the demand for case managers continues to surpass the supply, developing effective case management orientation programs becomes crucial. Healthcare organizations that have reputable orientation programs expedite the on-boarding and transition period of new case managers, have better alignment between what the new case managers do and what the organization needs them to do, and experience competitive case managers' engagement rates and lower turnover rates. The goals of using carefully orchestrated orientation programs for case managers include, but are not limited to, the following:

▶ Familiarize case managers with the organization's culture, structure, vision, mission, values, strategic initiatives, and history.
▶ Educate case managers about the organizational and departmental policies, procedures, clinical standards, corporate compliance program, human resources and compensation standards, position description and role expectation, and the "who is who" in the organization.
▶ Provide case managers with the opportunity to learn about equipment, devices, and health information technologies, and the departmental structure and functions; and gain an understanding of what is expected of them by the organization and what they should expect from the organization.
▶ Share with case managers the process of outcomes evaluation, quality and safety program, related value-based purchasing measures, and the performance review/appraisal process.
▶ Apply a consistent process for the on-boarding and transitioning of new case managers to the role, practice environment, and healthcare organization—one that assures the sharing of complete, accurate, and consistent information.
▶ Document adherence to accreditation and regulatory agency standards, including the Centers for Medicare & Medicaid Services, The Joint Commission, and the Occupational Safety and Health Administration.
▶ Prevent wastage of resources, maintain lower costs, and enhance the outcomes related to the transition period.

Successful case management program leaders recognize the value of the development and implementation of an orientation programs and plans that are competency based and flexible enough to meet the individual learning needs of the case manager, while supporting the mission and vision of the healthcare organization. The programs and plans are grounded in the case management scope of services and standards of professional practice. They also include an assessment of the case manager to identify her/his learning needs and assist with planning, implementation, and evaluation of learning. Effective orientation programs move from a global overview of the healthcare organization, to the case management department, and ultimately to the position-specific roles, responsibilities, competencies, and performance expectations. Case management leaders seek feedback from those who have participated in their orientation programs to improve these programs and the associated transition periods. One of the most important principles to convey to case managers during their orientation is the organization's commitment to them and to continuous improvement and ongoing learning. It is also as necessary to encourage the new case managers to feel comfortable with asking questions to obtain the information they need to learn, problem-solve, make decisions, and to assume an active and deliberate role in their own orientation and transition. Case management leaders can design realistic and meaningful orientation programs to meet the case managers' expectations and needs on the basis of inputs from case managers by asking what they want and need from orientation, and what they have or have not liked about it.

The benefits of well-designed and contemporary orientation programs are several. The following are some examples:

▶ *Promote a healthy and rewarding practice environment*: Effective orientation programs emphasize the importance of socializing the new case manager in the practice environment, are welcoming to new case managers, and provide a safe environment for them to speak up, verbalize concerns, ask questions, and inquire about performance and progress toward meeting the goals of the transition period. These programs promote practice excellence and professional development, and a healthy environment of care and practice (Cesta & Tahan, 2017).

▶ *Develop realistic role expectations and role engagement*: It is important that case managers learn as soon as possible what is expected of them, and what to expect from others, in addition to becoming knowledgeable about the culture and values of the organization. Most importantly, these case managers are given the opportunity to practice the competencies expected of them and to demonstrate satisfactory performance of these competencies. While they can learn from experience, they are at a much greater risk to commit many mistakes that are avoidable and potentially damaging.

▶ *Reduce anxiety related to the new practice environment*: Any healthcare professional, when assuming a new role, or put in a new and unfamiliar situation, will experience anxiety that can impede his or her ability to learn and master a new role or organizational environment. Thoughtful orientation programs promote optimal role adjustment and help reduce anxiety and stress associated with the unknown and lack of support.

▶ *Enhance retention, while reducing turnover*: One of the main reasons case managers may change jobs and/or employers is that they never feel welcome or part of the organization they join. Well-designed orientation programs and availability of support during the transition period to a new role or practice environment enhance case managers' morale, promote role engagement, increase motivation and positive attitude, and therefore result in increased retention and lower turnover rates. On the other hand, turnover increases when case managers experience ineffective orientation programs, disorganized transitional periods to new roles or practice environments, and lack of support. The poor quality of such programs may result in case managers feeling they are not valued by the organization, or inadequate when put in positions where they cannot possibly learn how to execute their responsibilities. Therefore, they may experience low morale, feel less motivated, and as a result may decide to leave the department or organization.

▶ *Save time of everyone involved*: The better the orientation program and the initial transition period, the less likely that case managers will need their peers, immediate supervisors, and/or other key healthcare professionals to spend time familiarizing them with the new environment and organizational expectations, and teaching them about their roles. When orientation programs effectively and efficiently cover the necessary information about the healthcare organization, the case management and other departments, the practice environment and services, and other characteristics, all that the immediate supervisor and other persons will need to do is only reinforce these factors.

▶ *Prevent failure*: The main reasons that orientation programs fail are: the programs are not planned; case managers are unaware of the position expectations and role requirements; case managers do not feel welcome and/or supported; and the transition period is disorganized and/or not enough in length (i.e., is rushed). Proactively managing these concerns prevents the risk for failure and wasted resources.

▶ *Reduce cost*: Proper orientation assists case managers get up to speed much more efficiently, therefore becoming productive more quickly and as a result reduce the costs associated with learning the new role. A well-thought-out orientation process takes energy, time, and commitment; however, it usually pays off for the individual case manager, the department, and the organization.

Orientation programs for case managers consist of three main components: (1) general orientation to the healthcare organizations, (2) orientation to the case management department and specialty, and (3) orientation to the specific area, unit, or patient population. Often, the general and specialty orientations are conducted in a central location such as a classroom or a learning laboratory if a computer-assisted or simulation learning approach is applied. The content of each of the three orientation components is decided on the basis of whether a competency can be learned in a classroom environment or on the actual patient care area in a real-world setting. For example, a knowledge area such as screening criteria for identifying patients who will benefit most from case management services can be discussed in a classroom setting; a case scenario can be used to demonstrate application of the criteria; and then the criteria can be used on a real patient situation on the patient care unit, which will provide the case manager with the opportunity to demonstrate the required learning and therefore the acquisition of the competency.

The unit- or patient population-specific orientation usually occurs in the actual practice environment (i.e., on-the-job) and with the assistance of an expert case manager who is competent in the case management role and feels comfortable with and knowledgeable about the department and organization. The expert case manager acts as a mentor to the new case manager, oversees the transition period, and ensures that the new case manager has acquired (or demonstrated an acceptable degree of comfort) the minimum knowledge, skills, and competencies required for safe and effective case management practice (Cesta & Tahan, 2017). Case managers learn best when they apply knowledge and information to real situations over time. Coaching and mentoring by expert case managers during the transition period, inclusive of discussions, debriefing, and feedback about performance, and reinforcement of training and expectations, help facilitate the success of the new case managers. Display 11-2 provides an example of the components of orientation programs, which is designed to primarily assist the new case manager to receive an individualized orientation to the new role and practice environment. Display 11-3 includes a list of topics (curriculum) suggested for inclusion in the training component of the orientation program. Display 11-4 shares an example or a template of a competency-based

---

display 11-2

COMPONENTS OF A CASE MANAGEMENT ORIENTATION PROGRAM

1. *General orientation to the healthcare organization*, especially for those new to the organization:
   - Regulatory and accreditation requirements to demonstrate compliance with the standards
   - Organization's mission, vision, and strategic objectives
   - Key policies and procedures, especially those related to human resources, code of conduct, organizational compliance, privacy and confidentiality rules and practices such as HIPAA, cultural diversity, and infection control
   - CMS-related mandatory training such as Medicare fraud, abuse, and waste, and others as appropriate.

2. *Departmental orientation* to familiarize the new case manager with:
   - The departmental structure and functions
   - Case management policies, procedures, and standards
   - The department's daily routine
   - Logistics, such as the use of technology, role expectations, customer service, and performance excellence.

3. *Unit- or service-specific orientation* which occurs on the job with the support of another peer who is a known expert in case management and trained as a mentor, coach, or preceptor:
   - The structure and dynamics of the unit or service
   - Opportunity to practice the application of organizational and departmental expectations and role

competencies in a real-life environment while being supported by a fellow case manager
   - Overview of the process to successfully transition to autonomous and independent practice
   - Use and completion of orientation checklist and competency assessment.

4. *Introduction to key personnel*
   - Case management department team
   - Nursing leadership
   - Medical affairs leadership
   - Physician organization representative (e.g., chairmen, chiefs, medical affairs)
   - Transfer/access center/admitting office/bed management
   - Patient advocacy services
   - Patient financial services
   - Managed care and health insurance contracts
   - Rehabilitation and therapies: physical therapy, occupational therapy, speech pathology, respiratory therapy
   - Onsite vendors and services: home care, skilled care, durable medical equipment, commercial insurer/payor representative
   - Revenue cycle
   - Clinical documentation improvement
   - Pastoral care
   - Ethics and ethics committee
   - Transportation vendors
   - Durable medical equipment vendors.

CURRICULUM FOR THE TRAINING OF CASE MANAGERS DURING ORIENTATION

1. Case management practice, standards, legal, and ethical
   - History of case management
   - Case management models
   - Case manager's roles and responsibilities
   - Case manager's competencies
   - Scope and standards of practice
   - Reimbursement methods
   - Ethical principles
   - Ethical decision making
   - Code of professional conduct
   - Advocacy
   - End-of-life care and palliative care
   - Related laws and regulations
   - Legal documentation
   - Health information systems and technologies: electronic documentation: computerized provider order sets, case management–specific systems
   - Event reporting system
   - Use of admission/discharge/transfer system
   - Review of the role of case manager versus social worker; working as partners
   - Case management accreditation.
2. Patient and family screening and assessment
   - Review of the patient's medical record
   - Risk screening and tools: medical/physiologic, social, functional, nutritional, financial, and so on
   - Screening and assessment tools
   - Review of assessments and plans of care of other disciplines
   - Initial screening versus comprehensive assessment
   - Patient and family interviewing
   - Use of the motivational interviewing method
   - Assessment of postdischarge needs
   - Readmission assessment.
3. Planning care
   - Identification of actual and potential problems
   - Determination of the care goals with the patient and family
   - Development and documentation of the plan of care
   - Identification of discharge needs and development of discharge or transition plans
   - Inclusion of various healthcare professionals
   - Integration of care needs into the case management plan of care.
4. Utilization review and management
   - Reimbursement methods
   - Determination of anticipated length of stay
   - Level of care and medical necessity assessment
   - Use of evidence-based criteria: InterQual and MCG guidelines
   - Mandatory utilization review requirements
   - 2-Midnights Rule
   - Observation status and patient notice of observation status
   - Documentation of clinical reviews and outcomes
   - Organization and presentation of review to payors
   - Gathering and maintaining knowledge of insurance/benefits

- Verification of insurance coverage; monitoring of benefit usage throughout the patient's stay
- Communication with physician advisor and other providers
- Obtaining authorizations for care and services
- Denials and appeals management
- Health insurance plans and contracts: Medicare/Medicaid versus commercial/managed care patients.
5. Transitional/discharge planning
   - Interdisciplinary care rounding and team meetings
   - Interprofessional practice and communication
   - Conditions of Participation
   - Use of criteria for screening patients for postdischarge services
   - Medicare Important Message
   - Discharge assessment and summaries
   - Handoff communication
   - eDischarge
   - Transitions of care
   - Review of health insurance benefits
   - Postdischarge follow-up
   - Physician organization and services
   - Transition to ambulatory care—Patient-Centered Medical Home
   - Medicare Notice of Discharge, refusal of discharge: HINN Letter
   - Readmission risk assessment
   - Personal instrument review (PRI) certification
   - Referral procedure: postdischarge services, social worker for complex needs assessment based on high-screening criteria; activation of social work based on triggers and use of automated tasking function/notification.
6. Quality and patient safety
   - Quality and safety program and goals
   - Value-based Purchasing
   - Evaluation of the case management program
   - Quality measures
   - Peer-review organizations/quality improvement organizations
   - Use of clinical pathways, deviations from pathways
   - Variance/delays management
   - Regulatory requirements and reporting
   - Risk management, escalation of quality of care concerns, serious safety events, reportable events
   - Readmission reviews—assessing for preventable versus nonpreventable causes
   - Case management dashboard: departmental, executive/organizational
   - Patient and family experience of care.
7. Leadership
   - Interprofessional practice
   - Team rounding and interdisciplinary collaboration
   - Skills: leadership, communication, negotiation, conflict management, managing resistance, critical thinking, problem-solving
   - Change management
   - Power
   - Empathy
   - Customer service.

Orientation Competencies	Self-Assessment (Code)	Method of Evaluation (Code)	Performance Rating by Mentor/Coach			Performance Improvement/ Development Needed (Explain)	Signature of Evaluator and Date
			Exceeds Expectations	Meets Expectations	Does Not Meet Expectations		
Case management process							
● Screening							
● Assessment							
● Opportunity identification and goal setting							
● Planning care							
● Implementation							
● Care coordination							
● Monitoring and reassessment							
● Evaluation							
● Conclusion of case management relationship and services							
Transitional and discharge planning							
Utilization review and management							
Ethical standards and patient advocacy							
Outcomes evaluation and management							
Quality and safety							
Interprofessional practice and communication							

(continued)

Orientation Competencies	Self-Assessment (Code)	Method of Evaluation (Code)	Performance Rating by Mentor/Coach			Performance Improvement/ Development Needed (Explain)	Signature of Evaluator and Date
			Exceeds Expectations	Meets Expectations	Does Not Meet Expectations		
Leadership skills ● Leading teams ● Communication ● Change management ● Negotiation ● Motivational interviewing							
Professional practice and behavior ● Customer service ● Role relationships ● Empathy ● Learning							
Classes attended:							

Note on Performance Development Plan:

Additional documentation required; include specific competencies requiring further development, plan for improvement, method of evaluation, timeline for completion, and professional responsible to follow-up and ensure successful achievement of the competencies

Self-Assessment Codes:

a. Competent and can perform independently
b. Familiar with, but need more practice and guidance
c. Aware of only, have observed before
d. Completely unfamiliar with, never practiced before

Method of Evaluation Codes:

1. Test
2. Direct observation in practice environment
3. Return demonstration/simulation
4. Discussion
5. Peer review
6. Medical record audit/quality review
7. Exemplar
8. Feedback from patients and families
9. Other, explain.

display 11-4

orientation tool. These examples are not comprehensive; rather they are mere examples that list suggested topics and elements for successful orientation of case managers. It is suggested that case management leaders and professional development specialists carefully review these suggestions and decide whether to include them in their orientation programs.

Cesta and Tahan (2017) also note that effective case management orientation programs must include three main content areas. One component is the theoretical and technological content which focuses on a review of case management programs and models and other materials such as policies, procedures, standards, positions description, roles and responsibilities, and departmental and organizational structure and functions. It also covers the type of devices and technology in use such as digital communication tools and electronic medical records. The second component is about orientation to the specific area of employment to facilitate immersion into the environment of practice. It promotes interprofessional teamwork and collaboration. It also enhances the case manager's ability to develop trusting relationships with members of the healthcare team. Additionally, this component familiarizes the case manager with the logistics necessary to feel a sense of belonging to the unit/area of work such as the office, laptop or desktop, telephone, mobile communication device, and other equipment necessary for job performance. The third component entails introduction to key personnel from various departments that directly or indirectly support the practice of case management. Sometimes, these personnel may include stakeholders who are external to the healthcare organization, such as patient intake coordinators from subacute care facilities, transportation and durable medical equipment vendors, and representatives from homecare agencies or payor organizations.

Case management orientation programs vary depending on the healthcare organization, practice setting, and the overall organizational culture. Any program, however, should provide case managers with a proper introduction to the organization, what is expected, and where they fit in to overall goals. Apart from the components of the orientation programs described earlier, here are some additional elements:

- Tour of the healthcare organization and key departments
- Introduction to peers and other team members
- Share and review a standard new hire handbook and paperwork
- Review of compensation and benefits
- Review of orientation goals, position description, and performance expectations
- Introduction to the mentor/coach and goals of the transition period
- Review of the transition period and evaluation process
- Process for filing a grievance or a complaint.

▶ COMPETENCY ASSESSMENT AND MANAGEMENT

Competency assessment and management (CAM) in case management practice is about creating a culture of ongoing competence that encourages, motivates, and supports professional advancement, learning, and skills development for the case managers and other professionals. Improving the performance of case managers through the application of CAM programs enhances the performance of the healthcare organization that employs them, which ultimately impacts the bottom line. High-performing practice environments and organizational cultures (and the cultures of the case management programs) rely on the competent and effective performance of case managers (and other professionals). Performance is the reflection of the competencies, traits, and characteristics that differentiate superior/optimal from average/suboptimal performers, a high reliability practice environment, a learning team, and exceptional leaders or leadership. Leadership and leaders, inclusive of case management leaders, are known to shape organizational cultures and the competence of the individuals/professionals who practice within the organization; competence, in turn, impacts organizational performance and therefore success.

From a case management perspective, competencies are the enduring traits and characteristics that determine the performance of case managers. They provide the foundation for an assessment process one may use in the selection of case managers for case management roles, provide a structure for the orientation of case managers who are new to the healthcare organization or the role, evaluate the performance of case managers against expectations and standards; and guide the development of performance improvement plans for those who require or are likely to benefit from them. CAM, on the other hand, is a leadership philosophy that focuses on performance. It is a practice that identifies and optimizes the skills, knowledge, abilities, attitudes, and behaviors required to deliver on a healthcare organization's business strategy inclusive of the case management program's purpose, goals, and strategic objectives. CAM also provides the foundation to lead and manage deliberate talent management practices such as workforce planning, acquisition of top talent, development of existing personnel to optimize their strengths and performance excellence, and supporting these personnel in their professional advancement and career goals. Moreover, CAM is essential for case management practice because it helps an organization to:

- Clarify performance dimensions, standards, and expectations.
- Enhance individual case manager's performance review.
- Evaluate group or team performance.
- Meet standards set by regulatory and accreditation agencies.

▶ Address problematic issues within the organization.

▶ Advance one's knowledge, skills, abilities, aptitude, and attitudes.

▶ Enhance the patient and family experience of care.

▶ Align the case manager's performance and expectation with the organization's vision, mission, goals, and business imperative.

▶ Provide a mechanism for directing and evaluating the competencies needed to assure provision of quality and safe healthcare services to patients/families.

▶ Identify areas of growth and development for the individual case manager or case management team.

▶ Provide opportunities for ongoing assessment and learning to achieve continuous performance improvement.

▶ Determine the needed learning resources and learning program offerings to advance performance.

▶ Identify talent pipeline and enhance succession planning.

Experts describe competencies as a cluster of related knowledge, skills, behaviors, aptitudes, and attitudes that are important for one's position and role in an organization—case manager. They are required to execute one's responsibilities and correlate with performance; they can be measured against known standards, and may be improved through training and development. Additionally, they are the case manager's capacity to perform his or her role functions and responsibilities against predetermined standards. Competencies are simply the "how to" that an organization expects the case manager to perform role responsibilities, in contrast to goals that are known to communicate the "what" a case manager is expected to accomplish. Competencies are concerned with whether the individual case manager possesses the required knowledge, skills, behaviors, and traits necessary to function well in a situation and perform in a way that demonstrates ability to meet or exceed the expectations. Some describe competencies as being whatever is required to do something adequately or successfully, or the ability to perform a task with desirable outcomes under the varied circumstances of the real world. Functional adequacy and capacity to integrate knowledge and skills with attitudes and values into the specific contexts of practice is also known as competence.

CAM is a strategic process that supports organizational and case management goals and initiatives. It should be regarded as a continuous process that is vital to case management operations to demonstrate adherence to regulatory standards, and to enhance a culture of safety and quality outcomes. It is important to assess and demonstrate the competence of case managers rather than simply assume its existence on the basis of past training and experience. This approach assures that case managers possess the required knowledge, skills, and competencies to manage role expectations. Successful CAM programs are usually fully integrated into day-to-day care processes, position descriptions, performance appraisal processes, and case management workflows, rather than expectations added to existing tasks. They are also dynamic, they change on the basis of fluid dynamics of the practice environment, and they meet not only current needs but also future expectations. Successful organizations and case management leaders support the case managers in their efforts to acquire and demonstrate competence by offering special learning programs. Expert case managers are then able to develop their competencies, skills, knowledge, and expertise through a sound educational base and a multitude of clinical experiences and learning activities. Through these offerings, case managers' expertise develops over time; skill acquisition and expansion of the case managers' knowledge for practice also evolve over time. Such dynamics allow case managers to remain current in their knowledge, skills, and abilities; to maintain their competence; and to adjust to the needs of patients and the evolving practice environment.

The concept of competencies is one way of breaking down the expected behaviors of case managers into explicit and concrete components. These are:

▶ *Task achievements*: also referred to as technical competencies. They are associated with performing one's role responsibilities: what one does and how one does it. These require case managers to apply their theoretical and experiential knowledge. An example is *identifies patients appropriate for case management services based on predetermined criteria and conditions, severity of illness, and resource utilization.*

▶ *Relationship building*: also referred to as interpersonal competencies. These are based on communication and interaction with patients/families, peers, and other healthcare team members. They also refer to the ability to relate positively and constructively with others (customer service), working well with others (teamwork, emotional intelligence), and meeting others' expectations (service orientation). An example is *collaborates with the provider and the interdisciplinary healthcare team to develop and implement a case management plan of care for a patient with complex and chronic condition.*

▶ *Personal attributes*: are competencies intrinsic to an individual. They relate to an individual's personality traits, aptitude, and character—how one thinks, feels, learns, and develops. They also reflect the traits and characteristics that relate to an individual's self-identity, and self-acceptance (integrity); decision-making ability (decisiveness); desire for ongoing learning (self-development); ability to deal with emotions and pressure (stress management); and use of logical, systematic reasoning to understand, analyze, and resolve problems (analytical thinking). An example is *follows through on commitment, agreements, and promises.*

▶ *Leadership*: are competencies of leading and managing an organization or people to achieve the organization's vision, goals, targets, and purpose. These relate to managing, supervising, mentoring, and developing people. These competencies also reflect communicating an inspiring vision, mission, and value system; executing an organizational or departmental strategy; taking well-calculated risks; guiding others through change and transformation; and building alignment to vision and mission. An example is *lead the interdisciplinary healthcare team through daily patient care management rounds.*

Competencies exist on a continuum that ranges from the requirements of a position (case manager role) to the ongoing needs; this categorization is based on the timing and chronology of the competency assessment (Display 11-5). Ongoing needs are of three types; they vary in complexity, and are time-bound. These are: (1) initial competencies that are achieved during an orientation program and role transition period; (2) needs that exist throughout one's employment and reflect the position characteristics and expectations; and (3) transitional ones that are situational in nature and required on the basis of specific events.

When developing case management competencies, it is important to ensure that they define the expected behaviors; provide a structure for enabling the identification, evaluation, and development of these behaviors; and communicate the required knowledge, skills, and attitude for the demonstration of these behaviors. Some of the competencies are required by everyone; these are core competencies and usually reflect the type related to relationship building, including communication, interpersonal skills, and organizational culture, values, and beliefs. Other competencies are role specific and reflect the position description and role responsibilities. Another way of looking at competencies is from the perspective of functional versus behavioral. Functional competencies are the technical activities that the case manager engages in, such as electronic documentation and use of the eDischarge system. The behavioral competencies, in contrast, are the soft skills that the case manager has, skills that reflect potential success in the role, for example, the conduct of the case manager during interdisciplinary rounding or

---

display 11-5

TYPES OF COMPETENCIES (DEVELOPED BASED ON WRIGHT, 2005)

1. *Hire competencies*: may also be referred to as on-boarding competencies. They start before a case manager is hired and reflect the qualification required by the position and documented in the position description. They are developed on the basis of regulatory and accreditation requirements and the position description articulated by the healthcare organization. Examples are licensure to practice one's health profession (e.g., nursing, social work), educational background (academic degree), and other credentials such as certification in case management or years of experience, and background check (good standing in the community).

2. *Initial competencies*: focus on the knowledge, skills, abilities, and competencies required during the first 6 months of hire and up to the first year of employment depending on the healthcare organization. These are referred to as orientation or probationary period competencies; these make a minimum requirement for a case manager to gain permanent employment and to become independent in the field of case management. Examples are those related to the case manager's role responsibilities of utilization review, utilization management, transitional and discharge planning, application of the case management process, and interpersonal communication. The initial competencies focus on safe and satisfactory performance rather than the mastery of skills and competencies.

3. *Ongoing competencies*: focus on the case manager's position requirements, standards, or policies. They are similar to the initial competencies. However, they are not a mere repeat of them; rather, they build on them. They are assessed on a regular basis such as annually. The ongoing competencies reflect the current nature of the case manager's role responsibilities, and the new, changing, high-risk, and problematic aspects (or problem prone) of the role. One key component of ongoing competencies is the inclusion of aspects of the role that are high risk but of low performance frequency. Examples are those related to case management standards of care (e.g., handoff communication during transitions of care), policies or procedures (e.g., conducting a concurrent clinical review with the payor representative), high-risk aspects of the role (e.g., readmission risk assessment and proactive action planning), and other aspects of the role that are rarely performed yet highly important (e.g., obtaining authorization for care for a patient from a country other than the United States and who requires clinical review with the country's medical attaché available at the country's embassy).

4. *Transitional competencies*: these are usually transient in nature. They focus on the problematic aspects of the case manager's role, a change in practice based on new evidence, or the launch of a new service or specialty. These competencies may also be identified on the basis of citations received because of an accreditation or regulatory survey. These may also reflect serious safety events, risk management issues, or quality management data and findings requiring improvement action plans. Examples are a review of the procedure of issuing Medicare Important Message to patients because of lack of compliance with a regulatory standard, the implementation of a readmission risk assessment on the day before hospital discharge as a corrective action plan for readmissions rate being much higher than the benchmark rate, etc.

when interviewing a patient or family to assess the case management needs. Thoughtfully developed competencies apply a process or a set of logical activities such as those described subsequently. These activities may vary on the basis of the framework or model that an organization uses.

- ▶ Reviewing the position description for the specific role: qualifications, roles, responsibilities, and purpose or goals;
- ▶ Studying the patient population served by this position to identify unique clinical and other needs;
- ▶ Identifying the behaviors expected for satisfactory performance including the essential knowledge, skills, and attitudes;
- ▶ Constructing competency statements and the associated measures;
- ▶ Developing detailed expectations, so that competencies are clear to case managers;
- ▶ Ensuring that the articulated competencies reflect the organization's or department's vision, mission, and business imperative;
- ▶ Reviewing the articulated competencies and making certain that they consist of core, functional, and behavioral types.

To measure competencies, the case management leader must consider each competency in terms of the behavior that defines it. This behavior can then be thought of in terms of knowledge, skill, and attitude. Such breakdown facilitates effective measurement of the competency. Knowledge reflects how the case manager uses the knowledge he or she has for optimal care provision. Skill refers to what abilities the case manager has and demonstrates in a situation and to what level. Attitude refers to the case manager's approach to performing a specific activity and the demeanor displayed during the activity. All three components are equally important and contribute to the overall performance of the case management department and organization. Refer to Display 11-6 for several examples of competencies. Generally speaking, CAM programs must be clear about the learning requirements of a competency (i.e., what needs to be done to demonstrate that a competency has been learned/acquired); the performance steps one must follow to successfully exhibit the expected competency; and the knowledge or skills one must have possessed to apply the competency and provide safe, quality care.

---

display 11-6

EXAMPLES OF CASE MANAGER'S COMPETENCIES

Screening for Patient Selection

a. Identify patients appropriate for case management services on the basis of predefined criteria.
   i. Identify high-risk patients through screening or assessment and engage them in case management services.
   ii. Gather relevant and comprehensive information and data through patient/family interviews and collaboration with other members of the healthcare team.
   iii. Determine the need for case management on the basis of actual or potential issues or concerns, resource utilization, severity of illness, and/or intensity of services.

b. **Knowledge:** Standard on criteria for case management services; case management process.

c. **Skills:** Motivational interviewing, interpersonal communication, and clinical judgment.

d. **Attitude:** Respect for the patient's culture and value system.

Care Coordination

a. Facilitate coordination, communication, and collaboration with patients/families and healthcare team to achieve target goals and maximize outcomes.
   i. Progress patient's care on the basis of test results and the patient's response to care interventions.
   ii. Implement the case management plan of care and facilitate service delivery.
   iii. Collaborate with the healthcare team to maintain appropriate levels of care and facilitate the transition of patients to the most relevant care setting across the continuum.
   iv. Negotiate service delivery and availability of necessary resources.
   v. Advocate for what is in the best interest of the patient and family.
   vi. Facilitate patient and family health education and instruction including the understanding of postacute services, health insurance benefits, and community resources.

b. **Knowledge:** Case management process, health literacy, health instructions using teach-back and ask-me-three tools, health benefits, and Medicare Conditions of Participation.

c. **Skills:** Collaboration, negotiation, advocacy, and teamwork.

d. **Attitude:** Attentiveness to patient and family preferences.

EXAMPLES OF CASE MANAGER'S COMPETENCIES (continued)

Discharge/Transitional Planning

a. Develop, implement, and evaluate the discharge plan reflective of patient/family needs and interests.
   - i. Engage patient/family and healthcare team in the development of the discharge/transition plan.
   - ii. Arrange for covered services to be provided by appropriate vendors and providers, especially those in the community.
   - iii. Negotiate for covered postdischarge services including durable medical equipment and medical supplies.
   - iv. Apply discharge or transition screening tools to identify potential concerns, such as risk for readmission to the hospital, and proactively manage them.
   - v. Coordinate follow-up care and services.
   - vi. Communicate patient status and needs to providers at the next level of care.
b. **Knowledge**: Transitions of care, discharge criteria, charity resources, and readmission risk assessment tools.
c. **Skills**: Brokering, negotiation, and communication.
d. **Attitude**: Responsiveness and attention to detail.

Utilization Management

a. Complete utilization review and management activities on the basis of procedures of health insurance plans and within expected time frames to enhance reimbursement and prevent financial risk.
   - i. Gather pertinent information from the patient and family, healthcare team members, health insurance plan representative, and others as necessary.
   - ii. Perform initial certification/authorization reviews with the health insurance plans using medical necessity criteria and plans of care.
   - iii. Convey complete and accurate information to the payor representative to support continued hospital stays.
   - iv. Communicate patient reimbursement information to the healthcare team such as continued authorization for services or denials of services.
   - v. Adhere to patient confidentiality laws, regulations, and standards.
   - vi. Verify in-network and out-of-network health insurance benefits and use such information for utilization management and resource allocation purposes.
   - vii. Collaborate with physician advisor on unresolved utilization management concerns.
   - viii. Maintain follow-up communication with the payor representative as indicated on the basis of contractual utilization management procedures.
b. **Knowledge**: Utilization management guidelines/criteria such as InterQual and MCG guidelines, medical necessity criteria, process for managing denials of services, and physician advisor role.
c. **Skills**: Negotiation, communication, conflict resolution, and denial.
d. **Attitude**: Responsiveness and attention to detail.

Legal

a. Adhere to relevant laws, regulations, and organizational policies governing all aspects of case management practice.
   - i. Maintain client's confidentiality and privacy throughout the case management process and provision of services.
   - ii. Obtain informed consent according to standards of practice throughout the case management process.
   - iii. Apply organizational policy related to the provision of case management services.
   - iv. Seek clarification from reliable expert resources when facing concerns regarding laws, regulations, and organizational policies.
   - v. Recognize and address situations of elder or child abuse and neglect; report these concerns according to laws and policy.
b. **Knowledge**: Healthcare laws and regulations such as patient's bill of rights and HIPAA, hospital policies and procedures, risk management, and chain of command.
c. **Skills**: Critical thinking, decision making, and accountability.
d. **Attitude**: Open-mindedness, decisiveness, and transparency.

Ethics

a. Adhere to the code of ethics for case management practice and other code(s) that underlie the professional credentials such as nursing—American Nurses Association code of ethics.
   - i. Adhere to the ethical principles and standards of case management practice.
   - ii. Provide care and services that are in the best interest of the patient and patient's family or caregiver.
   - iii. Recognize the patient and family as unique individuals with diverse cultural background, values, and belief systems.
   - iv. Respect the client's autonomy, cultural values, belief system, and the right to self-determination.
   - v. Address ethical concerns to the best ability or seek appropriate consultation as needed.
b. **Knowledge**: Code of Ethics, ethical decision-making process, principles of ethical practice, standards of case management practice, cultural diversity, and patient-centered care.
c. **Skills**: Critical thinking, ethical decision making, and competence cultural diversity.
d. **Attitude**: Transparency, cultural sensitivity, and nonjudgmental demeanor.

(continued)

Advocacy

a. Advocate in the best interest of the patient and family at various levels, including service delivery, health benefits, and policy making.
   i. Identify and address service gaps and act on service disparities to improve outcomes.
   ii. Educate and empower patient and family or caregiver to participate in decision making regarding care options and self-advocacy.
   iii. Communicate the patient's needs, goals, and strengths to healthcare providers and other stakeholders.
   iv. Influence the advancement of the patient's health and well-being.
   v. Identify opportunities for enhancing case management services and resources to meet the needs of the patient population served.
   vi. Advocate for health and social policy making and the enhancement of patient care, services, and funding at the local and national levels.
   vii. Maintain a firm patient advocate position all the time, regardless of the patient's health insurance or socioeconomic status.
b. **Knowledge**: Code of Ethics, principles of ethical practice, standards of case management practice, advocacy, health and public policy, and patient-centered care.
c. **Skills**: Critical thinking, influencing, decision making, and problem-solving.
d. **Attitude**: Empathy, acceptance, and fairness.

Professional Practice

a. Demonstrate personal responsibility for professional practice and growth in own practice, and the advancement of the general practice of case management.
   i. Identify and acknowledge own practice abilities and limitations and obtain supervision and mentoring as needed.
   ii. Demonstrate accountability for maintaining current knowledge, skills, and competencies for effective case management practice.
   iii. Act in accordance with the scope of practice relevant to one's profession and educational background.
   iv. Adhere to the code of conduct relevant to one's profession and organizational requirements.
   v. Apply the standards of practice for case management in own practice.
   vi. Evaluate best practice studies and apply evidence/findings to improve case management and service delivery.
   vii. Participate in case management training activities to acquire and share knowledge.
   viii. Serve as a resource to other members of the healthcare team and educate them through formal/informal learning activities.
   ix. Seek and achieve certification in case management.
   x. Engage in practice innovations and research activities, and disseminate findings to the case management community.
   xi. Participate in professional organizations and societies.
b. **Knowledge**: Case management professional organizations, evidence-based practice, case management standards of practice, and professional code of conduct.
c. **Skills**: Mentoring, professional development, and change management.
d. **Attitude**: Professional identity and image, inquisitive mind, and openness to learning.

Communication

a. Use effective communication methods and tools to enrich the patient/family's experience of care and enhance outcomes.
   i. Identify whom to communicate with (e.g., patient, patient's family or caregiver, healthcare providers, or other stakeholders) on the basis of the situation.
   ii. Apply effective listening skills and facilitate meaningful discussions.
   iii. Employ language appropriate to the patient/family or caregiver's health literacy level.
   iv. Apply effective verbal and nonverbal strategies during interactions.
   v. Provide information and respond to questions in a sensitive, timely, empathetic, and truthful manner.
   vi. Update patient, family, and healthcare providers on the patient's progress toward achieving care goals as appropriate.
   vii. Elicit and synthesize relevant information and perspectives from patient or family, healthcare providers, and other stakeholders.
b. **Knowledge**: Communication tools and models, health literacy, and health numeracy.
c. **Skills**: Interpersonal communication, relationships building, generous or active listening, and collaboration.
d. **Attitude**: Showing interest, sincerity, respectful manners, and empathetic presence.

▶ INTERPROFESSIONAL PRACTICE AND COLLABORATION

The practice of case management is interdependent; it relies on the collaboration of case managers with various members of interdisciplinary healthcare teams and on the basis of the needs of the individual patient/family and the healthcare setting. Interprofessional practice and collaboration has received much attention over the past decade, especially to meet the Institute of Healthcare Improvement's Triple Aim: better individual health (including the experience of care), better population health, and affordable care. Interprofessional collaboration is known to improve coordination of care and services, communication among diverse parties and stakeholders, and ultimately the quality, safety, and patient care outcomes. It utilizes both the individual and collective skills and experiences of team members, allowing them to function more effectively across professions to deliver a higher level of service than each one would have if working alone. To succeed in today's healthcare environment, interprofessional healthcare teams are essential for the provision of patient- and family-centered, safe, and effective care. Case managers have earned their presence as integral professionals on these teams. Such practice has gained increased popularity because of the Patient Protection and Affordable Care Act of 2010 which required the development of more responsive healthcare organizations and structures, such as accountable care organizations, integrated clinical care networks, patient-centered medical homes, health homes, transitional care models, and team-based care models.

Although the terms "multidisciplinary team or care, interdisciplinary team or care, and transdisciplinary team or care" are commonly used to describe successful healthcare teams, the application of a more contemporary term, "interprofessional practice," has been increasing. This term is more reflective of the context of practice in successful case management programs. Interprofessional practice occurs when individuals from two or more professions practice together to provide comprehensive services to patients/families, and to learn about, from, and with each other to enable effective collaboration and improve patient care and health outcomes. Eliminating silos and promoting mutual respect among the various healthcare professionals are critical to meeting the demands of value-based purchasing and pay-for-performance programs, as well as reducing the provider's financial risk as it relates to current reimbursement methods (e.g., prospective payment systems, bundled payment, and capitation). Collaboration across the various healthcare professionals, including case managers, help build relationships, partnerships, interconnections, accountabilities, and interdependencies to manage complex problems such as the provision of healthcare services for the management of chronic illnesses. To succeed in today's healthcare environment, interprofessional teams and practices are essential. Despite the value and increased popularity of interprofessional teams and practice, most healthcare providers today have not been trained to practice as integrated teams—a challenge case managers face daily, especially when engaged in interprofessional forums such as daily interdisciplinary patient care coordination and management rounds.

No one healthcare professional can possibly provide all the healthcare services and interventions a patient/family needs, regardless of the model of care or setting. Members of interprofessional teams are essential to meeting the diverse needs of patients. These teams usually consist of physicians, nurses, case managers, social workers, advanced practice clinicians (nurse practitioners and physician assistants), therapists (physical, occupational, and speech and language), dietitians, nutritionists, and pharmacists. Other team members may include mental health workers, health navigators, health coaches, community health workers, and payor specialists. Depending on the type of case management programs, the teams may also include vocational rehabilitation specialists, occupational health providers, workers' compensation specialists, life care planners, psychologists, and counselors. Most importantly, however, at the core of these teams are patients and their family members or caregivers. The healthcare professionals on the team integrate their knowledge, skills, competencies, values, and attitudes toward care provision for the benefit of patients and their families, and to improve health outcomes.

Effective interprofessional teams put patients and their families first and constantly advocate for them; demonstrate a commitment for transparency, shared consciousness, and open communication; they value the contributions of all professionals practicing at "the top of their license." This type of collaboration requires a culture that promotes commitment to building effective partnerships and shared accountability in care provision, especially to meet the health needs of the patient. Display 11-7 lists five core competencies of interprofessional collaborative practice.

Team-based care is a form of interprofessional practice; it supports the role of the case manager and provides an excellent context for case management success. Team-based care is defined by the National Academy of Medicine, formerly known as the Institute of Medicine, as "the provision of health services to individuals, families, and/or their communities by at least two health providers who work collaboratively with patients and their caregivers—to the extent preferred by each patient—to accomplish shared goals within and across settings to achieve coordinated, high-quality care" (Naylor et al., 2010). Effective implementation of team-based care improves the comprehensiveness, coordination, efficiency, effectiveness, and value of care, as well as the engagement and satisfaction of both patients/families and the various healthcare providers involved. Team-based care has witnessed increased popularity in the acute and primary care

CORE COMPETENCIES FOR INTERPROFESSIONAL COLLABORATIVE PRACTICE

1. *Values and ethics for the interprofessional practice*: Work with individuals of other professions to maintain a climate of mutual respect and shared values.
2. *Roles and responsibilities*: Use the knowledge of one's own role and those of other professions to appropriately assess and address the healthcare needs of the patients and populations served.
3. *Interprofessional communication*: Communicate with patients, families, communities, and other health professionals in a responsive and responsible manner that supports a team approach to the maintenance of health and the treatment of disease.
4. *Teams and teamwork*: Apply relationship-building values and the principles of team dynamics to perform effectively in different team roles to plan and deliver patient/population-centered care that is safe, timely, efficient, effective, and equitable. Interprofessional communication is especially important, as the exchange of information is a critical factor in all phases of collaborative patient care, and the impact of this exchange—or the lack of it—can be profound.

SOURCE: Interprofessional Education Collaborative Expert Panel. (2011). *Core competencies for interprofessional collaborative practice: Report of an expert panel*. Washington, DC: Interprofessional Education Collaborative.

settings. It has changed the culture and environment of practice in healthcare organizations to one that recognizes and rewards collaboration, cooperation, transparency, ongoing communication, and accountability for one's role and responsibilities, and for the optimal outcomes achieved because of the team approach to care provision.

Case managers are integral members of these teams. In most organizations, they are considered the linchpin that keeps the team integrated and performing as a solid unit. They also enhance the team's ability to maintain a patient-centered approach to care provision and decision making, while emphasizing the importance of team relationships. Team-based and patient-centered care provides many advantages such as the following:

▶ Expanded and enhanced patient access to care and services;
▶ Effective and efficient delivery of services that are essential to providing high-quality and safe care, such as patient education, behavioral health assessment, and patient counseling regarding engagement and self-management support;
▶ Optimal care coordination activities and processes;
▶ Provision of patient-centered care emphasizing the importance of relationship-based care where patients/families and healthcare professionals feel respected, appreciated for their contribution to the team, and engaged;

▶ Prevention of situations that present risk management concerns or a potential for litigation;
▶ A rewarding environment of practice where healthcare professionals and others are encouraged, and are able, to practice to extent of their licenses and abilities;
▶ Assurances that the expertise the various members of the team brings to patient care provision will result in meeting the patient/family needs and preferences;
▶ Empowered team where members own and support continuous quality improvement, effective intrateam and interteam communication, problem-solving, and decision making based on data;
▶ Prevention of harm to patients or the occurrence of serious safety events, and the elimination of duplication and fragmentation of services and resources because of enhanced communication and collaboration between healthcare team members;
▶ Better outcomes: increased patient experience of care scores, improved provider-patient communication and relationships, improved communication and relationships among team members, better patient/family engagement resulting in adherence to care, improved clinical and financial care outcomes, and enhanced reimbursement based on better outcomes (value-based purchasing).

The productivity, efficiency, and success of healthcare professionals engaged in team-based care are directly related to the personality traits, characteristics, knowledge, and competencies each professional brings to the team. These are also related to the strengths and weaknesses of the members, their professional backgrounds and experiences, their ability to carry out their responsibilities, and the openness to hold each other accountable. Teamwork skills are essential to the team's effectiveness; they determine a team's potential for conflict and suboptimal performance. To succeed, all members of the care team must be familiar with the team's (a) defined purpose and goals which are usually articulated by the healthcare organization on the basis of its vision, mission, and clearly articulated operational objectives; (b) understanding of the specific and measurable outcomes expected of the team and those used for evaluating performance; (c) familiarity with the organization's clinical and administrative systems and processes that support patient care delivery; (d) knowledge of the roles and responsibilities of the various professionals, especially those based on the member's health discipline, license, educational preparation, and assignment of roles; (e) training and preparation for the functions that each team member regularly performs and cross-training to substitute for other roles as appropriate; and (f) communication and relationship skills, especially familiarity with the communication structures and processes available in the organization. High-performing teams exhibit three teamwork-related competencies while demonstrating emotional intelligence skills and maintaining a positive attitude all the time.

1. *Knowledge*: understanding the behaviors needed for an effective team and how they are manifested in a team setting. These are related to a team member's ability to differentiate between optimal and suboptimal or empowering and disempowering relationships, interactions, and actions.
2. *Skills*: the learned capacity to interact with other team members demonstrating skills that promote team building, cohesiveness, unity, and optimal team presence.
3. *Attitudes*: internal states or individual capacities that influence a team member's decision to act in a certain way. These may include a team member's aptitude for emotional intelligence, empowering dialogue, ownership, and accountability.

▶ EXPERIENTIAL LEARNING

Experiential learning is not new to healthcare and case management. It has always been the practice where students in most health disciplines, such as nursing, medicine and social work, are required to complete a predetermined number of clinical practice hours before they graduate. Experiential learning has also been applied in employer-based settings in the form of orientation where a designated peer with greater experience acts in the role of a guide or coach to another who is less experienced or newly hired for support during the transition period to the new practice environment. Today, experiential learning has witnessed increased recognition and in forms beyond academic credits or orientation to a new role or organization.

Experiential learning is defined as the process of learning through doing and thoughtful reflection on doing. It focuses on the learning process where the learner observes an action (i.e., a concrete situation) and then practices its application (i.e., learning context). The process entails hands-on learning where case managers (learners) learn something new by experiencing how it feels like to do it and practice the way it is supposed to be performed. During this process, case managers may apply past experiences, knowledge, and skills to the action or situation being learned. Experiential learning is a desired form for training case managers especially during the orientation process of those new to the role. Examples of experiential learning are simulation, role play, use of case scenarios, return demonstration, role-shadowing, preceptorships, and internships.

Experiential learning is a cyclical process where the learner/case manager first engages in an experience; next, discusses and reflects on this experiencer to understand and grasp its cognitive, emotional, technical, and abstract aspects; then applies new concepts to the experience through discussion, reflection, and experimentation; and finally connects the experience to real-world application where during such application the case manager evaluates the learning and the experience. Being cyclical in nature, the results of the evaluation assist the case manager in determining the need to apply the process again. This repeated application may be warranted, especially in the case of a challenging or complex situation, until the case manager masters the expected behavior. There are many benefits for experiential learning; of special importance are two values: observation and interaction. Case managers involved in experiential learning observe an action and interact with the person demonstrating the action. They also interact with the experience of practicing the action—how to do it and how it feels while performing it. During this deliberate learning process, case managers make their own discoveries and experiment with the related knowledge and skills firsthand, instead of hearing or reading about others' experiences, thus, allowing a better understanding of the real-life environment and experience. This concrete experience requires the learner to physically experience the action, observe her/his performance, and reflect on the process and its outcomes, especially what has worked and which aspects require improvement. Therefore, the process enhances the learner's ability to make sense of the experience, draw meaningful conclusions, and gain confidence in performing the task—important steps toward skill acquisition and the development of competence.

Case management leaders, educators, and professional development specialists may apply Kolb's experiential learning model in the orientation and training of case managers, especially those new to the role. Kolb (1984) articulates four required elements that enhance learning and emphasizes them as integral to experiential learning. These are:

1. *Concrete experience*: the learner's engagement (active involvement) in the experience which requires hands-on practice. This element requires the learner to apply the concepts, facts, and information acquired through formal learning and past experiences.
2. *Reflective observation*: the learner makes meaning of the experience through reflective thinking and examination of the details of the experience. The learner explores the application of knowledge and skill to the real-world experience.
3. *Abstract conceptualization*: the learner's application of analytical skills to conceptualize the experience with special thinking about ways to improve future performance of the same action. The learner here focuses on the analysis and synthesis of knowledge, which may result in creating new knowledge and skill.
4. *Active experimentation*: the learner's application of decision-making and problem-solving skills to effectively use the new ideas gained from the

experience in real-life situations at a later point. Here the learner continues to engage in thought and reflection about the experience while practicing it repeatedly until reaching mastery.

Experiential learning is most effective when the learner (case manager) is motivated, demonstrates a desire to learn, takes the initiative to learn, and actively engages in concrete learning activities. Other essential activities of experiential learning include reflection, debriefing, and feedback. These are necessary for the reflective observation and experimentation elements of Kolb's model. When any of these activities is found lacking, learning outcomes suffer, and the learner becomes unable to master the acquisition of the new knowledge, skill, or competency associated with the action being learned. Debriefing and feedback are integral to reflective thinking and observation where the learner reflects on the physical, emotional, and cognitive experiences; recognizes changes in thought, judgment, decision making, feelings, skills, and knowledge; and identifies the optimal way(s) to retain what is learned and how to apply it in similar future situations.

▶ REFLECTIVE PRACTICE AND THINKING

Reflective practice is the intellectual and affective activities in which learners (case managers) explore their real-life experiences (their practice of case management) to gain new understanding, meaning, and appreciation. It is an important learning activity in which learners recapture their experiences, think about them, and mull over and evaluate them, often for the purpose of ongoing learning and enhancement of knowledge and skills for practice. Reflective thinking is an integral activity within reflective practice where the learner engages in critical and mindful reflection on a situation from his or her own practice by placing himself or herself into the experience and by exploring personal and theoretical knowledge to understand it, think about it, and view it in different ways seeking meaning. Miraglia and Asselin (2015) describe reflective practice as a deliberate process of critically thinking about a clinical experience to develop insights for potential practice change. The process requires the learner to build on existing knowledge, develop clinical judgment, promote optimal communication skills, and improve collaborative practice. Ultimately the process should contribute to improvement in one's performance and care outcomes for the patient/family including experience of care.

Reflective practice is a form of autonomous and self-directed learning that allows the learner to develop professional maturity and to shift practice from task orientation to purposeful presence and outcomes orientation. It promotes learning from experience and stimulates personal and professional growth. It also provides a strategy for the learner to:

▶ Embrace lifelong learning which encourages the case manager to maintain current practice knowledge.
▶ Improve the quality of care by closing the gap between theory and practice, thereby facilitating evidence-based case management practice.
▶ Encourage mindfulness, critical thinking, clinical reasoning, and clinical judgment—essential traits of the professional case manager.
▶ Enable greater ownership of the learning taking place—an approach that is of great fit for the case manager as an adult learner.
▶ Allow practitioners to avoid past mistakes in future situations, thereby promoting the provision of safe and quality case management services.
▶ Slow down activity, thereby providing time to process material of learning and link it to previous ideas and practices. This encourages the case manager to remain abreast of changes and new practices in the field.
▶ Enhance professional case management practice to improve patient care and healthcare organizational outcomes.

Case managers as effective reflective practitioners recognize and explore confusing or unique events, whether favorable or unfavorable, that occur during practice, and reflect on these events to enhance learning and ultimately improve their practice. In contrast, case managers who are ineffective as reflective practitioners are usually task oriented, engage in repetitive and routine practice, and neglect opportunities to think about the state of their case management practice or how best to seamlessly incorporate new standards into it. This suboptimal quality of reflection may then contribute to the case manager's feeling overwhelmed and unable to recognize practice gaps such as the application of outdated standards where existing knowledge does not reflect recent changes or evidence.

Reflection may be independent or shared. Independent reflection occurs when the learner engages in self-reflection and introspection. Shared reflection requires the participation of another person; often it is an educator/professional development specialist, peer, mentor (facilitator of learning), or a supervisor. Reflecting on one's performance is an attribute of a high-performance individual. Reflection is a powerful process in improving one's performance, and like any skill, it can be developed and mastered. Case managers as reflective practitioners and learners may engage in any of two types of reflection, each of which results in a somewhat different yet similar outcome—learning and knowledge acquisition.

▶ *Reflection On Action*: a retrospective process that occurs "after" an event has occurred. It involves thinking back on the event; that is, a practice situation of interest to the case manager whether because it was unique, confusing, or optimal. This process also facilitates the understanding of what has happened in light of the outcome(s), and allows for a new understanding, acknowledges practice acceptability, and often determines if any aspect of the practice needs to change and in what way is it necessary, for example, if any new necessary knowledge, skill, or a shift in attitude needs to be identified.

▶ *Reflection In Action*: a process of thinking about a practice situation while the case manager is "engaged in" the doing of a situation. It allows for reshaping of action while the action is actually taking place. This process of reflection leads to timely change in practice and acknowledges knowledge used which may be intuitive. For example, the case manager recognizes that he or she is facing an unfamiliar situation and seeks the support and guidance (i.e., a consult) of another experienced case manager (e.g., a peer or supervisor) for better management and resolution of the situation. Thus, this action results in learning.

For reflection to be effective, the case manager must engage in a deliberate *beyond reflection* type of thinking—an important aspect of reflective practice that is a must do, as otherwise the outcomes of reflection and learning are compromised. This is a reflective thinking process that facilitates purposeful learning and enhances the outcomes of learning. It prompts the case manager to create a learning action plan that must include the learning needs identified during the reflective practice process, and to overcome the identified practice gap(s): knowledge, skill, or attitude.

There are several frameworks for reflective practice one may apply. Regardless of the framework chosen, it must address three key action steps to maximize the case manager's learning opportunities and enhance case management practice. These are:

1. *Retrospection*: this is the "what happened" step. It includes thinking back on the event; what exactly happened including the decisions made, the actions taken to manage the situation, and the outcomes achieved.
2. *Self-evaluation*: this is the "so what" step. It consists of attending to the experience during the event and making sense of it with special focus on the feelings, emotions, thoughts, and behaviors. This activity should encourage an examination of whether the experience was optimal or suboptimal and the reasons why.
3. *Reorientation*: this is the "now what" step. It is the purposeful reevaluation of the experiences. This activity consists of the interpretation of what happened; drawing conclusions; identifying opportunities for improvement, advancement,

and growth; and implementing specific actions to improve performance in future similar situations.

For reflective practice to be successful, Taylor (2000) suggests several tips for those engaged in reflection to apply. These are essential for case managers especially because learning case management continues to primarily occur on the job; reflection enhances the quality of learning and the on-the-job experience.

▶ Be spontaneous; you do not need to apply strict academic practices to maximize the learning potential.
▶ Express yourself freely; it is from the frank and honest self that important insights arise.
▶ Maintain an open mind throughout the process; the more you share during the process, the better the learning will be.
▶ Take the time needed, do not rush; early conclusions can inhibit further insights and solutions, which ultimately may result in missed learning opportunities or unfocused learning.
▶ Avoid judgment or being critical; approaching the situation with self-blame is detrimental to the learning process. Always remember that although one of the keystone goals of reflection is to identify practice gaps that warrant the acquisition of new knowledge, skill, or attitude; reflection is also conductive to doing something better not because it was poorly executed in the first place.
▶ Involve a role model; an expert who reflects on his or her own practice and facilitates the other's reflection is instrumental in advancing your practice and its associated outcomes.

▶ SIMULATION

Simulation is a common and preferred method of learning today. It is the process of acting out or mimicking an actual or probable real-world condition, event, or situation in an environment that is void of risk such as a learning laboratory. The purpose of this approach to learning is primarily to better understand the event's occurrence and its conditions, circumstances, characteristics, context, players, processes, factors, behaviors, and consequences. It allows those involved in the simulation to practice the event and use the experience to forecast future performance (e.g., behaviors, decisions) and the effects (e.g., outcomes) of its assumed circumstances and factors when it happens in the real world. Whereas simulation is a useful tool that allows experimentation and repeated practice without exposure to risk, it is often a gross simplification of reality because it reflects only a predetermined number of assumptions or factors with a planned control over their behaviors during its operation and an anticipated control over their outcomes. However, in real-world situations, more factors and characteristics exist and the associated outcomes are virtually never ensured a priori. Despite these limitations and controls, simulation remains a highly desired and effective method of learning because of its ability to re-create an environment that is too close to the real world and one where inadequate or suboptimal performance does not compromise real-life results. For example, when case managers are practicing concurrent utilization reviews with a health insurance plan (payor) representative in a simulated environment and share limited information about a patient's case, resulting in the payor denying the requested service or continued hospitalization, such a decision does not impact outcomes for a real-life patient situation. However, such case managers can carefully examine their performance during the simulated interaction and identify where and how they were ineffective; they may then engage in a corrective action plan to avoid ineffective utilization management practice when caring for an actual patient.

Simulation usually feels so real because it is designed to look, feel, and behave as if it were a real-world occurrence. It is an imitated reality of a real-world system, process, event, or object including how it normally exists and behaves over time. Simulation can be used as a training and learning method to show novice or inexperienced case managers the eventual real effects of alternate conditions and courses of action. It can also be used as an adjunct to the on-the-job learning or observation experience. It is a helpful learning environment because of the challenges of learning in real-world situations where these situations usually involve a person's life and real healthcare services. Repeated practice in such situations by inexperienced case managers can be unacceptable, dangerous, and inaccessible. Simulation, then, provides an environment where the learner has the freedom to make unlimited number of mistakes to enhance learning. It also provides limitless opportunities for practice without assuming any risk before executing real actions in the real world.

When developing simulation scenarios or courses, it is important to include valid source information about the relevant selection of the situations of interest, key characteristics and behaviors, expected outcomes of the learning experience, and the approximation of assumptions to the real world. Seek the guidance of an expert and practice the simulation session a few times before it is finalized. It is also necessary to assess the fidelity and validity of the expected simulation outcomes. Fidelity is a term used in simulation to describe the accuracy of a simulation event and how closely it imitates its real-life counterpart. Fidelity is broadly classified as low, medium, or high. Low fidelity reflects the minimum characteristics required for the simulation event and participants to respond to it and experience how it is like if it were to happen in real life. High fidelity, on the other hand, reflects the simulation event and experience being nearly indistinguishable or as close as possible to the real world. Medium fidelity refers to moderate reflection of the real-world situation and is more favorable than the low-fidelity approach. For example, using a case- or problem-based scenario for learning is a form of low-fidelity simulation; a role-play scenario may reflect either low- or moderate-fidelity simulation depending on the accuracy of the role play; whereas using a standardized patient is a form of high-fidelity simulation. Standardized patient is an actor who is trained in acting as a patient in the simulated environment. Effective standardized patients have excellent memory, listening, and concentration skills. They respond during a simulation event exactly as a real patient would, and only as that patient, not as themselves. They also sustain not only the patient's character they are acting, but also their physical condition consistently throughout the simulation. Such characteristics enhance the learner's ability in exactly the way he or she otherwise would have acted in a real-world situation.

Training in case management practice using simulation is a bridge between classroom learning and real-life clinical experience. In nursing, for example, complex simulation learning events have been in use for a long time. These events rely on highly computerized mannequins that perform dozens of human functions realistically in a healthcare setting such as an operating room or critical care unit that is indistinguishable from the real world. Learning here may imitate the features and characteristics of a complex and risky procedure or intervention the learner uses to practice and master the procedure. Training in this case avoids putting actual patients at risk. Similarly, case managers may practice their challenging and complex responsibilities in a simulated environment before they apply their theoretical knowledge in a real situation with a real patient. Such is a desired approach for expediting the development of competence, thereby allowing the new case manager to gain confidence and develop "muscle memory."

▶ PROBLEM-BASED LEARNING

Issue-centered instructional methods are effective strategies used to prepare case managers for their roles and enhance their performance. They help individuals to expand their knowledge, acquire necessary skills and competencies, increase productivity, and ensure success. This section focuses on the problem-based learning (PBL) method and its application in case management to assist case managers, case management leaders, and educators in the application of the various key concepts discussed in this book to the practice of case management. We recognize that this is an effective strategy because it is learner-centered rather than educator-driven; it is educator-facilitated. It allows an "adult learning" approach to building one's knowledge for practice, improving existing skills and competencies, and developing necessary new ones. We consider it a valuable approach because case managers will find it flexible and easy to apply, whether formally in a classroom setting or informally during a roundtable discussion, conversation, or reflective thinking session.

PBL is simply the gaining of new knowledge and information through working with problems in groups wherein members reflect on their past experiences. It is a form of instruction where active learning is driven by using challenging situations and open-ended questions; learners work in small, collaborative groups; and teachers/educators assume the role of "facilitators" of learning. In PBL, learners confront contextualized, ill-structured problems and strive to find meaningful solutions by utilizing prior knowledge, experiences, and skills, or constructing new ones through literature reviews or consulting with experts (Duch, 2008; Gallo, 2008).

Active, experiential learning applies a "minds-on, hands-on" strategy and takes place in a group dynamic setting whereby through social interactions (e.g., discussions, knowledge sharing, questioning, challenging, and brainstorming) case managers probe deeply into issues searching for meaning and connections, grappling with complexity, and using prior (or new) knowledge to fashion suitable solutions. During the learning process, each member of the group of learners (i.e., case managers) may assume a specific role; that is, either a patient, another healthcare professional, administrator, payor, or vendor. The roles assumed by group members are usually relevant to the problem being addressed. In any case, one of the learners would need to assume the case manager's role. When roles are not assigned, group members will need to consider all aspects of the problem (from the perspectives of the various individuals involved in the problem) to effectively come up with a reasonable recommendation to solving the problem with the understanding that there is no "one right" answer.

Beginning the learning process using the PBL method puts learners in the driver's seat: to learn as they attempt to address the problem and at their own pace. They can use and explore what they already know, their hunches, and their wildest ideas to try for a solution. During this thinking process, they can develop an inventory of their already existing knowledge areas and at the same time identify what they need to know (knowledge or skill gaps). Once the learners get a sense of what they need to know, they can set off to question the facilitator of learning (e.g., educator, mentor, case management leader, or expert) and/or their groupmates, plunder the library, or surf the Internet seeking information and potential solutions to the problem (Study Guides and Strategies, 2008). What makes the PBL approach desirable by most learners is that they are not expected to simply memorize knowledge; rather, they apply knowledge to real situations. This approach to learning allows case managers a better understanding of what is being taught, instead of just the ability to restate facts.

When applying the PBL method to case management, before case managers learn new information, you (the individual who is assuming the role of educator or facilitator of learning) should present the group of learners (case managers) with a problem you have structured on the basis of a real-life situation, in a way that allows the learners to apply their theoretical and experiential knowledge and/or seek to acquire new knowledge and skills. As a rule of thumb, present them with some—not all—of the facts; enough to spur them to engage in a lot of talking—stating impressions, thoughts, and ideas; defending propositions; and criticizing possible solutions. To enhance the potential for learning, you must design and use problem scenarios that raise the bar for thinking and searching, and prompt the case managers who are learning to pursue the knowledge with which you would like them to become familiar. As a result of PBL, case managers should become effective problem-solvers, skilled practitioners, outstanding communicators, and successful managers of time, projects, meetings, delegating activities, and setting priorities.

The benefits of the PBL method are numerous. During the PBL group discussion and learning activities, case managers are able to (Duch, 2008; Gallo, 2008):

▶ Learn within the context of authentic tasks, issues, and problems that are aligned with real-world concerns.

▶ Act as if they were practitioners in real-life situations.

▶ Engage in reflective thinking and practice.

▶ Practice debriefing methods and techniques, and provision of feedback.

▶ Interact with peers and other healthcare professionals.

▶ Examine and try out what they know.

▶ Discover what they need to learn: knowledge and skill gaps.

▶ Pursue new knowledge and skills that are needed to handle the problem (e.g., literature review, consult with an expert, seek a mentor, etc.).

▶ Develop people skills necessary for achieving higher performance.

▶ Experiment with different leadership styles and discover how they react to successes and disappointments.

▶ Improve communication, teamwork, critical thinking/judgment, and problem-solving skills.

▶ State and defend positions (thoughts about plan of action) with evidence and sound argument.

▶ Recognize motivation for action.

▶ Explore emotional intelligence skills and traits.

▶ Become more flexible in processing information and meeting obligations.

▶ Collaborate with other learners while developing problem-solving skills within the context of professional practice.

▶ Engage in effective reasoning and self-directed learning, which increases the learner's motivation for lifelong learning.

▶ Practice skills needed for handling similar situations in the future.

There are seven key steps in the PBL process (Study Guides and Strategies, 2008). Although they are listed in a specific order, steps one through five are iterative and can be repeated any time the learning case managers feel the need to. The seven steps described herein are a guide for those interested in applying PBL to case management education, training, and learning. We suggest that you apply them to the case studies shared in this chapter. Before you start the PBL session, you will need to prepare a packet of materials to share with the case managers (the learners). The packet may include the key information about the problem or case scenario, a guide for the case managers to use to document their decisions about the problem, and a learning plan template that assists the case managers in recording the actions they intend to make to address the knowledge, skills, and competence gaps identified on the basis of the PBL scenario.

Before initiating a PBL activity, it is important to carefully design the case scenario and approach to learning. These involve the upfront efforts you exert to set the stage for the learning experience. At this stage, you thoughtfully design the learning objectives, the situation, or the central focus of the case to be used for learning, the activities you expect the learners to participate in, the identification of the key factors to facilitate learning, and the plan/approach for implementation. This preparation is essential for achieving success in the learning activity. The PBL process using the designed case, then, goes as follows:

1. *Introduce the problem and explore the issues.* As the educator and facilitator of learning, you begin PBL by an introduction of a "contextualized, ill-structured" problem to the group of learning case managers. Then discuss the problem statement and list its significant parts. The case managers may feel they don't know enough to solve the problem. Assure them that this is normal—that is the challenge and impetus for learning! The feeling of unknowing should prompt the case managers to generate hypotheses, identify the facts, gather information, and learn new concepts, principles, skills, or competencies as they engage in the problem-solving and learning process. Guide them in these activities and review the content of the PBL packet.

2. *Develop and write down the problem statement in your own words.* Formulate a problem statement on the basis of each member's opinion, the group's analysis of what is already known, and a consideration for what new knowledge or information may be needed to solve the problem. Ask the learning case managers to write the problem statement as they understand and agree on it as a group. When you are done with drafting their statement, ask them to seek feedback on it from you, (the educator or facilitator of the learning experience) or fellow learning case managers if the large group

is divided into smaller groups. Frequently revisit and edit the problem statement as new information is discovered, or "old" information is discarded. Inform the case managers that it is part of the PBL process to revise the problem statement, especially when they gain more knowledge about the problem being addressed.

3. *List possible solutions and actions.* At this time, the group of case managers has gathered what the problem is and is ready to start to develop an action plan for resolving the problem. They first brainstorm possible solutions to the problem and then order those possibilities from strongest to weakest. The group may use a consensus-building strategy to rank-order the possible solutions. One strategy is to analyze each solution for feasibility of implementation, likelihood to resolve the problem, need for resources, and time needed to complete the solution. Next, the group would choose the best one, or the most likely to succeed, as the most desired action. The following is a set of questions that would help the case managers to design the action plan and to identify their learning needs.

   ▶ What do we have to know and do to solve the problem?
   ▶ What outcomes do we expect to achieve?
   ▶ What are possible solutions?
   ▶ How do we rank the possible solutions?
   ▶ How do the solutions relate to the problem statement?
   ▶ Do we agree as a group on the solutions and their ranking?
   ▶ What modifications do we need to make?
   ▶ How long will it take to implement the solutions? To observe desired outcomes?

4. *Identify already existing knowledge, skills, and/ or competencies.* In this step, the learning case managers identify the knowledge areas, skills, and competencies they already possess that they consider helpful in solving the problem. This includes both what they actually know and what strengths and capabilities each group member has. Encourage the case managers to consider or note everyone's input, no matter how familiar or strange it may appear; it could hold a great possibility for managing or solving the problem. This step in the PBL process prompts the case managers to engage in reflective thinking, reflective practice, and sharing of knowledge among the group. As a result, this process guides them in identifying their knowledge, skills, and/or competency gaps.

5. *Determine the need for new knowledge, skills and/ or competencies.* The group members' already existing knowledge, skills, and/or competencies may not always result in generating an appropriate action plan for solving the problem. As a result, they will be required to research additional or new

information and gather data/evidence to support their solution. Such activities are necessary to fill in missing knowledge, skills, and/or competencies. In this step, case managers are expected to develop a learning plan and identify what possible additional resources are needed; they may interview experts, review books, conduct a literature review, surf websites, and so on, aiming to develop the most effective action plan. They are also expected to acquire the new knowledge, skills, and/or competencies. In some situations, additional knowledge may not be needed; in such cases, the above-mentioned activities are necessary to provide evidence that supports the action plan.

6. *Present and defend the plan of action.* Ask the learning case managers to share their plan of action in writing (e.g., prepare a report). An alternative, depending on the formality of the learning session (classroom or roundtable discussion), is a presentation of the findings and recommendations for action to other learning groups. The report or presentation must always include the problem statement, questions raised, data/information gathered, action plan, knowledge areas applied, decision-making processes, prioritization of the potential solutions, suggested evaluation plan, and support/evidence for solutions or recommendations: in short, the process and outcome of learning. The learning case managers should consider the following tips when they share their learning with others.

   ▶ State clearly both the problem and the conclusions.
   ▶ Summarize the process used, options considered, and difficulties encountered.
   ▶ Convince others; do not overpower them.
   ▶ Help others learn, as you have learned.
   ▶ If a challenge arises that you cannot respond to, accept it as an opportunity to be explored. If challenged, present your answer clearly. If you do not have an answer, acknowledge it and refer it for more consideration.

7. *Review performance.* An integral aspect of PBL is the opportunity to debrief about the process and its outcomes when a problem has been completely addressed. Part of concluding the process of learning is providing to and receiving feedback from those who participated in the PBL session(s). As a facilitator of learning, dedicate ample time for a review of performance and debriefing, which should apply both to individuals and to the group. This exercise provides an opportunity for the learning case managers and the facilitator of learning to take pride in what they have done well, learn from what they could have done better, and discuss possible options for improvement.

The PBL method is a form of experiential learning that applies a simulation-like approach to enhance the case manager's deliberate and active learning through the application of knowledge and skills to real-life problems. It emphasizes active or participative learning, relies on interactions, involves the whole person, incudes an element of surprise and variability, uses a structured context or exercise, and requires debriefing and feedback. This approach is different from traditional learning in that case managers as learners are not told what they need to learn, memorize it, and then be shown through an illustrative problem how to apply this knowledge in the management of the problem. Rather, it is a method where case managers as learners are given a problem to resolve, are expected to self-identify what they need to know to solve the problem, develop an action plan, and acquire the new knowledge, skill, or competency, with special focus on application to the situation. When carefully designed and executed, case managers as learners enhance their competencies in three main areas, with the understanding that the learners acquire new knowledge and skills to support these areas:

1. *Applied competence:* Case managers practice and demonstrate the ability to use organizational design and change management concepts and frameworks to identify and analyze variables that can influence case management practice and an organization's overall effectiveness. They test their theoretical and experiential knowledge, skills, and competencies that are relevant to the PBL scenario. Ultimately the applied competencies enhance one's case management practice.

2. *Skills competence such as critical thinking, clinical reasoning, problem-solving, collaboration, and communication:* Case managers identify problems and/or opportunities in organizational contexts or individual patient situations, and make specific recommendations, supported by theory, to improve the situation. They accurately and competently use theoretical frameworks from organization design, change literature, case management program structures and functions, emotional intelligence, and interprofessional practice to interpret and solve business problems, and effectively communicate the analyses made to others in a variety of professional contexts. Additionally, they plan the implementation of the identified solutions and other problem-solving activities with a commitment to quality, safety, and enhanced patient and family experience of care.

3. *Interprofessional collaboration and leadership competence:* Case managers collaborate as members of a project team (a PBL group), taking the initiative in identifying and solving problems or pursuing opportunities for learning and improvement within the group. Through the process of solving PBL scenario, they practice interprofessional collaboration and act as leaders in problem-solving, decision making, and assuming accountability for improved care delivery processes and systems.

▶ CASE STUDIES/PROBLEM-BASED LEARNING SCENARIOS

The following case studies reflect real-life situations and dilemmas. In case management, answers are neither right nor wrong; the case management field is a fluid, creative process tailored to the immediate, individual, and changing needs of the patient. No two patient situations are alike; each patient is a kaleidoscope of medical, biologic, financial, physical, emotional, and psychosocial components. Therefore, no "answers" will be given at the end of this chapter. These cases are included for discussion, teaching, learning, and practicing case management by proxy, especially for applying the PBL method, whether formally in a classroom setting or informally in a roundtable discussion.

Not a day goes by in which we lack interesting or challenging situations. Sometimes the outcomes are so well orchestrated that everyone is satisfied. At other times, our hands have been so tied by the magnitude of needs and lack of financial, social, or health insurance support that the outcomes cause sleepless nights. Although these instances are rare, most case managers with any longevity have had their share of them.

Case management by proxy is suggested for many levels of education, and in various practice settings. We cannot say why any better than with this anonymous verse:

Tell me. . ..I'll forget

Show me. . ..I'll remember

Involve me. . ..I'll understand.

Consider the case of Chuck. All the nurses were fond of Chuck, nicknamed Chuckles because of his bright and positive attitude. Chuck, in his twenties, suffered from a form of leukemia that seemed intractable to all therapies attempted. The only hope for his survival was bone marrow transplantation.

In the mid-1980s, his state's Medicaid plan did not include bone marrow transplantation in its list of covered services. Nonetheless, his case manager delivered a barrage of telephone calls over a 6-month period, and physicians wrote several letters to Medicaid on Chuck's behalf. However, Medicaid's stance was firm—no bone marrow transplantations. Suddenly a letter was received from Medicaid stating that, in 3 months' time, autologous bone marrow transplantations would be added to its list of covered services. Chuck's case manager quickly made all arrangements and scheduled Chuck's appointment, so that on the first allowable day Chuck would be ready to go.

On the day preceding his appointment, Chuck went into grand mal seizures. His disease had spread, and he had central nervous system involvement. The transplantation procedure was postponed. An Ommaya reservoir, chemotherapy, and two further bone marrow transplantations were planned, but each time Chuck was too ill to attempt the surgery. He died a short time later.

This experience with Chuck was his case manager's first big revelation about the inequities in the healthcare system, and for a time she felt somewhat bitter that Chuck was denied timely access to a procedure for a possible cure. The case manager can have an impact—positively—on a case-by-case basis. Although it was too late for Chuck, the case manager could not help feeling that all the telephone calls and letters helped identify a major problem and eventually change Medicaid policy. Therefore, as you manage your cases, broaden your scope and look for ways that case managers can effect future changes in the healthcare system. To further illustrate the benefit of case managers, the case of Travers described next demonstrates how case management intervention can change the course of a person's illness curve. The patient in this case was readmitted into the acute hospital level of care within 2 weeks of discharge. This case was selected for case management for the following three reasons:

1. The condition of the patient on admission indicated poor care at home.
2. The home health agency liaison reported that the patient's significant other felt exhausted and totally overwhelmed with the care required.
3. The diagnosis included a recent tracheostomy with a fistula formation, pneumonia, and malnutrition—all red flags.

Travers (58 years old) was admitted to a medical floor with a primary diagnosis of cancer of the larynx (squamous cell) with metastases to the lymph nodes and neck. His admitting diagnoses included right lower lobe pneumonia, a fistula leaking into his tracheobronchial tree, extreme swelling of the neck, and malnutrition. On hospital day 2, the home health liaison referred this case for case management, stating that Travers' mate was exhausted and overwhelmed with his care. Afraid of "causing more damage," she wanted the patient placed in an extended care facility. However, Travers, being alert and oriented, did not want to be placed in a nursing home; he wanted to maintain his independence at home.

A review of the patient's history revealed that approximately 3 weeks before this admission, Travers had gone to the doctor's office with a 2-month history of hoarseness. He underwent endoscopy, a massive tumor was found, and a tracheostomy was immediately placed to relieve airway compromise. The following day, the surgeons performed a total laryngectomy, partial pharyngectomy, and a left radical neck dissection. His postoperative course included fever and major swelling of the neck after the removal of two Jackson-Pratt drains, necessitating a reopening of the neck wound and reinsertion of one drain.

Travers remained in the hospital for 10 days. During this time, a home health agency was consulted and met with him and his mate. A speech therapist referred him to the American Cancer Society for support and a "loaner" electrolarynx; she also conducted a brief session on stoma care and recommended one or two speech therapy visits at home. However, the electrolarynx was not obtained, and Travers' health insurance plan would not pay for home speech therapy visits on the grounds that "he is ineligible and did not meet criteria."

During the first hospitalization, nurses performed all stoma care, changing of inner cannulas, and tube feeding care. The day before discharge, a nurse reported that Travers' mate refused to learn tracheostomy care. This was the first time anyone had broached the subject, and the mate was fearful, stating that she preferred an extended care facility stay. On the day of discharge, the physician's orders were the following:

▶ Discharge home with Jackson-Pratt bulb suction.
▶ Discharge to home health or extended care facility.
▶ Needs: tracheostomy care, tube feeding, empty Jackson-Pratt bulb each day, and office visit in 4 to 5 days.

On the day of discharge, the discharge nurse instructed the patient and his mate in the following:

▶ Various aspects of tracheostomy care
▶ How to change the inner cannula
▶ How to clean the stoma
▶ How to redress the stoma
▶ How to flush the feeding tube with water
▶ How to empty the Jackson-Pratt drain.

Written instructions were given and a home health nurse was authorized for two to three visits for the purpose of tube feeding. No equipment other than a feeding pump and oxygen was obtained for this patient, and no social services were requested.

Travers received no teaching. He did not know how to suction himself, clean and dress his tracheostomy, or set up his tube feedings and pump. He did not even know how to cough correctly; he covered his mouth (as was his habit since childhood), and sputum was expelled out of his tracheostomy. Although his mate was very supportive, she was unsure of herself and needed more help.

Travers was readmitted to the hospital with the tracheostomy grossly infected; suctioning revealed significant amounts of bloody sputum with clots. Treatment contained the following: IV antibiotics, frequent suctioning every 2 to 4 hours, IV fluids, chest percussion therapy, small volume nebulizer (SVN) procedures every 2 to 4 hours, and tube feedings for malnutrition. A social service consult was placed.

This time the nurse case manager assessed Travers' needs and self-care management capabilities with the medical staff, the social worker, the patient, and the patient's mate. They came to an agreement that the hospital days would be used for intensive teaching in addition to healing the fistula and treating the pneumonia. If Travers could become independent in self-care, his mate might not feel so overwhelmed.

After the infection started subsiding, orders were written for respiratory therapists to teach all aspects

of self-suctioning. Travers quickly became proficient at suctioning, along with tracheostomy cleaning and redressing. Another order was written for nurses to teach the patient to administer his own tube feeding independently; again, Travers quickly learned to do this.

The speech therapist requested that a barium swallow study be performed near the day of discharge, which showed only one questionable, tiny fistula remaining and little or no aspiration. Puréed foods were added, which the patient had no difficulty swallowing. The dietary department helped him by teaching nutritious combinations and incorporated some of his favorite foods in puréed form. Because Travers had lost about 30 pounds before his initial surgery, the physician chose to continue tube feedings at 75 mL per hour from 9:00 PM to 7:00 AM each day, in addition to his puréed diet. Again, Travers was encouraged to obtain the electrolarynx from the American Cancer Society, because his Medicaid plan would not cover the cost of one for him. Home health visits were reinstated.

During the hospitalization, a catheter was inserted into the fistula and placed to suction. The fistula gradually closed, allowing the discontinuation of that catheter before discharge. Travers' pneumonia cleared up, and he was discharged with liquid antibiotics. The following items were set up or ordered for Travers on discharge:

▶ A hospital bed;
▶ A bedside commode (from the American Cancer Society);
▶ A shower chair (from the American Cancer Society);
▶ Feeding bags, tubing, and feeding solution were ordered. Travers was given his new feeding schedule. A tube feeding pump was already in his home.
▶ A portable oxygen tank to allow more mobility and an aerosol setup for the tracheotomy wound to reduce the chance of infection and bleeding from dryness. (Oxygen was already in the home.)
▶ A suction machine and catheters were ordered because Travers still required intermittent suctioning.
▶ Tracheostomy and stoma supplies including dressings, tracheostomy ties, peroxide and normal saline solutions, and cleaning brushes. (Travers' type of tracheostomy was changed during this admission, and he no longer required inner cannulas.)

This time, when Travers was discharged, both he and his mate were comfortable doing the tasks required. Because Travers was independent in his self-care, his mate did not feel solely responsible. In addition, Travers felt more in control of his situation and less depressed.

At a certain point in Travers' disease process, a short stay in an extended care facility was needed for strengthening and finishing up a course of IV antibiotics. At this point, a hospice referral was initiated because of his advanced stage of cancer. Through the care of the hospice attendants, Travers was able to return home, as was his wish. He died shortly after, with hospice and loved ones present.

Without case management, Travers and his family experienced exhaustion, frustration, and a preventable deteriorating condition. Case management added the element of self-care and independence to his life, allowing the remainder of his life to be lived at home, which was his wish. This patient received quality care. Because the family and patient provided the remainder of his care at home with intermittent home health and finally hospice visits, his care was also cost-effective.

We have seen many patients who were not provided with the skills of a case manager. In general, such patients stay in the hospital too long because the diagnostic and treatment portions of their care are drawn out; they often contract nosocomial infections, which further extend their stays.

Examples of poorly managed care—in hospitals and extended care facilities or in the community—are common. For example, patients may be subjected to two operations (one for a foot and bone debridement and one for a long-term IV access) when one operation may suffice. Perhaps home healthcare is ordered when the skills and emotional support of hospice case management are more appropriate. Conversely, perhaps more support is ordered than was required merely because a thorough psychosocial assessment was not performed. This assessment might reveal a strong formal and informal patient support system, which could easily have met all the unskilled needs that the patient required. Subjecting the patient to professional agencies, often at a high premium for the patient, may not be in the patient's best interests.

An analysis of cases that received case management, compared with those that have been poorly managed, reveals that quality care *is* cost-effective care. A case that has been skillfully assessed and creatively planned should translate into the two main goals of case management and managed care: quality of patient care and the wise use of healthcare resources.

▶ DIRECTIONS FOR PRACTICING CASE MANAGEMENT BY PROXY

The remainder of this chapter contains several case studies that can be used for further training and education purposes and for practicing case management by proxy. We suggest that the case management expert facilitating the learning experience modify the case studies as necessary to meet the desired learning objectives as well as the needs of the learning case managers group involved in PBL. Although it may not be necessary, we also suggest that the expert facilitating learning develop a set of case study–specific questions on the basis of the case circumstance to be used, in addition to the general questions listed in the following paragraphs under seven main areas of case management practice.

We advise you to approach each case study as a PBL or simulation opportunity; therefore, experiential learning events. Discuss the case study in a group and apply the seven key steps of PBL described earlier, as well as attempt to answer, to the degree they are applicable, the questions listed in the following seven major aspects of learning case management. You may also apply the reflective practice process described earlier in this chapter. Be sure to ask the case managers involved in the learning activity to recall similar situation(s) from real-world practice and share how similar or different; what they did in the real-life situation; what were their experiences like—feelings, thought processes, problem-solving approach, decision making, and so on; what were the outcomes; would they do anything differently if the situation were to occur again.

1. Look at role definitions, skills, and knowledge.
   ▶ What might the case manager do in this situation?
   ▶ What value might the social worker be in this circumstance?
   ▶ What might the case manager–social worker team share or do together?
   ▶ What value might other health professionals be in this circumstance?
   ▶ What knowledge and skills are necessary to effectively manage the situation?
   ▶ Do you already possess the knowledge and skills required to solve the problems?
   ▶ What new knowledge and skills might you need to effectively handle the situation?
   ▶ Where and how will you make sure you acquire the new knowledge and skills?
2. Assess strengths in each case study.
   ▶ Is there a strong support system? This may include family, significant others, friends, neighbors, and any informal support that can be tapped.
   ▶ Are the patient and/or family able to handle the situation?
   ▶ Does the patient or family have the financial ability to provide himself or herself with the optimal circumstances?
   ▶ Is the insurance policy adequate to meet the needs assessed for medical care and discharge or transitional planning?
   ▶ Are the patient's own emotional, mental, social, psychological, and spiritual resources positive?
3. Consider the limitations in each case.
   ▶ Assess any knowledge deficit, in the patient, family, and in any caregivers.
   ▶ Assess the limitations of insurance coverage.
   ▶ Assess limitation or lack of social support.
   ▶ Assess housing or homelessness.
   ▶ Assess limitations because of poor medical status that cannot be changed or improved.
   ▶ Consider the limitations resulting from nonadherence to the medical regimen.
   ▶ Assess limitations from poor financial status.
   ▶ Assess which limitations might be improved and how this can be best accomplished.

4. Think about the case management plan during hospitalization.
   ▶ Actualize a comprehensive case management/medical plan.
   ▶ Determine appropriate utilization of resources.
   ▶ Evaluate the patient's financial status, including the presence of health insurance.
   ▶ Examine the appropriateness of the level of care on the basis of acuity of the patient's condition and the needed healthcare resources.
   ▶ Determine whether authorizations, by payor for services, were obtained. Discuss the necessity of authorizations.
   ▶ Actualize a tight transitional/discharge plan.
   ▶ Assess for quality of care and use of standardized medical guidelines.
   ▶ Assess the status of advance medical directives.
5. Consider the patient's needs for posthospital care or across the continuum of health and human services.
   ▶ Determine placement and discharge needs.
   ▶ Determine the need for authorization by the payor for services, level of care, transitions, and so on.
   ▶ Assess the availability of insurance coverage, either private insurance or Medicaid/Medicare.
   ▶ Assess the availability of public community resources.
   ▶ Determine the level of rehabilitation needed. This may range in scope from in-home physical, speech, or occupational therapies to acute (inpatient) or subacute rehabilitation.
   ▶ Assess the home environment for safety.
6. Consider other miscellaneous issues.
   ▶ Are there any psychological issues, such as mental capacity/competency, grave disability, danger to self, and danger to others?
   ▶ Are there any substance abuse issues?
   ▶ Are there any adult or child abuse issues?
   ▶ Assess the need for ethics committee involvement.
   ▶ Determine any legal and risk management issues that need attention.
   ▶ Finally, ask the question, "Is this a case in which everything that could be done was attempted but still failed?" If so, do not be discouraged. Remember that sometimes the dragon wins.
7. Take time to evaluate and reflect.
   ▶ Examine whether the interventions worked; if not why? if yes, offer rationale.
   ▶ Explain your views of the situation. What would you have done differently? Provide a rationale for your actions.
   ▶ Think about what you already know that is applicable to the case study and what areas for additional learning were brought out by the case study.

CASE STUDIES

CASE STUDY 1: TIMMER

Timmer, age 76, arrived at the emergency department on a Thursday evening complaining of chest and abdominal pain. Although generally a poor historian, he did manage to convey to the staff that he had suffered gunshot and bayonet wounds and malaria as a POW during World War II. He also stated that he has had pneumonia.

The ECG taken in the emergency department showed an acute anterolateral myocardial infarction (MI). Because he was not eligible for a primary angioplasty, tissue plasminogen activator was immediately started with effective results. His chest radiograph revealed cardiomegaly and questionable congestive heart failure. His breath sounds were described as tubular; no pedal pulses could be appreciated.

In questioning Timmer, emergency department personnel found his living situation to be transient; currently, he was residing in a motel. He had two children but did not know where they were or how to get in touch with them. They had not spoken for a few years.

Timmer was admitted to the ICU, where tissue plasminogen activator was continued, along with heparin, Tridil, and lidocaine drips as well as IV methylprednisolone (Solu-Medrol). An echocardiogram, abdominal ultrasonography, and cardiac catheterization were ordered.

On hospital day 2, the ultrasound examination showed cholelithiasis. On day 3, Timmer was moved to a telemetry floor level of care. A cardiac catheterization, originally scheduled for Monday (day 5), was rescheduled for Tuesday (day 6) because of conflicts arising out of scheduling the catheterization laboratory.

The cardiac catheterization revealed the need for a triple coronary artery bypass graft (CABG X3). Surgery was performed the following day, day 7.

Timmer was on an intraaortic balloon pump until day 9 (postoperative day 2) and went to the telemetry floor on day 11 (postoperative day 4).

Day 12. Timmer complained of being too weak to ambulate; cardiac rehabilitation was ordered. His oxygen was increased from 2 to 4 L per nasal cannula. SVN treatments were added for diminished breath sounds and egophony in the left base.

Day 13. Timmer again refused to leave his room to ambulate.

Day 14. He still refused to cooperate with cardiac rehabilitation staff. A social service consultation was ordered.

Day 15. Complaints of weakness continued. A chest radiograph revealed atelectasis and small pleural effusions. A multigated acquisition (MUGA) scan was performed.

Day 16. Arterial blood gases with the patient on 2 L of oxygen showed an oxygen saturation of 97%; therefore, Timmer's oxygen was discontinued. He still refused to leave his room for cardiac rehabilitation.

Day 17. The MUGA scan taken 2 days previously was read, and it revealed an adequate ejection fraction of 48%. A transfer for the following day to an SNF was requested. Social service personnel saw the patient and began working on a transfer to a veterans' facility.

Day 18. On the planned day of transfer, Timmer complained again of chest pain. Because of the patient's sedentary postoperative course, physicians felt the need to rule out pulmonary emboli and ordered a ventilation/qualification (V/Q) scan.

Day 20. The V/Q scan was negative. An adenosine cardiolite stress test was performed; it showed no MI or ischemia. Still, the patient complained of chest pain. The chest radiograph showed atelectasis without any change from the last radiograph. Timmer began to ambulate 40 feet with a minimum assistance of two people. He was told he would be transferred the next day. On hearing this news, the patient expressed suicide ideation but refused to speak to a psychiatrist for a consult.

Day 21. The patient was transferred to a respite center.

CASE STUDY 2: JIMMY

Twelve-year-old Jimmy was normal and healthy until 3 years ago. At that time, Jimmy developed a severe, unsubsiding headache. MRI scanning performed 3 months later showed carotid and basilar aneurysms. Several months after that, Jimmy suffered a brain-stem stroke. A basilar aneurysm clipping was performed, but the basilar artery remained thrombosed postoperatively.

A long and stormy course followed surgery, with vocal cord paralysis and pneumonia manifesting as complicating factors. Jimmy worked tirelessly in an inpatient rehabilitation unit and was eventually able to return to school, where he was a well-liked "A" student. Nearly 2 years later, Jimmy suddenly developed seizure activity. A residual right-sided weakness in this right-handed adolescent was disconcerting. A CT scan again revealed the carotid aneurysm. A carotid repair and bypass were performed. According to records, Jimmy did well postoperatively and was discharged home.

The day after discharge, a fever and recurrent seizure occurred. An electroencephalogram (EEG) and MRI were both abnormal. Herpes viral titers proved to be high; Jimmy was treated with the appropriate medication, acyclovir, and restarted on dexamethasone for presumed herpes encephalitis. Urinary tract infections and gastrointestinal (GI) problems were also identified. Inpatient rehabilitation was again provided, and soon Jimmy "graduated" to a day rehabilitation unit. Because of constant GI upsets and frequency of urination, the day hospital could not continue to provide care.

Multiple urinalysis cultures, with occasional exceptions, were negative. Jimmy responded well to an oral antibiotic prescribed for the presumed urinary tract infection.

Jimmy's GI symptoms persisted. GI workups were performed several times, with few conclusive returns.

An esophagogastroduodenoscopy showed mild gastroparesis. Jimmy showed a low iron level on laboratory tests, but his mother stopped his iron at home because of GI complaints.

Jimmy is now readmitted 3 months after his last cranial surgery. The mother's stated concerns for her son are his persistent nausea, abdominal pain and vomiting, fevers to 102°F, urinary frequency every 3 minutes, constant seizures (low voltage), blackouts, head deviation, and facial twitching.

Another thorough workup is being performed. Jimmy's dilantin level is low and IV dilantin is started. On hospital day 4, his potassium level drops to 2.9 mEq/L (normal levels, 3.5 to 5.5 mEq/L) requiring IV boluses. He is afebrile much of the time, with low-grade fevers to 101°F noted. Occasional small emesis (75 ml) is charted, although Jimmy is frequently complaining of nausea. Urinary frequency every 3 minutes has not been noted. His iron level remains low at 14 mg/dL (normal level, 36 to 150 mg/dL).

Neurologic findings are nystagmus, perhaps a little more than Jimmy's chronic state, which is consistent with his old brain-stem stroke. Cognitively, Jimmy remains stable, according to neurologists. He does have a significant short-term memory loss.

Following are the hospital tests and their results for this admission:

▶ MRI—no acute changes; some atrophy that may be from the recent herpes infection.
▶ 24-hour Holter EEG—no acute changes; essentially negative for anything new.
▶ Urinalysis—one of four was positive for leuko esterase.
▶ UGI-SBFT (upper GI, small bowel follow-through)—negative.
▶ Barium enema—negative.
▶ CT of abdomen and pelvis—normal.
▶ Lumbar puncture—negative, no growth of cultures.

There are many unresolved issues between Jimmy's mother and the physicians. According to the physicians, these range from unreasonable demands by the mother to nonpayment of medical bills. Doctors claim that insurance reimbursement checks sent to the mother were never paid to the physicians. The nursing staff states that they are under attack from Jimmy's mother for not charting mental status changes that she deems are occurring (and for not noticing them) and for not knowing all details about Jimmy when she asks.

Jimmy's mother is angry because she feels that no one is in charge. Her request for one doctor to give her overviews is granted; however, she is displeased with him. The same day she requests two more specialists: a hematologist and an endocrinologist. The request is carried out, although it is explained to the mother that this type of consultation can be provided on an outpatient basis because the patient is stable.

The mother now demands a multidisciplinary team meeting immediately, and the social worker sets it up quickly—with only 2 hours' lead time. The mother announces that she will be tape-recording the session and clearly states, "This is not just a threat but a promise that everyone involved in this case will be going to court."

During the 1.5-hour meeting that follows, Jimmy's mother demands a diagnosis for all of Jimmy's problems before discharge or she will refuse to pick up her son and take him home. She also wants to know why her son was like his "old self" after a lumbar puncture.

CASE STUDY 3: MICHAEL

Michael is 24 years old with an extensive history of suicide attempts and substance abuse. Methods of suicide gestures have included one attempted hanging, one self-inflicted knife wound of a superficial nature, and several drug overdoses, some of which he claimed were accidental. His use of drugs includes alcohol, LSD, marijuana, cocaine, and amphetamines.

Precipitating factors focus on dysfunctional relationships and episodes of major depression. Each admission has lasted 2 to 3 days, because Michael quickly stabilizes medically and each time renounces any further plans to harm himself.

Michael is now readmitted after ingesting a handful of cold medicine tablets and the remainder of his prescription for fluoxetine (Prozac), about 22 pills. The precipitating event is a date with a man, which occurred 1 week ago. He enjoyed the experience and is feeling immensely distressed because of it.

After 24 hours in the ICU, Michael is medically stable and ready for another level of care. He has again been diagnosed with major depressive episodes and multidrug abuse. Because Michael's condition is now stable and he has been eager to go home for 2 days, discharge orders have been written. Discharge will occur pending a social service referral to appropriate outpatient counseling and support groups. (Outpatient care is limited for this patient because of inadequate psychiatric insurance coverage, which includes only 72 hours of emergency inpatient care for episodes such as suicide attempts.)

The social worker has assessed available options and is discussing with Michael the appointments that have been made and the support groups available. In a surprising turn of events, Michael now states that he wants to remain in the hospital and that if he cannot be an inpatient, he will do further harm to himself when he leaves.

The discharge is being held to allow psychiatrists to reevaluate the patient. While waiting for his psychiatric interviews, Michael again turns the tables, announcing that he wants to leave the hospital immediately, before any additional evaluation takes place.

CASE STUDY 4: ETHICS

As a case manager for a large Medicaid plan, you feel ethically imbalanced as you perform your gatekeeper role in the following two cases:

Case Study A: Mrs Varo

Mrs Varo is 46 years old with advanced metastatic breast cancer. She finished a course of chemotherapy that left her with intractable nausea and vomiting. She has not vomited for 24 hours but is very weak and nauseated. She lives alone with little social support. She has no intensity of service with which to authorize any further hospital days. The physician advisor of the insurance plan felt that she could be managed at home.

Later the same day, you perform an initial review on the following case:

Case Study B: Ciro

Ciro's admitting diagnosis was suicide attempt. He was placed in an ICU bed for close observation. Ciro had called 911, saying he had just swallowed most of a bottle of diazepam (valium) and had drunk a fifth of whiskey. His toxic screen showed very little drugs or alcohol. However, it did test positive for cocaine. Later that day, Ciro told a social worker that he had spent his last dollar on cocaine and that he considered the weather to be too hot (it was August in Phoenix) to sleep outside, so he feigned suicide. On physical examination, the physician finds cellulitis on both of his legs from cocaine injections. His hospitalization is authorized for initiation of IV antibiotics for bilateral cellulitis.

CASE STUDY 5: MRS BROWNELL

Mrs Brownell, age 77 and widowed, lives in a supervisory care setting where she has her own room and bathroom. The minimum requirement for living in this setting is the ability to get to and from the bathroom and dining room independently. Before this admission, Mrs Brownell was alert and oriented and able to ambulate independently with a walker.

Mrs Brownell's history is as follows: gastrointestinal bleeding from ulcers, non–insulin-dependent diabetes mellitus, hypertension, breast cancer with bilateral mastectomies 12 years earlier, atrial fibrillation, a cerebral vascular accident 5 years earlier, and alcohol abuse with hepatic cirrhosis and hepatic encephalopathy. She now presents to the hospital with a cough with brown sputum, diarrhea, mental status changes, and a decreased ability to ambulate because of weakness, falling at home, and anorexia. A left facial droop and right-sided weakness are also noted.

Mrs Brownell was admitted with bilateral pleural effusions noted on chest radiograph, specifically *Klebsiella* pneumonia found by sputum culture. Her blood urea nitrogen (BUN) was 50 mg/dL and her white blood cell count was 19.5 TH/UL. She was immediately hydrated and given IV antibiotics. A CT scan of the head revealed no irregularities except for some ischemic small vessel disease. Radiographs revealed the possibility of metastases; therefore, a bone scan was ordered. Uptake was noted in the thoracic and lumbar areas, but these findings were more consistent with degenerative or osteoarthritic changes.

During the course of hospitalization, Mrs Brownell's mental state and weakness improved. Physical therapy was instituted.

It is the anticipated day of discharge, because all antibiotics are oral and her temperature has remained normal for 24 hours. She is eating 100% of her diet, and her laboratory values are within normal limits. She can walk 20 to 40 feet with minimum assistance but cannot get up and out of bed independently, secondary to severe back pain.

CASE STUDY 6: COLLINS

Collins, age 52, has been a diabetic since 1973. In 1989, he had a left below-knee amputation at ankle level. His history includes retinal macular degeneration, which has rendered him nearly blind. He also has pulmonary edema from severe valvular insufficiency.

Collins is admitted with multiple bilateral leg ulcers; one of them is huge with foul-smelling drainage. He states that this condition, along with a steadily increasing abdominal girth, has been ongoing for nearly 4 months. A physical examination reveals anasarca. Bilateral above-knee amputations may also be necessary.

Collins has several nonmedical problems: a recent nasty divorce, impending loss of his private insurance, and current unemployment. He also recently lost his home. He has five sons, none of whom he feels he can turn to for help. They have not been in contact for more than 5 years. Collins refuses to contact any of his sons and insists that he can handle his situation without any help.

Although Collins is very ill and is facing the possibility of losing both his legs, he is fixated on nonhealth matters. His physician feels that he is in maximum denial of his illness (as evidenced by his waiting 4 months to seek medical assistance) and has some "paranoid ideation."

CASE STUDY 7: LUBER

Luber, age 31, disappeared from his girlfriend's home 4 days before admission. On his return he was shaking, seemed disoriented, and then fell in a parking lot. Paramedics were called. Emergency department doctors found to be agitated, combative, and verbally inappropriate. The emergency department assessment showed blood pressure, 130/86 mm Hg; pulse, 130 beats per minute; respirations, 40 breaths per minute; and temperature, 103.3°F (39.6°C). A toxicology screen was positive for cocaine and marijuana. This patient also has a history of alcohol abuse.

A chest radiograph revealed a left lobe infiltrate; Luber was admitted for pneumonia (probably aspiration), fever, and confusion, and to rule out meningitis. The results of a lumbar puncture proved unremarkable, and Luber was given appropriate IV antibiotic therapy for pneumonia.

Luber claims he has had amnesia for the past 2 years; physicians have conflicting opinions about this. He says he remembers driving a truck cross-country 3 years ago but does not remember that he has lived with his girlfriend for the past 18 months. The neurologist on the case feels his amnesia is "fictitious," whereas the psychologist feels that it is a possible dissociative state or psychoactive substance-induced organic mental disorder.

Luber's girlfriend says that he currently makes a living making bottles at a manufacturing plant. He lost both parents when he was 12; they died 6 months apart. His mother may have had amnesiac states. He has two children who live 800 miles away. He has served several jail sentences for driving under the influence and assault and battery. Luber has no support system other than his girlfriend, and no medical insurance.

CASE STUDY 8: QUINLAN

This is the third admission in 6 weeks for 46-year-old Quinlan, who is developmentally delayed and living in a training center. Each admission diagnosis has been for dehydration, acute renal failure (BUN 50 mg/dL, creatinine greater than 3.0 mg/dL), thrombocytopenia, anemia, and mental status changes. His history also includes seizures.

During the first two admissions, dehydration, renal failure, and mental status changes returned to normal by the time of discharge. It was believed that his seizure medication was causing the thrombocytopenia, and it was changed to another agent. Still, his problems returned and compounded.

Quinlan had been independent in self-care and living in a cottage on the center's grounds with other "high-functioning" persons. Because his condition began to deteriorate, he was moved to the center itself, where more care could be provided. The training center attendants reported that Quinlan's condition had been going downhill for the past 4 months. Recently, he started refusing food and was losing a considerable amount of weight. When questioned, the attendants said they believed this behavior could be related to a temper tantrum reaction.

The patient had many bruises on admission. The caregiver told the clinicians that the patient had fallen against a railing. The staff nurses were aware of Quinlan's thrombocytopenia and knew that he bruised easily. The staff nurses also reported fearful cries of, "Don't hit me," when the patient was incontinent. When asked who was hitting him, Quinlan consistently named the training center attendants.

This time, the hospital course has been very complex and without clear answers as to a cause of his symptoms. It started much like the previous two hospitalizations, with the symptoms of renal failure and dehydration resolving quickly.

IV medications were needed, but no IV access could be obtained because of the patient's poor vein status. Because a percutaneous endoscopic gastrostomy feeding tube placement was believed to be in the patient's best interests, a central line was to be inserted at the same time. The patient was at times wildly agitated, so the procedures were obtained under general anesthesia. Quinlan did not resume spontaneous breathing, and a postoperative chest radiograph showed right-sided "whiteout" with questionable pleural effusions versus aspiration. Two IV antibiotics were initiated while the patient remained ventilated. A nasogastric tube insertion produced a heme-positive return, and his anemia deteriorated to a hemoglobin of 6.7 g/100 mL and a hematocrit of 19.0, requiring transfusions. Three days later, Quinlan masterfully extubated himself and was able to resume spontaneous respirations.

Quinlan was sent to floor status with IV antibiotics, a nasogastric tube (still draining bile-colored secretions), and orders to start physical therapy. Tube feedings were initiated after 5 days of attempts because of intolerance and vomiting of the formulas. Several competent physicians, including pulmonary, gastrointestinal, and neurology specialists, are still unsure of the cause of the patient's diagnosis.

CASE STUDY 9: VAQUERO

Vaquero, age 26, has a history of insulin-dependent diabetes mellitus. Consistently noncompliant with his medical care for most of his life, Vaquero developed retinopathy, neuropathies, several diabetic foot ulcers, and chronic renal failure. He is now legally blind. A year ago, Vaquero's renal function became so impaired that hemodialysis was initiated.

Vaquero lives in the country, almost 50 miles from the nearest hemodialysis unit. His parents live next door, but his mother is blind and his father has advanced Alzheimer disease. He has only one friend, and this friend is unable to help. There is no public or volunteer transportation to help him get to and from hemodialysis thrice every week, and no other social support is acknowledged.

Vaquero has been in the acute care setting many times in diabetic ketoacidosis and with dangerously elevated BUN, creatinine, phosphorus, and potassium as a result of inadequate dialysis treatment. He has also been hospitalized for several foot problems, resulting from carelessness and not wearing shoes. His injuries include nonhealing cuts and cellulitis and second-degree burns from hot pavement. Vaquero has private insurance, but the policy has no long-term care or SNF benefits.

CASE STUDY 10: MRS OLIVER

Mrs Oliver is 58 years old. Her medical history is as follows: lupus erythematosus, insulin-dependent diabetes mellitus, diabetic neuropathies, neurogenic bladder requiring an indwelling Foley catheter, chronic bladder yeast infections, chronic renal failure, congestive heart failure with cor pulmonale, and recurrent episodes of shortness of breath resulting in frequent emergency department visits. Mrs. Oliver has also gained hundreds of pounds over the past several years, making her morbidly obese. She now weighs approximately 550 lb. This raises the question of Pickwickian episodes. The abdominal skin folds frequently break down, making abdominal cellulitis another recurring problem.

Two months earlier, Mrs Oliver was able to get out of bed and use her walker to get to a bedside commode or chair. Now she is totally bedbound and requires the maximum assistance of two physical therapists to "stand" her for 5 seconds.

Mrs Oliver habitually requires a lengthy hospitalization every few months, often on a telemetry unit. Her first hospitalization of the current year was in February for congestive heart failure and pneumonia in addition to her other chronic problems. Her husband, age 70 and 135 lb, is very supportive but is finding it almost impossible to care for his wife at home any longer. Nevertheless, each time the issue of an SNF is broached, Mrs Oliver bursts into tears and begs her husband to take her home. To complicate matters, at the end of a previous hospital stay (after discharge orders were written), the home health agency previously helping with her care declined her case on the grounds of serious safety issues. No other home health agency could be found to take the case.

There seems to be only one alternative now. Mr Oliver convinces a protesting and teary Mrs Oliver to go to an SNF for physical therapy in an effort to get her back to baseline.

Two weeks later, Mr Oliver is calling the case manager because the latter informs the former that Mrs Oliver insists on leaving the SNF. Then, a home health agency is found to take her case. Unfortunately, the agency is not providing enough help. Mrs Oliver is on a waiting list for an SNF with an excellent reputation for rehabilitation/physical therapy, but while waiting for a bed to become available, Mr Oliver finds himself at his outermost limits. He does not feel that he can handle his wife's care any longer.

The bed in the SNF did not manifest soon enough. After two more emergency department visits for shortness of breath, Mrs Oliver was readmitted with pneumonia. The long-awaited SNF bed became available, and Mrs Oliver was transferred while finishing her last days of IV antibiotics.

Six weeks later, Mrs Oliver is still not making progress in physical therapy at the SNF. Her insurance company will pay for up to 50 skilled home health nurse visits and 100 days of SNF skilled care for 1 year. Mrs Oliver has too many assets to qualify for the state's long-term care and too few assets to privately pay for all the care she requires. No one else in the Oliver family will help.

By June, Mrs Oliver has been bounced from the SNF to the hospital several times with severe respiratory distress, congestive heart failure, and pulmonary edema. Her CO_2 has reached the middle 70s and BiPAP ventilation has been tried. She now has 3 weeks of SNF coverage remaining.

CASE STUDY 11: SIMMS

Seventy-two-year-old Simms has a history of schizophrenia and chronic obstructive pulmonary disease. The emergency department report states that she has been extremely schizophrenic, delusional, and paranoid for the past 1 week. Her chief complaint is shortness of breath. Her physical examination reveals some expiratory wheezes after an SVN treatment, but no respiratory distress, rales, or rhonchi and no use of accessory muscles. She is speaking in full sentences. Simms is afebrile; blood pressure, 143/90 mm Hg; pulse, 96 beats per minute; and respirations, 26 breaths per minute. The emergency department diagnoses rule out paranoid schizophrenia and chronic obstructive pulmonary disease. She is admitted to a medical floor.

Simms is very frightened. She feels the Vietnamese, the Chinese, and the Germans are out to get her and her family. She believes she is not safe anywhere and will not make it out of the hospital alive. The Asian resident assigned to the case had to make himself scarce because Simms exhibited severe fright, accusing him of following her and planning to transfer her out of town to be tortured.

Simms wishes to go to the state hospital, although she is sure the staff will rape her and put her into a machine that will crush her.

Simms never married. She lived in a convent many years ago, but her bizarre behaviors made it impossible for her to become a nun. She trusts the Catholic priests and states that God has talked to her.

Simms has a twin. When her sister is out of town, as she is during this admission, the schizophrenic exacerbations intensify. Her niece and grandnephew are sympathetic and willing to help, but when they visit they are physically attacked by their aunt.

Simms has been taking appropriate psychotropic medication, but there is some question about her compliance. A transfer to an inpatient mental health unit has been arranged, but she refuses to sign the conditions of admission forms.

CASE STUDY 12: MRS LING

Seven years ago, Mrs Ling, who was on hemodialysis, received a kidney from her son, one of her 10 children. The kidney transplantation was a success, and for many years under the meticulous care of her husband, she maintained a serum creatinine level of 0.8 mg/dL. Mr Ling closely monitored his wife's complicated medical requirements for diabetes, chronic urinary tract infections, anemia, coronary artery disease, hypertension, and medications to maintain the kidney. She also had a history of a left cerebral vascular accident and underwent laser surgery to her eyes because of diabetic complications.

About 6 months ago, Mr Ling suffered a cerebral vascular accident and was no longer able to care for his wife. The adult children took over the care of both parents, but their care proved to be haphazard. Cyclosporine was not listed among Mrs Ling's medications, and azathioprine was being given incorrectly.

Mrs Ling was admitted to the hospital with intractable nausea and vomiting; she was unable to keep down food and was intolerant of any medications. Her critical admission laboratory values were the following:

BUN, 178 (normal, 5 to 25),

Creatinine, 17.5 (normal, 0.7 to 1.5),

Potassium, 7.8 (normal, 3.5 to 5.5), and

Phosphorus, 12.3 (normal, 2.5 to 4.5).

The degree of kidney failure indicated that the rejection was not acute. Mrs Ling's physicians had not seen her in more than 6 months; this was in contrast to the careful way Mr Ling made and kept physician appointments. It is difficult to say how long the rejection had been occurring. After 10 days of receiving heavy IV methylprednisolone (Solu-Medrol) doses and frequent hemodialysis, the creatinine was still around 6.5 mg/dL. Outpatient hemodialysis was set up. The patient has Medicaid and, although only 61 years of age, will soon be eligible for Medicare because of hemodialysis.

CASE STUDY 13: MS JOHNSON

Ms Johnson is a 36-year-old divorced woman with a long history of multiple hospital admissions for medical and psychiatric problems. She lives with her 15-year-old daughter. Her mother had bipolar disorder, and her father was schizophrenic. Her insurance coverage is Medicare and Medicaid. She is unemployed and on disability.

She also hospital-hops, so that it is difficult to assess true hospital admission numbers. In 1 year, Ms Johnson entered one hospital 18 times—6 times in 1 month. It is not known how many times she was also admitted to various other hospitals during the same period. Medically, Ms Johnson's history includes asthma with frequent exacerbations, bowel obstructions, seizures, bladder incontinence, and an appendectomy. Psychiatrically, Ms Johnson meets criteria for chronically mentally ill, with the diagnoses of borderline personality and psychotic depression. She has had several inpatient hospital stays at five different mental health facilities.

Ms Johnson's behaviors are superficially slashing her wrists (at one point thrice in 1 week), overdosing on carbamazepine and other pills, hallucinating, consuming excessive amounts of alcohol, and manipulating. Her "usual" admission can be psychiatric, medical, or a combination of both, and is very short. If presented with a plan that Ms Johnson finds distasteful, she leaves against medical advice (AMA). She often shows up in an emergency department within 1 or 2 days of the AMA episode.

After several such events, one psychiatrist deemed Ms Johnson severely mentally ill, and a petitioning process was initiated. She was court-ordered into treatment (she fired that particular psychiatrist). After her court-ordered "incarceration," she resumed her previous behaviors of multiple suicide gestures, asthma exacerbation admissions, and leaving AMA.

Ms Johnson has learned that it is easier to leave AMA when she "voluntarily" agrees to a psychiatric admission than when the involuntary "court order" is initiated, so now she rarely, if ever, refuses a psychiatric admission.

CASE STUDY 14: PAINE

Thirty-two-year-old Paine was diagnosed with HIV 5 years ago. Three of her eight children have died of AIDS. The remaining five children, the youngest of whom is 3 months old, live with relatives or are in foster care. Paine earns her living through prostitution. This supports her polysubstance abuse habit, which includes the use of cocaine (inhaled and injected), alcohol, and whatever else will keep her "drugged out." She practices no regular birth control and does not practice "safe sex." She is currently homeless. Her mental status is assessed as lethargic, alert, and oriented, but she is inconsistent in her answers to different examiners. For example, she changes her occupation from prostitute to burglar when the issue of "safe sex" is broached.

Paine has a history of being admitted to hospitals and leaving AMA—she actually "disappears" when specific issues are raised. She is savvy about the system and knows she cannot be deemed incompetent or incarcerated involuntarily in a mental health unit unless she "threatens her own life or the life of someone else in this state."

On her first admission to a particular local hospital, Paine appeared cachectic, ill-kempt, and disheveled. She had not had anything to eat or drink for 3 days, secondary to frequent smoking of crack during this time. Her left foot had obvious cellulitis. She was admitted for dehydration, cellulitis (rule out osteomyelitis), and electrocardiographic T-wave abnormalities, and bradycardia. She has a history of severe oral thrush and pneumonia. On this admission, Paine's thrush was severe and her chest radiograph was clear, but she had a persistent dry cough. IV antibiotics, IV fluids, and supportive care were initiated.

In addition to treating Paine's obvious physical problems and checking her toxicology screen (positive for cocaine during the hospitalization) and pregnancy test (negative), the attending physician used the time to address the many psychosocial needs and issues of this case. The attending physician felt that Paine was definitely a public health concern and ordered a psychiatric evaluation.

The psychiatrist deemed Paine competent with antisocial tendencies. The recommendation was to explore petitioning on the grounds that she showed definite judgment impairment, that she was "acutely and persistently disabled," and that she was unable to safely care for herself. However, this psychiatric status could not be court-ordered, because the patient knew of alternate options for taking care of herself (she can live with relatives) and she had no previous documented psychiatric history.

Hint: Ethical and legal issues define and also limit the possibilities and probable outcomes for this case.

CASE STUDY 15: JENSEN

Jensen was a pleasant but persistently noncompliant patient known to every hospital emergency department in the metropolitan area. He was an unstable diabetic (even during hospital admissions) with a lifetime of poor diabetic control. His blood sugar levels would routinely register HHH or LLL on the glucose monitors, and yet he was able to sit up and carry on a full conversation with a blood glucose level of 18 mg/100 mL. It is no surprise that Jensen suffered from every diabetic "-opathy" in the medical literature.

In his late thirties, Jensen underwent several angioplasties to his lower extremities for severe artery disease. He had chronic, extensive leg ulcers and partial foot amputations, but he managed to maintain self-care with the use of a wheelchair.

Jensen had an impressive IV drug abuse habit, and after injecting a large amount of cocaine one day, suffered an MI, necessitating an emergency four-vessel coronary artery bypass. Jensen's drug use did not decrease, and many more hospital emergency department visits and admissions were needed to treat his congestive heart failure, chest pain, diabetic ketoacidosis, pneumonia, endocarditis, and out-of-control diabetes. Most emergency department visits included the complaint of chest pain; he knew just how to manipulate the nurses and doctors at these emergency departments. Although Jensen's assessment revealed drug-seeking behaviors, it is also likely that he did have pain and that his tolerance for pain medications was high.

Jensen's insurance coverage was fairly thorough; he had both Medicare and Medicaid. Nevertheless, with all his extensive hospital utilization, he was dipping heavily into his Medicare lifetime reserve days. When not residing in the hospital, emergency department visits would range from a few times per week to daily.

Jensen has lived with his girlfriend for many years. She is much healthier than he physically, but several times she had to be escorted off hospital units for abusive behavior toward the staff. She was also an "aider and abettor" during several episodes when Jensen went "downstairs for a smoke." A two-pack-a-day guy, Jensen often returned to the floor glassy-eyed and with positive toxicology screens.

Jensen received maximum social service, psychiatric, and case management attention but never followed through on medical or community suggestions and referrals.

Discharge planning was complicated by several factors. Although home IV therapy would have shortened hospital lengths of stay, no physician could safely send Jensen home with an easy IV access because of his IV drug abuse. Home nurses were ruled out because those who visited him at home refused to go back, scared because of all the drug paraphernalia and hard-core addicts hanging around his apartment. Eventually, no home health agency would touch this case.

Extended care facilities soon became out of the question, too. When sent to an SNF for endocarditis, which required several weeks of IV antibiotics, Jensen would (as in the hospital) go outside where someone would meet him, and he would come back stoned. He was even caught trying to sell drugs to other SNF residents. Nips of alcohol would be supplied freely to these residents. SNFs, like home health agencies, are no longer an option for Jensen.

DISCUSSION QUESTIONS

1. Reflect on how you learned the case manager's role and share how the process of preparing case managers has evolved since. Discuss how the process is similar or different from what is shared in this chapter.

2. On the basis of the topics of a case manager's training program listed in this chapter, would you change or modify the training program at your healthcare organization? How would you go about achieving that? Why?

3. Compare the orientation program at your healthcare organization with the content of this chapter; what opportunities do you see to enhance your orientation program? How would you integrate experiential learning and simulation into your program?

4. Review your CAM program and identify its strengths and opportunities for improvement. Discuss the competency framework of your CAM program; what areas of knowledge, skills, and attitudes your program seems to emphasize? Why do you think these areas are essential to the practice of case management?

5. How may you implement the PBL approach to practicing case management by proxy at your healthcare organization? How may you implement reflective practice and reflective thinking in your own practice as a case manager?

6. Review the case studies shared in this chapter and identify the strengths found in each. Recognize the weaknesses or concerns found in each. Determine effective approaches to addressing the issues identified in each of the case studies.

7. Examine your current practice from an interprofessional perspective; how do you contribute to interprofessional practice and collaboration? How do you not contribute? What can you do differently to enhance interprofessional practice on your unit? In your practice? At your healthcare organization?

▶ REFERENCES

Cesta, T., & Tahan, H. (2017). *The case manager's survival guide: Winning strategies in the new healthcare environment* (3rd ed.). Lancaster, PA: DEStech Publishing, Inc.

Duch, B. (2008). *Problems: A key factor in PBL.* Retrieved October 20, 2008, from http://www.udel.edu/pbl/cte/spr96-phys.html

Gallow, D. (2008). *What is problem-based learning?* Retrieved October 20, 2008, from http://www.pbl.uci.edu/whatispbl.html

Kolb, D. (1984). *Experiential learning: Experience as the source of learning and development.* Englewood Cliffs, NJ: Prentice Hall.

Miraglia, R., & Asselin, M. (2015). Reflection as an educational strategy in nursing professional development. *Journal for Nurses in Professional Development*, 31(2), 62–72.

Naylor, M. D., Coburn, K. D., Kurtzman, E. T., Prvu Bettger, J. A., Buck, H., Van Cleave, J., & Cott, C. (2010). *Inter-professional team-based primary care for chronically ill adults: State of the science*. Unpublished white paper presented at the ABIM Foundation meeting to Advance Team-Based Care for the Chronically Ill in Ambulatory Settings, 2010 March 24–25, Philadelphia, PA.

Study Guides and Strategies. (2008). *Techniques and strategies for learning with problem-based learning*. Retrieved October 20, 2008, from http://www.studygs.net/pbl.htm

Tahan, H., Watson, A., & Sminkey, P. (2015). What case managers should know about their roles and functions: A national study from the commission for case manager certification: Part 1. *Professional Case Management*, 20(6): 271–296.

Taylor, B. (2000). *Reflective practice: A guide for nurses and midwives*. Buckingham, Open University Press.

Wright, D. (2005). *The ultimate guide to competency assessment in health care* (3rd ed.). Minneapolis, MN: Creative Health Care Management, Inc.

CHAPTER 12

Strategies for Success in Case Management Practice

"The function of Leadership is to produce more Leaders, not more followers."

RALPH NADER

LEARNING OBJECTIVES

Upon completion of this chapter, the reader will be able to:

1. Recognize subtle approaches to effective time management.
2. Explain the importance of self-care.
3. List three strategies for avoiding role conflict.
4. Illustrate five strategies for effective communication.
5. Recommend techniques for enhancing emotional intelligence skills.
6. List three effective approaches to transdisciplinary collaboration.
7. List three essential components of effective leadership.
8. Discuss the role of the case manager as a change agent.

ESSENTIAL TERMS

Accountability • Authentic Leadership • Change Agent • Charismatic Leadership • Collaboration • Communication • Conflict Management • Critical Thinking • Delegation • Emotional Intelligence • Empowerment • Humor • Interprofessional Collaboration • Intuition • Leadership • Participative leadership • Problem-Solving • Professional Development and Advancement • Quiet Leadership • Role Clarification • Self-Care • Servant Leadership • Situational Leadership • Succession Planning • Support System • Time Management • Transactional Leadership • Transformational Leadership

▶ INTRODUCTION

On most days, being a successful case manager takes all the tools and techniques you can muster. In the first three editions of this book, this chapter was called, "Job Stress and Success Factors in Case Management Practice." As our knowledge of the factors and strategies for success has evolved, so too have the concepts highlighted in this chapter.

Some concepts, however, are not time-limited and will be left in for the use of newer case managers who will benefit from them. Expansion of the themes includes those on leadership, accountability, emotional intelligence, and critical thinking. We case managers are no longer the "new kids on the block"—we are fundamental, vital, and respected members of the interprofessional healthcare team; and demonstrating leadership in our roles and influence on our team is critical. Such ultimately impacts the patient experience of care and quality outcomes.

All "helping" professionals can succumb to job stress and burnout, and case managers are certainly no exception. This chapter will include those factors that can considerably reduce stress associated with case management practice. It highlights specific areas case managers must pay closer attention to if they desire to succeed in their role and overcome, reduce, or prevent job-related stress.

At its most basic level, *stress* is the perception of threat or an expectation of future discomfort that arouses, alerts, or otherwise activates the individual's affect or behavior in an undesirable way. Stress itself is not harmful. However, the way you react to stress or cope with it may result in untoward consequences. It is so important for us case managers to be aware of their reactions to stressful stimuli because it is inherent in our roles that we handle delays in care or treatments, prevent undesirable outcomes (both organizational or patient related), resolve conflict, negotiate solutions, address ethical dilemmas or risk-management events, and advocate for what is in the best interest of patients and their families. Indeed, our roles involve the mindful scrutiny of the performance of the interprofessional team; identify issues before they escalate to serious concerns; address them; and ensure optimal clinical care outcomes, quality of services, patient safety, and care experience. Without a doubt, these functions do not occur free of stress.

Too little stress can leave you listless and apathetic, whereas a small dose of stress can provide an edge, a positive boost to action. Volumes have been written on the havoc stress imposes on a person's physical, psychological, emotional, social, and mental health. An optimal level of stress is the perfect motivator and is essential for success. Finding this optimal level is an individual matter and entails being able to read your own personal stress meter. Through self-awareness, it is possible to notice when the reading gets close to the stress overload level. The actual red flag indicators are different for various people: poor judgment, bursts of anger or frustration, depression, forgetfulness, preoccupation with worrying, nonproductive time, isolation, feeling the urge to quit your job immediately, or an inability to make decisions. On the other hand, feeling good about outcomes achieved, content with what you do every day, satisfied with your job, and energized to come back to work the next day, among other positive things, are signals that stress is under control. Recognizing these reactions, not only in yourself but in others, allows you the opportunity to anticipate how to interact with them as well as recognize when it is appropriate to act as their support system if needed. We all have been in the situation when our coworkers exhibit certain subtle cues that signal to us how they feel (sad, angry, withdrawn, or happy), and on the basis of these cues, we decide how to approach them. For example, a coworker whose voice gets quieter and her handwriting larger when she is approaching "stressed out"—her response to feeling overloaded—indicates that it is time to step in and ask if you can help. However, someone else who exhibits the same cues may signal to us "leave me alone," and we know that is not the opportune time to offer assistance.

How one handles perceived insurmountable stress is an individual matter. Scarlet O'Hara would affirm, "Think about it tomorrow." Some call on a peer to help process stress; others may seek spirituality. Others quit or find other healthcare positions or completely change their profession, as in the following case.

Consider this story from Biller (1992):

> In the early 1990s, administrators at a 350-bed, non-teaching hospital in Southern California decided to make some changes at their facility. Their goals were to decrease lengths of stay, improve quality of care, and escalate nursing retention. They felt that instituting nursing case management could best accomplish these goals. Three case managers were selected and told they would be in-charge of decreasing the lengths of stay and ensuring that patients received high-quality care. At first, the nurses felt privileged and excited in their new roles. Within 2 months, they felt overworked, unprepared, unheard, and unsupported. They all abandoned their case manager roles because of unrelieved frustration and burnout. We all know that similar situations continue to occur even today. Case managers are still being prepared for their roles on the job; often not sufficient enough to acquire necessary theoretical and foundational knowledge and skills for successful performance.

That the administration goals were positive really did not matter. Because these nurses were essentially thrown into their new roles with little preparation, education, or support from staff or management, they were doomed to fail. Unfortunately, similar events still happen today despite the existing expansive knowledge base and evidence of case management practice; there seems to be a lack of academic preparation of case managers for success in their roles. Although we have learned much from the early 1990s, some still insert a "case management role" into a current workflow. When there is little orientation or education, it is no surprise that these professionals are stressed out and often unsuccessful. In this case, the leadership finally came to the conclusion that "preparation is the key to success" (Biller, 1992, p. 146).

▶ ROLE CONFLICT, CONFUSION, AND CLARIFICATION

No matter how much clinical expertise a new case manager has, the case management role requires many new skills, knowledge areas, associated competencies, and learning curves. It is essential that a case manager has support from the healthcare facility's upper management, nursing staff, physicians, and other professionals, and most importantly, from fellow case managers. It is also imperative that the novice case manager receive some training (both in the classroom and on-the-job with a mentor/experienced case manager). The hospital administration in the aforementioned case example learned the hard way that case management support and training are important for the case manager preparation and professional development; these are also essential for meeting the goals of case management. This chapter offers usable suggestions that will assist in a successful professional case management career.

When designing and implementing a case management program, it is necessary to clearly define the case manager's role, including its required qualifications and reporting structure. Often, healthcare leaders mistakenly assume that the role of the case manager is clear just by virtue of implementing one; or that the role will become clearer over time as case managers practice their roles, interact with other professionals, and build their role relationships.

This is an erroneous assumption that sometimes may cost an institution its case management program as well as unnecessarily waste of resources (funds and personnel), efforts, and reputation, and create resistance to having case management. Such approaches compromise rather than enhance the value of case management to patients and their families, as well as to the organization's bottom line.

Each job has certain key roles; these roles include accountabilities and responsibilities with which come authority. Responsibilities, on the other hand, involve multiple activities that are usually required to satisfy the assigned responsibility. Each activity, in turn, involves specific behaviors for its effective execution. When implementing the case manager's role, it is important to clarify the level of authority you assign to the role. To accomplish this, the job description should explicitly describe the role responsibilities and accountabilities, stated in a simple manner, preferably in the form of functions, activities, concrete tasks, required knowledge, role relationships, and behaviors. Job descriptions should also include required educational background, knowledge, skills, and competencies that make up the qualifications for the role. The role descriptions and qualifications are essential for overcoming role confusion or conflict. Chapter 2 discusses this in more detail. Always remember that there is a legal and regulatory component (see Chapter 8), and an ethical component (see Chapter 9) as well.

Role clarification is often required for a team's productivity, especially when new members are added, or critical changes have occurred. Effective role clarification can help avoid redundancies in jobs, empower staff, foster effective relationships among staff, increase productivity, enhance job satisfaction and engagement, and improve outcomes. One strategy found helpful in defining a case manager role is periodically setting aside time to give and receive feedback (i.e., deliberate reflective thinking and practice session). This can be done either in an individual meeting between the case manager and the case management program leader or during a regularly scheduled staff meeting. Either way, during the session the case manager can describe how he or she is executing the role, using clear and concrete examples of activities, feelings, and/or behaviors. On the basis of the examples shared, the leader can then suggest to the case manager which role statements he or she should perform more and which ones less. During this exercise, the case manager may also share the feeling(s) experienced during the shared situation and how he or she handled them. The leader may then suggest, as necessary, more effective ways of handling emotions (i.e., focus on emotional intelligence). It is important to avoid labeling the role statements or emotions shared "good" or "bad" as such an approach may result in resentment and role dissatisfaction, in turn, leading to disengagement. The ultimate goal of this session should be validation of what the case manager should be doing; that is, activities, behaviors, feelings, and relationships.

There is no question that the case manager's role is an interdependent one. It is executed best when there is clearly communicated authority and in an environment where teamwork and cross functional/departmental relationships are effective. Role confusion and conflict surface when the case manager's role, including responsibility, authority, and accountability, is not clearly defined and it is left to members of the healthcare team to interpret the existence of the role as they rightly or wrongly understand it. A prerequisite to role clarification is role perception. An organization can have the clearest and best-written job descriptions, but continue to experience role conflict or confusion. The reason for this most likely lies in the case manager's perception of his or her role (may result in role misconception or confusion). Other reasons may relate to the roles, functions, and responsibilities described in the job description are not discrete enough (may result in lack of role clarity) or they are same as those of other healthcare team members (may result in role conflict). Case managers will exercise their roles the way they understand and perceive them. If their perception is faulty, the result is either role confusion, conflict, or both.

One example of role confusion can be when there is a mismatch between the role definition and the role perception. Suppose the case manager identifies a variance/delay in care, documents the variance, but does not manage the variance or institute action to resolve it, assuming that it is someone else's role to manage variances. Over time, the variance or delay will continue to occur, the case manager may perceive that the documentation is busy work, and the patient outcomes will never improve. This type of scenario will provide its own type of stress.

During the preparation period (i.e., training and education) of case managers for their roles, it behooves an organization and case management leader to spend ample time discussing role perception and expectations with the case managers in practical and concrete terms. A favorable approach is the use of role-play, case-based scenarios, and problem-based learning techniques. These sessions provide an opportunity for case management leaders to clarify what the case manager's role is all about, correct misconceptions, explain what authority means, demonstrate how one can best execute case management activities, and evaluate whether the case managers clearly understand their role and related expectations.

To avoid role confusion or conflict, communicate with all members of the healthcare team and with all departments impacted by the implementation of the case management program and the case manager's role. This should be done as a training and education session, in newsletters, as well as in departmental or organization-wide reports. Regardless of the format, the communication should, at a minimum, include model design, goals and expectations, table of organization, job description (e.g., role responsibilities, concrete examples of activities, and qualifications for the role), impact on the other members of the healthcare team, and how each staff member can assist in the success of the case management program. Answering the "what is in it for me" or "how does this affect me" questions during these communications is necessary.

▶ Accountability

Now, once role clarification issues have been explained, the concept of accountability steps in. Accountability is feeling that you are responsible and willing to perform what you signed on to do: to act with a true sense of obligation toward others, one's role, and organization. Sometimes managers just call it a good "work ethic." Case managers cannot influence others without accountability. If one does not do what one says one will do (also known as "follow-through"), that person gains a reputation that is difficult to change, or worse, a negative outcome for a patient may occur.

Some examples of how case managers can exhibit role accountability include (CMSA, 2017):

▶ Accepting responsibility to act.
▶ Owning their actions and their impact on achieving desired outcomes.
▶ Expressing willingness to collaborate with the patient/client/support system/family and other members of healthcare teams.
▶ Showing obligation to answer, respond to, or report on the outcomes of their own actions.
▶ Safeguarding the patient/client and public interest: quality, safety, cost-effectiveness, advocacy, and timely access to necessary healthcare services.
▶ Taking initiative, identifying opportunities for improvement in the systems of care, and effecting desirable change.
▶ Advocating for patients/clients and their families/support systems.

▶ UNDERSTANDING OF ALL THE PARTS OF THE UBIQUITOUS CASE MANAGER

The subtitle is said "tongue in cheek," but it really could not be truer. To decrease stress in one's job, the case manager must be accountable to learn all the various nuances associated with the work . . . and that includes a wide (ubiquitous) amount of knowledge. Fortunately, there is a fountain of knowledge for professional case managers readily available today (not so much in the 1990s), ranging from textbooks, certifications, classes, conferences, journal articles to university courses.

To understand the ramifications of a diagnosis-related groups' reimbursement method (or prospective payment systems) compared with a per diem reimbursement; to know the utilization management modalities; to grasp the goal of holistic, quality care for an ill person and his or her family; to identify the unique knowledge and skills needed for your type of case management practice—are all essential for you to be a confident and successful case manager. Maintaining the most current knowledge base in your area of clinical expertise allows intelligent discussion with physicians and managed care representatives, which increases the case manager's credibility. The mental and emotional preparation also ensures the development of a proper care plan for the patient. It will take some homework time to do this but, as former stellar UCLA basketball coach John Wooden says, "It's what you learn after you know it all that counts."

Ideally, you will be service based and working with patients in your area of clinical expertise. Knowledge of evidence-based standards/treatments, guidelines, and expected outcomes allows the case manager to anticipate the patient's length of stay and facilitate an appropriate course of treatment. This gives the case manager a handle on how much time is needed to manage the case. Keeping current on ever-changing tests, medications, and medical breakthroughs gives the case manager the sharp clinical edge.

Often times, case managers may deal with other types of patients, other than those you are most familiar with. Sincere questions to specialty nurses or attending physicians usually elicit enough information to allow the case manager to speak to families and insurance company representatives and to plan alternative levels of care. If you are routinely asked to cover an area with which you are less familiar or knowledgeable, time spent in learning more about it will be time saved in apprehension and asking questions, ultimately experiencing less stress. Also, remember that having a comprehensive handoff from the case manager you are to cover for will bring you one step closer to having a manageable degree of stress, or a time completely stress-free.

Take some time to identify your individual case management assets and limitations. Accept both while you turn your limitations into strengths. Do not underestimate the great strengths of your peers. Their guidance and support can be invaluable.

▶ EARLY INTERVENTION

You may have noticed that early intervention in cases has been emphasized repeatedly. This is because it is so important to the formulation of a good care plan and to the mental health and satisfaction of a case manager. If you were the type in high school (or college) who waited until the day before the term paper was due to start it and are still a last-minute type of person, use caution. Crisis case management—cases that need intervention *now*—occurs all too frequently anyway. With too many of these, you run the risk of work and stress overload, poor judgment, inability to prioritize competing demands, disempowering feelings, and possibly suboptimal care plans. Avoid procrastination and mismanagement of time.

Starting your cases (planning and implementing the care your patients require) "early" is somewhat a thing of the past; lengths of stay are stunningly low, but the complexity of patients is high. "Immediately" is the name of the game today. However, should you have the luxury of this "early" phase, you are free to assess a possible discharge or transfer plan without pressure and time constrictions. Unless a case is very strong for the first plan assessed, it is suggested that you have and "try on" a Plan B. This approach allows you to remain ahead of the game and to avoid surprises or events you are not otherwise prepared to handle. Evaluate Plan A, looking for possible areas of failure, and solve problems in advance. If Plan A does fail, then Plan B is already considered and ready to be put into action; 98% of the time one of these plans, or a modification, is usable. This alleviates scrambling for ideas at the last minute when an unforeseen change in your patient's condition occurs, warranting modification in the case plan.

▶ DEVELOPING AND MAINTAINING THE PRESENCE OF A SUPPORT SYSTEM

Maintaining a positive and healthy attitude is not always easy when working with difficult or tragic human predicaments every day. Add to that an insurance atmosphere that is squeezing us tighter with every new idea or criteria that managed care can throw at us—sometimes it feels downright unmanageable.

Remember the three case managers mentioned at the beginning of this chapter? They were placed in the role of case manager lacking more than knowledge about managed care and the case management process or clear role responsibilities—they lacked support from upper management (senior leaders) and their peers—and had no way to "phone a friend" (a peer case manager). Upper management gave them no specific role definition to work with, and hard feelings emerged between the case managers and the other primary nurses on the units because the staff felt as if they were losing their autonomy. No one in the organization acted as support or mentors for these fledgling case managers, and this hospital's initial attempt at case management failed swiftly and miserably. This would have been easily prevented if the case managers' support was evident from the start and the needed resources, knowledge, and training were made available to them.

Today, this is not an unlikely scenario and we get calls, texts, and emails from case managers at other organizations, even in other cities. There are few case managers, no matter how new, who do not have an area of expertise that makes them worthy of being called mentors to others less knowledgeable in that area. Each of us came to the case management profession with a pocketful of information that others may lack. We frequently call on our peers for ideas on cases in which we are insufficiently knowledgeable, especially about clinical areas or resources, and we are grateful that there is someone to whom we can turn. Sometimes we just need a sounding board to vent frustration. Reciprocally, we are mentors to others in our specific areas of expertise. This mutual support system is a fortunate and effective means of reducing stress and enhancing a positive attitude.

▶ PROBLEM-SOLVING TECHNIQUES

There are times when a case seems to be "stuck," and no amount of rational thinking produces the magic answer to the tenacious problem; it is time (or beyond time) for a case conference. The teams that comprise the case conference have various names with nuances that extend beyond the group of experts/professions that comprise them: multidisciplinary, interdisciplinary, transdisciplinary, interprofessional, cross-disciplinary, or interprofessional to name a few. Essentially, you will be involved in two types of case conferences: a multidisciplinary team-based case conference made up of those who can assist with the bottleneck. A second type is a patient-/family-focused case conference. This team should include those on the healthcare team directly involved in the patient's care, plus the family and/or the patient; and perhaps an ethicist or a patient advocate if warranted.

The multidisciplinary team-based conference is needed when disagreements exist about the patient's plan of care, the discharge or transition plan, or when the payor denies (lack of authorization) certain treatment options or procedures that the healthcare team views as otherwise necessary. The focus of the case conference in this instance is mainly on resolving conflict, on ensuring that members of the healthcare team are all on the same page regarding the patient's plan of care, or on strategizing how to appeal the denial. The patient-/family-focused case conference is needed when the patient has agreed with the plan of care proposed by the healthcare team but the family has not, or vice versa; or when both the patient and family have expressed their disagreement with the healthcare team. The main purpose of the case conference in these situations is reaching agreement or consensus on the plan of care.

There are many guidelines for problem-solving when variance, delay in care, or disagreement exists. This one was formulated for case managers and includes the following steps: (1) performing variance (or delay in care) analysis, (2) focusing on desired outcomes, (3) brainstorming alternate strategies or approaches, (4) finding the next best intervention, and (5) evaluating the plan (Zander, 1989). Despite it not being recent, it still applies today and considers easy to use.

▶ Step 1: Performing Variance (or Delay in Care) Analysis

The first step in problem-solving is to identify the problem. It is important to have a clear idea of what you are solving before you can solve it. If possible, break it down into smaller issues or concerns. This strategy makes resolution more manageable. When more than one problem is identified, assess whether there may be a common denominator at the root of the problem or problems. This may require further data collection and exploration; it will certainly require the gathering of all the facts and checking with the appropriate parties. Using a case conference or a multidisciplinary team meeting to discuss variances, delays in care, or other problems encountered is essential for identifying how best to proceed and to ensure the collaboration of other healthcare professionals in resolving the problem. Sometimes it may be important to interview other healthcare professionals or team members to gather the facts and understand the problem from every possible angle.

▶ Step 2: Focusing on the Desired Outcomes

Identifying the type of data needed to understand the problem is necessary for effective handling of the problem and ultimately resolution. As a case manager, it is important to focus your data collection first on those data that are directly related to the problem or outcome and then on those that are indirectly related to it. First and foremost, include the patient/family preferences. If the issue is a delay in care/variance, identify what contributed to the variance or delay in treatment. Was it a medical error committed by a healthcare team, a member? Was it a patient refusal? Or was it a denial of the treatment/procedure from the payor? To be more focused in your approach, it is necessary to seek the opinions of other members of the healthcare team, whether formally in a case conference forum or informally by discussing the situation one-on-one. When you develop a satisfactory understanding of the problem at hand, you can then begin to effectively develop your goals for resolving the problem. What do you, as a group, feel would be the best end result to the problem (or problems) assessed in Step 1? What short-term goals are possible? What long-term goals are possible? Are there limitations that must be overcome (e.g., limited social, financial, or insurance support; limited desire from the patient to manage the illness; limited mental capacity to learn and handle self-care; or denial from the payor)? Can the limitations be overcome successfully or at least diminished? Can a thorough and detailed utilization review activity solve the problem?

▶ Step 3: Brainstorming Alternate Strategies or Approaches

Brainstorming is a strategy often used by case managers during a case conference to resolve a problem and reach agreement, decide how best to approach a conflict, or tackle denial of service. Anything goes during brainstorming sessions. Participants are encouraged to be as creative as possible to explore new ideas and ways of looking at the problem, potential resources, and possible interventions (Zander, 1989). The primary rule during a brainstorming session is that all suggestions are acceptable and all judgment is withheld until all suggestions are squeezed out. Judgment often arrests the creative flow, and many potentially useful suggestions may never be spoken. Once all the participants have no further suggestions, the ideas can be listed in order of feasibility. Those that have the greatest potential to provide the solution are discussed in further detail. Remember that the alternate solutions or strategies must be appropriate to manage the problem. Examine each for feasibility of implementation, complexity or intensity, reliance on additional personnel, cost implication, and time period for execution and showing potential results.

▶ Step 4: Finding the Next Best Intervention

The brainstorming session often elicits potentially workable interventions that may be attempted. This intervention must be realistic and take into consideration all the strengths and weaknesses of the individual case. If no promising intervention is found, ask whether the problem needs to be redefined (Zander, 1989). It is likely that the focus was inappropriate; perhaps issues that are indirectly related to the problem were being handled first instead of those that were directly related. If this is the case, do not worry; just modify your approach accordingly, refocus, and try again. Remember to identify a plan A and a plan B; and sometimes a plan C. Knowing the priority sequence of your alternate solutions ahead of time is a step toward resolving the problem in an efficient and timely manner.

▶ Step 5: Evaluating the Plan

Sometimes, you may not be certain that you have identified the best strategy to resolve the problem. In such an event, try it out and evaluate its effect on the situation. Some problems may require testing more than one strategy until one works. If your first attempt does not work, try your other alternate solutions. Your brainstorming session must have resulted in identifying at least a few relevant alternate solutions. Usually at the close of the case conference, it is hoped that a new, realistic, practical, and individualized plan for the problem or case has been defined. This plan compensates for weakness and fills in needed gaps. The case's strengths are assessed and used to their fullest capacity.

Occasionally, a case comes along that remains tenaciously difficult; the solutions to the problem remain elusive. Then the case conference may serve as a support system for the dejected case manager, who will realize that he or she is not alone, uncreative, or incompetent.

The good news is that although some cases seem basically unresolvable, you will never have a case that did not eventually come to closure. As Will Rogers said, "Things will get better despite our efforts to improve them." The support system around you is essential; seek the assistance or guidance of another case manager who has experienced similar situations in the past or who has more experience than you.

▶ CRITICAL THINKING

Critical thinking is a vital part of any decision-making process or technique. Critical thinking is purposeful, outcome-directed thinking that aims to make judgments on the basis of facts and scientific principles (Alfaro-LeFevre, 1999). It is a creative, active practice, which supports and advances all the components comprising the case management process. In professional case management practice, critical thinking equates with the global thinking necessary to appropriately put all the pieces of the client/patient puzzle together (Powell & Tahan, 2008). More than merely finding a single solution to a problem, it is—in healthcare—referred to as clinical reasoning.

There are some variables that can affect critical thinking:

1. Thinking styles;
2. Personal factors, such as age, gender, and education; and
3. Situational factors, such as available time, resources, peer support, and administrative support.

Personal assessment of your thinking styles and mindfulness of situational factors are important to consider when the conversations get heated. One critical thinking process that case managers may apply in their roles consists of the following action steps (CMSA, 2017):

1. Analyze all the problems or issues in a situation.
2. Determine the expected outcomes.
3. List all possible alternatives and solutions to the problems.
4. Select the best or highest-priority alternative.
5. Determine if the plan worked (i.e., were the outcomes met?).

Critical thinking is one of the most sought after skills in a case manager. Often employers assess for this skill during a job interview and ongoing performance evaluations. It is an in-demand asset of a case manager. Critical thinking is a self-guided, self-disciplined form of thinking that occurs at the highest level of quality in a fair-minded manner. It is a process that involves the evaluation of information and its source(s) such as data, facts, observations, and other available evidence, to support the making of effective decisions, or designing a successful approach to resolving a concern. The critical thinking process is characterized by assessment, analysis, identification of key aspects, reconstruction, and conclusion on which ultimately improves one's thinking. Case managers who are effective critical thinkers can draw reasonable conclusions from a set of information and discriminate between useful and less useful details for solving a problem (e.g., delay in care) or for making a necessary decision. They can present coherent reasons for adopting a position and decline or reject unrealistic reasoning regarding a potential alternate solution. For example, a competent case manager uses critical thinking when analyzing the information available in a patient's medical record to strategize how to approach a concurrent review before engaging in such a utilization management activity with a payor representative. This case manager is astute at determining in advance of the concurrent review whether the payor representative will authorize the patient's hospital stay, deny it, or ask for more information. He or she doesn't rush to pursue the concurrent review until after gathering the essential information and has determined what the potential outcome is likely to be. Often this case manager has a plan A and an alternate plan B in mind to use as a response on the basis of the decision the payor representative shares during the utilization review conversation.

There are several behaviors that demonstrate that a case manager is a critical thinker such as the following:

- ▶ *Clarification*: the ability to not only restate information, but to state it in a way that is easy to understand and facilitate decision making and prevent conflicting thoughts or impressions.
- ▶ *Evaluation*: activities that are related to assessing or judging the validity of an idea, strategy, alternate solution, or a decision. Taking the time to think about the potential impact of an action before it is executed allows the case manager to avoid unintended consequences. One may also refer to this behavior as *judgment*.
- ▶ *Explanation*: like clarification, and refers to the ability to clearly state information, and even add one's own perspective to that information. This is essential to avoid misjudgment and misinterpretation of information. An astute case manager asks for clarity on vague issues rather than assuming their meaning and intents.
- ▶ *Inference*: behaviors that pertain to the ability to draw conclusions on the basis of the available information or one that is given (which may be limited). The critical thinker case manager exercises caution when engaging in inference to avoid miscalculation or focusing on the wrong issue by assuming something exists when in reality it does not. Asking for clarification about the issue or validating the inference with those concerned before action is important.

▶ *Interpretation*: the understanding of information; it often refers to communicating the meaning of information in a format that is clear for a particular audience. An example here is a case manager developing a transitional care plan for a patient and identifying the need to educate the patient and family about the health insurance benefits available to them to better understand their options for postdischarge services and the impact of these options, perhaps from a financial perspective. Often, language about such benefits in a health insurance plan or policy may be unclear to the lay person and interpretation by a healthcare professional such as a case manager is necessary. When engaged in interpretation, the act of *explanation* is usually necessary.

▶ *Objectivity*: being objective means that you evaluate an idea fairly, free of criticism or judgment, and without bias. Case managers who are astute critical thinkers demonstrate ethical behavior and adherence to ethical standards and principles. For example, respecting a patient's independence, autonomy, self-determination, right to choice, and cultural values and beliefs demonstrate objectivity in the care provision process a case manager is engaged in.

▶ *Reflection*: a higher order of thinking that requires relating new knowledge to prior understanding. It is to think about an approach, technique, or an action one has implemented, assimilate it, relate it to other aspects of the situation or prior experiences, and to change or adapt it as necessary. Case managers who demonstrate reflection (or reflective thinking) apply such thought processes in their practice and when executing an action(s). For example, a case manager explains to a patient and family the need to transition the patient to an acute care rehabilitation facility and discusses the goals and how the specialized care provided in such a facility will enhance the patient's independence in activities of daily living. Later, the case manager takes the time and thinks through the interaction he or she had with the patient and family, approach to the interaction, how it flowed, outcomes of the interaction, and so on. Such review and thinking demonstrates an act of reflection which may result in the case manager changing course or affirming that the one taken was the most appropriate. Key aspects of the critical thinker demonstrating reflection is distancing oneself from any pressures, taking a different perspective, making independent judgment, and taking responsibility for one's actions.

▶ *Reasoning*: refers to thinking logically about a question, situation, or problem to form a conclusion or judgment. It involves the use of inference and interpretation to arrive at a conclusion. Objectivity

and understanding are also characteristics of the case manager who demonstrates critical thinking abilities.

▶ *Validating*: sharing conclusions and inquiring whether they are accurate, relevant, and appropriate. An example is when a case manager has completed an assessment of a patient and identifies the important issues the plan of care will focus on; he or she shares these issues with the patient and family seeking their opinions about whether they are accurate and their impression whether these are indeed their priorities as well.

▶ *Problem-solving*: is another important behavior that demonstrates critical thinking; it involves analyzing a problem, generating a solution, implementing a key action plan, and assessing the impact of the plan. Effective problem-solving involves almost all the behaviors that demonstrate critical thinking described earlier. On the basis of the situation, an astute case manager identifies the key activities (e.g., inference, validation, explanation, or reflection) needed to resolve or improve the situation of concern.

Case managers who are critical thinkers usually understand the logical connections between ideas; identify, construct, and evaluate arguments or alternate plans; detect inconsistencies and common mistakes in reasoning; solve problems systematically; identify the relevance and importance of different ideas or approaches; and reflect on the justification of beliefs and values. They are aware that critical thinking is not merely a matter of accumulating information or having a good memory for details, or knowing a lot of facts; it is rather the act of deducing consequences from what one knows, using the available information in solving problems, and seeking relevant and diverse sources of information to inform decision making and achieve the desired outcomes.

Some people believe that critical thinking hinders creativity because it requires following the rules of logic and rationality, but creativity might require breaking rules. This is a misconception. Critical thinking is quite compatible with thinking "out-of-the-box," challenging consensus, and pursuing less popular approaches. If anything, critical thinking is an essential part of creativity because we need critical thinking to evaluate and improve our creative ideas.

▶ EMOTIONAL INTELLIGENCE

One simply cannot practice critical thinking without an element of emotional intelligence. Emotional intelligence (EI), also called emotional quotient, describes an ability, capacity, or skill to perceive, assess, and manage the emotions of one's self, of others, and of groups. This is a critical trait to possess in very many areas of professional case management practice, from choosing the use of humor to leadership. The concept is that emotions play a greater role in thought and decision making than previously perceived; in fact, high EI has been positively correlated with job performance, job satisfaction, job engagement, and stress management (Treiger & Fink-Samnick, 2016), and all the concepts discussed in this chapter that equate with success in case management.

EI is one of the necessary skills for successful leaders. Those who possess EI characteristics make better leaders. Because case managers are also leaders in their organizations, EI skills are necessary for their success and for influencing optimal outcomes for all: the patient and family, the healthcare providers or organization, the payors for healthcare services, and other case management stakeholders. These skills are even more important given that the case manager's role is built on the notion that to be effective, one must be an excellent communicator—better yet, an outstanding communicator. EI skills ensure this quality of communication. As you may have thought, the term has something to do with the effective management of emotions. EI is the case manager's ability to sense, understand, control, steer, and use one's and others' emotions (both whether verbally or nonverbally expressed) as sources of information for effective communication, decision making, negotiation, building relationships, resolving conflict, critical thinking, and instituting actions (Tahan, 2000).

Feelings and emotions, whether negative (disempowering), positive (empowering), or neutral (void of impact), influence the case managers' thoughts, opinions, perceptions, and experiences about a situation, which ultimately influence their decisions, actions, and behaviors in response to the situation. These emotions also affect how the case manager connects with him- or herself and others when developing relationships. The case managers' success in establishing effective relationships with other healthcare professionals, patients, and families depends on three essential things (Tahan, 2000):

1. Perception and awareness of one's feelings and emotions
2. Perception and awareness of others' feelings and emotions
3. Perception and awareness of the effect of these feelings and emotions on the situation at hand.

Self-awareness of emotions and feelings raises a case manager's consciousness to his or her strengths, capabilities, and challenges. This allows the case manager to have better control over actions, reactions, and interactions (Tahan, 2000). Control can best be demonstrated when, for example, the hospital-based case manager knows that the payor-based case manager is "annoying," "dismissive," or always "late" to respond, but does not allow these negative emotions to interfere in his or her relationship, and still continues to communicate with the payor-based case manager in a respectful and courteous manner,

share information as needed, and negotiate resolution on denied services. He or she controls any destructive impulses, regulates his or her mood in effort to prevent stress, and maintains focus on the needs and interests of the patient and family.

Awareness of others' feelings and emotions means that the case manager is attuned to the subtle signals others send through their verbal communication, body language, written words, actions, and behaviors. Such awareness allows the case manager to better understand others' needs, emotions, and perspectives; this is empathy in action. Awareness of others' emotions also enhances understanding, teamwork, decision making, engagement, and satisfaction (Tahan, 2000). In the above-mentioned example, the hospital-based case manager could have easily confronted the payor-based case manager, argued about the exhibited behavior, or expressed concern that such behavior is not acceptable; however, he or she chose not to escalate the situation and remained focused on the goal of quality and safe patient care. Such empathy ensures better outcomes. The hospital-based case manager must have recognized that the timing was not right to discuss the disruptive behavior and thoughtfully ignored the behavior at that time.

Being aware of the effects of feelings and emotions on the situation at hand is essential for their effective management and for preventing their negative impact on the situation, including the relationships between the case manager, the patient or family, and other healthcare professionals. To be successful at managing the effects of emotions and feelings, the case manager must possess social skills that enhance his or her ability to build influential relationships. Social skills are making others feel welcome, part of the team, and at ease, especially during stressful events; controlling one's own emotions and feelings; adeptness at inducing desirable responses in others; interpersonal effectiveness; having a nurturing attitude toward oneself and others; group work and synergy; and thinking "outside the box" and looking for nontraditional approaches to solving problems (Tahan, 2000). In the aforementioned example, the hospital-based case manager demonstrated social skills that allowed him or her the ability to control the situation, focus on the task, and manage the issue without compromising the existing relationship with the payor-based case manager.

EI allows the case manager to establish effective role relationships. These can be demonstrated through a therapeutic relationship with the patient and/or family, and an empowering relationship with oneself and with others such as team members. Getting along well with the patient and family can best be achieved through careful attention and understanding of their needs, interests, desires, and goals. In addition, developing a care plan that is patient-/family-centric and culturally sensitive demonstrates that the case manager listened to them, has their interests "at heart," respects their cultural background, and works as their ally and advocate. Examples of how a case manager develops a successful relationship with the patient and family may include respect for their values and belief system, right to self-determination, and safeguarding their dignity and well-being. Not being able to understand and manage one's and others' emotions and feelings could lead to an ineffective relationship that ultimately may trigger deviation from the care plan or delays in achieving the desired outcomes.

Developing an effective relationship with yourself is as important as the relationship with the patient/family. In your role as case manager, it allows you to recognize when you feel sad, happy, angry, or anxious; with such recognition comes the ability to control these emotions and prevent them from interfering with your ability to work well with the patient/family and fellow healthcare professionals. An example of building relationships with yourself is knowing yourself, becoming aware of the disempowering triggers, proactively managing these triggers to prevent suboptimal consequences, and taking the time to engage in self-care activities such as taking long walks and deep breathing exercises, or listening to relaxation music (especially when under stress) to reenergize or revision yourself.

Establishing effective relationships with others is essential to achieving desired case management outcomes and being satisfied in the case manager role. Examples of behaviors that demonstrate the ability to develop relationships with others are expressing respect and appreciation for team interdependence and the uniqueness of each team member, and recognizing that team achievements are dependent on every member's contribution. Others include building a culture of learning, mutual support, respect, critical thinking, reflective practice, and creative problem-solving. Case managers with effective relationships with others inspire those others and make them comfortable in social situations, especially when conflict or disagreements exist.

▶ TIME MANAGEMENT

There is a story about a strapping young man who wanted to be a lumberjack. On his 18th birthday, he set out to get a job in the logging industry. Being young, strong, and healthy, he quickly got his wish. He was given his axe and set out to work. On the first day, he single-handedly felled 12 trees. The boss was very pleased and commended him on his energy and strength. On the second day, the young man seemed to work just as diligently but cut down only 10 trees. On the third day, he cut 7 and on the fourth day, still trying very hard, only 3 trees came down. By the fifth day, with all the effort he could muster, no trees were cut.

The young man went to his boss, feeling terrible, and explained he had not cut one tree that day. The boss asked why. "I am working as hard as I can. I'm really

trying, sir," was the reply. Then the boss asked, "Have you taken the time to sharpen your axe?" The boy had not. He had been working so hard that he did not take the time to work smart.

Sharpening your axe, or your time management skills, or your critical thinking skills, or your EI savvy, saves time and effort. Time is a limited commodity, and case managers usually have much to do in their allotted time frame. Some people seem to be naturally disorganized, but like any skill, time management can be learned. Articles, books, seminars, and college courses are available on this subject. The time spent sharpening the axe—learning organizational skills—will be rewarded many times over in reduced stress and frustration. Here are some work efficiency tips.

▶ Assess the Time Robbers

The time robbers include anything that stops us from reaching our objectives most efficiently (Charlesworth & Nathan, 1984). Each person has individualized robbers that he or she allows, ranging from minor distractions and problems with attitudes to the inability to make basic decisions in a reasonable amount of time. Once these problem areas have been recognized, the next step is to work to make them strengths.

▶ Make Lists

Lists are security blankets. They can be electronic, on paper, or using post-its. After a task goes on your list, do not waste energy worrying that you might be forgetting something. Lists are the perfect tool for the essential time management skill of prioritizing. They can be labeled, starred, numbered, dated, and crossed out, and details can be added to the main subject—whatever works for the individual case manager. Lists also help you make sure that you are not forgetting any important tasks, activities, follow-ups, and so on. Coupled with time management savers, you should be able to manage keeping your list at an appropriate length. You should be crossing out or deleting completed tasks as you add new ones to the list.

Using lists is not enough for managing your time effectively. Examine your progress periodically; if you find that you are adding more to your list than crossing out, it means that having a running list of tasks to help manage your time better and be more organized is not working. Look in other places and see why is it that you are unable to get your tasks done. Perhaps you are not focused on the right thing; you are not delegating to others; or you are assuming others' responsibilities. If you are taking on more than your time allows, you should look for ways to engage other members on your team. For example, instead of assuming responsibility for patient and family education yourself, have the registered nurse participate. You can supervise instead of completing the actual task.

▶ Sharpen Prioritizing Skills

Establish clear-cut goals, both short term and long term. Ask what has to be done this hour, this morning, this afternoon, this day, tomorrow. Do those first (in that order). "This hour" priorities may include a meeting, finalizing a priority case that will be picked up very soon, or the unexpected "now" situation that suddenly occurs. A Code Blue on one of your patients may be a priority for the patient or family; other priorities fall a step below. "This day" priorities may include insurance calls, confirming tomorrow's discharges, or finding resources for patients who will need them in a few days. "Tomorrow's" priorities may be those decisions that are awaiting a response from a payor or a patient's family member to confirm a transition to a postacute care facility.

Making the priority list is the first thing you should do in the morning; it is how you can plan your day. Refrain from assigning item numbers indicating the order of priorities because this can be too rigid. Order of priorities changes throughout the day; you should be flexible in shifting gears as the need at that moment in time demands. Stars are put on the most pressing cases, but often new situations arise and cases not on the original list are put on and starred. This may include situations such as a new patient who needs attention immediately or an unexpected need for a family meeting or case conference, or a last-minute warranted change in a patient's disposition/transitional plan.

▶ Be Succinct

If you ask certain people what time it is, they will tell you how to make a watch. Rambling and going off on tangents are major time-wasters and are annoying to the busy recipient of the verbosity. This is not the same as small talk, which in measured doses adds to camaraderie and job satisfaction and engagement. When you are on the phone with a managed care organization–based case manager sharing a concurrent review, be clear, to the point, and succinct in your delivery of information. Be prepared and certain of the message you deliver. If you ramble on and go in circles, your inability to be clear in your information may result in a denial of service for a patient. Additionally, a few minutes interaction may result in a half-hour question and answer. Being well-prepared cuts down on the time you need to complete a task such as a concurrent review. Tools such as SBAR (Situation, Background, Assessment, Recommendation) have been used successfully in many organizations.

▶ Be Efficient

One way to be efficient is to be proactive and plan ahead. Case managers may spend a good deal of time on the telephone and on hold. In this instance, you can make a choice: (A) bring something to do in case you are placed on "eternal hold" (this might be a case to review or your list to go over and possibly reprioritize) or (B) use the time to take a breath and recharge. Choice A eliminates the frustration of wasting valuable time when a lot needs to be done. Choice B is useful and necessary for reducing stress and increasing production. The important point is that by planning ahead you have made a conscious choice of how you will use your time; you are in control of the situation. No "terminal hold" stress reaction will be initiated.

Efficient use of time also includes not wasting time pursuing avenues that have been closed or are in need of major reconstruction work. For example, if you feel a patient needs a special piece of equipment that you cannot negotiate from the insurance company, take another route. Know when persistence may work or when to look elsewhere. Know the limitations of a case early on, and use your time and energy on more viable possibilities.

▶ Delegation

Some individuals try to be all things to all people. Not only is this impossible, it is a time robber and is often not in the best interests of your patients. If the patient needs a minister, rabbi, social worker, or any variety of ancillary services, provide that person. Initial processing may be needed to ascertain what is needed, but then it is time to delegate. Delegation is a process of assigning tasks to another qualified person and supervising that individual as needed. You are not a team of "one." There are others on your team who should assume responsibility for certain tasks or intervention on the basis of their role and scope of practice. You may delegate certain tasks that are clerical, administrative, or transactional in nature to a case management support staff member or assistant. For example, a case management assistant may call a transportation provider to confirm the time and modality of discharge transportation for a patient. This assistant can then report back to you about the outcome.

Some people see delegation as a loss of power and control. Be conscious of this possibility and put your patient's needs first. Some simply do not trust others to do the job correctly; they live by the credo that if you want something done correctly, do it yourself. If this is true and backup people cannot be relied on to do a good job, then this issue should be addressed. If you happen to see delegation as a loss of power or control, you need to start now to change your perception; remind yourself that delegating to others does not mean that you are no longer involved, or even that you have relinquished your responsibility. You are still accountable for following up on the outcome. You will need to make sure that the delegated activity has been completed and the expected outcome or goal has been achieved. An effective delegator is someone who does not feel tangential to a delegated task; on the contrary, someone who feels intimately involved, in control, accountable, and responsible for ensuring that the desired outcome has been achieved regardless of who physically completes the actual activity.

It is important to distinguish your own job responsibilities, which are the case manager's responsibilities, from those responsibilities that can or should be delegated. The best interests of the patient should always be the deciding factor. Some case managers feel a legal liability when delegating responsibility. This is not without merit, but there are a few delegation standards that will minimize risk:

1. Always act in a reasonable and prudent manner.
2. Assign tasks that are within the person's scope of training, practice, and responsibility.
3. Provide proper supervision to the person to whom the task was delegated.
4. Use job descriptions as a guide to delineate who on your team can do what.
5. Follow up on the delegated tasks and evaluate the outcome achieved.
6. Keep the delegated task on your list of things to do, indicating that you are to go back and oversee the outcome achieved.
7. Provide to the person to whom you delegate a time frame when you expect him or her to report back to you on the outcome. This is essential in keeping the delegated person closer to you. Over time, it builds effective relationships.

What is delegated and how it is delegated must be given careful attention. Consider the following recommendations for effective delegation, whether you are working as a supervisor or as a team leader:

▶ Stress the potential results, not the details. Make it clear that you are more concerned with the final outcome than with the day-to-day details. This provides autonomy to the one who is responsible for producing the results.
▶ Do not always become the solution to everyone's problems. Teach others how to solve problems, rather than just providing the answer. Again, this builds confidence and independence, and provides autonomy.
▶ When an employee or coworker comes to you with a problem and a question, ask him or her for possible solutions. Be there to brainstorm when needed.
▶ Establish measurable and concrete objectives. Make them clear and specific. This is the road map that others can follow.
▶ Develop reporting systems. Obtain feedback from written reports, statistical data, and planned face-to-face meetings. This does not always work in case management if a particularly tough problem arises; teach employees when to come to you with details, and when to come to you after exhausting other avenues.
▶ When appropriate, give strict but realistic deadlines. This gives the task credibility and gives the person accountability.

▶ Keep a delegation log. This is especially important for very busy people or those with many employees.
▶ Recognize and utilize the talents and personalities of the people you work with. Being a good delegator is very much like being a good coach.

▶ Trust Your Hunches/Intuition

Let's move from the left, logical side of the brain to the right side for a moment. Balancing the logical and intuitive sides of your personality can prevent all types of headaches. Nurses have cultivated "nurse's intuition" since the days of Florence Nightingale. As staff nurses, we could sense that a patient's condition was going to deteriorate. That intuition should still be used when negotiating an additional hospital day from an insurance company or when you have a "gut feeling" that the discharge plan you put in place is going to fail and resort to "Plan B" instead. You are there with the patient and can see subtle changes that sound alarms in your data bank. Once, a case manager did not listen to her intuitive feeling, and the patient was back in the emergency department in 3 hours with pulmonary emboli.

Perhaps your hunch says that the discharge plan may fail in whole or in part. Try to put your finger on the disconcerting feeling and have a modified Plan B available for use. This action most likely will avoid an impending disaster from happening. It may also prevent being caught off guard at the last minute when "Plan A" did not work.

Sometimes it behooves the case manager to listen to the patient's intuitions and not waste valuable time making elaborate discharge plans that will never come to pass. Do not underestimate the power of a patient to predict the timing of his or her death. One 92-year-old asked for help to the bedside commode early one morning, then promptly said, "Oh, please help me back to bed. I'm going to die now." Within minutes, she was unresponsive; within 30 minutes, she had died.

It is surprising how often hunches become reality. Listening to that small voice called intuition can be a truly efficient time management ally. In a recent editorial, Powell stated:

Intuition is a component of our healthcare life—whether yours or the patient's/family's. When you receive intuitive information from any source, check it for validity, use your decision-making skills, and above all use common sense. We cannot simultaneously talk about "activating patients" in their own care and disregard what they are feeling or telling us about their experiences. (Powell, 2008, p. 192)

Intuitive knowing is knowledge about a fact (past, present, or future) without the conscious knowing of why it surfaces to consciousness at that moment in time. One may not be certain that it is a fact; however, one perceives it as a truth. When you as a case manager experience such knowing, it is advisable not to dismiss it, rather investigate deeper what might be going on, identify whether parts of the truth were missed in the first round, and act on it by revising a plan, offering more teaching, or reassessing and monitoring the patient's and family's responses to the implemented actions (case plan).

To summarize: be efficient; work smarter, not harder; and keep your case management tools (including your intuitive thinking skills) sharpened.

▶ JUDGMENT DAZE

Critical thinking and use of critical (and clinical) judgment are essential when matching laboratory data, radiology results, and the patient's symptoms to the care plan. No case manager should leave home without them. However, being critically judgmental when it refers to a patient's life choices has little place in our profession. A large number of hospitalized patients or patients in rehabilitation facilities are there because of their life choices: alcohol, poor diet, noncompliance versus nonadherence, illegal drugs, high-risk sexual practices, and smoking. We have seen excellent clinicians and case managers burnout through excessive condemning and sitting in judgment. They became so miserable (and made others miserable) that they felt they needed to change jobs. We all can share stories of watching individuals go through multiple job changes; unfortunately, they took their judgmental attitude with them and were no happier with the changes. In the end, a miserable person is miserable no matter which job such a person holds or pursues. It is the personality and attitude, not necessarily the job, which needs changing.

Being judgmental seems to be a universal human trait. When you find yourself criticizing someone else, take the time to remind yourself that you have no right to do so because you have no way of knowing the whole story. Someone wrote to Ann Landers (America's famous advice columnist for 47 years) once, angry that taxpayers' dollars in the form of food stamps were being used frivolously. It seems this writer was a cashier at a grocery store when she observed a woman purchasing a $32 bag of shrimp and a $17 birthday cake with her food stamps. The grocery clerk railed against this use of food stamps for luxury items, and in support of her stance an onslaught of angry letters ensued applauding the courageous complainer. Then came another letter from the "perpetrator of the crime." The shrimp and cake purchaser remembered the withering look of the store clerk. What the clerk did not know was that the expensive birthday cake and the shrimp (a favorite food) were for her little girl who had terminal bone cancer. She was not expected to live out the year; this birthday would be her last. Judging without having access to all the details is problematic; it is similar to identifying a problem when assessing a patient before you complete your assessment and gather all the necessary data. It leads to a faulty case plan and case managers do not have the time or efforts to waste. Minimizing judgmental behavior will definitely lower the incidence of "foot-in-mouth" disease and burnout.

▶ HUMOR

One case manager hung a picture of a disgruntled-looking little guy saying, "God put me on this earth to accomplish a certain number of things. Right now, I am so far behind I will never die." We suspect most case managers will live a long, long time. Taking oneself lightly certainly lifts burdens, but what about the use of humor with patients, families, physicians, and peers? Are "needling" patients and going for the "jocular" vein in good taste?

Like other treatments, humor can be assessed using the "rights" learned in school; assess the right timing, the right recipient, the right approach, and the right dose (not too much). Some patients and families relish a lighter perspective and a break in the focus on illness and anxiety.

> Mrs. Farris' esophageal cancer had progressed to the point where she needed a permanent feeding tube. After an 8-day hospitalization with a variety of medical complications, she had become quite confused. Because this was her third visit on the same unit, the staff and family had become well acquainted with each other. As yet another day ended with Mrs. Farris still confused, her husband pleaded with the charge nurse to give her something for sleep so that he could get some rest. "She's been calling me every 15 minutes from Las Vegas asking for money," he related. The charge nurse, deadpan, asked, "Tell me something, Mr. Farris, has she won anything?" "No!" he responded. "That's why she keeps calling me for money!"

After the mutual laughter, the walls tumbled down. The laughter allowed Mr. Farris a moment of release, and he was able to share his fear about his wife being so ill; explained that in 50 years of marriage he had never seen her in such a state. The ability to laugh during bleak times sends a message that life is tolerable, even now. Often the family needs that healing message as much as the patient.

Studies have shown that humor and that universal means of communication, laughter, have a wonderful array of positive benefits when used judiciously. Humor and laughter can:

▶ Help keep stressful situations in perspective.
▶ Reduce stress and tension. Some educators rely on humor and games during the teaching process, feeling it allays fear and anxiety related to serious diseases.
▶ Help facilitate more serious communication, and in some situations neutralize conflicts.
▶ Build and maintain group morale and bonding by promoting a sense of affiliation and cohesion.
▶ Provide a catharsis and release pent-up energy.
▶ Increase heart rate, increase oxygenation to rates seen in aerobic activity, release endorphins (the morphine-like biochemical responsible for "runner's high"), and exercise hundreds of muscles throughout the body.

Humor and laughter are not just for patients. No matter how stressful the day is, laughter and humor cut through the stress like a laser and make the job worth doing again. Laughing at our own profession also levels the playing field. The following are actual medical documentations gathered by an unknown source, likely a professional who can laugh at him- or herself. It is difficult to know if these were typographical errors, exhaustion, stress, or anatomically incorrect medical terminology, but they are fun:

▶ "While in the emergency department, she was examined, X-rated, and sent home."

▶ "M.D. at bedside attempting to urinate. Unsuccessful."

▶ "The baby was delivered, the cord clamped and cut and handed to the pediatrician, who breathed and cried immediately."

▶ "Patient complains of indigestion since last night when he ate a stake."

▶ "Rectal examination revealed a normal-size thyroid."

▶ "She is numb from her toes down."

▶ "The patient lives at home with his mother, father, and pet turtle, who is presently enrolled in day care three times a week."

▶ "The patient had waffles for breakfast and anorexia for lunch."

▶ "On the second day, the knee was better, and on the third day, it had completely disappeared."

▶ "The patient was to have a bowel resection. However, he took a job as a stockbroker instead."

▶ "Both breasts are equal and reactive to light and accommodation."

▶ "The test indicated abnormal lover function."

▶ "Indwelling urinary catheter draining large amount of urine the color of American beer."

▶ "She stated that she had been constipated most of her life until 1989, when she got a divorce."

▶ "Examination of genitalia was completely negative except for the right foot."

▶ "Bleeding started in the rectal area and continued all the way to Los Angeles."

The Norman Cousins story about how he managed a rare disease with vitamin C and laughter is common knowledge. A lesser-known study shows what happened in a burn unit. An enterprising physician created a humor room and filled it with comedy tapes, funny books, and funny toys. The burn patients were encouraged to recall humorous moments in their lives and to laugh as often as possible. The result: a 13% to 33% increase in cell regeneration over the average (Braverman, 1993).

The Hawaiian Hunas have a saying: "Where your attention goes, energy flows." In essence, this is because joy and sadness pathways cannot operate simultaneously (White & Hows, 1993). Humor and anger, for example, are antithetical; try holding onto anger during a prolonged belly laugh!

Although some nurses have difficulty with the use of light-heartedness when it comes to patients, consider the following story about a young mother of four who was dying of cancer.

> Once, in a workshop she was attending, the woman asked the group how it felt about a 28-year-old mother with four young children who was dying of cancer. The participants responded with a barrage of joylessness, anger, pity, sadness, and horror. Then she asked, "How would you feel if you were that 28-year-old mother and everyone who came to visit you felt that way?" (Braverman, 1993)

For everyone to focus constantly on illness does not always serve the patient. As a patient advocate and a human being, try to maintain a balanced perspective that includes joy, hope, support, and whenever possible, the gift of laughter.

▶ CASE MANAGEMENT SELF-CARE

Case managers give, and problem-solve, and give some more. It is like always breathing out and never breathing in. If this sequence continues, there will be a point at which the case manager is all used up (usually referred to as burnt out); it is as detrimental to life as never breathing in. We teach self-care to our patients, but we do not always practice what we preach.

▶ *Just ask*: In work, if lack of training is causing stress, ask for what you need. Be specific with requests to supervisors: if you specialize in medical case management and receive a case that requires workers' compensation expertise, you would probably feel unsure and stressed. You may ask your supervisor, "Can I attend a seminar for this specialty or can you suggest good reading material?" If requests are denied, find out why. Were they unrealistic or was the timing wrong? Is there another way to obtain what you feel you need that can be supported? If ethical situations are more than you can bear, find a support team—even if it is online. If every diplomatic attempt to improve working conditions has failed, consider updating your resume; sometimes, it is a cue to move forward.

▶ *Get a life*: This is not meant colloquially but rather literally. Every case manager must have priorities outside the stressful world he or she works in. This is not always easy; everyone is well aware of what it takes to survive. However, finding something that is enjoyable to you—no matter how small—is critical to your health. One case manager comes home from work, makes a cup of tea, and listens to her favorite musician for 15 minutes; she is recharged. It is a small thing, but to her it is essential and she looks forward to it. A case manager with interests outside of case management and beyond caregiving, who can find joy and excitement in life, has a gift to give to patients. Instead of presenting a tired and weary plan, such a case manager brings vitality and creativity. Make self-care a priority in your life.

▶ *Engage in reflective practice*: When you face a challenging or stressful situation, take the time to discuss it with a fellow case manager or supervisor. Share the details of the situation, explain your actions, and discuss the outcomes achieved, whether optimal or not. Make sure to also focus on sharing your thought process about the situation—how did you arrive at your decisions, how did you go about executing your plan, and what critical thinking or judgment went into your action planning. Most importantly, however, be transparent about the feelings and emotions you experienced during the process. Reflective practice brings your critical thinking and EI alive; these significant processes become more concrete and tangible. Through the reflective practice process, you are better able to understand your case management knowledge, skills, and competencies. This process also allow others to share their experiences related to similar situations; perhaps such sharing establishes opportunities for mentoring, psychosocial or emotional support, and further guidance.

▶ COMMUNICATION AND INFORMATION-GATHERING TECHNIQUES

Communication is critical in every aspect of the case management process; skillful communication and interpersonal skills are required to perform effective case management. Without these skills, case management job responsibilities will certainly become extremely stressful. Within the case management process is the need at times to conduct an interview to gather data. This activity has been elevated to the form of "art" and has made several talk show hosts a healthy living. Like any skill, it takes practice. Asking sensitive, personal, and sometimes disturbing questions cannot always be avoided in case management, but there are some basic steps to take and some paths to follow to make it less intimidating and more productive.

▶ *Introduction*: Introduce yourself and explain why you will be asking a lot of questions. Reasons may include helping the patient to regain independence and assisting him or her by providing a safe treatment and discharge plan. Ask permission to proceed.

▶ *Empowerment*: Allowing others to make decisions with support from the leader or manager is a key tenet in case management. Let the patient do most of the talking. Be patient if he or she has a memory block or an inability for self-expression. Allow the patient to finish all sentences.

▶ *Trust*: Establishing trust is not always easy in sensitive or vulnerable situations, especially if this is a first meeting. However, trust is essential to best help the patient. Using layman's terminology avoids a language barrier and puts the patient more at ease. Self-disclosure (in small doses) often makes you appear more human. Reassurances that you can manage this case and conveying commitment to it are necessary.

▶ *Respect*: Maintain a level of respect and empathy. Being judgmental can be picked up in nonverbal body language.

▶ *Body language*: Observe the patient for general appearance: nervousness, withdrawal, avoidance, and congruence. Use all the senses. Body language is a form of communication and should not be ignored during your interaction with a patient. Sometimes body language cues are more telling than spoken words. Eye contact is necessary for establishing a connection and for communicating that the person you are interacting with is the most important individual at that moment.

▶ *Active listening*: Listening, in contrast to hearing, is an active cognitive process requiring sensitivity and focused attention. Hearing is what adolescents do with their parents; it does not require paying attention, and not much sinks in. Active listening is deliberate; it requires real participation and uses attending behaviors such as facial gestures, head nodding, and reflecting about what is said. You are an active listener in a situation if you are interested in understanding, rather than mentally creating a response or crafting your come back while the other person is speaking.

▶ *Data collection*: Use a pad and pencil as a tool to prevent omissions, but avoid taking too many written notes during the interview, because it is distracting and can promote suspicion about what you are writing. If you decide to take notes during the interview, ask permission and explain what you will be jotting down and why.

▶ *Questioning*: Ask about the major problem first (if appropriate). Explain the purpose of the interaction you are about to pursue. The more detailed, delicate questions may be answered without asking as the patient talks about other topics. Use open-ended questions whenever possible; these require more than a "yes" or "no" answer. Too many "why" questions may sound accusatory. Attempt to combine several questions into one, so that you are not "firing" short questions at the patient. Example: "Tell me about your family, employment, and what you do to relax and enjoy yourself." However, be careful how you do this. With some patients, combining several questions into one may be distracting, a source of anxiety, or a stressful task. Some patients may have problems remembering a lengthy question. If they forget the details, they may be embarrassed to share that with you or may feel upset about it. Be sensitive during questioning. Understand your patient and act accordingly. Ask for clarification when appropriate and validate your understanding before you assume your conclusion is accurate and final.

▶ *Testing discrepancies*: Sometimes patients' words do not match their body language. In general, words are easier to change than the way they are expressed. If the words are positive but the expression is not, consider the message negative. If the words are negative but the expression is positive, consider the message positive. When you notice discrepancy, it is best to clarify your observation with your patient. Be sensitive, objective, and nonjudgmental in the way you clarify.

▶ *Avoid distraction*: With today's mobile communication technologies and electronic health records, it is unlikely that you are in a patient's room or engaged in an important discussion with a patient and family and your mobile telephone rings. Reflexively you look at your phone to see who is trying to reach you or to read a text message. These behaviors communicate to the patient that you have been distracted or perhaps you view checking your mobile phone more important than the discussion you were having with the patient. Sometimes, you may be using the mobile computer workstation and while talking to the patient your eyes are fixated at the computer and your hands engaged in navigating the health record or typing information. Having no eye contact with the patient at that moment may indicate to the patient that the computer is more important than the former. These are natural behaviors and are usually common traps that indicate distraction and may unintentionally communicate to the patient or family that they are the most important individuals at that moment. Be mindful of your habits around the use of mobile technologies. Remember to silence the mobile phone or do not bring it with you altogether. When using the mobile computer workstation, engage the patient. For example, explain to the patient what you are doing; share with the patient what you are reviewing in the record; and ask the patient to validate information you are reading or to clarify it.

Close the interviews with a verbal summary that captures the essence of the interview. This allows the patient to add or correct the summary. It also shows that you have been listening, especially to understand. Interviews are influenced by both internal factors, such as anxiety, and external factors, such as noisy rooms. For some case managers, the interview can take place in the patient's home. This is often ideal because the patient usually feels less anxious. Some patients reside in a skilled nursing facility or are temporarily in a hospital, making privacy more difficult. If the patient does not have a private room, interview him or her while the roommate is having a procedure done or is out of the room for some other reason. Attempt to have as few distractions as possible. Let the staff know you will be conducting an interview and time it between medications or tests. Turn off the television or radio and close the doors or curtains. Make sure the patient is as comfortable as possible. Always ask permission first. For example, asking the patient's permission to turn off the television or radio is necessary to show that you are courteous and respectful. Such gestures allow you to establish trust and build effective relationships.

▶ Interviewing Tools—Motivational Interviewing

Several tools are available to guide the case manager on the process of interviewing. For example, assessment guides, screening criteria for case management services, and case management standards of practice. One important tool every case manager must develop competence and proficiency in applying is "Motivational Interviewing." Referred to as MI, it is a technique in which you become a helper in the change process and express acceptance of your patient/client. We know that helping others to make positive changes can be challenging. The case manager who practices MI does so with five general principles in mind:

1. Express empathy through reflective listening.
2. Develop discrepancy between clients' goals or values and their current behavior.
3. Avoid argument and direct confrontation.
4. Adjust to client resistance rather than opposing it directly.
5. Support self-efficacy and optimism (Miller & Rollnick, 2012).

There are several courses on MI and the Case Management Society of America has incorporated them in its "*The Case Management Adherence Guidelines*."

MI is an essential skill case managers apply in their care delivery processes to enhance patient activation, engagement, and self-management abilities. It assists case managers in communicating with the patient and family, understanding the patient's condition and lifestyle behavior, identifying sensitive information that stands in the way of adherence to health regimen including medications management, and determining what is of utmost importance to the patient and family. MI employs a style of communication that is supportive, counseling-like, and empathic. It promotes understanding and respect, while facilitating the patient's motivation to change. To be effective case managers:

> listen to patients and families/caregivers instead of telling them what to do; evoke deep and meaningful self-exploration, identify areas of strengths or opportunities for change rather than requiring them to alter unfavorable behavior; and approach them from the perspective of 'you have what you need, and together we will find it,' rather than 'I have what you need and this is what I think you ought to do.' (Cesta & Tahan, 2017, p. 218)

As case managers apply MI for the improvement of patient care outcomes, they focus on the patient's engagement in own health and healthcare. They also ensure the application of the following strategies to achieve success and meaningful change for the patient and family.

▶ Using culturally sensitive and patient-centered bidirectional communication that is in the form of counseling rather than something that is evaluative and judgmental.

▶ Engaging in a goal-oriented and collaborative approach to care planning that respects the patient's autonomy and self-determination.

▶ Avoiding authoritarian interactions or those that are commanding in nature; rather guiding patients and families toward targeted change so that they successfully overcome ambivalence and fear.

▶ Allowing or encouraging patients to make their own decisions and determine incremental improvements.

▶ Being deliberate in gaining insight about the patient's behavioral (e.g., impact of health status on adherence to the plan of care), cognitive (e.g., skills and knowledge in assuming self-management), and emotional (e.g., awareness of feelings especially anxiety, apprehension, and stress) states.

▶ Bringing the patient and family to a state where they recognize they are able to change and understand the potential benefit of such change.

▶ Assessing the patient's and family's readiness for change and shifting readiness to actual change behaviors, while providing support and counseling throughout the process.

▶ Monitoring and evaluating the patient's progress toward meeting target goals such as independence in assuming self-management. Upon demonstrating effective change, case managers begin to partner with the patient and family about sustaining these gainful improvements (Cesta & Tahan, 2017).

▶ Perceptions in Communication

Perhaps one of the most essential components to understand when communicating with others (be it a patient, your boss, members of the multidisciplinary team, your children, or your spouse) concerns perception. Consider the definition of stress at the beginning of this chapter: stress is the perception of threat or an expectation of future discomfort that arouses, alerts, or otherwise activates the individual. What is stressful or painful to you may be no problem to another. Perceptions are totally subjective, and true communication cannot occur unless the case manager at least understands "where the person is coming from"; stated another way, how the person perceives the situation.

Dr. Stephen Covey and his seven habits of highly effective people can be helpful to the case manager (Covey, 1989). One of the habits is to "seek first to understand, then be understood." It sounds so simple; however, underneath it, is one of the most difficult of skills. Most people seek first to be understood, then maybe, to understand. To truly understand another's perception—which is often the cause of the problem, misunderstanding, perceived stress, or behavior—the case manager must listen and determine the perceptions behind the words; we must be able to see through that person's eyes. One of Dr. Covey's methods for doing this is to give the person "emotional air." Essentially, this means let the person talk! Just as humans require the exchange of oxygen to live, they require the exchange of emotions—the giving and the receiving. The case manager may find a different definition of health, or success, or grief, or hope than the definitions he or she harbors. Because venting often precedes rational discussion, giving "emotional air" is critical to getting to the deeper issues. Therein lies the key to the goal of matching the patient's perceptions to the plan of care. By doing this, the case manager may observe greater compliance because the other person's perceptions and capabilities have been acknowledged and respected. Understanding the patient's and/or family's perceptions is essential for establishing a case management plan that reflects their interests, wishes, problems, and goals.

▶ Communication Skills for Quality and Patient Safety

Poor communication skills can have ramifications that range from stressful working environments, as mentioned earlier, to unsafe patient environments, and ultimately to poor outcomes, or even a patient's death or permanent injury. The communication difficulties may take many forms and have many causes.

Clear communication plays a huge role while dealing with patients, and communicating accurately and thoroughly is essential. Consider the following (CMSA, 2017):

1. The transfer of timely and accurate information across settings (e.g., transitions of care and hand-offs) is critical to the execution of effective care transitions.

2. One definition of care transfers includes transfers to or from an acute hospital, skilled nursing or rehabilitation facility, or home with or without home healthcare.

3. Not all patients undergoing transitions are at high risk for adverse events; however, those with poor transitional care plans are particularly likely to "fall through the cracks" (HMO Workgroup on Care Management, 2004).

4. Processes for accurate and complete transitions of care must be developed by healthcare organizations and case management programs. However, at this time, there is often a lack of agreement about what comprises the core clinical information that all practitioners require irrespective of setting.

5. The Care Transitions Measure (CTM) was developed by researchers at the University of Colorado Health Sciences Center to assess the quality of care transitions from the perspective of the patient or his or her proxy. CTM scores have been shown to be significantly associated with a patient's return to a hospital or emergency department after discharge (HMO Workgroup on Care Management, 2004).

Looking at communication from a different angle, poor communication—coupled with lack of emotional intelligence—can lead one to "act out," rather than "talk it out" when the topic is one of high stress/high stakes (Patterson, Grenny, McMillan, & Switzler, 2002).

In the "Silence Kills" study, it was found that the ability to hold crucial conversations is key to creating a culture of safety in healthcare; conversely, the prevalent culture of poor communication and faulty collaboration among health professionals relates significantly to continued medical errors and patient complaints.

Crucial conversations occur when the stakes are high (as often is in healthcare), opinions vary (common in healthcare), and when emotions are strong (Patterson et al., 2002). When responsibility and accountability are also missing (e.g., this is not my job), something important may not get done at all or in a timely manner.

On the positive side, dialogue skills are learnable and can be used in nearly every case management encounter. For positive dialogue, case managers may apply the following specific strategies (Patterson et al., 2002):

1. Figure out what you really want: for yourself and for others.

2. People often act out (go to "silence or violence") when they do not feel *safe*. Learn to notice when the other party does this.

3. Make it safe. Conditions/dialogues that promote *mutual respect* is one place to start.

4. Apologize when appropriate. Agree when appropriate.

5. Consider that what YOU think is happening, may not be exactly correct (i.e., What "story" are you telling yourself?). If you are telling a negative "story" about the other person, go back to "just the facts." And ask what part you play in the scene.

6. *Ask* others questions, and consider that they have good information to add to the pool of knowledge.

7. Seek *help* and *support* when you face a situation you are unable to resolve alone.

8. Understand and recognize your limitations and do not *overcommit or over promise.*

▶ CASE MANAGEMENT AS LEADERS

Once all of the points stated earlier have been mastered, or at least enhanced—accountability, delegation, conflict resolution, collaboration, consultation, coordination, communication, critical thinking, motivational interviewing, EI, and documentation—it is time to realize that case managers are no longer just managers of care. Case managers are leaders, and there is a difference. *Managers manage systems; leaders lead people.* Case managers do both; they manage cases (a number of patients or clients) and lead, or guide, people. Leadership is one step up the ladder of professional growth and development. As case management responsibilities continue to grow, leadership qualities will necessarily be presumed (Powell, 2000).

Leadership is about the ability to influence people (e.g., clients, healthcare professionals) to accomplish goals. Leaders can be *formal* (by their position in the organization or society) or *informal* (by the amount of influence they have on others). Case managers are constantly in a position to influence people to accomplish their healthcare goals.

Leadership can be defined as a process where the "leader" exerts influence over others. This leader inspires, motivates, and directs others' activities to help achieve group or organization goals. Within this definition of leadership, there are six core components that expand on the description (Shortell & Kaluzny, 2000):

1. Leading is a *process,* an action word, a verb.

2. The *locus* of leadership is a person; only individuals (as opposed to corporations or inanimate objects) can lead.

3. The *focus* of leadership is other people or groups. This connection must exist for leadership to take place.

4. Leadership necessitates *influencing.* It is the leader's ability to influence others that sets apart an effective leader from an ineffective one. This may be the most critical of the leadership components.

5. The object of leadership is *goal accomplishment.*

6. Leadership is *intentional,* not accidental.

To describe these components in practical case management language, case management is a process where the case manager (the leader) must assess multiple variables that relate to the patient, the family, the disease process, the treatment, the health insurance plan, the psychosocial situation, the desired goals and outcomes, and the interdisciplinary healthcare team. The goals chosen are the roadmap for the creation of the best outcomes, as the case manager must intentionally influence the situation to bring about the best outcomes for the patient and family, and for the healthcare organization or provider. While these are true, the ability to influence others may be the case manager's "center of gravity" and most critical skill. Influence is a multipronged concept, and, on a daily basis, case managers intentionally influence patients/families to take appropriate medications, to think carefully about possible treatment choices, or to eat a diet that is best for their disease state (for example). Case managers influence insurance companies and other important healthcare team members (CMSA, 2017).

Different case managers use various leadership styles and choice is often based on a combination of beliefs, values, personal traits, and preferences, in addition to the leader's organization's culture and norms, which will encourage some styles and discourage others. Sometimes the leadership style is dependent on the situation (or even "who" is the recipient). There are several styles of leadership. Case managers use these styles differently, depending on the situation and the role they are playing at the time. However, personality traits may make one or two styles predominant (or nonexistent).

- Authentic leadership
- Charismatic leadership
- Participative leadership
- Situational leadership
- Transactional leadership
- Transformational leadership
- Quiet leadership
- Servant leadership

Authentic leadership is defined as an approach to leadership that emphasizes building the leader's legitimacy through honest, open, and transparent relationships with followers, who value their input and are built on an ethical foundation. Generally, authentic leaders are positive people with truthful self-concepts who promote openness and vulnerability. Authentic leaders are characterized by Kruze (2013):

Self-awareness and a genuine attitude. They are self-actualized individuals who are aware of their strengths, their limitations, and their emotions. They also show their real selves to their followers. They do not act one way in private and another in public; they don't hide their mistakes or weaknesses out of fear of looking weak.

- They are mission-driven and focused on results.
- They lead with the heart, not just with the mind. This does not mean authentic leaders are "soft." In fact, communicating in a direct manner is critical to successful outcomes, but it's done with empathy; directness without empathy is cruel.
- They focus on the long-term goals and vision, and are future-oriented in actions and plans.

- They focus on maintaining objectivity, seeking out pertinent insights, and ensure nothing important is missing before making final decisions.
- Authentic leaders adhere to ethical and moral standards, and demonstrate integrity, self-regulation, and alignment of own behaviors with personal values to ensure that their actions are consistent with their spoken words (Shirey, 2015).

Charismatic leaders sense that charm and grace are all that is needed to create followers and that people follow others that they personally admire. They often pay a great deal of attention in scanning and reading their environment, and are good at picking up the moods and concerns of both individuals and larger audiences. Then they will hone their actions and words to suit the situation ("Leadership Styles," 2006). The word *charisma* is derived from a Greek word meaning "divinely inspired gift." This leadership style flourishes when the leader is genuinely focused on connecting with people, understanding them and accepting where they are, developing successful relationships with them, and inspiring them to improve or unleash their potential including innate power and abilities.

Participative leaders believe that involvement in decision making improves the understanding of the issues concerned by those who must carry out the decisions. Further, they believe that people are more committed to actions when they have been involved in the relevant decision making, and are less competitive and more collaborative when they are working on joint goals ("Leadership Styles," 2006). Participative leaders value the input and feedback of those on their teams or integral to the situation. They encourage them to speak up and prompt to hear from everyone. They are free of judgment and demonstrate respect and acceptance to wherever the individual is at.

Situational leadership uses a range of actions and styles that depend on the situation. This style may be *transactional* or *transformational* (see in the following paragraphs) or any of the leadership styles discussed. Situational leaders are astute at understanding the situation and exercise an approach to action that is most appropriate and relevant.

Transactional leadership is based on the belief that people are motivated by reward and punishment. Social systems work best with a clear chain of command. When people have agreed to do a job (the transaction), a part of the deal is that they relinquish all authority to their manager. The prime purpose of a subordinate is to do what his or her manager orders ("Leadership Styles," 2006).

Transformational leadership focuses on creating a vision and innovation, and inspiring others to follow. While transactional leadership attempts to preserve and work within the constraints of the status quo, transformational leadership seeks to subvert and replace it, and looks at the greater good (Shortell & Kaluzny, 2000).

- Transformational leaders believe people will follow a person who inspires them, has vision and passion, and can achieve great things. The way to get things done is by injecting enthusiasm and energy.
- Transformational leadership starts with the development of a vision (by the leader or by the team)—a view of the future that will excite and convert potential followers ("Leadership Styles," 2006).
- Transformational leadership is about the leader developing other leaders from the followers and creating opportunities for them to expand and recognize their potential.

Quiet leadership believes that the actions of a leader speak louder than his or her words. People are motivated when you give them credit rather than take it yourself. Ego and aggression are neither necessary nor constructive ("Leadership Styles," 2006). Quiet leaders promote a sense of calm, peace, and comfort in their environment and people around them.

Servant leadership believes that the leader has responsibility for the followers and toward society and those who are disadvantaged. The servant leader serves others, rather than others serving the leader ("Leadership Styles," 2006).

▶ Leadership Skills

There are specific actions that successful leaders share, regardless of the type of organization or team they lead or their unique style. Note the similarities between effectively working with patients/clients and the qualities of effective leaders (another way to say that case managers are, indeed, leaders). Effective leaders:

- *Hold their staff (team members) accountable,* but also let them do their jobs.
- *Promote empowerment* by emphasizing the strengths and utilizing the talents of others. Leaders share decision making with others, allowing those people at the point of care or service to be the key decision makers. Then, they share in the success and give credit where it is due.
- *Communicate a vision.* People need a vision of where they are going. Leaders provide this vision ("Manager's Intelligence Report," 1997).
- *Follow the golden rule.* Anyone who has been demeaned or treated with disrespect knows what effect that treatment has on the work ("Manager's Intelligence Report," 1997).
- *Admit mistakes. Praise others in public.* And criticize others only in private.
- *Stay close to the action.* In case management, this is the administrator who goes to the "front lines" occasionally to stay in touch with the reality of the working situation. This also means that the leader is visible and accessible (Powell & Tahan, 2010).

- Say "*I don't know*" when confronted with a case management problem, then assist with a solution (Powell & Tahan, 2010).
- Focus on *what* is right, not *who* is right (Powell & Tahan, 2010).
- *Empower others to lead* and use their utmost potential.
- Create opportunities for others to *become leaders.*

▶ CHANGE AND CASE MANAGERS AS CHANGE AGENTS

As leaders, case managers are also fundamentally "change agents." In the late 1990s, the first edition of this textbook stated, "We seem to be living in an age of instability. The face of healthcare is changing so rapidly that in a few years we may scarcely recognize it." This statement is as true today as it was when initially. And case managers have certainly been in the lead as healthcare has changed.

Although some people embrace change, most find it intimidating; it is change that is at the core of stress. Case management is more important than ever before to manage change and transition in the best interests of the patients and their families; case managers are "change agents." New and fast-changing financial constraints must also be managed to keep necessary institutions fiscally healthy. Staff nurses feel squeezed from unrelenting downsizing, experienced, trained, and competent case managers are scarce, and many physicians cannot play by the new rules; they want the "good old days" back. The present situation will not go back to the way it was. We cannot change this. Nevertheless, "Strangely enough, this is the past that somebody in the future is longing to go back to" (Ashleigh Brilliant). When looking at change from this future perspective, perhaps the state of healthcare today is worthy of another assessment. Compare your current job duties with those of the nurses of 1887 (Display 12-1).

Change gets a bad rap. People are suspicious of change. Substitute the word "change" for the word "truth" in the first line to reveal a recurring phenomenon:

Every truth passes through three stages before it is recognized:

- First it is ridiculed.
- Then it is opposed.
- And finally, it is regarded as self-evident.

Physicians washing their hands before assisting in childbirth; the earth is round; women are smart enough to vote—these were once blasphemous beliefs, but everything changes, even death and taxes. Fifty years ago we did not have the technology to hold human beings on the threshold of death, and taxes change every year. We cannot do much about the fact that change happens. We can do quite a bit about our response to change. Because of the

NURSES' DUTIES IN 1887

Nurses' Duties in 1887

In addition to caring for your fifty patients, each nurse will follow these regulations:

1. *Daily sweep and mop the floors of your ward, dust the patient's furniture and window sills.*

2. *Maintain an even temperature in your ward by bringing in a scuttle of coal for the day's business.*

3. *Light is important to observe the patient's condition. Therefore, each day fill kerosene lamps, clean chimneys, and trim wicks. Wash the windows once a week.*

4. *The nurse's notes are important in aiding the physician's work. Make your pens carefully; you may whittle nibs to your individual taste.*

5. *Each nurse on day duty will report every day at 7 A.M. and leave at 8 P.M., except on the Sabbath, on which day you will be off from 12 noon to 2 P.M.*

6. *Graduate nurses in good standing with the director of nurses will be given an evening off each week for courting purposes or two evenings a week if you go regularly to church.*

7. *Each nurse should lay aside from each payday a goodly sum of her earnings for her benefits during her declining years so that she will not become a burden. For example, if you earn $30 a month, you should set aside $15.*

8. *Any nurse who smokes, uses liquor in any form, gets her hair done at a beauty shop, or frequents dance halls will give the director of nurses good reason to suspect her worth, intentions, and integrity.*

9. *The nurse who performs her labors and serves her patients and doctors faithfully and without fault for a period of five years will be given an increase by the hospital administration of five cents a day, providing there are no hospital debts that are outstanding.*

SOURCE: Cobb Memorial Hospital, Phoenix City, AL.

unpredictable nature of change, some people respond to it with fear. Others, realizing that inherent in change is the need to give up something (exchanging one thing for another), react with anger or grief. More positively, still others choose to reframe the situation. Changing how you look at the situation mentally often changes how you respond to it. Here are some ideas to bear in mind when changes occur that may have you feeling frustrated or off-balance.

▶ *Sometimes the dragon wins*: You have worked hard with the case and used the clinical pathways. Then it seems that the case is falling off the path at every turn, and variances (or dragons) are winning. The MRI machine breaks down; there is still barium in the patient's colon necessitating another bowel preparation before proceeding with the test; the family refuses to pick up Mom after she has been discharged (why did they not mention anything on the telephone this morning?); the patient refuses every other test and there is still no definitive diagnosis; the patient who insisted on going home rather than to an extended care facility is back in the emergency department within 24 hours. Every case manager can add his or her own story. There is no shortage of dragons. First, assess whether you could have done anything differently for a better outcome. If so, learn from it. If not, realize that sometimes the dragon wins.

▶ *Choose your battles*: Once, during an extremely frustrating case, a wise physician counseled a case manager with this pearl of wisdom. Many aspects of case management are completely out of the case manager's realm of control. Assess whether the problem is something on which you can make an impact. If not, save your battle energy for more productive endeavors.

▶ *Remember this wise adage*: Dr. Robert Eliot, a cardiologist at the University of Nebraska, developed two rules for keeping things in perspective. Although it is not meant for us to take our responsibilities lightly, from a cardiologist's perspective, the present problem is probably not worth having a coronary over. Then you are in the hospital with a case manager managing you!

1. Don't sweat the small stuff.
2. It's all small stuff (Charlesworth & Nathan, 1984).

▶ *Change is risk*: According to Ray Bradbury, the alternative to never taking risks is not very appealing. "If we listened to our intellect, we'd never have a love affair. We'd never have a friendship. We'd never go into business, because we'd be cynical. Well, that's nonsense. You've got to jump off cliffs all the time and build your wings on the way down." Instead of spending time and energy fighting change, build your wings and plan how you can succeed within the changing environment. Remember, control is overrated; trying to control a situation that is generally not controllable is a waste of effort.

▶ *It is OK to disagree*: Not everyone has to be in agreement to move forward. One continuous quality improvement technique (consensus) is built on this assumption.

▶ *Anticipate changes and transitions*: Do not wait for changes to happen. This has been said in many different ways. Be proactive. Have a Plan B ready when a change in the patient's condition or the family's attitude occurs. By anticipating changes, you remain poised and alert for them. This allows you to refocus quickly, often without missing a step, rather than becoming flustered. This rapid refocusing necessitates a certain degree of flexibility and spontaneity. Here you stand at the crossroads between what is and what is not in your control. You could not control the change in plans, but you could quickly redirect the case in a new direction.

We cannot direct the wind. . .But we can adjust the sails. (Author Unknown)

▶ The Eight-Stage Change Process

Successful transformations are neither easy nor linear. Still, some change experts believe that a general sequence of change *does* occur, that no steps should be missed, and that—at times—multiple phases occur at once. The Eight-Stage Change Process (Display 12-2) (Kotter, 1996) includes timeless concepts that can help case managers in many aspects of their work (both at the patient level and at the corporate level) (Kotter, 1996).

▶ Change and Grief

The insecurity and fear associated with change may be one of the greatest causes of stress. In fact, change reactions have been likened to the reactions one has to grief. In "The Ten Stages of Change," the phases of change are compared to Elisabeth Kübler-Ross's grief stages from her famous book, *On Death and Dying* (Pearlman & Takacs, 1990). The 10 stages of change are (Pearlman & Takacs, 1990, p. 30) the following:

1. *Equilibrium*: Here, the staff, employer, or manager is comfortable and content with the organization. Balance is the keynote of this stage.
2. *Denial*: Pressures become strong, and the ability to maintain equilibrium is no longer on solid ground. Personal energy is used to resist change.
3. *Anger*: There is blaming taking place as well as demands that someone "fix" what is going on.
4. *Bargaining*: The staff and employees attempt to prevent the inevitable from happening. Often, negotiations demonstrate unrealistic solutions and little concrete data.
5. *Chaos*: Diffuse energy, insecurity, and feelings of powerlessness appear. Nothing seems to make sense, and people feel like there is no direction.
6. *Depression*: Self-pity and sorrow characterize this stage.
7. *Resignation*: Acceptance of reality starts to occur.
8. *Openness*: Growth in new directions occurs.
9. *Readiness*: For the change.
10. *Reemergence*: Energy increases to the point that the individual becomes more proactive and willing to take chances. There is a more realistic sense of what can be controlled.

Change does cause grief. Life will never be the way it was, which often leads to fear and insecurity. However, life always remaining exactly the same does not leave room for growth and anticipation (which is oftentimes the most fun part of looking forward). Deepak Chopra, an American author, public speaker, alternative medicine advocate, puts it another way and guides us through some of these stages:

The search for security is an illusion. In ancient wisdom traditions, the solution to this whole dilemma lies in the wisdom of insecurity or in the wisdom of uncertainty. This

EIGHT STAGES OF KOTTER'S CHANGE PROCESS (Kotter, 1996)

Stage of Change	Highlights
1. Establish a sense of urgency.	This can be accomplished by examining the market and competitive realities or the patient's clinical trajectory, identifying crises or potential crises, and/or identifying major opportunities.
2. Create a guiding coalition.	Put together a group of professionals with enough power to lead the change; then, get the group to work together like a team (leadership is needed here). In case management, this may be the essential patient care team.
3. Develop a vision and strategy.	The vision created will direct the change effort. Then, develop strategies to achieve the vision. What does the team want? More importantly, what does the patient/family want? Consider how the strategy will potentially achieve desired outcomes.
4. Communicate the change.	Use all vehicles to communicate the vision and strategies. Have the guiding coalition to role-model the behavior.
5. Empower broad-based action.	Remove obstacles (from the team, the patient, the case, if possible). Change systems or structures that undermine the change vision. Encourage risk-taking and nontraditional ideas.
6. Generate short-term wins.	Plan for visible improvements early in the process. Visibly recognize and reward the people who made the "win" possible. From a patient perspective, this may help the patient/family become more autonomous. An example is the patient demonstrating adherence to a healthy lifestyle behavior such as quitting tobacco consumption.
7. Consolidate the gains and produce more change.	As the patient/family becomes more knowledgeable or independent, use this progress to instill more sense of autonomy and produce more results.
8. Anchor the new approaches in the culture.	Last step and perhaps most important for a department/organization. Create better performance through customer service and excellent leadership. Articulate the connection between new behaviors and organization success. And develop ways to ensure leadership development and succession.

means that the search for security and certainty is actually an attachment to the known. And what's the known? The known is our past. The known is nothing other than the prison of past conditioning. . . . Without uncertainty and the unknown, life is just the stale repetition of outworn memories. . . . Relinquish your attachment to the known, step into the unknown, and you will step into the field of all possibilities. In your willingness to step into the unknown, you will have the wisdom of uncertainty factored in. This means that in every moment of your life, you will have excitement, adventure, mystery. You will experience the fun of life—the magic, the celebration, the exhilaration, and the exultation of your own spirit. . . . When you experience uncertainty, you are on the right path—so don't give up. You don't need to have a complete and rigid idea of what you'll be doing next week or next year, because if you have a very clear idea of what's going to happen and you are rigidly attached to it, then you shut out a whole range of possibilities. (Chopra, 1994, pp. 86–88)

Building a safe harbor to cope with job (and life) stresses is no easy task. Display 12-3 shares eight truths about change you may find insightful as a case manager. As Grace Hopper (1906–1992) was an American computer scientist and United States Navy rear admiral. As she so eloquently worded it, "A ship in port is safe, but that's not what ships are built for." The healthcare field is constantly changing and is showing few signs of slowing down. Change is the force

THE EIGHT TRUTHS OF CHANGE

1. To gain, you must first give up. Every transition begins with an ending. We have to let go of the old before we can take up the new . . . not just outwardly, but inwardly too.
2. Every transition is an ending that prepares the ground for new growth and new beginnings. The curtain drops so the stage can be set for a new scene.
3. The more you leave behind, the more room there is to discover something new.
4. Distress is not a sign that something is wrong but a sign that a transition is taking place.
5. The lesson in all experiences of transitions is when we are truly ready to make a beginning, an opportunity will come.
6. The only way to get rid of the fear of change is to go directly into the change. "The doing it" comes before the fear goes away. Fear of change situations dissolve when they are confronted.
7. You are not the only one to experience fear when in unfamiliar territory. Feeling inadequate is a universal response to change.
8. Living through the fear of change takes far less effort than living the emotional turmoil and negative consequences of resistance.

SOURCE: Collaborative Consulting, Inc.

that creates, destroys, and re-creates. Remember that stress is often "in the eye of the beholder," and how one *perceives* occurrences in their lives can determine whether it is an adverse venture or an adventure. The Chinese symbol for change consists of two symbols: danger and opportunity. Change *is* dangerous; it often destroys systems and structures. Change also re-creates, and therein lies the opportunity.

DISCUSSION QUESTIONS

1. Take a moment to remember when you first became a case manager. Describe your perception of your role then. Compare it with your perception of your role today. Did role confusion or conflict exist then? Do they exist today? What do you attribute this to? (Note: if you are about to assume this role, use your perception of the role to answer these questions.)

2. Picture a recent day where you had too much to do and not much time to achieve it all; describe how you went about prioritizing your day/activities? How did you use time management to effectively complete your tasks? How did you feel at the end of the day? Could you have done anything differently?

3. Describe a recent event where you either supported a fellow case manager or a fellow case manager supported you. How did it feel? Describe another where support was lacking. How did it feel? What lessons did you learn from both encounters?

4. Describe a situation of conflict where too many feelings and emotions were exhibited. How did you handle the situation? Did your behavior reflect EI skills? Why? How could you have handled the situation if you were emotionally intelligent?

5. Describe a situation where you did not follow your intuition and there was a negative patient consequence/outcome. What made you not listen to your intuition? How could you have acted differently?

6. Describe a day when you utilized leadership skills. What type(s) of leader were you? What skills were used? How can you have mitigated the challenge more appropriately (or not)?

7. Identify a situation from your case management practice, whether patient- or healthcare team–related. Engage in reflective practice about the situation. Explore your leadership approach to it, critical thinking skills or strategies, and your EI behaviors. Examine opportunities for improvement and determine an action plan for effective advancement or change.

▶ REFERENCES

Alfaro-LeFevre, R. (1999). *Critical thinking in nursing*. Philadelphia: W.B. Saunders.

Biller, A. M. (1992). Implementing nursing case management. *Rehabilitation Nursing, 17*(3), 144–146.

Braverman, T. (1993, August). *Warning: Humor may be hazardous to your health* (p. 14). The Arizona Light.

Case Management Society of America. (2017). *Core curriculum for case management* (3rd ed.). Philadelphia: Author.

Cesta, T., & Tahan, H. (2017). *The case manager's survival guide: Winning strategies in the new healthcare environment*. Lancaster, PA: DEStech Publications, Inc.

Charlesworth, E., & Nathan, R. (1984). *Stress management: A comprehensive guide to wellness*. New York: Atheneum.

Chopra, D. (1994). *The seven spiritual laws of success*. San Rafael, CA: Amber-Allen Publishing.

Covey, S. R. (1989). *The 7 habits of highly effective people*. New York: Simon and Schuster, Inc.

HMO Workgroup on Care Management. (2004). *One patient, many places: Managing health care transitions*. Washington, DC: AAHP-HIAA Foundation.

Kotter, J. P. (1996). *Leading change*. Boston, MA: Harvard Business School Press.

Kruse, K. (2013). *Forbes: What is authentic leadership*. Retrieved April 11, 2015, from http://www.forbes.com/sites/kevinkruse/2013/05/12/what-is-authentic-leadership/

Leadership styles. (2006). Retrieved March 19, 2006, from http://changingminds.org/disciplines/leadership/styles/leadership_styles.htm

Manager's intelligence report. (1997). Chicago: Lawrence Ragan Communications, Inc.

Miller, W. R., & Rollnick, S. (2012). *Motivational interviewing* (3rd ed.). New York: Guilford Press.

Patterson, K., Grenny, J., McMillan, R., & Switzler, A. (2002). *Crucial conversations: Tools for talking when the stakes are high*. New York: McGraw-Hill Publishers.

Pearlman, D., & Takacs, G. (1990). The ten stages of change. *Nursing Management, 21*(4), 33–38.

Powell, S. K. (2000). *Case management: A practical guide to success in managed care*. Philadelphia: Lippincott Williams & Wilkins.

Powell, S. K. (2008). Intuition: Believe it or not. . .but place it in your toolbox. *Professional Case Management, 13*(4), 191–192.

Powell, S.K. & Tahan, H. A. (2008), *Case management society of America (CMSA) core curriculum for case management* (2nd ed.). Philadelphia: Lippincott Williams & Wilkins.

Powell, S. K., & Tahan, H. A. (2010). *Case management: A practical guide for education and practice*. Philadelphia: Lippincott Williams & Wilkins.

Shirey, M. (2015). Self-awareness: Enhance your self-awareness to be an authentic leader. *American Nurse Today, 10*(8). Retrieved August 17, 2015, from http://www.americannursetoday.com/enhance-self-awareness-authentic-leader/

Shortell, S. M., & Kaluzny, A. D. (2000). *Health care management: Organization design and behavior* (4th ed.). Albany, NY: Delmar Publishers.

Tahan, H. (2000). Emotionally intelligent case managers make a difference. *Lippincott's Case Management, 5*(4), 162–167.

Treiger, T., & Fink-Samnick, E. (2016). *Collaborate for professional case management: A universal competency based paradigm*. Philadelphia: Wolters Kluwer.

White, C., & Hows, E. (1993). Managing humor: When is it funny—and when is it not? *Nursing Management, 24*(4), 80–92.

Zander, K. (1989). Case consultation: Determining the next action. *Definition, 4*(1), 3841.

INDEX

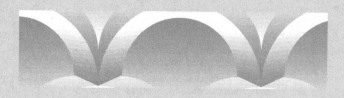

Page numbers in *italics* denote figures; those followed by t denote tables